The Gluten Cure

Scientifically Proven Natural Solutions to Celiac Disease and Gluten Sensitivities

By Case Adams, Naturopath

The Gluten Cure: The Scientifically Proven Natural Solutions to Celiac Disease
and Gluten Sensitivities

LOGICAL BOOKS
Wilmington, Delaware
http://www.logicalbooks.org

Printed in USA
Cover Images: Wheat field: © Narimbur. Bread: Paola Sucato
Wheat image page 20: GrainChain

Publishers Cataloging in Publication Data
Adams, Case
The Gluten Cure: Scientifically Proven Natural Solutions to Celiac Disease
and Gluten Sensitivities
First Edition

1. Medicine. 2. Health.
Bibliography and References; Index

ISBN-13 paperback: 978-1-936251-48-3

Other Books by the Author:

ARTHRITIS – THE BOTANICAL SOLUTION: Nature's Answer to Rheumatoid Arthritis, Osteoarthritis, Gout and Other Forms of Arthritis

ASTHMA SOLVED NATURALLY: The Surprising Underlying Causes and Hundreds of Natural Strategies to Beat Asthma

BOOSTING THE IMMUNE SYSTEM: Natural Strategies to Supercharge Our Body's Immunity

BREATHING TO HEAL: The Science of Healthy Respiration

ELECTROMAGNETIC HEALTH: Making Sense of the Research and Practical Solutions for Electromagnetic Fields (EMF) and Radio Frequencies (RF)

HEARTBURN SOLVED: How to Reverse Acid Reflux and GERD Naturally

HAY FEVER AND ALLERGIES: Discovering the Real Culprits and Natural Solutions for Reversing Allergic Rhinitis

HEALTHY SUN: Healing with Sunshine and the Myths About Skin Cancer

NATURAL SLEEP SOLUTIONS FOR INSOMNIA: The Science of Sleep, Dreaming, and Nature's Sleep Remedies

NATURAL SOLUTIONS FOR FOOD ALLERGIES AND FOOD INTOLERANCES: Scientifically Proven Remedies for Food Sensitivities

ORAL PROBIOTICS: The Newest Way to Prevent Infection, Boost the Immune System and Fight Disease

PROBIOTICS – Protection Against Infection: Using Nature's Tiny Warriors To Stem Infection and Fight Disease

PURE WATER: The Science of Water, Waves, Water Pollution, Water Treatment, Water Therapy and Water Ecology

THE ANCESTORS DIET: Living and Cultured Foods to Extend Life, Prevent Disease and Lose Weight

THE CONSCIOUS ANATOMY: Healing the Real You

THE SCIENCE OF LEAKY GUT SYNDROME: Intestinal Permeability and Digestive Health

TOTAL HARMONIC: The Healing Power of Nature's Elements

Table of Contents

Introduction

Imagine for a moment the promise of taking just one pill to eliminate every ache and adverse health condition we have. Just one pill.

Now imagine this same pill will also increase cognition, boost energy, help us dream better, remove our headaches, and help us lose weight.

Yes – just one pill.

Would you take it?

And what would this be?

A *panacea*.

Now imagine that instead of taking a pill, we could accomplish all of the above simply by removing one type of food from our diet. Yes, by eliminating just one element of our diet we would no longer experience headaches, fatigue, indigestion or intestinal difficulties. Just by eliminating this one compound we'd have more energy and better sleep. We would dream better, have increased cognitive skills and have a greater capacity to learn and remember what we learned.

Would we do it?

Absolutely. In a heartbeat.

But this proposal – giving up just one type of food – would still fall into the same category as defined above: A *panacea*.

Panaceas – a word taken from the Greek demi-goddess of medicine *Panakeia* – have provided significant impetus in healthcare for thousands of years. Famous *panaceas* that have traveled through cultures via word of mouth or otherwise have included *the fountain of youth, the philosopher's stone, the emperor's (Samarcand) apple, the dulse of Guiodin, the balsam of Fierbras, the sap of the elephant tree* and others. Even the health-promoting *Panex ginseng* and *Maitake mushrooms* have been considered *panaceas* at times.

Today we are finding a new type of *panacea* spreading through our culture: The *gluten-free panacea.*

This doesn't mean gluten sensitivities don't exist. It also doesn't mean there aren't good therapeutic reasons for going gluten-free for certain people at certain times. Just as *Panex ginseng* and *Maitake mushrooms* have been clinically shown to be effective for certain conditions, a gluten-free diet has been shown to eliminate symptoms among celiac disease patients, wheat allergy sufferers and a percentage of those who suspect they are otherwise sensitive to gluten or wheat in general.

But just as all the other *panaceas* have eventually been found out for what they are, this text will unfortunately illustrate that our modern gluten-free *panacea* won't provide the cure-all many are hoping and purporting it will accomplish. Yes – unfortunately. In other words, it would certainly be nice if it was the *panacea* it is being purported as.

This doesn't mean there isn't a problem. The evidence, in fact, supports the fact that there is a problem affecting millions of people.

What we know is that gluten sensitivities appear to be dramatically increasing, with phenomenal growth among wealthier nations – especially among Western countries. We also know that more people are trying to eliminate gluten foods from their diets – with varying results – than ever before in the history of our species.

Gluten sensitivities – even if they are not related to celiac disease or wheat allergies – have been associated with symptoms of bloating and indigestion, along with fatigue, headaches, brain fog and others.

For this reason, the term *gluten-free* has become ubiquitous among health food stores and consumers.

Yet, as this book will show, wheat-based foods have been part of the human diet for over a million years, and some of the healthiest diets according to research – including the Mediterranean diet and others – contain generous servings of whole wheat-based foods. This adds to the research showing that dietary fiber provided by whole wheat grains reduce heart disease, diabetes and related metabolic disorders.

The evidence of these points will be clarified within this book.

Furthermore, the cornerstone of the diets of many traditional societies – ancestors to a majority of the world's populations, some known for their long life spans – have been gluten-containing foods. Some of these cultures are known for their advancements in writing, science, math, language and other technologies. In other words, these weren't idiots. They were some of the world's most intelligent societies and cultures. And there is no mention of gluten-related disorders among the ancient medical texts.

This bears the logical question posed by the gluten-free hypothesis: Has humanity been poisoning itself with wheat and other gluten-containing grains (including wheat, barley, rye and others) for thousands – even millions of years as humans advanced in language, culture and science?

This doesn't mean there is no problem occurring with gluten sensitivities over the last few decades. And this book is not intended to deny or evade the problem.

However, there are some questions to be answered:

- Is gluten the cause of sensitivities to wheat-based foods?
- Are gluten sensitivities increasing or is there a greater awareness of its possibility?
- Similarly, are doctors diagnosing gluten sensitivity more now because there is more gluten sensitivity or more awareness?

- Are the new diagnostic tests such as ELISA IgG testing producing more awareness?
- Not to mention: Are these new diagnostic tests accurate or do they have too many false positives – as discovered by many allergy professionals?
- And the most obvious question – could there be something else at the root of the increase in gluten sensitivity complaints?

Certainly these are complex questions to be answered, along with sorting out the different types of gluten sensitivities, how they are diagnosed, the root causes of gluten sensitivities and the potential strategies to reverse them.

Therefore, much of the early part of this text will cover not just the basic facts about gluten sensitivity, but the facts about food sensitivities in general. Why? Because in fact, gluten sensitivities are food sensitivities.

And just as it is apparent in most food sensitivities, there is a distinct physiological difference between food intolerance and food allergy. Thus we will focus on distinguishing between gluten allergies such as celiac disease and other wheat allergies, and gluten intolerance as we elucidate their symptoms, diagnosis, causes and solutions.

Most importantly, the aforementioned questions are not only raised by this text: The text will attempt to answer these with clarity and scientific objectivity.

This is, in fact, part of the "cure" being offered with this text. While certainly the text will address strategies to resolve gluten sensitivities of different types including celiac disease and wheat allergies, one of the major problems – or diseases – presenting itself in the case of gluten sensitivity is the lack of objective and clear information about what gluten is and what it does, along with the rest of wheat's components; the history of gluten sensitivity; how celiac disease and wheat allergies are related and so on.

At the same time, some of the most important information being presented here is the newest research that tests some of the conclusions that have been made from earlier research – conclusions that have created the notion of the gluten-free *panacea*.

This is the crux of the matter because research done two, three, four and more decades ago primarily investigated the effects of gluten among celiac disease patients – people with a seeming genetic autoimmune disposition that makes them allergic to some gluten proteins. And certainly, going gluten-free resolves their condition to the greater extent. So for a celiac sufferer, a gluten-free diet is somewhat of a *panacea*: At least with respect to the symptoms related to this condition.

The problem occurred when many of the discoveries made along the way towards understanding celiac disease were applied – even if certainly well-intended and sometimes applicable – to those without celiac disease.

Some of these discoveries about gluten's effects on celiac physiology led to the potential that those who were otherwise seemingly sensitive to gluten may also suffer some of these physiological effects.

And for some who were gluten sensitive, it may be true.

But then some of those findings taken from research on celiac patients were extended to healthy individuals – indicating the possibility that gluten was a health concern for everyone.

This is when things got real serious.

What followed was a myriad of isolated laboratory research, research on animals and those with and without celiac disease. Different conclusions were drawn from these, sometimes with and sometimes without understanding the context of the study. And sometimes without understanding the limitations of the study and how far the study could be applied. Or without understanding the scope of application for the study.

This doesn't mean those conclusions were wrong. Certainly there are opinions and conclusions that have come from those with impeccable credentials. Who is the author to doubt these opinions?

But over the past five years or so, those conclusions have been further clinically tested to determine whether they could be applied to the general populace – those without celiac disease or wheat allergies or with other disorders such as IBS.

This text pays close attention to the careful examination of this recent clinical research, because this research answers many of the questions posed by earlier studies.

The combination of research evidence and application also takes us further – indicating viable solutions for not only gluten intolerant people, but for those with celiac disease and other wheat allergies.

The presentation of the scientific data – without opinionated or anecdotal presumption and without a stake to gain – provides the best "cure" for the misinformation circulating – though well-intended – through our media and through word of mouth.

But this isn't the only "cure" being offered by this text.

A detailed and scientific description of not only how our immune system works, but how hypersensitivity develops within the body is pursued in this book.

It doesn't stop there. The text discusses the relevant science regarding the underlying causes of not just gluten sensitivities but food sensitivities in general. These causes are revealing because they allow us to trace back to those things we have done with food production and processing, our lifestyles, our environment and our medicine that have contributed to this growing problem of sensitivity to gluten and other mainstay food proteins.

The picture is not pretty. In fact, it paints the possible scenario that if we continue to neglect the health of our food supply, our environment, our medicine and our inner microbiome we may end up not being able to eat many of the foods that assure our future survival as a species.

These points raise crucial questions about gluten, grains and intolerance. Should we settle on gluten-free diets without finding the answers to these questions? Should we just assume our ancestors ate poison for thousands – even millions of years – and be done with wheat?

While some may settle for the avoidance strategy of a gluten-free diet with good reason, along with the assumption that those gluten-containing foods such as wheat, rye, barley and spelt are simply toxic; to dismiss a collection of foods that has fed our species for thousands of years without a proper trial would be short-sighted.

Such an assumption – the edict of these foods being toxic – especially in the face of significant evidence showing whole wheat foods are nutritious and provide disease reduction – would be unheard of in any objective court of law. Such an assumption would certainly contradict our human intelligence and our quest for knowledge along with survival: It would contradict our history of intelligently solving problems by discovering their causes and devising solutions, even in the midst of challenge.

And it is not as if a gluten-free diet is easy, either. One study (Do-Nascimento *et al.* 2014) surveyed 91 celiac disease sufferers and found that 71% had difficulty finding gluten-free foods, and nearly all were dissatisfied with their choices of gluten-free products.

The question this creates:

Why – in this modern world full of technology and advanced medicine – are we copping out so easily on the topic of celiac disease, wheat allergy and gluten intolerance? Why are we so easily ready to drop a staple food that has nourished us and kept so many of our ancestors from starving in centuries past?

One word: *Panacea.*

Today the gluten-free trend is having a great impact on the food industry. An NPD Group survey states that 30% U.S. adults are attempting to eliminate or cut back on gluten foods, and a *Nutrition Business Journal* report states that in 2012, 63 percent of special diet sales were gluten-free foods.

Yet many of our brothers and sisters throughout the world do not have this luxury of giving up wheat-containing foods. Currently, the very grains that contain gluten proteins many are trying to eliminate from Western diets actually feed much of the world. In fact, much of the world's populations – especially among poorer countries – eat wheat foods as a mainstay of their diet.

Frankly, this is because whole grain breads and other whole grain flour products contain numerous nutrients, including minerals and proteins necessary for human survival.

Gluten-containing foods are not only an important part of our past survival: They are a critical part of our future survival. Population research estimates that by 2050 the world's population will grow from seven billion to over nine billion. How will we feed this population?

According to an analysis done by National Geographic and the University of Minnesota Institute on the Environment (Foley 2014), if humans continue our current shift away from traditional plant-based foods such as wheat, we will have to figure out how to double the amount of crops we grow around the world by 2050.

Food scarcity is not just an idea bantered back and forth by environmentalists. It is a reality. Millions of people around the world today are hungry. And charity organizations are shipping in – you guessed it – wheat, in order to prevent starvation. How come wheat is preventing starvation? Because of its significant content of protein, vitamins and minerals.

As we will discover from this text, the story of wheat runs far deeper into our ancestry than we have considered – far longer than the 10,000-12,000 years purported to humanity's consumption of wheat.

We will find that our oldest ancestors ate wheat and other grains, millions of years ago.

And this text will also prove that wheat is an essential food for our intestinal microbiome.

This science, the reader will find, changes the very landscape of the question of whether gluten is a toxin.

The challenge the author made to himself, and makes to anyone who has given up or is considering giving up wheat: *Let's investigate* – from all sides – the facts about gluten and wheat, and then discover what is actually occurring physiologically in gluten sensitivity.

This challenge is not just an important medical concern. It is important to the survival of the human species. Why? If we cannot discover why we are becoming sensitive to the very foods that fed our species for over a million years, then we have a critical problem:

We have a problem that will inevitably lead to increasing food scarcity among our descendents.

And here is another important gauntlet: If we continue down this path of eliminating the foundation of our former diet without determining the real cause of gluten sensitivity or intolerance, gluten-based foods will not be the last foods we will have to eliminate from our diets.

As this text will prove, the metabolic problems causing our gluten intolerance also produce multiple food sensitivities. Furthermore, these metabolic issues will lead us and our future generations toward becoming increasingly intolerant to many other foods we also need for survival.

So before you dismiss the contents of this text before reading it: Consider these consequences carefully.

After we eliminate the food feeding much of our species at the present time, humanity will be limited to producing those foods we are not yet intolerant to. That would require a major food production shift that would certainly result in economic and populace upheaval.

And then – if we do not solve the cause of gluten and other food sensitivities – we will have to one day also eliminate those new foods we shifted to – foods that have greater environmental and economic impact than wheat does. What will we eat then?

In such a scenario, we cannot assume everyone will become intolerant to the same foods. In fact, this is already occurring, as people are becoming increasingly intolerant and sensitive to a variety of foods from dairy to nuts to seafood. What are the ramifications of multiple food sensitivities increasing among our species?

Are we ready for such a world? Just consider a localized scenario. Just consider what would happen at a dinner table made up of dinner guests and family members who are variously sensitive to gluten and/or other common foods. What would the dinner look like?

Could one dinner even be produced? No. That kitchen would become quite the nightmare delicatessen. It will take on a completely different appearance than today's kitchen.

Such a kitchen would need to produce a variety of dishes and side dishes to appease the different food sensitivities among its guests and family members. It would likely double or triple the variety of foods required to handle the various intolerances. And such a kitchen could not serve one main dish and a few other side dishes. It would have to serve a myriad of main dishes with different ingredients in order to satisfy the various sensitivities among the dinner guests and family. Such a kitchen would look more like a restaurant than a home kitchen.

Now just imagine this scenario among a larger crowd. Typically, restaurants and cafeterias are set up to accommodate a large crowd of people with dishes containing common foods. But what happens as the myriad of sensitivities and intolerances expands as it is doing today? Practically every order would require a special 'made-to-order' dish. Picture the overload upon those businesses and organizations that feed large numbers of people. Many would collapse under such a scenario.

Now expand these scenarios into cities, states and countries.

The bigger picture is that humanity as a whole will begin to starve. Economies would collapse. As a species, humanity will by necessity be hit with a scarcity of food that will impact the survival of billions of people around the world, resulting in world-wide food shortages the likes of which we have never seen.

So the objective of this book is broad-reaching. A sensitivity to gluten might seem trivial when compared to cancer or heart disease or Alzheimer's disease – conditions plaguing and killing hundreds of millions of people every year. But food – this is something that effects every one of us. Every single one of us will starve without enough food to eat.

And certainly food sensitivity feels trivial. *'Get over it'* might be the response of members of a poor family who must eat bread or starve.

But this instruction to *'get over it'* will feel insulting to a person experiencing some of the symptoms of gluten sensitivity, which can include bloating, vomiting, diarrhea, inflammation in various parts of the body and/or chronic fatigue when they eat wheat-based products.

This doesn't mean the author is against a gluten-free diet. As this text will lay out, there are solid therapeutic reasons for gluten elimination at certain periods of time for certain people and certain conditions.

As a result of these considerations, gluten-sensitivity is not being approached simply in this text. That would not be good enough given the consequences. It would simply not be responsible.

Sure, it would be easier to just say, *'stop eating wheat.'* But that's too easy. And it's a cop-out.

Anyone who has read any of my other books knows: I don't lay down on a topic. I don't settle for the commonly accepted approach on many conditions.

And I haven't on this condition. In my sense of things, a person who has become intolerant to gluten-containing foods deserves the right to know the whole story. The story behind the anecdotes. The story behind the headlines. The story behind the fad. The real story steeped in the science and the research. The story that runs consistent with our metabolism and physiology, our history as a human species, and the natural world around us.

Thus the reader will find some complex discussions in this text that involve the immune system, the digestive system and nutrition in general. While I try to simplify the science to embrace the layperson, the science must be illuminated in order to understand the underlying facts and relationships.

Basic questions the reader might ask: Are the conclusions of this text the anecdotal opinions of the author? *No.* Did the author start with a hypothesis and then try to prove it? *No.*

The conclusions of this text are the logical assessments calculated from a deep investigation of the evidence, together with a foundation of understanding of the body's anatomy and metabolism.

And the research I conducted to write this book has also opened my eyes in many ways – and changed my opinions on more than a few elements of this topic. It even changed some of my own dietary habits.

I clarify this because there are many who have jumped on the gluten-free bandwagon without knowing even the most basic facts. Facts that could hurt their bodies in the long run. Facts related to our metabolism and our food supply. Facts related to nutrition and the digestive tract.

And none of these can be isolated from the others.

With this I hope the reader can weather through some of the technical jargon used in order to arrive at the understanding for the real causes of gluten sensitivity along with practical strategies that can help clinicians and laypersons alike: Strategies that incorporate the wisdom of nature with the latest research and technology.

To compile the conclusions of this text, the author has drawn facts and evidence from over a thousand research papers, including hundreds of controlled, randomized and double-blind clinical studies; along with numerous case histories and historical practices of traditional medicines.

Furthermore, much of the research data presented here has come from medical schools, prestigious universities, hospitals and/or government agencies from around the world. When combined, these present a variety of clear and proven procedures that can be applied to wheat allergies and intolerances.

In addition, a number of medicinal herbs and formulae specific to food sensitivities are presented together with their research. This includes clear evidence from clinical research along with documentation by physicians, credentialed traditional doctors, naturopaths and herbalists from around the world. As the reader will find, these herbs come with medicinal benefits that produce increased tolerance and strengthen the immune system.

The reader should know, however, that the information presented here is not meant to present a thesis that gluten intolerance does not exist or that a gluten-free diet is not a healthy diet. And it does not present a thesis for the status quo in terms of the kind of gluten-containing foods we have been eating within the typical Western diet.

Rather, the information presented will unfold new, practical solutions for gluten sensitivities. In other words, gluten sensitivity is not a foregone condition that cannot be reversed. And if a person decides to utilize the nutritional benefits offered by including whole wheats, barley and rye into the diet, there is a pathway for reversing gluten sensitivity.

Yes, the evidence reveals the radical conclusion that even celiac disease and wheat allergies can be resolved. The evidence does not indicate a *panacea*, however. It indicates a therapeutic process that can – to the degree it is applied – lessen the severity of a celiac sufferer's condition, if not completely eliminate the sensitivity altogether.

While these two conditions will be discussed throughout and often considered together, gluten intolerance – a non-allergic negative response to gluten – will be focused upon concurrently. This is because, as will be shown, some but not all gluten sensitivities may in fact be pre-allergic conditions – conditions that may one day develop into an allergic disorder.

Unless, of course, something is done to intercede its progression.

Perhaps we should discuss the nomenclature used here for clarity: Food sensitivities typically cover both food allergies and food intolerances, and the phrase *gluten sensitivity* is a general term that includes all three possibilities – celiac disease, wheat allergy and gluten intolerance.

To separate the other two from celiac disease, the phrase *non-celiac gluten sensitivity* will be used to clarify their distinction.

Furthermore, the phrase *gluten intolerance* will be used to exclude wheat allergy and celiac disease. And the phrase *non-celiac non-wheat allergy gluten sensitivity* will be used to refer to a sensitivity that is either gluten intolerance or some unknown intolerance or sensitivity to other components of wheat foods.

Also, for the purposes of simplicity, the word *wheat* will be used to describe gluten-containing foods including barley, rye and wheat. Barley and rye can be considered generally as wheat, but they can also be referred to as cereal grains. Nevertheless, these will be identified here generally as *wheat*.

All CAPS will be used to indicate words appearing on food labels.

For one who recently suspects having a gluten sensitivity or intolerance, the multitude of recommendations in this book might seem onerous. Certainly ones personal health professional should be consulted before making radical changes, especially if the person has any diagnosed medical conditions.

But as the reader – whether clinician or layperson – assesses the curative information offered in this text, the practical application of that information will still need to meet ones particular metabolism and physiology. While numerous generalized and specific tools are offered here, the reader must realize we each have a slightly different metabolic physiology. As such, application must accompany the context of our general health, the health of our immune system, the health of our digestive tract, the health of our liver and so-on.

For this reason, having a personal health professional who knows our history and relative metabolic idiosyncrasies is tantamount to the success of the curative strategies introduced and discussed in this text.

Chapter One

Just the Facts Please

The name of this chapter defines the attempt to lay out the basic facts about gluten sensitivity without opinion or anecdotal theory. This will serve to provide the framework for laying out the evidence throughout this text with a thoroughness that can allow the reader to make an informed decision.

First a bit of history. Celiac disease as a wheat-related condition is a fairly recently discovered disorder. An intestinal disorder being linked to wheat consumption was first described in a 1950 dissertation by Dutch pediatrician Dr. Willem Karel Dicke. Dr. Dicke proposed that eating wheat was the culprit for a rare infantile intestinal disorder. Dr. Dicke co-opted the word "coeliac" to describe the disorder, and it stuck.

The word "coeliac" – translated from the Greek word κοιλιακός (koiliakos) – is thought to have first been used to describe an intestinal disorder in 250 A.D. by Aretaeus of Cappadocia – a Greek physician. However, the word κοιλιακός (koiliakos) – which was translated to "coeliac" in 1856 by Francis Adams as he translated Aretaeus' works – actually translates more specifically to "abdominal" – and makes no reference to wheat.

Furthermore, there was no mention of wheat sensitivity in Aretaeus' description of an abdominal disorder. There was no mention of wheat whatsoever, which was a staple during those times. Furthermore, the condition was described as not affecting children, but mostly women, and related to the consumption of cold water.

As we now know that celiac disease does affect men and women alike and often occurs in children, we can rule out that Aretaeus was describing what we now know as celiac disease.

It should be noted that Aretaeus' description of the abdominal disorder could well describe a number of different abdominal ailments, including the more likely dysentery – often caused by drinking water tainted by microorganisms.

In 1888, Dr. Samuel Gee described an abdominal disorder using the same term "coeliac," but this time describing children with abdominal pains. However, we see again that the condition was unrelated to celiac disease, because Dr. Gee described a curative diet that included slices of bread.

Once again, the disorder being described was unrelated to a sensitivity to wheat, so we can rule out the word utilized was describing what we know today – what was first described by Dr. Dicke – as celiac disease.

Thus we can conclude that celiac disease is a relatively modern condition, first described in the mid-twentieth century, long after the industrial revolution began.

Furthermore, the condition was only described in modern Western medicine. There is no mention of a disorder relating to eating wheat among the various traditional medical texts of Chinese, Ayurvedic, Arabic, Greek or any other recent or ancient medical texts dating back over the centuries into the thousands of years.

And given medical journal documentation, non-celiac non-wheat allergy gluten sensitivity is an even more recent condition. It was first described in the 1980s (Catassi *et al.* 2013) by doctors who found that a few patients reporting sensitivity to gluten-containing foods had no signs of celiac disease. This gave birth to the new term a decade later, "non-celiac gluten sensitivity."

Celiac disease and wheat allergies can be serious conditions, causing immediate and life-threatening episodes such as anaphylaxis – a seizing of the airways almost immediately after eating a wheat-based or gluten-based food. While certainly possible, it appears improbable that such a disorder would go undiscovered for thousands of years, as wheat has been a staple of many diets.

Today, both of these conditions – celiac disease and wheat allergy – can be diagnosed with clarity using one or multiple tests as we will discuss later.

Gluten intolerance – or non-celiac gluten sensitivity – however, is a different animal altogether. In fact, as we will explore, diagnosing gluten intolerance is quite difficult, requiring the physician to rely primarily upon the patient's own experience of symptoms, even when food challenges are instituted. And for this reason, unfortunately most medical insurance companies will typically not cover medical treatment for gluten intolerance.

Yet there is a growing legion of circumstantial evidence and clinical observation that gluten intolerance is a real medical disorder and its incidence is growing substantially, as we will illustrate in this chapter.

And many who have eliminated gluten foods from their diets report feeling better. They report fewer digestive problems, increased energy, fewer headaches and other positive effects.

At the same time, as we'll illustrate, research has found that among many, a gluten-free diet does not reverse their symptoms. Others have reported that a gluten-free diet lessens symptoms but doesn't eliminate them.

Before we dig in to the research behind these and other facts, let's look at a couple of fairly typical scenarios that involve gluten sensitivities:

Bobby

Bobby is an optimistic teenager, except when it comes to eating. After years of digestive discomfort, Bobby's mom took him to a doctor who specializes in food intolerances. After being tested for food sensitivities, Bobby was diagnosed with gluten intolerance along with an intolerance to 113 other foods.

No one knows exactly what caused it, but Bobby's digestive difficulties seemed to have started about a year after Bobby went to hard foods as a baby.

The diagnostic test shows Bobby's food intolerances range from serious to not-so-serious. As a result, Bobby's mother has taken Bobby off of gluten and does her best to avoid the other 113 foods in Bobby's meals. It goes without saying that this provides significant difficulty for a mother of three other children.

Bobby's intolerances began to worsen a few months after a childhood cold got worse and moved into his lungs. He had an ear infection concurrently. His doctor prescribed a course of antibiotics.

The diet Bobby mostly eats is a typical Western diet. He particularly likes French fries and cokes.

Bobby and his parents have not reliably found whether or not Bobby is intolerant to all 114 foods. But a previous doctor – an allergist – tested Bobby and found he had no known allergies to any foods.

This doctor conducted a skin prick analysis – one of the more reliable tests. The allergist also conducted a test for IgE antibodies – and found Bobby had no IgEs to foods.

This was after Bobby and his parents have visited no less than three other doctors over the past decade. At each of those visits, Bobby's parents were told he was probably under stress and just not digesting his food well. They suggested he take his time eating and chew his food better.

Bobby often has bloating, indigestion and diarrhea, along with occasional headaches. And they seem to come after he eats a big meal – often with gluten-containing foods such as breads and pancakes.

After his diagnosis with food intolerances, Bobby has gone on an elimination diet: A gluten-free diet.

Bobby feels a little better, except he can't find much to eat at the school cafeteria or a restaurant – or most other places. He also can't go out with his friends to eat without feeling pretty embarrassed.

As a result, Bobby doesn't go out with his friends much anymore. He is now pretty much a loner because he is embarrassed that he cannot eat what his friends are eating.

And Bobby is not a starter on the basketball team anymore, primarily because he has been feeling like an outsider. This started when the coach passed around pizza during the bus ride home from a game and Bobby was ridiculed by his teammates because he refused the pizza celebration from his coach.

Then the last birthday party Bobby went to he had to sneak away when they started cutting the cake. He also can't have sandwiches when he goes on a picnic or to a game. He can't find much at all to eat at a ballgame. Or at his favorite pizza parlor. Or practically any other place. Including the school cafeteria.

Bobby lost his best friend when his friend asked him over for dinner and a sleep-over and Bobby turned him down. His friend thought he just didn't want to be friends anymore.

Sam

Sam is 52 and he's been a good eater most of his life, and always considered his digestion as 'solid as a rock.' He ate pretty much anything and everything his parents gave him as a child. Then as a college student he relished all the greasy cafeteria food.

After marrying, Sam's wife carried on the tradition. For dinner he ate sirloin, grilled burgers, fries, ham, hot dogs, mashed potatoes – the typical Western diet – and his breakfasts and lunches also included some of the same foods, except alongside or inside some slices of white bread, biscuits, waffles and pancakes. And then there were the slices of cakes and let's not forget the donuts.

Sam is a retired policeman but still working as a part-time security guard. So donuts – and bear claws – have been his staple break snack and sometimes-breakfast food for decades.

Sam felt healthy until he turned 50. After that, he started getting constipated a lot. Then he would feel bloated and have indigestion after eating a big meal. After some time he found he could hardly finish a meal because he seemed to feel so full so quickly.

Sam weighs about 250 pounds and stands well over six feet. So finishing a meal was never difficult for him. In fact he usually had seconds or finished up others' plates.

But now Sam is reduced to picking through his food and leaving half on the plate. The gurgling and bloating he had in the beginning has now turned to cramping at times. At least every week or two Sam will have a major cramping situation, often after a stressful day, but always following a meal.

And more recently Sam has started having headaches.

One day Sam was complaining to a co-worker about his digestion and headaches and the co-worker suggested he probably had gluten intolerance. His friend said that he read on the internet that gluten intolerances are now causing all sorts of conditions, even schizophrenia.

Freaked out, Sam decided to give it a shot. After all, he didn't want to get schizophrenia. He stopped eating toast or biscuits or pancakes in the morning. He stopped eating sandwiches on his lunch break. And he stopped eating donuts.

He also had to start refusing the donuts brought into work and skipped the company July 4th picnic because he was embarrassed about not being able to eat any breads or buns.

And then Sam was invited out to lunch by his boss and he had to refuse. He didn't want his boss knowing that he couldn't eat a sandwich. Especially since he hadn't been given a diagnosis. He was just guessing.

But Sam says he feels a little better on his new diet. He seems to have a little less bloating and cramping, but he still has major – now worse – constipation. He's still waiting to see if the gluten-free diet will stop his headaches. And his relationship with his boss is still a little strained after he refused the boss' invitation to go to lunch.

Who Gets Food Sensitivities?

Gluten sensitivity is a food sensitivity. Thus understanding gluten sensitivity requires understanding food sensitivities. We might compare this to getting the larger perspective on a map before focusing in on the street details.

The latest analyses show that food allergies affect from 5-8% of children and 3-4% of adults within the United States, and are increasing in incidence. And food sensitivities appear to affect about 12% of the general population in developed countries. (Railey and Burks 2010, Wang 2010, Pons *et al.* 2005, Woods *et al.* 2001, Sicherer and Sampson 2010).

While developed Western countries lead the world in food sensitivities, the U.S. numbers appear to be some of the highest, following the U.K. Combined research data from developed countries around the world have indicated that food allergies occur in 3-8% of children under six years of age, and about 2-3% of adults (Cingi *et al.* 2010, Moneret-Vautrin and Morisset 2005, Rodríguez-Ortiz *et al.* 2010).

Britain's food sensitivity stats are off the charts. British researchers (Walker and Wing 2010) estimate that 25% of Britain's population may suffer from one kind of food sensitivity or another.

Most of the above studies and others concur that among undeveloped countries, food sensitivities are much less prevalent. Furthermore, in countries such as South Africa, where there is a significant difference between those living in cities and those living in the countryside: those in the urban areas have significantly higher rates of food sensitivities (Hooper *et al.* 2008).

It appears this is related to both diet and environment. Studies in Italy (Cataldo *et al.* 2006) on rates of food allergies among immigrants from developing counties indicate that the immigrant allergy rates were lower before moving, yet become similar to Italy's rates following their immigration.

Confirming an environmental association, researchers from Sweden's University (Böttcher *et al.* 2006) tested 30 Estonian and 76 Swedish infants and found that the environment during the first two years of life predicated an increased risk of food sensitivities growing up.

Among developed countries, those with more sunlight exposure appear to have less food sensitivities. In a large-scale international study, 17,280 adults between the ages of 20 and 44 from different countries were studied by researchers from Australia's Monash Medical School (Woods *et al.* 2001).

Natives of Northern European countries such as Scandinavia or Germany, had higher levels of food sensitivities when compared with Southern European countries such as Spain and Italy. In other words, countries closer to the equator had lower food sensitivity rates.

This geographical relationship has also been seen among food sensitivities and urgent care treatments throughout the U.S. For reasons we will discuss more in depth later, those living in Southern states had lower incidence of food sensitivities and far fewer hospital room visits for food sensitivity reactions (Rudders *et al.* 2010).

French researchers (Rancé *et al.* 2003) found that a child's first allergic reaction becomes evident at about two years old. This depends, of course, on the type of food allergy. It is also recognized that atopic dermatitis allergies and food sensitivities occur more frequently among infants and younger children. Hay fever, or allergic rhinitis and allergic asthma tend to develop throughout adolescence among children.

University hospital researchers from Northern Mexico (Rodríguez-Ortiz *et al.* 2010) studied 60 patients with food allergies during 2007 and 2008. Fifty-one percent of them were under five years old.

Also, many children with food allergies tend to outgrow them. In a study by the Food Allergy Research Program of London, the food allergy rate was 5.5% in children before the age of one. This was reduced to only 2.5% of six-year-olds with food allergies.

Furthermore, only 2.3% of the 11- and 15-year-olds had food allergies (Venter *et al.* 2006; Pereira *et al.* 2005).

We might also point out that more food sensitivities seem to occur among females. In the Italian study of 25,601 allergy patients mentioned earlier, 64% of the patients were women.

Who Has Gluten Sensitivity?

Many pathology texts estimate that celiac disease appears in about one in 5,000 people. But real incidence appears to be higher. Researchers from the University of Maryland School of Medicine (Fasano *et al.* 2003) found in a blood screening of celiac antibodies of 13,145 U.S. persons that one in 133 people in the U.S. may actually suffer from celiac disease when looking at the disorder from a diagnostic basis – rather than from a symptomatic basis.

Later research showed the possibility that as many as one in 100 might now be celiac (Leffler and Schuppan 2010). Again, this is immunologic diagnostic testing rather than symptomatic diagnoses.

Some allergy specialists have gone on record indicating the symptomatic occurrence is far less – possibly among one in 250 or more.

There is a strong possibility that celiac disease is on the rise. One study (Rubio-Tapia *et al.* 2009) illustrated that celiac disease has increased by four to five times over the past fifty years.

Another review – this from the University of Maryland (Catassi *et al.* 2010) indicates that celiac disease prevalence may have been 1 in 501 in 1974, and 1 in 219 in 1989. This also indicates a five-fold increase in celiac sprue in the U.S. between 1974 and today's levels.

It is important to note the variance with celiac disease occurrence around the world. Among Europeans, the highest occurrence comes from Western Ireland. However, celiac disease occurs rarely among African and Asian countries (Laghi *et al.* 2003).

Occurrence of gluten sensitivity in general may well be much higher, at least among Europeans and Americans.

But a more real indicator of serious gluten sensitivity may well be in how many people are avoiding gluten – by eating a gluten-free diet.

As far as people reporting being on a gluten-free diet, Columbia University researchers (DiGiacomo *et al.* 2013) surveyed 7,762 people as part of the Continuous National Health and Nutrition Examination Survey (NHANES). They found that of the entire population studied, only 49 non-celiac people reported maintaining a gluten-free diet. This worked out to 0.55% – less than 1%.

They concluded:

> *"The estimated national prevalence of non-celiac gluten sensitivity is 0.548%, approximately half that of celiac disease."*

Yet we find anecdotal evidence suggesting that the number of gluten intolerant people is significantly greater. Why?

In interviews with the media, Dr. Alessio Fasano from the University of Maryland has stated that he believes gluten sensitivity may affect between six and seven percent of the U.S. population. This would mean that some 20 million people could be gluten sensitive. Dr. Rodney Ford believes the condition affects many more – he thinks between 10% and 30%, and possibly up to 50% of the population. Half of the population?

Interviews with an owner of a leading gluten sensitivity testing lab (name withheld for confidentiality) indicate he also believes gluten sensitivity affects half the population. This, he has stated, relates to positive IgG testing – though he suspects 10% to 15% of Americans have either IgA or IgG anti-gluten antibodies (see the ELISA IgG section later for more information on IgG testing).

The testing lab owner also estimates that between 60% and 65% of those with irritable bowel syndrome also test positive in IgG testing for anti-gluten antibodies.

But he also estimates that between 20% and 25% of those without any self-ascribed symptoms of gluten sensitivity will also test positive for IgGs to gluten. This is called a false-positive. Why so high?

In fact, many of these later statistics are actually based upon a combination of positive IgG tests for gluten proteins and the patient's own self-ascribed report. See the last section in this chapter regarding IgG testing.

It is this self-ascription that has also been used in an attempt to support IgG testing. The two are thus irreparably tied it seems.

The question now is, how many of those who self-describe themselves as sensitive to gluten sensitivity are really gluten sensitive?

This is a big question, and a current controversy we will investigate with the evidence later on.

What kind of person will become intolerant to gluten?

A 2014 study from Australia's Monash University (Biesierkierski *et al.*) conducted a survey of Australians with gluten intolerance. Of the 248 survey respondents, 147 completed the gluten survey. Eighty-eight percent were women, and the average age was 43 years old.

Interestingly, a full quarter of the respondents or 24% were restricting gluten consumption yet still had "uncontrolled" symptoms – meaning they were not managed. About 56% of the respondents were on a gluten-free diet after the advice of a health professional, while 44% took it upon themselves to eliminate gluten from their diet.

A full 65% of those with a verified non-celiac gluten sensitivity also had other known food intolerances.

The researchers also found that only one of four of those claiming gluten sensitivity actually fulfilled the criteria for non-celiac gluten sensitivity. The others didn't have a gluten sensitivity. Most were nonetheless believing they had a sensitivity to gluten and had eliminated it from their diet.

This of course represents many who are currently on gluten-free diets.

Are Food Sensitivities Increasing?

Many researchers agree that food sensitivities are increasing globally. Others have questioned whether the increase may be related to an increase in diagnosis, or an increase of awareness.

The research clearly supports increasing incidence, however; especially among developed countries.

For example, researchers from New York's Mount Sinai School of Medicine (Sicherer *et al.* 2010) exhaustively studied cases of peanut, tree nut, and sesame allergies in 2008, 2002 and 1997. They found that among 5,300 households and 13,534 subjects, 1.4% reported peanut allergy, tree nut allergy or both in 1997. In 2002, the rate was 1.2%. Peanut and tree nut allergies in children (less than 18 years old) was 2.1% in 2008, compared with 1.2% in 2002, and 0.6% in 1997. Tree nut allergy alone increased from 0.5% in 2002 and 0.2% in 1997, to 1.1% in 2008.

Many government agencies, such as the United Kingdom's Department of Health, have announced that – based on recent statistics – food sensitivities were increasing (Waring and Levy 2010).

For example, food allergy hospital admissions increased five times in the fifteen years between 1990 and 2005 in Britain (Gupta *et al.* 2006). Increased awareness could not be the only culprit for this sort of increase.

British and American researchers (Venter *et al.* 2010) studied peanut allergy prevalence among children born on the Isle of Wight, UK between 1989 and 2002. The records were reviewed at three or four years old, and a total of 4,345 subjects were studied. They found that children born in 1989 had the lowest incidence, at 1.3%. Those born between 1994 and 1996 had the greatest incidence, at 3%. Those born between 2001 and 2002 had 2% incidence. Clinical diagnosis also grew in the same way, from .5% to 1.4% to 1.2%.

However, we should mention that the last group was only surveyed at the age of three years old, a full year younger than the first group and much of the second group. As other studies have shown, many peanut allergies tend to develop between three and five years of age. So it is likely that if four year olds had been included in the third group, the rates may have continued to increase linearly from the second group.

Scientists from Poland's Military Institute of Health Sciences (Bant and Kruszewski 2008) found that among the 41% of people living in towns and cities in Poland, IgE sensitivities to atopic allergens increased 52% in the 16 years from 1986 to 2002. This means that on the average, allergen sensitization increased at a rate of about 3.25% per year.

Australian researchers (Poulos *et al.* 2007) studied the prevalence of critical allergic reactions such as anaphylaxis, angioedema, and urticaria, resulting in hospitalization among developed countries. They analyzed data for three periods – 1993-1994, 2004-2005 and 1997-2004. During the three periods, hospital admissions for angioedema (swelling of mucous membranes and submucosal tissues) have increased an average of 3% per year. Allergic urticaria (skin rashes) has increased an average of 5.7% per year. More significantly, hospitalizations for the sometimes-lethal anaphylaxis allergic response increased a whopping 8.8% per year. Increases in anaphylaxis hospitalization were highest among children under five years old.

A number of other studies from a variety of international agencies and universities have reported significant increases in food sensitivities around the world, particularly among Western societies and developed countries. Increases in hospital admissions and emergency room treatments have also increased among these countries (Gillman and Douglass 2010).

While studies report increasing rates of food sensitivities among industrialized countries, children and young adults are not the only victims of increasing food sensitivities. A phenomenon called *immunosenescence* occurs among the aging when the immune system must adjust to new or even repetitive environmental or dietary inputs. For this reason, as we'll discuss more later, the rates of adult food sensitivities among industrialized societies have been increasing as well.

At least among wealthier countries, specific food sensitivities typically depend upon the food most consumed. More than 170 foods can cause IgE-reactions. Among the developed Western countries, for example, dairy consumption is quite high. As would be expected, most research illustrates that milk is the most prevalent food allergen in the United States and Britain. This is followed by eggs, peanuts and walnuts (del Giudice *et al.* 2010).

Hugh Sampson, M.D., a pediatric immunologist and researcher with nearly thirty years of experience with food allergies, points out that about 2.5% of U.S. children under the age of three have allergies to cow's milk, while 1.5% have allergies to eggs, and 0.8% have allergies to peanuts. Other foods, he states, affect far fewer children and tend to develop later (Charles 2008).

University of Helsinki researchers (Salmi *et al.* 2010) found that cow's milk allergy (CMA) is the most common form of food allergy, affecting 2.5% of children in Finland. We should also note that Finland also enjoys the highest consumption of milk products compared to the rest of the world.

In the Mexican University hospital study mentioned earlier (Rodríguez-Ortiz *et al.* 2010), most had allergies to dairy products, eggs, seafoods, beans, soy, chili, mango, cacao and/or strawberry. Dairy, eggs and fish allergies caused the most allergies in this study.

Researchers from Turkey's Karadeniz Technical University (Orhan *et al.* 2009) found that among 3,500 6-9 year olds from urban areas, 32% were sensitive to beef, 18% to cow's milk, 18% to cocoa, 14% to eggs and 14% to kiwi (14%) were the most prevalent allergies. Other allergens reported with lower levels included soy, wheat, peanuts, fish, and hazelnuts.

In the Asero Italian study mentioned earlier, pollen-related food allergies were the highest, with 55% of all food allergies in Italy. The majority (72%) of those were from fruits and vegetables. Of those with Type I allergies, 96% lived in Southern Italy, where most of Italy's urban populations (such as Rome) are located.

Peanuts are a very popular food among developed Western countries. As a result, approximately .6% to 1.5% of the population in the United States, Britain and Canada are allergic to peanuts (Morisset *et al.* 2005, Boyce *et al.* 2010). Using the food allergy rates of 6-8% for children and 3-4% of adults, this means that peanut allergies make up somewhere in the neighborhood of 10-20% of all food allergies in these countries.

As would be expected, due to the varied diet of Western countries, there are many other foods that people are becoming increasingly allergic to.

Researchers from the McGill University Health Center in Montreal, Quebec (Ben-Shoshan *et al.* 2010) surveyed 10,596 households in 2008 and 2009 – with 3,613 household responses covering 9,667 people. Of those surveyed, they found an increased prevalence of food-allergies and an increased occurrence of peanut, tree nut, fish, shellfish, and sesame allergies and anaphylaxis over the one year period. Shellfish allergies made up 1.6%; tree nut allergies were 1.2%; peanut allergies were 1%; fish allergies were 0.5%; and sesame allergies were 0.10%. This means that seafood presented the largest allergy levels, at 2.1% among Canadians. Not surprisingly, Canadians are big seafood consumers.

We should also add that people who contract food sensitivities often have multi-food sensitivities.

Fruit and vegetable allergies, for example, are typically related to pollen sensitization or latex allergy (Moneret-Vautrin and Morisset 2005). These typically occur among adults.

In a review of 934 worldwide studies by researchers from London's King's College (Rona *et al.* 2007), food sensitivity rates were reported to be anywhere from 1.2% to 17% for cow's milk; 0.2% to 7% for eggs; up to 2% for peanuts; up to 2% for fish; and up to 10% for shellfish.

In a study of specific IgE allergens among primary school children in Taipei, Taiwan, hospital researchers (Wan *et al.* 2010) found different allergens than those found among Western countries. A total of 142 primary city schools and 25,094 students 7-8 years old were screened by survey, and then tested with the IgE Pharmacia CAP system. 1,500 students (6%) had confirmed allergic sensitivities (including food). Of these 1,500, 88% had crab allergies. 23% had milk allergies, 24% had egg white allergies, and 22% had shrimp allergies. Wheat allergies were not listed.

Other sensitivities among these same children were also apparent. These included various species of dust mites, including *Dermatophagoides pteronyssinus, D. farinae* and *Blomia tropicalis*. Allergies to dust mites ranged from 85% to 91% among the food allergenic children. Other concurrent allergies among food-allergenic children included dog dander, cat dander and cockroach allergies. Once again, the rates were higher among more industrialized areas.

Discrepencies still exist in this data, however. Danish researchers (Zuidmeer *et al.* 2008) found that among 36 studies of more than 250,000 children and adults, few used the gold standard of food challenge. Those that did showed only 0.1% to 4.3% allergies for fruits or tree nuts; only 0.1% to 1.4% for vegetables; and less than 1% for wheat, soy, and sesame. Meanwhile, IgE testing for wheat ranged as high as 3.6% and 2.9% for soy. This range of discrepancy simply indicates that food intolerance is thoroughly being mixed in with food allergy rates, and that IgE testing tends to report higher allergy rates than do food challenges.

What is Gluten?

The word *gluten* is drawn from the root "glut," derived from the Latin word gluttīre – meaning 'to fill up or feed to satiety.'

One of the reasons gluten intolerance is misunderstood is because many of us simply do not understand what gluten is. Let's get clear on this before we go much further.

First of all, every part of the wheat berry will contain proteins of various types. This includes the bran, the endosperm and the germ of the wheat berry. This means that all types of wheat foods – including white flour which has little if any bran and germ – will also contain protein.

But gluten proteins are primarily contained within the endosperm of the grain, as we'll discuss further.

In general terms, gluten is a collection of proteins that together will become gooey or glue-like as they combine with water.

In a broad sense, we might compare gluten to a category of any type. Let's say instead of proteins, we are speaking of kitchen tools. In the kitchen there are pots, pans, forks, knives, bowls, plates, glassware and so on. In this case, gluten might be considered the same as utensils – which would include both forks and knives, as well as other utensils such as spoons. Now it is not as if there is a single thing called "utensils." Rather, "utensils" is a category of implements. The individual implements – the individual knives, forks, spoons and others fall within the category of utensils.

And so it is with gluten proteins – which can be compared with a category such as utensils.

As a group, gluten proteins can be separated from wheat flour by washing the ground up flour with water. This was first documented in 1728 by Dr. Jacopo Beccari, a professor of physics and medicine at the University of Bologna.

Around 1820, Johann Taddel separated a portion of these gluten proteins using alcohol as a solvent. The portion that was soluble in alcohol he named "gliadin." The portion of gluten not soluble in alcohol soluble he named "zymom."

Later laboratory work separated other protein types from gluten – including what was considered "plant albumin" and "plant-gelatin."

Today gluten is considered a category of proteins, as mentioned above, which includes gliadins and glutenins. But gluten is not – as detailed by some – a single entity composed of gliadin and glutenin.

The reality is that wheat grains contain various gliadin proteins and they contain various glutenin proteins. These are types of proteins, and these two – glutenins and gliadins – can be summarized as gluten proteins.

Now if we look at the entire protein makeup of wheat, then each of these two types of proteins can be considered fractions – gliadins are the water-soluble protein fractions of gluten, and glutenins are insoluble.

In this language, we have to see these wheat proteins as a lab scientist would see them: As part of a mixed slurry of ground up wheat.

When a laboratory determines the components of a particular food or other compound, it will typically grind the food into a slurry. This might be compared to putting the food into a blender.

But then the slurry is centrifuged. This centrifuging will separate the components of the food, as the most dense parts of the food will head to the outside – away from the center – and the less dense components will remain closer to the center. This will produce different sections of components, divided by their density – these sections are called *fractions.*

Without getting too much into the technical details, laboratories will employ different speeds to centrifuging to separate different components within a mixture. Different speeds will separate different types of components.

For example, carbohydrates would be separated from proteins at one speed, and different proteins from others at another speed.

As these proteins become separated, the proteins that have similar densities will become part of the same fraction.

Putting this in the context of wheat: Wheat contains thousands of different poly-peptides called proteins. And a series of centrifuging speeds will separate these proteins from the polysaccharides (carbohydrates) and other elements of wheat because proteins have different densities than these other elements.

These different proteins then can be separated and centrifuged. This centrifuging will separate the types of proteins into different fractions. One of the fractions – which contain the gliadins and glutenins within the wheat – can therefore be called the gluten fraction. This gluten fraction may contain hundreds of different proteins.

But then when the gluten fraction is centrifuged, it will separate the different gliadin and glutenin proteins into their own fractions.

Each of these fractions can be further centrifuged to separate the different protein types – which can then be identified using gas chromatography or other molecular analysis instruments to identify the molecular formula of the protein.

Thus, when lab scientists discuss the different protein makeup of the different proteins that together makeup wheat, they will detail that gliadins and glutenins are each fractions. But this does not mean that gluten is one protein – made up of gliadin and glutenin as it is often described.

One of the problems here is molecular identification. Again, there are thousands of different protein molecules in a particular wheat berry, and there are tens of thousands of different varieties of wheat. Such a situation creates an incredibly difficult task of identification: One that simply doesn't have much funding to perform.

While a pharmaceutical company will pay a group of researchers millions of dollars to collectively identify chemicals that can be used to make a drug, the funding to identify every type of gliadin and glutenin protein is simply not there.

Adding to this is another complexity: Wheat berries contain many different types of proteins. These include glutelins, albumins, prolamins and globulins.

Gliadins are prolamins: A prolamin is a protein that has a higher content of the amino acid proline.

Meanwhile, glutenins are glutelin proteins. Glutelin proteins are not exclusively glutenins, however. Glutelin proteins exist in other foods, including rice.

In a wheat allergy, one may develop a sensitivity to any or a mix of the four types of proteins mentioned above.

But in celiac disease, the immune system becomes sensitive to gliadins. Currently, most accept three gliadin protein molecule types:

- alpha-/beta-gliadins
- gamma-gliadins
- omega-gliadins

These different gliadin types are related to their different – yet similar – peptide chain configurations. In other words, their amino acid and molecular make up may be very similar, but there will be different orientations and order of molecules between each.

A celiac sufferer may be sensitive to any combination of these three types of gliadins.

Along with these gliadins there will be many different types of glutenin proteins in different wheats – and the type of glutenins may vary depending upon the variety of wheat.

A wheat allergy sufferer might become sensitive to any of these glutenins as well as any of the gliadins. A wheat allergy sufferer may also become sensitive to other components within the wheats, including other proteins, or starches, or lignans.

For example, researchers from The Netherlands (Graveland *et al.* 1985) isolated five different protein fractions in the Sicco wheat variety – which they creatively named glutenin I, IIa, IIb, IIIa and IIIb.

Each of these protein fractions had different molecular weights, and this allowed the researchers to differentiate between them using an identification process called gel filtration chromatography.

Yet these different protein molecules were similar in that they shared what are considered molecular subunits, In proteins these are peptide sequences – a distinct series of amino acids. Two different types of proteins may have the same subunits while the rest of the molecule is different.

Or molecules may be the same except they may stack the same subunits in a different order or configuration. In other words, they may contain many of the same sequences, but the sequence of their sequences are not the same.

Gliadin proteins are quite large and complex, but certainly not the largest or most complex proteins we consume. Research from Boston University (Helmerhorst *et al.* 2010) analyzed 58 alpha/beta gliadins, 110 gamma-gliadins and 8 omega-gliadins. They found that alpha/beta-gliadins contain an average of 288 amino acids, gamma-gliadins contain an average of 276 amino acids, and omega-gliadins contain an average of 356 amino acids.

In comparison, some animal proteins will contain thousands of amino acids. Of course these are not different amino acids. Some 21 amino acids typically make up edible proteins.

There are more than 25,000 different cultivars among so many different wheat varieties. Each of these contains a different mix of proteins – slightly different from others. These proteins, along with their different starch and polysaccharide molecules, will make one wheat taste slightly different from the other. They will also make different types of flours.

DNA and Proteins

Why is this important? It is important to know that pinpointing the particular protein that one may be sensitive to or intolerant to can be difficult because there are many different proteins with different amino acid configurations.

Yet because they share some of the same subunits, these proteins may all be recognized by the immune system as foreign. Or one particular configuration might. It depends.

What's it depend upon? How well any of these proteins are broken down by the digestive tract.

The digestive tract is not designed to absorb large, complex proteins like glutenins and gliadins. And the body's cells are not designed to utilize such large proteins. The digestive tract is supposed to break these complex proteins down into their amino acids or very small combinations of amino acids called peptides.

Why? Why can't the body utilize large proteins?

Because proteins are what makes our body unique from others. Our proteins are even unique among us humans – except perhaps among identical twins. Each of us has a slightly different genome.

What is our genome? Our genome is our body's blueprint of protein assembly – a combination of sequences within our 23 chromosomes, which define the types of proteins our body will assemble within our cells.

Why is this important and what's this have to do with gluten intolerance? Everything. You see, our genome – the composite of our DNA – consists of the major instructions – the navigation map for doing all of the body's functions. These include:

- ✓ *Cellular metabolism:* Our DNA provides the instructions for what our cells do and how they function.
- ✓ *Organ and tissue metabolism:* Our DNA provides the instructions for how groups of cells function.
- ✓ *Cell division:* Our cells are able to divide before they die. Our DNA provides instructions for cell division and our DNA is handed over to the next cell, giving our cells continuity.
- ✓ *Protein assembly:* Our DNA also provides the instructions – typically resolved through RNA – for building proteins within the body.
- ✓ *Reproduction:* The DNA in our chromosomes determines – along with the DNA of the opposite sex – the DNA of our offspring.

While all of these functions of our genome are vital to the notion of gluten intolerance, protein assembly is one of the most important, and it determines how DNA governs much of our metabolism.

What is this? The DNA contains the blueprints for our cells to produce the proteins they need to function.

What are these proteins? They include everything from enzymes that perform all sorts of functions to structural parts for muscles, bones and other tissues to messengers such as signaling cytokines and ligands to hormones. They also include the enzymes – proteases – that help break down the proteins we consume in our diet.

The varied proteins the cells assemble are unique to our metabolism because our DNA is unique. And the proteins in our foods were created from the DNA blueprint – an altogether different blueprint – within the plants we eat – such as wheat.

Each of us carries approximately 20,000 gene sequences that determine the makeup of our body's proteins. In all, this means about three billion pairs of genes – called base pairs. A base pair is made up of two nucleotides – for example, guanine-cytosine – whose assembly provides the instructions for making the body's proteins.

Typically, protein assembly takes place utilizing RNA, which are mapped from the body's DNA. The RNA is like a messenger in the process of assembly.

Proteins are very complex in themselves. Some can be huge when considered from a chemical standpoint. Every protein is made up primarily of amino acids, and there are only 20 amino acids in our DNA give or take a few unique aminos. But it is the combination and the molecular structure of these amino acids that counts.

A single protein molecule may contain thousands of some or all of these 20 amino acids, stacked together into a unique sequence and formation. For example, the connectin protein that helps provide muscle elasticity contains up to 33,000 amino acids chained together. Most other proteins are smaller, from 3,000 to 6,000 amino acids long.

So where does the body get these complex protein assemblies? It makes them. It stacks these amino acids together by virtue of the cellular RNA – mostly from within regions in our cells called ribosomes. The assembly line created by the RNA is not only complex: it is intelligent.

In other words, the proteins that a plant uses are distinctly different than the proteins that our bodies use. And the same goes for animals and other critters. Even among humans we have major protein differences: Yes, we do use mostly similar proteins and for this reason we can share blood and certain organs. But even in these cases, the immune system will recognize – because it is coded by our DNA – that a transplanted organ or blood or other set of proteins is not ours. This is called tissue rejection, but it is really *protein rejection*.

For this reason, doctors typically expect a rejection response from a blood or tissue recipient. The new blood or tissue may save their life. But this will be because the immune system will often tolerate or accommodate new tissues and proteins from similar donors.

The immune system will realize those proteins from the new tissue or blood can be used by the body, so its rejection-inflammation process will be more manageable.

But if we transplanted some plant cells into our tissues the rejection would likely be a lot worse. This is because those plant proteins are obvious foreigners.

They have no function within the body. They will simply be seen as toxins in that form. This would especially be the case for those proteins the plant uses to protect itself. These would likely stimulate a larger response, because just as we try to protect ourselves from danger, plants produce some proteins that are difficult for animals and humans to utilize. Yes, plants are smart that way, as we'll discuss further.

The same with transplants from animals. The level of tissue rejection will typically be consistent with the level of differences in the proteins that make up those tissues. Many of these differences are specific to the immune systems of that particular animal. This is why animal transplants to humans rarely last long.

So what happens when we eat proteins?

Okay, we are skipping a little ahead in terms of the physiology of food sensitivity. But let's get the process of protein digestion clarified right away.

Many imagine that we simply absorb proteins from our foods into our bloodstream and start using them immediately. This is why many talk of eating lots of protein. As if our body absorbs protein.

Remember above how large proteins can get – with thousands of amino acids chained and stacked together in complex arrangements.

Just as our immune system will reject transplanted tissues, the immune system will also reject any long chains of complete proteins that make contact with our tissues or our bloodstream.

These tissues include our intestinal walls. Should large proteins come into contact with our intestinal tissues – those cells that make up our intestinal wall – our body's immune system can react with a rejection response. Okay, that's a little generalized. But we will discuss the mechanisms in more detail later.

What the body needs – and does not react to – is the amino acids, along with simpler and smaller (recognizable) chains of amino acids. The body does not want these large protein chains.

So how do those large proteins get broken down before they come into contact with our intestinal walls? Special cells and our intestinal bacteria produce a special category of proteins called digestive enzymes, which break down our foods.

And in order to break down the proteins in our foods, the body and its gut microorganisms produce a special type of digestive enzyme called *proteases*.

We will discuss enzymes more completely later on, but for now, know there are many types of proteases, simply because there are many different types of proteins.

What proteases do is called *proteolysis*. The word *lysis* means to break apart, and of course *proteo* refers to protein. So what proteases do is break apart protein molecules.

This process of proteolysis is also typically referred to as hydrolysis, because the enzymes utilize water during their process of breaking down the proteins.

They break off the individual amino acids and recognizable small peptide chains that the body can use.

These amino acids and small peptides become the building blocks of our body's own protein production – which takes place within the ribosomes of the cells.

Now back to gluten. The various gliadin and glutenin proteins within the grains of wheat plants fall in the category of these very large proteins. They are huge, and complex. They must therefore be broken down by the proteases before they come into contact with the blood or the intestinal cells.

This goes for practically any protein or large unbroken molecule from the foods we eat. But some food proteins are more complex than others. And some require specific proteases to break them down, while other more simpler proteins might be broken down by a variety of different proteases within the digestive tract.

But those more complex proteins in some foods are often the proteins the body becomes sensitive to. Because they don't get broken down as easily.

What happens if they are not broken down?

This is where rejection – intolerance or allergic reaction – comes into play. Either the immune system will completely reject that protein and mount an inflammatory response to rid it from the body, or it will signal in other ways that the food is not acceptable.

Now an inflammatory response can be a major one or a minor one. We will discuss the different types of inflammatory responses later, but for now it should be clear that if the large proteins within our foods are not properly broken down by proteases in the digestive tract, then the body will respond. It might respond through an immunity response or a less critical tissue inflammatory response, depending upon the protein and the state of our immune and digestive system.

The bottom line is that when we are talking about gluten sensitivity, we are not speaking of one single protein or a single type of response. We are talking about a host of different possible proteins, all of which must be properly broken down by proteases within the digestive tract. Those that are not broken down may cause an inflammatory or other response.

And we are not speaking of just the gluten proteins needing to be broken down. Every protein we eat must be broken down by proteases before the building blocks – the amino acids and small polypeptide chains – can be utilized to conduct the body's metabolism.

Wheat and Flour

Wheat can grow with very little other attendance. A couple of waterings during the summer will usually suffice in dryer areas. Winter wheats can produce nice crops without being watered at all.

Once the mature wheat is ready for harvest, the typical commercial wheat farmer drives large combine harvesters through the field and cuts the wheat. The combine is equipped with blades that cut the wheat and threshers that strip the chaffs off the stalks and separate the wheat berries.

Before the combine was used – named because it combined the process of cutting and threshing the wheat – farmers cut wheat by hand. Farmers used scythes to cut the wheat, and hand-threshed the wheat with flails on a wheat threshing floor – basically by whacking it against a hard surface to knock out the wheat berries.

Once the wheat berries are separated, they are typically brought to a grain elevator, where they are stored until needed for shipment to a mill which will grind the wheat berries into flour. Once the mill is ready, truckloads of grain will be delivered from the elevator. The mill is equipped with various roller-grinding machines called millstands, which grind up the grain to the specifications needed in the flour.

Let's get a closer look at the wheat berry and its essential parts:

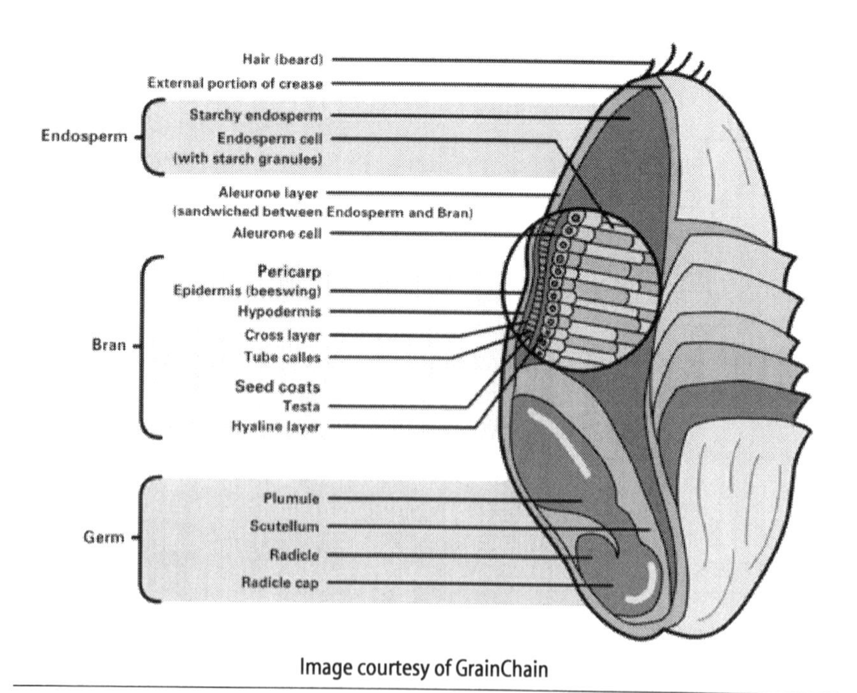

Image courtesy of GrainChain

As the image illustrates, there are three primary elements of the wheat berry: The endosperm, the bran and the germ. Within each are sub-elements that relate to the nutrient and protein content – including gluten proteins.

The wheat berry is essentially a seed. Its primary purpose is to procreate – or grow a new wheat plant. The inner wheat germ – fairly typical among most plant seeds – has the primary components from which a new wheat plant can grow. It is therefore the embryo of the seed. Of the three components, wheat germ contains the most protein and oil.

In fact the wheat germ contains a dense source of nutrients – one of the most nutritious foods known. (See nutrition discussion later). Wheat germ oil is often pressed from the wheat germ – derived mostly from the plumule and the radicle.

Common wheats and durum wheats do not contain husks, as does spelt and some other wheats – such as einkorn. Rather, wheat kernels are packed into chaffs – organized into stiff packets called rachis, or glumes. These hold the kernels together onto the chaff, which can easily be separated during threshing. What comes off the separated chaffs are called spikelets – pointed semi-coverings which hold the wheat berry in place.

The outer layer of the wheat kernel is the bran, and this is composed of several layers. The outermost bran layer is called the pericarp, which covers the testa – the seed coat. The seed coat covers the hyaline coat and the hyaline coat covers the aleurone – which makes up 6.5% of the total wheat kernel by weight. Within the aleurone is the endosperm – which makes up 83% of the wheat kernel's contents by weight.

The bran is the rough outside layer of the wheat berry and the upper part of the bran is covered with small hairs. The bran protects the rest of the wheat berry – allowing the wheat germ and endosperm to virtually stay fresh long after the wheat has been harvested. In fact, the bran will allow a wheat kernel to remain intact until the next sprouting season – a good nine months from its maturity.

The wheat germ – along with most of the rest of the wheat berry – also contains lectins called wheat germ agglutinins (WGA). We will discuss these more specifically later.

Wheat germ separated from the bran and endosperm will go rancid quickly because of its oil content – which can become oxidized. Millers that retain separated wheat bran will typically refrigerate it to keep it from going bad. Even then, it can go rancid within a week or so. Outside of refrigeration, most wheat germ suppliers will toast or roast the wheat germ. This has the effect of neutralizing much of the lectin content as well as gives wheat germ a longer shelf life. We'll talk lectins later.

While the wheat germ contains much of the vitamin content of wheat, the endosperm of the wheat berry is where much of the wheat's carbohydrates are stored. This section of the berry also has less nutrient density than the other two parts of the wheat berry. For this reason, white flour will spike blood sugar more than whole wheat flour.

All of these components of the wheat berry will contain protein. But the bran will contain more than double the protein content of the endosperm (at 16% versus 7%), while and germ will contain triple the protein content of the endosperm (at 23% versus 7%).

However, the gluten proteins – the gliadins and glutenins – are contained within the endosperm. This means the endosperm contains the starchy and gluey portion of the wheat. And the bran and the germ contain higher amounts of fibrous oligosaccharides and waxy phytonutrients. We will discuss these in depth in the next chapter.

Making Flour

Milling companies make flour by first tempering the wheat berries with water to soften up the bran layer. This allows the bran layer to be more easily separated from the endosperm during milling.

Using different rollers, the bran, endosperm and wheat germ layers are practically shaved away from each other as the wheat is run through a series of repetitive grinding passes through the mill. Before the berries are fed through millstand rollers, the miller adjusts the rollers to separate off the different parts of the wheat berry before it is finally ground into flour.

These three parts (bran, endosperm and germ) and their fractions are often separated from each other and then blended back together to make the various grades of flour.

Refined flours have both the wheat germ and the bran separated and not added back. Most of these are then bleached with oxidizing agents to make them "white flour."

What are they bleached with? There are several types of bleaching agents used, depending upon the mill and processor. These include:

- Chlorine dioxide (CiO_2)
- Benzoyl peroxide ($[C_6H_5C(O)]_2O_2$)
- Calcium peroxide (CaO_2)
- Nitrogen dioxide (NO_2)
- Potassium bromate ($KBrO_3$)
- Azodicarbonamide ($C_2H_4O_2N_4$)

As far as azodicarbonamide goes, this has been banned for use in flours in the EU and Australia, and many food manufacturers have voluntarily eliminated it from their products. It will degrade to urea and semicarbazide when baked with.

However, the other additives are used frequently to oxidize flour, making it easier to bake with and cake. Caked flour is extremely fine, and as such is a favorite among confectionary bakers who produce cookies, cakes and biscuits.

Most manufacturers who utilize these bleaching agents will be quick to state they mostly disappear during the baking process. This may be debatable in some cases, and many labels will list those bleaching agents on the labels of the final bread, so this would make their disappearance questionable. What cannot be removed, however, is the oxidation of some of the nutritional components in the flour by these bleaching agents.

As a result of much resistance to the bleaching process, many mills and their bakery customers have elected to use unbleached refined flour. This is typically identified on the label as UNBLEACHED ENRICHED FLOUR.

On the other hand, flour that has been refined and bleached will typically be listed on the label as ENRICHED FLOUR.

In other words, neither will a bread nor other bakery label typically utilize the words 'BLEACHED, WHITE or REFINED. Why not?

Because these words are considered derogatory to consumers. Bread manufacturers want to put the best face on their labels.

And what is enrichment anyway? Because the more nutritious bran and germ have been removed, refined flour is mandated in most countries to be enriched with some of those nutrients lost due to the elimination of the bran and germ. These typically include:

- Iron
- Thiamine
- Riboflavin
- Niacin
- Folic acid

Note these are added back because whole wheat is known to be rich in these nutrients.

Among modern mills, whole wheat flours will have the wheat germ and the bran added back. This also means the amount of germ and bran added back can be formulated. Different grades of wheat flours will thus contain more or less bran and germ according to the formulation of the mill. Brown flour, for example, will have about 85% of the germ and bran added back.

The mix of the flour the miller makes is often determined by the customer of the flour – the baker. Protein levels are often targeted to accomplish certain types of baking. Large bakeries will often have a custom blend of flour with protein and gluten ranges that will be designed specifically for the bakery application.

Our ancestors utilized large round stones to grind wheat into flour. And many smaller mills still maintain grinding stones. In contrast to most modern millers, a 'stone ground' flour typically utilizes stone mill stones, whereupon they might make only one or several passes over the wheat berry, depending upon the grade of flour preferred. Here the protein specifications will depend upon the grain brought in, though the fineness of the flour can be defined by the number of passes through the mill.

Stone grinding is often identified as a more natural process, but a modern mill that blends back all parts of the grain virtually accomplishes the same thing.

The difference in the end, however, may be in the extent of the grinding. Depending upon the mill, a stone mill may not grind the flour as completely as a modern mill might, leaving more partly-whole kernels. This is often called cracked flour.

Cracked wheat flour may also be done by a modern mill, however.

One critical concept here is that while the endosperm contains the least amount of protein by weight at around seven percent – a good portion of those proteins in the endosperm are gluten proteins.

Meanwhile, the higher level of proteins contained in the germ and the bran are not glutinous. This means that white flour will contain a significantly greater content of gluten as a percentage of total weight compared with whole wheat flours.

Furthermore, there is evidence that the epicarp hairs (see illustration – labeled "hairs, beard") and the outer bran components provide a limiting balance to the effects of gluten, at least during dough making. This should certainly translate through to digestion, as we'll discuss further. Research from King's College London (Gan *et al.* 1989) revealed that the epicarp hairs disrupt the "gluten-protein matrix."

These effects are connected to the bran, and the sizeable portion of the bran called the aleurone. The aleurone's components protect the nutrients within the grain, and balance its pH. These components include plant hormones such as auxin and gibberllin, which provide antioxidant properties as well as protective properties to the grain and its embryo.

We'll discuss aleurone further in the next chapter.

Foods With and Without Gluten

Gluten proteins are contained in many but not all grains. Here is a quick list of those plants and foods known to contain both gliadin and glutenin proteins:

Gluten-containing Foods

Common Name	Botanical Name	Foods Often Found In
Wheat	*Triticum* species	Bread, flour, cookies, cakes, biscuits, breakfast cereals, crackers, tortillas, sprouts, muffins, naan, noodles, bulgur, pancakes, cooked dishes, pastries, bagels, vegan/vegetarian foods
Rye	*Secale cereale*	Cooked dishes, bread, cakes, muffins, crisps, seeds
Spelt	*Triticum spelta*	Cooked dishes, bread, flour, muffins
Barley	*Hordeum vulgare*	Whole, cooked, flour, cereals
Kamut	*Triticum turanicum*	Bread, flour, muffins, crackers
Durum	*Triticum durum*	Pasta, couscous, noodles
Einkorn	*Triticum monococcum*	Whole cooked, pasta, bulgur
Blue wheat	*Triticum aestivum*	Pasta, flour, breads, muffins
Rivet	*Triticum turgidum*	Bread, flour, muffins

The most common wheat by far is *Triticum aestivum.* There are at least 20,000 varieties of this wheat being grown around the world today and in the recent past. Different varieties will grow during different seasons or different climate regions. Some will vary by the altitude.

Major seasonal varieties include winter wheat and spring wheat. Beyond these will be soft wheat and hard wheat. For example, a hard winter wheat will be a dramatically different plant with different nutritional qualities than a soft winter wheat or a soft spring wheat. Hard wheats typically have higher protein and gluten content, and are thus typically used for bread making.

The wheat food list above presents the reality that many of our humanity's most popular foods contain gluten. These are foods served at nearly every kitchen, cafeteria, food court, restaurant, community breakfast and party – not just in Western countries, but throughout the world.

Gluten-containing foods are eaten among both the richest and poorest peoples of the planet. In Western countries, gluten foods are used in breads, muffins, pancakes, cereals, muffins, pasta, noodles and more. In the Mediterranean and Middle Eastern world, gluten is used in traditionally-made pasta, bulgur, couscous and breads.

In Asia, gluten is contained in noodles, breads, naan, chapati, cakes and others. In Central and South America, foods containing gluten include wheat tortillas, breads, muffins and cereals. Among island peoples of the South Pacific, glutun-containing wheat flour is a staple used to make breads, cakes, chapatti, naan, cookies and others.

Rich or poor, wheat is the mainstay of many traditional diets. It is a central component of subsistence diets and gourmet meals alike.

In addition to these basic foods, many other popular foods utilize or blend some of these gluten-containing foods as ingredients.

Foods that contain gluten include soy sauce, beer, granola bars, processed meats and others. Because gluten is often used as a stabilizer, it can also be contained in any sort of soft food or condiment.

The food industry uses gluten-containing grains to make wheat starch, vital wheat gluten and just plain gluten, which can be added to breads or other foods to give them density and baking vitality. Here are some foods that vital wheat gluten is used in:

Baking mixes: Gluten may be added during milling or manually by the baker. It gives flours strength and increased baking tolerance, while improving absorption and fermentation tolerance. Any specialty bread, multigrain, high-fiber or grain texture breads can benefit greatly from gluten.

Pasta: Gluten can improve the cooking quality of pasta by improving breakage resistance, maintaining optimum texture and reducing cooking loss.

Retorted products: Gluten helps improve the structural integrity during retort processes.

Vegetarian meat replacements: Gluten can be added to increase the protein levels, texture and structure of a variety of meat replacement recipes. Gluten is known to simulate meat texture by binding to and restructuring starches and proteins.

Breakfast cereals: Gluten adds protein and flavor compatibility without adding fat levels.

Breading and batters: Gluten improves adhesion, provides barrier properties and controls greasiness.

Wheat starches are also used in a variety of foods. Wheat starch is known for its ability to withstand cooking and processing extremes. It can form a soft tender paste or gel, and is more reliable than other starches for this function.

Wheat starches are thus used as thickeners, extenders, ingredient carriers and stabilizers in products such as noodles, soups, cereals, coatings, bakery mixes, cakes, pie fillings and others; and are commonly used in meal-solutions and convenience foods. Here are some uses of wheat starch:

Cookies: Controls thickness and spread

Pie Crusts: Retains tenderness and reduces shortening requirement

Cakes: Improves batter viscosity, volume, structure, tenderness, and fat absorption

Cereals: Flake strength and puffing
Frosting and glazes: Improves spreadability.
Sauces and Soup Bases: Increases solids and thickening control
Pancake/Waffle Mixes: Controls spread and provides volume
Pudding/Dessert Mixes: Assists in body softness
Spice Mixes: Gives bulk and flow without flavor

Note that in the above descriptions, there is no opinion being made with regard to the healthiness of these foods. Don't worry, this will be covered later on.

What about wheat grass?

As for whether wheat grass, barley grass; and grass of the other wheat varieties mentioned contain gluten, this is a bit tricky to answer. Strictly speaking, these grasses do not contain the gliadin proteins typically associated with gluten intolerance. So in most people allergic to gliadin proteins, there should be no allergic response.

However, these grasses will contain proteins that can contain some of the same polypeptides that may be recognized by antibodies on immune system cells. This may trigger an allergic response in a person who is either celiac or otherwise has a wheat allergy.

The author reviewed a laboratory test of gliadin content within a commercial wheatgrass juice powder. This Neogen Vertox® test found that gliadin content in wheatgrass juice was below the limit of detection. The detection limit was 10 parts per million (ppm). One ppm is equal to one milligram of gluten per kilogram (about 2.2 lbs.) per food.

We can thus conclude that wheatgrass should not disturb a gluten intolerant person, and likely not even a person allergic to wheat.

What about foods that share facilities?

The above foods only provide the tip of the iceberg. There are many other grain foods, including corn, oats, flax and many others (listed below) that are stored at the same grain facilities that also store wheats, and transported by the same trucks that transport gluten-containing grains.

Just consider the case of a typical grain elevator. A grain elevator is in the business of storing those grains that farmers in that region grow. During the wheat harvest they will take in – some of them – hundreds of truckloads of raw harvested wheat berries. The wheat berries will be dumped from the back of the truck onto a conveyor that carries the grain up to a silo inlet. Here the grain will be offloaded down into the silo – the storage bin.

But during this offloading process, grain can spill off the side of the truck and off the side of the conveyer. It can also spill out through the various gaps of the silo. Now we're not talking a couple of grains here and there. We're talking about pounds – even hundreds of pounds – that can become intermingled with other grains in that elevator.

And this doesn't include the dust carried by the movement of all this grain into the silo. This grain dust is typically great enough for grain elevator operators to be required to wear masks to protect their lungs from all the dust. And what does this dust contain? Naturally, it will contain the glutens and gliadins from the wheat, along with various other particulates.

In fact, as we'll discuss, there are a number of allergies – including gluten allergies – that working in a grain mill or elevator increases the risk of contracting.

When it comes to moving the wheat out, these grain elevators will use conveyers or vacuum blowers to load the grain onto trucks or railcars for transportation out. At this point once again grain can leak onto the floor of the elevator and around the train or truck.

Then, once the silo is empty of grain, another type of grain may be loaded into the same silo. And it is not as if these giant silos will necessarily be sterilized. Some of them are hundreds of feet tall.

The walls of the silos are typically made of a metal of some sort. Often it will just be galvanized steel – or sometimes but rarely, stainless steel. As most metals can, galvanized steel becomes easily magnetized when any material is whisked by it. Thus the steel will attract the gluten and gliadin proteins that have filled up that silo.

This is for a grain elevator that will carry different grains at different times. The elevator may attempt to sweep out the grains at the bottom of the silo or bin between shipments. But outside of that, there can be a lot of intermingling. While some elevators will maintain only one type of grain, many elevators would go out of business if they tried to do this.

Some grain elevators will carry different grains at the same time. They might have a silo of wheat, a silo of durum wheat, a silo of corn and a silo of oats all at the same time.

This issue of commingling has become an issue for consumers who now demand labels are marked with whether the facility also packages foods that are known allergens such as nuts or soy.

Warning consumers that the facility also packages some products containing gluten might seem easy, but a food-packing facility may not know whether the elevator commingles grains.

And many food facilities – certainly the majority that bake or pack any other grain food – will pack gluten foods in addition to packing gluten-free foods.

Furthermore, there is the transportation issue. Nearly every trucking company that transports grains will transport both gluten grains and gluten-free grains, often in the same trucks. These trucks will typically do a "wash-out," but contamination with gluten protein dust is very difficult to remove completely.

As such, these facilities and trucks maintain a strong likelihood of cross-contamination between grain proteins simply because farmers grow different types of grains. And often a medium-sized farmer will grow a combination of different types of grains at the same time because the soils benefit from rotating crops. So they might rotate wheat with oats for example, or even corn with wheat.

This doesn't mean that there aren't farmers, facilities, truckers and distributors who are dedicated non-gluten grains. These may be careful not to mix bins or loads or silos and may carefully wash their trucks. However, the risk of cross-contamination is always still there.

Thus practically any grain can have some level of a crossover gluten-type protein fraction. Some grains will certainly have less, albeit. But it is a very hard road to hoe, as it were.

For example, in a study published in the *Journal of the American Dietetic Association* (Thompson *et al.* 2010), 22 grains, seeds, and flours that were supposedly inherently gluten-free – including flours from sorghum, buckwheat and millet – were analyzed for gluten-type protein fraction content in a laboratory in June of 2009. The lab found that nine of the 22, or 41% of the supposedly gluten-free samples contained more than the limit considered as quantification for gluten-free, of five ppm (parts per million). In addition, seven of the 22 samples, or 32%, contained gluten levels that averaged more than 20 ppm.

Under the FDA's proposed rule for gluten-free labels, these supposedly gluten-free grains would not qualify to be labeled as "gluten-free."

The Food Allergen Labeling and Consumer Protection Act (FALCPA) took effect in January 1, 2006. This act, passed in 2004, says that food labels from products that contain one or more of the major food allergens must state the allergen either on the ingredient panel or elsewhere on the label in plain English. The major allergens in the law include milk, eggs, fish, shellfish, peanuts, tree nuts, wheat and soy.

The Food Allergen and Consumer Protection Act is also being updated for gluten-free products. Within the language of the currently proposed rule, many foods are considered gluten-free. Millet is a good example. However, a millet label cannot, under the new rule, be labeled as "gluten free" without stating that all millet foods are inherently gluten-free. For example: ALL MILLET IS GLU-

TEN FREE. In addition, the limit for being able to describe the product as gluten-free under the new ruling is 20 parts per million.

Liquid chromatography-mass spectrometry (LC-MS) based assays, and the enzyme-linked immunosorbent assays (ELISAs) are the best methods of analyzing grain foods for their gluten or allergen content.

Potentially Gluten-free Grain-type Foods

Yes, given this risk of contamination, there are many foods that theoretically do not contain gluten. For starters, all fruits and vegetables do not contain gluten. As far as foods that can be used like grains, below is a basic list of non-gluten grains and other foods sometimes used in breads and other flour- or oil-based foods. Note this is neither an exhaustive list nor an exhaustive description of how each can be used:

A Few Gluten-free Foods

Food	Uses (outside of whole)
Amaranth	Flour, sprouted grain
Beans	Flours and cooked
Buckwheat	Flour used for noodles and pancakes
Cassava/Tapioca	Roots are used to make flour
Chickpea	Makes gram flour – used in Asian/Med dishes
Corn/Maize	Whole, flour or oil or polenta (cornmeal)
Flax seeds	Flax can be eaten whole or in flour or oil form
Hemp	Used to make flour or oil
Hops	Medicinal herb and fermented
Linseeds	Can make flour, oil or eaten whole
Millet	Boiled, steamed or porridge; also flour
Mustard	Seed or oil, bitter flour
Nuts	Tree nuts and legumes (peanuts)
Oats	Groats, cereal, granola bar, meal and flour
Potato	Whole, flour, mashed
Pulses	Beans and legumes – flours and oils
Quinoa	Cooked whole, flour and bread
Rice	Whole grain and flour
Sesame	Seeds, flour and oil
Sorghum	Flour and oil
Soybeans	Oil and flour, whole, many uses
Teff	African cereal grass – flour, cooked

The choices for gluten-free foods are considerable. But many of these foods are not readily available in restaurants and many stores. Frankly, some are difficult to find outside of a health food store in the U.S., Australia or Western Europe.

As a result, in those localities that do not have a health food store, finding prepared gluten-free grain-based foods will prove quite difficult.

One of the reasons is because many of these specialty grains require selective environments. Some – not all – are more temperamental to grow and/or to store or prepare.

Yes, there is quite simply less supply of many of these grains because they are more difficult – or specialized – to grow. As far as retail prices for the end consumer, this creates the triple-whammy of more expensive seeds, farmers needing to charge higher prices for their crops, and the distributors/retailers having to add their typical markups to their higher distributor pricing. We'll discuss this in a moment.

Not that the author doesn't like health food stores. Health food stores provide the key to the future prevention of a myriad of health conditions. Most also insist upon carrying organic products and GMO-free products, which is good for the planet and our health. Unfortunately, many in the world have no access to health food stores. Many people are limited to buying foods from small corner shops or open village markets.

In the U.S. and the U.K., an increasing number of stores are offering gluten-free foods across the board. For a price, of course.

As such, the difficulty of maintaining a gluten-free diet is great.

We are not speaking just of inconvenience here. We are speaking of hard work. It takes some real dedication and hard work to maintain a diet that is gluten-free. This is why studies have shown – as we'll illustrate, that many who start a gluten-free diet do not maintain it for long.

Especially when traveling, visiting friends or family – during holidays – or even going to restaurants or trying to find gluten-free foods at the local supermarket.

What about cost?

Reduced supply of seed and specialized growing conditions results in significantly greater food costs to consumers who attempt to eat gluten-free. There is more than a convenience issue to discuss here.

A marketing study found the average gluten-free customer will have an average grocery bill of more than three times that of the average American consumer (NFM 2014). This means that a gluten-free consumer's food shopping bill will be $300.00 for every $100.00 spent by the average consumer.

As we will clarify in this text, a gluten-free diet plays a useful and important part in a strategy to reverse a gluten intolerance or allergy. But a permanent strategy of gluten-free is not only impractical – it is costly and not affordable for most people.

As such, it simply is not a viable permanent solution for gluten intolerance, along with – as we will show – celiac disease and wheat allergies.

What is Celiac Disease?

Celiac disease is a type of allergic response to the gliadin protein fraction and possibly – in some cases – to certain glutenin proteins.

Celiac disease has been traditionally classified as a genetic autoimmune disorder. We will prove there is more involved.

Put it this way: Celiac disease has been linked to heredity and particular gene sequences, and it often appears in families. A 2003 study (Fasano *et al.*) found that a first-degree relative of a celiac sufferer has about six times more risk of having celiac disease.

The genetic link in some celiac sufferers has been seen in the HLA class II D-region of chromosome 6 in the DNA. It has been estimated that about 90-95% of sufferers have genetic markers for celiac disease haplotypes (Heap and van Heel 2009).

Yet having the genetic marker for celiac disease does not guarantee a person will have the condition. Like any genetic marker for a heretic condition, those genes will still have to be switched on to execute the condition. This is the subject of epigenetics, which relate to the effects of environment, consumption, and lifestyle, which can produce genetic mutations as the body adapts to current conditions.

A study from Sweden's Umeå University (Myléus et al. 2012) in fact found those Swedish children who developed celiac disease before the age of one year had more early infections and gastroenteritis in their first year. Did the infections trigger their genetic susceptibility? We'll discuss this study and others more specifically later.

Other research (Forsbert *et al.* 2004 and others) has found that celiac disease patients (inactive and active) have greater incidence of rod-shaped bacteria. We'll dig in deep on this point later as well.

Nonetheless, celiac disease is still considered an autoimmune disorder. And it does not typically involve immunoglobulin E antibodies as do wheat allergies and most other food allergies.

In celiac disease, the body forms immunoglobulin A (IgA) antibodies to tissue transglutaminase (tTG) and deamidated gliadin peptides (DGP). This has been seen as the result of a genetic abnormality – and an associated autoimmune condition as mentioned.

Autoimmunity relates to the immune system attacking normal tissues – a simplistic definition that we will investigate further in this text. Other medical scientists have questioned celiac disease as an autoimmune disorder (Sollid and Jabri 2005; and others).

Celiac disease occurs among both infants and adults, and more often among Caucasians. It is characterized by scarred lesions (sprue) and inflammation within the small intestines, which produce a variety of symptoms.

Celiac disease typically produces an intense inflammatory response when the celiac sufferer eats any food containing gluten. This also includes inhaling some dust with gluten, and sometimes even having skin contact with gluten-containing foods.

People in advanced stages of the condition typically have what is called villous atrophy. This is when the villi of the small intestines become deranged to the point where they have become flattened. This condition exposes the entire intestinal membrane to foods eaten – without the protection of the villi and the mucous membranes that coat them. As a result, many celiac sufferers are also sensitive to other foods.

In other words, signs and symptoms of celiac disease can be pretty intense – and hard to miss. See the section later in this chapter describing and listing common food sensitivity symptoms.

Celiac disease is no laughing matter. In a 2007 study (Anderson *et al.*), out of 13,338 people who underwent testing for the endomysial antibodies and anti-gliadin antibodies in Northern Ireland between 1993 and 1996, 490 people tested positive and were diagnosed with celiac disease. In their follow-up of these patients, they found that death incidence was increased among them compared to the general North Ireland population. However, cancers – especially lung and breast cancers – were lower among both celiac and wheat allergy patients.

The fact that celiac or wheat allergies appear far less among Africans and others in second- and third-world countries may indicate genetic predisposition, but aggravations by epigenetic variables including diet and local environment are also likely. This is because celiac mechanisms are comparable to the inflammatory intestinal response that takes place in other food sensitivities. We'll discuss this in depth later.

This response is seen in lesions along the villi and cells of the small intestines. These lesions disrupt nutrient absorption and produce a variety of metabolic symptoms around the body caused by macromolecules entering the bloodstream and tissues. Thus, higher risks of diabetes and other metabolic diseases are common among celiac sufferers.

Celiac sprue are the inflamed and damaged epithelial cells inside the intestines. They are often worse in the jejunum. As mentioned, the cells become flattened, and this will deform the villi. The intestinal wall will also often become thickened, and will be teeming with a variety of immune cells, cytokines and plasma cells ready to react on a hair-trigger.

This is consistent with the fact that the symptoms of celiac disease are extremely variable. They can range from weight loss, fatigue, diarrhea, flatulence, irritable bowels, malabsorption issues (nutrient deficiencies) and so many others. Upon examination, celiac patients may have high cholesterol, anemia, hypocalcaemia, high albumin levels, blood clotting issues and elevated liver enzymes. Gluten ataxia may also result. This can cause disorientation, headaches, fevers and other issues.

Adults can contract celiac disease at any age. The middle ages are most prevalent. This poses the question of why the late onset if the disease is hereditary? Celiac disease also occurs among children during the first three years of life, but typically after the first year. The symptoms will often include ongoing diarrhea, slow growth and a large belly.

These symptoms sometimes go away during the teenage years.

Adults might suffer severe weight loss and nutrient absorption problems, which can in result in bone loss, rickets, osteoporosis, eye problems, hormone disruption, seizures, ataxia and infertility. Worse, celiac disease increases the risk of stomach cancer, intestinal cancer or lymphoma by forty to one hundred times compared to the general population. Celiac children also have an increased risk of Down's syndrome. Nutrient deficiencies and their symptoms are common among celiac patients, and depression is also prevalent.

ELISA-derived tests for gliadin-specific IgA, IgG and antigliadin antibodies (AGAs) often clearly indicate celiac disease. AGAs may not be present during a gluten elimination diet, however. So this test has to be taken after an episode or after gluten consumption.

Summarizing, celiac disease is basically a food allergy. It is a little different than a wheat allergy, but if a person is sensitive to gluten this possibility should be eliminated early on to prevent the potential of a life-threatening reaction.

What is Non-celiac Gluten Sensitivity?

A non-celiac gluten sensitivity must first be distinguished from celiac disease as mentioned. It must also be separated from a wheat allergy.

In other words, gluten intolerance is not celiac disease and it is not a wheat allergy. It is a non-allergic response to the wheat proteins categorized as gliadins – typically classified as gluten.

Typically a proper gluten intolerance diagnosis will be tested for celiac disease and wheat allergy in order to remove those possibilities.

Repeated research over the years has found that gluten intolerance does not produce inflammation among the intestinal mucosa as it does in celiac disease. In one of many of these studies, researchers from Italy's University of Salerno (Bucci *et al.* 2013) studied 119 people at two medical centers. Of these, 69 were found to have celiac disease, 16 had non-celiac gluten sensitivity. The researchers also tested 34 healthy adults as control subjects.

The researchers conducted biopsies and endoscopy testing with gluten-gliadin proteins. They were tested for markers of inflammation. Their blood was drawn and their blood immune cells were tested for inflammation response.

Mucosa samples from all the patients with celiac disease had inflammation markers when tested with gliadin proteins. Of the 16 patients, only three of the patients with non-celiac disease gluten sensitivity had any inflammation markers for intestinal inflammation or blood-borne inflammation. This matched with three showing similar inflammation markers among the healthy controls.

The researchers concluded:

> *"Unlike the duodenal mucosa from patients with celiac disease, upon incubation with gliadin, mucosa from patients with non-celiac gluten sensitivity does not express markers of inflammation, and their basophils are not activated by gliadin."*

This means gluten intolerance is extremely difficult to diagnose independently of a patient's complaint that they don't feel well after eating gluten. When a patient complains of gluten sensitivity, and celiac disease and wheat allergies have been eliminated with testing, gluten intolerance will often be assumed.

But there are few if any tests that absolutely indicate gluten intolerance – even the highly-sensitive IgG-C3d immune complex test. We'll discuss this more in the testing section near the end of this chapter.

Non-celiac gluten sensitivities do indeed exist. This has been shown repeatedly among clinical researchers. For example, clinicians at Italy's University La Sapienza (Picarelli *et al.* 1996) investigated 10 non-celiac patients who did not immunologically seem to have celiac disease. Out of the ten, four tested positive for the genetic marker HLA known in celiac disease. Out of the remaining six, three showed some inflammation among intestinal cells after performing biopsies. While some were clearly pre-celiac in that they had the genetic marker but not the immune response, it became evident to the researchers that at least some of the patients had a non-celiac gluten sensitivity of some sort.

And in a study (Sapone *et al.* 2011) of celiac disease and non-celiac gluten sensitive patients, researchers found that anti-gliadin antibodies (AGA) were not associated with non-celiac gluten intolerances.

Research from Italy's University Hospital of Palermo reviewed the (Marsueto *et al.* 2014) research on non-celiac gluten sensitivity to date, and found that most gluten intolerance patients report both digestive and non-digestive symptoms.

Most have also stated that a gluten-free diet reduced those symptoms.

Furthermore, patients reporting gluten intolerance report a variety of symptoms – according to University of Bologna (Volta *et al.* 2012) researchers who studied 78 patients with non-celiac gluten sensitivity, their symptoms included:

> *"abdominal pain, bloating, diarrhea, constipation, foggy mind, tiredness, eczema/skin rash, headache, joint/muscle pain, numbness of legs/arms, depression, and anemia."*

However, these symptoms have been difficult to trace to any particular mechanism that might drive the sensitivity.

Let's use an example. To diagnose diabetes mellitus type 1, a blood test will reveal abnormal levels of glycated hemoglobin. This is also called an HbA1c test, as higher levels of HbA1c glycated hemoglobin indicate a lack of glucose control, and a diabetic metabolism.

In the HbA1c test there is a clear metabolic link between diabetes, and higher levels of glycated hemoglobin are clearly linked with a lack of glucose control because there is a metabolic pathway connecting the two. When blood glucose increases, glycated hemoglobin also increases because of a metabolic process called the glycation pathway – or non-enzymatic glycosylation. In glycation, lipids become bound to glucose.

When there is too much glucose in the bloodstream there is an increase in glycated hemoglobin because of this tendency of glucose – as well as fructose – to undergo glycation.

In gluten intolerance there is no known pathway between the markers of the currently popular diagnostic test – increased levels IgGs for gliadin peptide antibodies IgGs – and the symptoms correlated with gluten intolerance. This fact was confirmed in the Volta study mentioned above – where the researchers tested IgG DGP-AGA antibodies as well as IgA tTGA and IgA EmA (will explain these later) on both the 78 non-celiac gluten sensitive patients and the 80 celiac patients.

They found 89% of the celiac patients tested positive for IgG DGP-AGA while only 1 of the 78 non-celiac gluten sensitive patients tested positive. And none of the non-celiac gluten sensitive patients tested positive for IgA tTGA or IgA EmA.

Again, this doesn't mean that non-celiac non-wheat allergy gluten sensitivity is nonexistent.

But in many non-celiac non-wheat allergy gluten sensitivity patients, there are multiple food sensitivities.

In a study from Italy's Hospital of Sciacca (Carroccio *et al.* 2012), researchers tested 276 patients that had been diagnosed with wheat sensitivity using a double-blind placebo-controlled food challenge. They utilized patients with IBS as control subjects.

Many of the wheat-sensitive patients had multiple food sensitivities.

The researchers then tested the subjects for IgGs, IgAs and cytometric basophil activation. The researchers found many of the wheat sensitive patients had higher levels of anti-gliadin IgG and IgAs, and basophil activation.

But primarily only those with wheat allergy symptoms had these higher activations.

And the main physiological element common among the wheat sensitivity patients was: *"eosinophil infiltration of the duodenal and colon mucosa."*

Eosinophil infiltration is a condition whereby the walls of the intestines and/or colon are damaged. The condition is technically known as eosinophilic gastroenteritis. It is characterized by symptoms such as diarrhea, weight loss, bloating, nausea and abdominal pain.

These of course are some of the same symptoms reported by those who report they are sensitive to gluten. So there is more than coincidence.

But as to antibodies among those with non-allergic wheat intolerance: There is currently little consensus that an immune response – e.g., antibodies – are associated.

What is a Wheat Allergy?

Food allergies such as celiac disease are reactions of the immune system to molecules of food – called allergens. A wheat allergy is a similar condition, but it is not genetically based as is celiac disease.

Also a wheat allergy can include other proteins in wheat besides the gliadin proteins. It can be an IgE sensitivity to any number of proteins within wheat. These can include the wheat's globulins, albumins, prolamins and/or glutelins.

An allergen is a portion of a food molecule that the immune system considers foreign to the body. In other words, the immune system is threatened by part of the food. Once an allergen is marked as a threat, it will be remembered as such for some time.

Once the immune system considers any molecule a threat, it stimulates a process to remove that substance from the body. Normally this is a quite docile and automatic process that happens without our perception. However, if the immune system is weakened, imbalanced and/or otherwise overactive, the response can be out of proportion with what would ordinarily be required to remove such a molecule from the body.

As we will discuss in more detail later, most food allergy reactions occur using a part of the immune system called immunoglobulin E, or IgE. Ordinarily, foreign molecules are removed using immunoglobulin A (IgA), which line our mucous membranes. By using IgA, the immune system can remove foreigners before they can gain access to the body's tissues.

In an IgE or other non-IgA immune response, the foreign molecules have penetrated further into the body than they would have normally. This makes them a potential threat. Once the molecules come into contact with the IgEs, the IgEs will stimulate the release of inflammatory mediators such as histamine, prostaglandins and leukotrienes. These will produce allergic reactions around the body such as rashes, wheezing, sinusitis, watery eyes and so on.

As we've discussed, gluten is not a single protein. It is better described as a category of proteins. Rather, the gluten proteins in wheat are primarily either gliadins or glutenins. Within these two types are many different specific proteins. Furthermore, the types of glutinous proteins in wheat are not like the glutinous proteins in most other grains. In fact, between these two types, gliadins are considered the most prevalent allergen – common in both baker's asthma and wheat allergies (Ueno *et al.* 2010).

There also many other possible wheat allergens. They include alpha-amylase inhibitor, peroxidase, thaumatin-like protein (TLP), lipid transfer proteins (LTPs) such as LTP2G and low-molecular-weight glutenins. These allergens are heat resistant and do not readily cross-react with grass pollen allergens (Pastorello *et al.* 2007).

Noting this, it appears the reason why people react to proteins in wheat and other grains is through cross-reactivity among similar strings of amino acids, called peptides. While the full proteins (complex strings of hundreds of amino acids) will be different between wheat, barley and oats, for example, they will often share similar peptide strings. These are also sometimes referred to as protein fractions.

French researchers (Bodinier *et al.* 2007) found in a laboratory study that hydrolyzed omega5-gliadin fractions and lipid transfer proteins could penetrate a monolayer cultured with intestinal cells. Most other wheat peptides were blocked by the monolayer, in contrast.

These common protein fractions may be present in wheat, rye and barley. But lipid transfer proteins (LTPs) are quite common among other plants and foods. However, LTPs will greatly differ in molecular arrangement from species to species. A person sensitive to one plant's LTPs will likely not be sensitive to another plant's. But as research has illustrated, their susceptibility to becoming allergic to that LPT will nonetheless be increased.

In the same way, wheat sensitivities may leave one more sensitive to foods that use wheat proteins such as blue cheese, bouillon cubes, chocolate, curry, food colorings, starches, grain alcohols (including beer, ale, rye, scotch, bourbon or grain vodka), gum base, hydrolyzed vegetable protein, malts, marshmallows, modified food starches, monosodium glutamates, non-dairy creamers, processed meats, pudding, wheat/soy sauce, and even distilled vinegars.

While many of these will not contain the complete allergen in its full configuration, they may contain traces of certain peptide sequences.

This of course may significantly change the perspective most people have as they consider wheat sensitivities.

Certainly other foods can be allergenic outside of those mentioned above for a person who is wheat sensitive. And it is often assumed that ingredients are clearly stated on the ingredient panel. This is not always the case, however. Many processed foods will contain known allergens without the allergen being listed. This not only presents a danger for those who are sensitive, but for food processors, because the list of food allergens has been growing significantly over the past few years.

Spanish researchers (Palacin *et al.* 2010) found that wheat allergies are rising. They also found that the wheat flour lipid transfer protein (LTP) Tri a14 appears to be the key allergen responsible for baker's asthma and wheat sensitivities among their test population. And because cross-reactivity is common among the LTPs, there is often a transference between asthmatic bakers so that they become allergic to eating bread at some point. This has been termed *LTP syndrome*. The researchers confirmed this effect among eight adults who suffered from anaphylaxis after eating wheat foods.

Many children with wheat allergies become tolerant as they get older. Multiple studies have found the average age for becoming tolerant to wheat is about seven years old.

What's the Difference between Allergy and Intolerance?

In order to distinguish the difference between a gluten intolerance and a gluten allergy – celiac disease or another type of wheat allergy – we need to focus in on food allergies, and why they are different from food intolerances such as gluten intolerance.

Food intolerances such as gluten intolerance may seem like allergies sometimes, but they are not. This is because the body may also be reacting to what it considers a foreign molecule – usually a protein. But the response is not the same. The body may simply utilize its general detoxification systems to break down the foreigner. Or it may launch an inflammatory process to rid the foreigner.

The difference is that the body simply does not know how to handle the foreigner, so it produces physiological symptoms related to its inability to handle the food.

People typically confuse food intolerances with food allergies because they consider any sort of negative physiological response to food as an allergic reaction.

An intolerance is usually the result of the body not managing or digesting a food properly – and thus not breaking down at least some of the proteins. If the food is not properly managed and the proteins not broken down by the body's digestive system, the food can disrupt the body in a variety of ways. This may include digestive discomfort, headaches, fever, and a host of other symptoms, as we've talked about with gluten intolerance. This response is significantly different than an allergic response.

In food intolerance, the food molecule is not being targeted specifically by the immune-inflammatory system. The body is simply reacting negatively to a food molecule that it finds in regions that molecule is not normally found.

One might wonder what is the big difference. In both occurrences, the body is reacting to a foreign molecule or group of molecules. And yes, there is a lot of similarity between the two reactions sometimes. But inherent in the word "allergy" is the existence of a particular "allergen."

In an allergy, the allergy is caused by the intrusion of an allergen that is identified as a threat to the body. This allergen (or epitope) – often a protein or a portion of a larger protein molecule – produces *a specific type of immune response* when it binds with an immunoglobulin atop an immune cell such as a mast cell or basophil.

A food intolerance does not involved this binding system. Nor does it produce the same type of inflammatory response.

For example, food intolerances do not produce anaphylaxis. Anaphylaxis is a sometimes life-threatening reaction that sometimes requires an urgent medical response to prevent fatality.

Because of this increased risk of mortality, many confuse the urgency of food intolerances with that of food allergies.

For example, one might have heard that a tiger can be dangerous – it can cause serious injury and even kill a person. Would it be logical to put that same sense of urgency regarding tigers upon a house cat? Certainly not. But a person who was uneducated on the differences between tigers and house cats might.

As a result of this sense of urgency regarding a reaction to foods, there are far fewer food allergies than most believe. For example, in one Italian study (Asero *et al.* 2009) of 25,602 allergy clinic patients, 12,739 of them had allergy skin symptoms but only 1,079 (4.2% of the whole group and 8.5 of those with skin symptoms) were found to have IgE-mediated clinical allergic reactions: A true allergy in other words.

In a food intolerance, there is a imbalance between the food's makeup and the ability of the body to process and metabolize the food. In some cases, this means that the food contains proteins, sugars or other nutrients the digestive tract cannot properly break down. In other cases, the food may contain some constituent that the body reacts negatively to. In these cases, the food constituent may be given access to the walls of the intestine or stomach and specifically irritate those cells. Or the constituent may gain access to the bloodstream, where the liver or other metabolic process in the body may have to work to remove it.

Illustrating the distinct difference between gluten allergy and gluten intolerance in terms of metabolism, researchers from Italy's Second University of Naples (Sapone *et al.* 2010) took intestinal biopsies from 13 adults with celiac disease, 11 adults with gluten intolerance and seven healthy people (controls).

Food allergies including celiac disease are known to activate the cytokine interleukin-17 (IL-17) among T-cells as they stimulate inflammation within an autoimmune process. So the researchers tested the biopsy samples from the subjects' small intestines and tested them for IL-17A expression. The researchers found that the celiac group had significant expression of IL-17A (one type of celiac does not utilize IL-17) while none of the gluten intolerant subjects had markers for IL-17A, as did the healthy control subjects.

The researchers stated clearly:

> *"We conclude that gluten intolerance, albeit gluten-induced, is different from celiac disease not only with respect to the genetic makeup and clinical and functional parameters, but also with respect to the nature of the immune response."*

This is the crux of the matter. "the nature of the immune response" relates to how the immune system handles the food constituent.

Nearly any food can cause intolerance, but foods often causing intolerance include dairy, soy, wheat and gluten-containing grains, nuts, seeds, particularly acidic foods such as vinegar or orange juice, and a variety of processed foods. Nightshade foods such as tomatoes, eggplants, potatoes and peppers have sometimes caused intolerances. Normally healthy glycoalkaloids such as solanine can irritate intestinal cells in an already-damaged intestinal tract (Shimoi *et al.* 2007). In a healthy person, glycoalkaloids are antioxidants that help prevent cancer (Lu, *et al.* 2010).

Again, the research has shown that people tend to self-diagnose themselves as allergic to a food when it may be a case of food intolerance, or even something else. To this confusion we can add mild food poisoning cases, which can result in years of intolerance to a certain food.

We will discuss the specific causes of intolerance later.

Credible research, including Woods *et al.* (1998) and Pereira *et al.* (2005), have suggested that actual food allergies are a quarter of the levels perceived by many in the media and population. The remainder are likely food intolerances or symptoms of other conditions.

Illustrating this, researchers (Orhan *et al.* 2009) found in a study of 3,500 6-9-year-olds that food allergies reported by the children's parents among from urban area schoolchildren were 5.7% of the total population. However, using the (gold standard) double-blind, placebo-controlled food challenge method, only 0.8% of the children actually had clinical allergies.

As mentioned earlier, we will be using the word *sensitivity* to cover both food intolerance and food allergies. In either case, because the body is reacting to the food, the body and/or the person has become sensitive to it.

What are the Symptoms of a Wheat Allergy?

This is important for anyone considering they possibly have some sensitivity to gluten. Why? Because unlike a simple gluten intolerance, an allergy to gluten or some other part of wheat can be lethal if not managed.

Food allergies in general can cause a variety of symptoms, which can include any part of the body, including the skin, digestive system, cardiovascular system, respiratory system, nervous system and even urinary and reproductive systems. They can also cause anaphylaxis and heart conditions.

The most common allergic symptoms are hives, itching, redness, sinusitis, congestion, wheezing, inflammation and puffiness of the skin. Itchy lips or mouth is often the initial reaction in an allergy. After that, the cheeks may become swollen and red. The arms may become covered with hives and rash. The legs may become itchy and inflamed.

Skin reactions are seen as one of the highest-occurring symptoms of food sensitivities. In the Italian study mentioned earlier (Asero), nearly 50% (12,739) of the entire group had skin reactions.

Rodríguez-Ortiz *et al.* (2010) reported that 58% of the Mexican food allergy population had symptoms related to skin rash and hives. Digestive and respiratory symptoms followed in prominence. Coexistent conditions included urticaria angioedema (in 38%), allergic rhinitis (in 20%), atopic dermatitis (in 15%), and asthma (in 6.6%). To clarify, urticaria angioedema is an allergic rash that occurs underneath the skin, while allergic rhinitis is a sinus-related allergic reactions and atopic dermatitis is an external skin-related allergy reaction.

Digestive responses include irritable bowels, GERD, constipation, diarrhea, bloating, flatulence, ulcer and others. Many of these tend to be the result of food intolerances, but they can also be the result of allergies.

Allergic rhinitis is a frequent symptom of wheat allergies. Here we see watery eyes, runny nose, sneezing, stuffy nose, scratchy throat or any combination thereof. Rhinitis is frequent among peanut, shrimp and milk allergies.

Respiratory allergy symptoms related to allergic rhinitis will include lung congestion, breathing passage congestion, sinus congestion and in general, difficulty breathing. This may seem like asthma, a cold, hay fever or even being choked or gagged. The latter occurs when the wind pipe becomes swollen and the breathing passageways narrow. This typically occurs in anaphylaxis.

The chart below summarizes symptoms that can occur in a wheat allergy, compared to wheat intolerance:

Wheat Allergy Symptoms

Symptom	Food Allergy	Intolerance
Hives	Often	Rarely
Airway constriction	Often	Rarely
Asthma	Often	Rarely
Wheezing	Often	Rarely
Itching	Often	Rarely
Drop in blood pressure	Often	Rarely
Shock	Sometimes	Rarely
Weak pulse	Sometimes	Rarely
Rapid pulse	Sometimes	Rarely
Dizziness	Sometimes	Rarely
Watery eyes	Often	Rarely
Runny nose	Often	Rarely
Skin rash	Often	Rarely
Skin eruptions	Sometimes	Rarely
Swollen tongue	Sometimes	Rarely
Irritable bowels	Rarely	Sometimes
Abdominal cramping	Often	Sometimes
Vomiting	Often	Sometimes
Diarrhea	Often	Rarely
Nausea	Often	Rarely
Fainting	Sometimes	Rarely
Itchy mouth	Often	Rarely
Lightheadedness	Sometimes	Rarely
Drooling	Sometimes	Rarely
Inability to swallow	Sometimes	Rarely
Change in voice quality	Sometimes	Rarely
Redness	Often	Rarely
Fever or warmth (flushing)	Often	Rarely
Gastritis	Rarely	Rarely
Diarrhea	Sometimes	Sometimes
Ulcers	Rarely	Sometimes
Bladder infections	Rarely	Rarely

Ear infections	Sometimes	Rarely
Joint pain	Rarely	Rarely
Low back pain	Rarely	Rarely
Migraine	Rarely	Rarely
Headaches (non-migraine)	Sometimes	Sometimes
Sinusitis	Often	Rarely
Itchy Throat	Often	Rarely
Sore Throat	Sometimes	Rarely
Constipation	Rarely	Sometimes
Irritable bowels	Rarely	Sometimes
Panic attacks	Sometimes	Rarely
Fatigue	Rarely	Sometimes
Anxiety	Sometimes	Rarely
Depression	Rarely	Rarely

Hives are the most frequent response to IgE-mediated food hypersensitivity according to research from Italy (del Giudice *et al.* 2010).

Rhinitis (watery eyes, sinusitis and so on) due to food allergies typically does not usually occur alone. Rather, it will likely occur with other symptoms, including eczema, asthma, urticaria, oral cavity ruptures, and various gastrointestinal problems.

What is Atopy?

Atopy is used frequently among doctors and scientists to describe food sensitivity symptoms. What is atopy anyway? Atopy is derived from the Greek word meaning *"unusual"* or *"not ordinary."* Atopic is used to describe the condition where a person is reacting to a substance in a way that is unrelated to the contact with the substance.

For example, a normal response to breathing in some dust is to sneeze. This response is normal, and will act to remove the dust from the sinuses. But if suddenly a rash breaks out all over the body including the legs, the reaction is more than a normal physiological response. It is an extraordinary response that has engaged mechanisms outside of the realm and proportion of the exposure. In the case of most allergies, the body engages antibodies such as immunoglobulin E, or IgE. This engagement with IgE produces what is called a *mediated response*. Again this response is outside of the ordinary IgA response that expels the foreigner before it penetrates the body's tissue systems. Once within the tissues, the allergen is identified by IgE, which stimulates the production of inflammatory mediators such as histamine, prostaglandins and leukotrienes. These produce the various atopic symptoms listed above.

If a person has atopic allergies, they will most often have hives, rashes, itchiness and respiratory issues. Atopic reactions are typically related to the mucosal membranes. These are expressed as asthma, allergic rhinitis, conjunctiva rhinitis, and even eosinophilic esophagitis. Some digestive symptoms are considered atopic, but here the response must be considered out of proportion with a typical response to a foreigner – such as indigestion, a little diarrhea or constipation or a slight stomach ache.

In other words, an intense period of abdominal cramping immediately after eating might be considered atopic or it might not. It might simply indicate a lack of enzymatic digestion or an intestinal infection of some sort.

Eczema or dermatitis of the skin is considered atopic when the substance is not being consumed through the skin. In other words, if eating a food produces a skin irritation; this is likely an atopic response. While atopic skin responses can appear anywhere on the skin, atopic skin rashes will often occur on the hands, elbows or knees. These areas can become itchy and very uncomfortable in an atopic condition. Over a few days of an outbreak, they can also become scaly and crusted. These lesions can also worsen with by the use of chemical soaps or certain types of clothing.

On the other hand, a skin reaction to a chemical lotion we just spread onto the skin would not be considered an atopic condition. In fact, such a response would be quite normal considering the many chemical lotions on the market today.

Diseases Related to Food Allergies

Food allergies including those to wheat have been associated with a number of disorders. The list can be very long, depending upon who you talk to.

This does not necessarily mean allergies are isolated from other conditions. To the contrary, a number of conditions have been associated with food sensitivities – especially those related to the gastrointestinal system and inflammatory conditions.

For example, in a study by Polish researchers (Grzybowska-Chlebowczyk 2009), 95 children between two to 18 years old with various disease diagnoses were given IgE immunity tests for food allergies. Food allergies were found among a third of children with urticaria (skin conditions). Food allergies were also found among 21% of Crohn's disease patients.

Here is a list of common disorders that have been clinically linked to food allergies (note: correlation, not causation):

- Rheumatoid arthritis
- Colitis
- Irritable bowel syndrome
- Sinusitis
- Asthma
- Crohn's disease

- Migraines
- COPD
- Constipation
- Ulcers
- Urinary disorders
- Cardiovascular disease
- Mental conditions
- Immunosuppression
- Diabetes

There are many others that have been otherwise linked. In some cases, the association with the conditions listed above is considered causative. In others, it may be the other way around. In fact, many of these conditions are classified as autoimmune diseases. As a matter of association, food sensitivities might be, and often are considered autoimmune. This is supported by the fact that autoimmunity is defined as a condition where the immune system begins to attack its own cells.

In the case of the food sensitivity, the body is responding to the consumption of food molecules that should otherwise provide nutrition to the body – and thus become part of the body's cells and tissues. That is, if the digestive tract handled the food properly.

What is Anaphylaxis?

An anaphylactic response is considered a severe response to an allergen. And wheat allergies have been known to produce anaphylaxis.

Practically any symptom of a food allergy can become anaphylactic – or life-threatening. This can range from a skin response, a gastrointestinal response, a cardiovascular event, or most commonly, a respiratory event. In the latter, the throat can constrict and reduce the ability to breathe.

In the 12 years between 1993 and 2005, there were 17.3 million emergency room visits for acute allergic reactions in the United States. These represented 1.3% of all emergency room visits (Rudders *et al.* 2010). In other words, about 13 out of every 1,000 emergency room visits are for anaphylaxis.

The Food Allergy and Anaphylaxis Network (FAAN) has established through randomized phone surveys that approximately 12 million Americans – about 4% of the U.S. population – have severe allergic reactions to either peanuts, tree nuts such as cashews or pistachios, or seafood. This indicates that about two-thirds of these people are self-managing their severe allergic responses at home or without frequent urgent care responses. Many allergy sufferers or their parents carry an epinephrine injection kit, for example.

Allergy specialists report that there are generally three different types of anaphylaxis responses:

1) *Uniphasic* – a onetime rush of symptoms.
2) *Biphasic* – an initial reactive rush of symptoms, followed by another reaction later, sometimes several hours later.
3) *Protracted* – an ongoing rush of symptoms that do not abate for several hours. This is somewhat rare, but it does sometimes occur in extreme anaphylaxis.

People with food allergies and asthma have a higher risk of anaphylaxis than people who suffer from food allergies without asthma (González-Pérez *et al.* 2010). About half the deaths from anaphylaxis come from allergic responses to tree nuts or peanuts.

Researchers from California's Kaiser Permanente (Iribarren *et al.* 2010) found that the incidence of anaphylactic shock among allergic responses occurred in about 109 person-years out of 100,000 person-years, primarily when food allergies were associated with asthma. From a patient population of 526,406 cases over ten years, about one-fifth of anaphylactic shock cases (20 per 100,000 person-years) occurred in cases of asthma without food allergies. In other words, asthma sufferers with food allergies are five times more likely to experience anaphylactic shock than those with asthma alone. Other population studies have found food anaphylaxis occurs between one and 70 of every 100,000 people (Boyce *et al.* 2010).

A collaborative multicenter study from the researchers from the Massachusetts General Hospital in Boston (Clark *et al.* 2004) accumulated data on emergency room visits for food allergy complications. These visits included airway obstruction (anaphylaxis), rashes and other acute care situations. They found that 55% of the ER visits were life-threatening. Urgent care food allergy suffers had an average age of 29 years old. Emergency room visits were about 57% female. About 40% of the allergy sufferers were Caucasian.

Among the allergens that provoked the urgent care, 21% of the visits involved nut allergies, 19% were caused by eating shellfish, 12% were cause by fruit, and 10% were caused by fish.

Wheat didn't make it to the list, but that doesn't mean wheat doesn't cause anaphylaxis. In a study (Cianferoni *et al.* 2013) 93 children, researchers found that a child that tested positive in an oral challenge for a wheat allergy had more than double the risk of having an anaphylactic attack.

How do doctors treat anaphylaxis? In the Boston hospital study above, doctors gave 72% of the anaphylaxis patients antihistamines. Forty-eight percent were given corticosteroids. Sixteen percent were given epinephrine. In addition, 33% were given respiratory treatments such as albuterol (inhalant). Among those with severe reactions, only 24% were given epinephrine. In all,

16% of patients were given self-injectable epinephrine to use. Twelve percent were further referred to an allergist.

It is also important to note that research has shown that anaphylaxis from food allergies has been fatal in about 1% of severe anaphylaxis cases (Moneret-Vautrin and Morisset 2005). If we consider how rare severe anaphylaxis is among the general population, we can see how rare death is. Still it does happen and those who suffer from anaphylaxis should remember this.

Most food anaphylactic deaths have co-existent asthma. Most occur among adolescents and young adults (Gillman and Douglass 2010).

Researchers have found that factors that increase the risk of severe allergic anaphylaxis include agents that tend to cause increased intestinal permeability. These include aspirin, beta-blockers, angiotensin-converting enzyme (ACE) inhibitors, and alcohol (Moneret-Vautrin and Morisset 2005). We'll discuss this topic in more depth later.

Multiple Food Sensitivities

Single food sensitivities are a dying breed. Multiple food sensitivities are increasingly occurring. And those with wheat sensitivities are not immune to becoming sensitive to multiple foods.

This was found in a study of 920 irritable bowel syndrome patients, including 276 patients who had been diagnosed with a wheat sensitivity at some point using a double-blind placebo-controlled challenge. Of these 276 wheat-sensitive patients, only 70 were sensitive only to wheat. The other 206 patients had multiple food sensitivities.

The growing consensus among clinicians is that whether it is an allergy or intolerance, having one food sensitivity dramatically increases the likelihood of having multiple sensitivities.

When children present with multiple sensitivities, doctors attempt to find which allergy was primary to the others. The primary allergy is typically the one the child became sensitized to first. The primary allergen sometimes produces a cross-reactivity that causes the second sensitivity, but sometimes they are unrelated. In other words, once there is an initial food allergy, subsequent allergies tend to follow.

In an attempt to understand this better, researchers from Germany's Charité University Medical Center (Matricardi *et al.* 2008) followed 1,314 children for up to thirteen years from birth. They found that sensitization to milk and eggs decreased over years, from levels of about 4% at two years old to less than one percent at ten years old. On the other hand, allergies to soy and wheat increased as the children got older: From about 2% at two years old to about 7% at 13 years old for soy; and from 2% to 9% for wheat allergies.

When the children were ten years old, confirmed allergies to grass pollen were from 97% to 98% of those children who were also allergic to soy and wheat. In addition, allergies to birch pollen among the soy and wheat allergy children occurred in 86% and 82%, respectively.

The researchers concluded that the pollens were the primary allergens in most cases. They found that soy or wheat allergies were primary to grass or birch pollen in only 4%; and 8% among participants sensitized to soy and wheat, respectively.

How do I Know if I Have a Wheat Sensitivity?

Diagnosing Wheat Allergies and Celiac Disease

Wheat allergies and celiac disease have reliable and clear ways to diagnose. There is also a clear metabolic relationship between the test results and symptoms of these conditions.

The most assured test for celiac disease called the endomysial antibody test. This test measures the antibodies that bind with transglutaminase within the endomysium, which is part of the bodies connective tissue system. This is also referred to as tissue transglutaminase (tTG) which we have discussed. Antibodies to tTG are called anti-endomysial antibodies or EMA.

The test was confirmed for its accuracy in a number of studies, including a study (Ferreira *et al.* 1992) of 117 celiac patients along with other groups of patients that had intestinal issues or gluten issues that were non-celiac, including healthy control subjects. The researchers found the test was 100% accurate, even for those celiac disease sufferers not previously diagnosed.

Celiacs can also be tested for stage of the condition by testing their villous atrophy. An endoscopy test can send a camera into the small intestines to visualize the condition of the small intestines and their villi. A biopsy of a small part of the small intestines can also be taken and analyzed.

The results of such an analysis yields a Marsh Score. This indicates the degree of atrophy among the villi. The worst score is Stage Four – which indicates not only atrophy – flattening of the villi – but villi crypts. These crypts are pockets within the intestinal wall around the villi. This indicates significant intestinal wall damage.

As far as wheat allergies go, as mentioned earlier, many studies have shown that only a small percentage of those who believe they have food allergies actually have food allergies. This is especially true for parents. Many more parents believe their child has a food allergy than do. Manchester hospital researchers (Nicolaou *et al.* 2010) studied 933 children, 110 with reactions to peanuts. They found that of these 110, only 24% were found to be clinically allergic to peanuts.

Furthermore, in a study from Dutch researchers (Hospers *et al.* 2006), out of 43 children diagnosed with food allergies by a physician, only 68% were confirmed as having an allergy using double-blind challenge testing.

So what is the best way to determine whether we have a food allergy? The first thing is to consider our symptoms and their severity. See the chart earlier in this chapter. Do one or more of these rated "Often" or "Sometimes" take place within a half hour of eating? Or are the symptoms less severe and occur several hours after eating? The former, according to the research, will more likely be a food allergy, while the latter will more likely be a food intolerance.

Most of the science on diagnostic tests has focused primarily upon IgE-related food allergies, as these are most likely to cause life-threatening anaphylaxis. We should remember that there are other types of food sensitivities, such as eosinophilic gastrointestinal diseases and food protein-induced enterocolitis. Outside of these, there are a variety of sensitivities to different constituents of foods.

Regardless, we should consider getting tested to at least screen out the possibility of an IgE allergy. There are several diagnostic tests now in use:

IgE Immunoassays

Blood may be drawn and submitted to what some refer to as a *radioallergosorbent test* (or RAST). This is more accurately called the *immunoassay for allergen-specific IgE,* however. This test will measure the content of allergen-specific immunoglobulin Es in the bloodstream.

When we say allergen-specific IgEs, know that an IgE responsive to wheat protein will not be the same as an IgE that is responsive to milk proteins. This means that the immunoassay may determine whether an food allergy exists, and if so, what the allergen might be.

A well-respected immunoassay test for accuracy is the CAP-RAST test. Because CAP-RAST immunoassay tests determine the level of an allergen-specific IgE in the blood, they are considered more accurate. Typically the test comes with a level on a 1-to-100 scale, with 100 being the highest level and one being the lowest. A score of 75 will typically produce an allergy diagnosis. On the other hand, a level that is, say, 10 or 15, might be problematic to diagnose. At this level, there may be tolerance to a food that was previously considered an allergen to the body.

Indeed, one of the problems of immunoassay testing is the fact that different people have different levels of tolerance at the same IgE levels. The immunoassay test also does little to indicate the severity or type of allergic reaction a person might have. A person, for example, might have a high immunoassay IgE number but have a strong immune system that manages the response quite well. On the other hand, an immunosuppressed person with a lower IgE level might have severe reactions to the food.

On the other hand, one of the benefits of obtaining such a clear number is that from successive tests, a person can find out whether their sensitivity is dropping or increasing with time. A higher number can indicate increasing sensitivity, while a lowering number can indicate increased tolerance. This can be truly helpful with some of the strategies we'll discuss later on.

Skin Prick Tests

In skin prick testing (often referred to as SPT), a small amount of a food that the allergist thinks we are sensitive to is inserted underneath the top layer of skin by a pricking of the skin. The skin is then monitored for response. If the skin responds with a *weal* (a small circular mark or welt), this indicates the existence of a sensitivity to that food.

There are typically three methods used to apply this skin prick test. A skin prick instrument may be soaked in the food before the skin is pricked with it. The diagnostician may also place a drop of the food onto the skin before pricking the skin underneath the drop with a needle or probe.

The diagnostician may also inject the allergen underneath the skin with a needle. This is rarely employed for food allergies.

Once the prick is done, it usually takes about 10-15 minutes for the weal to come up. It will often look like a small pimple. It is the histamine response that makes this happen. A salt water prick test is often deployed to test for skin sensitivity to the pricking alone.

Skin prick testing has proven to be one of the least accurate forms of testing, however. While a negative response (no weal) usually confirms no allergy to that food, a positive response may not indicate an actual food allergy or intolerance when the food is eaten. Research has revealed that up to 60% of positive results can be false *(false positives)*.

Food Challenges

If there is a strong suspicion of a food allergy, the allergist may invoke a food challenge by feeding the patient with first a tiny amount, and then increasingly larger doses of a food while they watch for reactions. This can be a painstaking and extensive test. And for someone who is showing signs of allergies, this test should only be performed by or in the presence of a trained health professional prepared to react with medical care should anaphylaxis result.

There are a number of different types of food challenge tests, but the most employed method is giving the patient a capsule of the allergen (or a placebo). When a placebo is employed, it is called a *double-blind, placebo-controlled food challenge.* In other words, neither the diagnostician nor the patient will know whether the capsule contains the allergen or the placebo. This can eliminate results produced through the inclinations of either the health professional or patient.

As mentioned earlier, the double-blind, placebo-controlled food challenge is considered the gold standard among diagnostic tests for food allergies and most food sensitivities.

The Difficulty of Diagnosing Gluten Intolerance

Outside of the resistance many of us have to going to a doctor in general, the reality is that gluten intolerance is extremely difficult to diagnose. Wheat allergies and celiac disease are much easier to diagnose as we've illustrated above.

As we will also illustrate, there is currently no clear and medically acceptable diagnostic tool that will confirm a gluten intolerance outside of a patient's subjective assessment. And more importantly, there is little that will ascertain that gluten intolerance is causing negative physical symptoms being attributed to a gluten intolerance.

The issues of correlation and causation, which will be discussed shortly, are critical in this discussion. This is not just regarding the condition of gluten intolerance: This relates to a particular person's ability to correlate their symptoms with gluten intolerance, and a clinician's ability to determine with accuracy whether their symptoms are being caused by the gluten intolerance.

Having a negative physical reaction occurring some time after we have eaten a meal containing gluten might give us the assumption of a gluten intolerance – especially if we have read on the internet or heard from a friend that it is a possibility. (Note: in medicine, *symptoms* are subjective assessments from patients while *signs* are objective observations by clinicians and others.)

The question posed: Can a doctor make a valid diagnosis of a gluten intolerance outside of the subjective assessment of the patient? Certainly, we could complain of bloating, headaches, fatigue and other issues that seemed to disappear after we stopped eating gluten. And certainly that would sound like a pretty airtight case of gluten intolerance.

But could there be other ingredients within those gluten-containing foods that could be causing the symptoms? Or could there be a psychological – a placebo – effect at work? Indeed, the placebo effect is so great that at least a third of research subjects have been known to report success when they know they are taking what others consider is a therapeutic treatment.

Or could something else relating to ones diet or food combinations be the cause of their symptoms?

We are not proposing these necessarily: We are making the point that a patient's statement that removing gluten foods from their diet made them feel better is not a scientific means of making an accurate diagnosis.

Rather, a clinician would likely record something like, "patient reports symptom clearance post gluten elimination. Possible gluten intolerance."

But could the doctor – knowing human physiology – make an absolute cause-and-effect physiological relationship between the gluten and the symptoms we had? Currently no.

Why? Because there currently is not a known physiological mechanism for gluten producing those symptoms. There are a few theories, as we will discuss later, but there are no absolute diagnostic tests.

Yes, there are antibody tests for immunoglobulin G – typically done using enzyme-linked immunosorbent assay (ELISA) – but as we will show below, this test does not confirm the existence of a gluten intolerance. It might confirm the possibility, but as we'll show below, the IgG test has a huge probability of false negatives. There is also reason to believe a positive IgG result can just as easily indicate past exposure and subsequent tolerance.

In other words, we will illustrate with credible scientific research that while a positive IgG test may often correlate with gluten intolerance, a positive IgG test for any particular food may also indicate a history of eating that food often in the past and subsequently becoming tolerant to the food.

While a number of smaller studies have landed on this possible conclusion, a large study tested 21,306 adults with ELISA IgG testing (Zeng *et al.* 2013) has offered a more conclusive result. We'll discuss that research in detail below.

This doesn't mean all IgG antibody testing is irrelevant. For example, studies have linked IgG antibodies specific to tissue transglutaminase to many cases of celiac disease. This is a different case, however, compared to having positive IgGs specific to foods that have been commonly eaten.

This doesn't mean that gluten intolerance doesn't exist. Nor does it mean that there isn't a real correlation between gluten intolerance and symptoms of gluten sensitivity. And it does not mean that gluten intolerance cannot be diagnosed, at least utilizing patient feedback.

In fact, the most scientifically reliable means of diagnosis for gluten sensitivity, accepted by most experts in food sensitivities, is something called a double-blind placebo-controlled food challenge.

This means that the patient is tested with gluten-containing foods and placebo foods – foods that do not contain gluten. The patient will eat both and indicate whether they had symptoms to either. If a patient reports symptoms to the gluten foods and not the placebo foods, this is considered a more reliable means of establishing a diagnosis of gluten intolerance.

As we will show, this test does eliminate many who complain of a gluten intolerance but actually do not have one.

But this process is still a correlation. It still does not solve the issue of whether the gluten is causing the problem or whether there is something else being reacted to within the foods being tested. Or whether there isn't something altogether different going on – which we will discuss at length.

And none of this information is a condemnation of gluten-free strategies. There is certainly a place for elimination diets in a sound strategy to resolve the real problem, as we'll discuss further.

Enzyme-linked Immunosorbent Assays (ELISA)

This test and its relative, the ALCAT test, have been met with significant resistance and criticism from many medical researchers and physicians. The complaint of most is quite simply that ELISA testing has not been proven to be reliable for food allergy diagnosis.

This was illustrated by researchers from India's Post Graduate Institute of Medical Education and Research (Sharnan *et al.* 2001). The scientists gave skin prick tests and ELISA tests to 64 children with food allergies previously confirmed through food challenges, along with 32 control subjects. They found that the ELISA tests had greater specificity than the skin prick tests (88% versus 64%). And the ELISA provided some reliability for a lack of allergy. But the ELISA testing generally did not provide a reliable basis for determining an allergy was present. They concluded that ELISA provided no useful advantage over skin prick testing.

New ELISA procedures for testing protein-specific IgEs using ELISA are emerging, however. Researchers from the Fujita Health University School of Medicine (Nakamura *et al.* 2014) tested the protein-specific IgE ELISA assay and found it to show consistent testing results for the HWP-IWA wheat allergen among 19 wheat allergy patients.

One of the issues with ELISA testing (and some say its advantage) for food sensitivities is its use in testing other immunoglobulins such as IgG and IgG4. Some research has indicated that IgG4 is indicative of a hidden food allergy (Shakib *et al.* 1986), but other research has shown that allergen-specific IgG4s can also simply indicate a recovery from a prior food sensitivity (Savilahti *et al.* 2010). We'll discuss this further below.

One of the issues some have with ELISA IgG testing is that some of the IgG lab assays will document a huge list of foods that tested positive for IgG levels from the patient's blood. We mentioned this in the case of Bobby earlier. It is not uncommon for a patient to receive an IgG test that shows dozens if not hundreds of foods that the patient is supposedly sensitive to.

More puzzling is the fact that many of these foods will have been part of the patient's diet for many years without any signs of sensitivity.

Were they sensitive even without signs or symptoms? To this, some clinicians will say that must be the case. The problem is that if they are relying upon the IgG test as an absolute measure for sensitivity, they cannot explain positive results for those foods that produce no sensitivity symptoms.

Nevertheless, these IgG ELISA test results often convince the patient that their suspected food sensitivity to gluten is actually food intolerance to a host of other foods. It is quite a difficult thing to swallow, and the author has worked with many patients with such a perplexing situation.

The difficulty of this conclusion is the patient is typically advised to eliminate all those foods from their diet – forever.

As a result of this and other science, the conclusion of many clinicians and food allergy/intolerance experts is that there is little evidence IgG antibodies are linked to delayed allergic symptoms or intolerance to foods.

IgG ELISA Testing

As indicated, over the past two decades the use of IgG testing to determine food intolerances has continued to be met with controversy. There is good reason for this. Research now proves that IgG testing offers little in the way of concrete diagnostic accuracy for food intolerances and food sensitivities.

To be fair, one of the studies that many proponents of IgG ELISA testing have leaned on is a study solely-authored by the Chief Executive Officer of an IgG testing lab, Immunosciences Laboratory, Inc. (Vojdani 2011). This well-designed study tested the blood of a total of 96 subjects. Of the entire group of 96, 48 of them were healthy with no signs of any sensitivity to gluten, wheat and so forth.

Of the 48 remaining persons, 24 had received a previous diagnosis of celiac disease. The remaining 24 persons had been diagnosed with Crohn's disease.

The study illustrated those with either Crohn's disease or celiac disease had a greater likelihood of having a positive IgG result for gliadins and wheat proteins. About half the celiac patients tested positive for wheat sensitivity, and about half – not necessarily the same half – tested positive for a range of other gliadin proteins, glutenins, as well as TG and WGA.

But the study also found that the blood of many of the healthy persons also tested positive for IgG to gluten and wheat proteins: Nearly a quarter of the healthy subjects (11 out of 48) tested positive to glutenin 21 IgG. And about the same amount (10) tested positive to gluteomorphin IgG, while nine tested positive to wheat IgG. Other healthy individuals tested positive for alpha-gliadin-33, gliadin-17, gliadin-TG, and WGA.

These all represent what is called a false positive. In all, there were 34 false positives among the 48 persons for one or another wheat component – if we assume that IgG indeed indicates a gluten sensitivity. This is 34 false positives from 48 patients. While some may have had multiple sensitivities, that still is a lot of false positives.

Yes, the study shows that celiacs and Crohn's patients have a greater likelihood of IgG positive testing. But can the converse be proven from this? That positive IgGs definitely mean gluten sensitivities? This certainly isn't the case for the 34 positive results among the 48 healthy patients with no signs of any sensitivity. Or is this a matter of a hidden sensitivity?

The real question is whether gluten sensitivity even produces an IgG result. Or is this a marker indicating the body's attempt to produce tolerance to a particular food that may have provided some challenge earlier in life?

This would be more likely, given the serious number of false positives.

This notion that IgG may relate to tolerance is not a new one, nor is it the speculative opinion of the author. It has been suspected for many years by immunity researchers. We'll discuss this further later on.

This study and many others have shown similar instances of false positives among IgG testing, as illustrated by reviews of the research from food allergy societies such as the European Academy of Allergy and Clinical Immunology and the American Academy of Allergy, Asthma and Immunology (AAAAI) and others (see below). These have warned against using IgG testing to diagnose food sensitivities.

Despite this, numerous clinical practices regularly diagnose food sensitivities using IgG testing offered by diagnostic labs under a variety of names and trademarks. Recently drugstore pharmacies have joined the fray, offering in-store blood draws with follow-up test results.

IgG stands for Immunoglobulin G – an antibody protein produced by the immune system's B-cells. As we've discussed, food allergies are typically diagnosed with the presence of IgE antibodies, and other issues such as celiac disease can be diagnosed with IgA testing. IgG's link to food sensitivities has yet to be scientifically established.

Medical boards of the above mentioned allergy academies have surveyed the evidence. They have documented that positive IgG results can just as easily indicate a food that has been eaten regularly as much as it might indicate a food intolerance. But the evidence has still allowed some room to maneuver for IgG testing proponents. Until now.

The controversy was recently put to a clearer test in the form of a very large study from researchers at the International Medical Center of Beijing's PLA General Hospital. The researchers (Zeng *et al.* 2013) conducted a multi-center study of 21,306 adults from around China.

The researchers stated this about the importance of their study:

> *"Although commercial laboratories worldwide are currently offering broad-scale testing for serum levels of food-specific IgGs to the public, to our knowledge, the study described here is the first representative cross-sectional study to address the distribution of food-specific IgGs and its relationship to chronic symptoms in a large population."*

The study population composed of both healthy people and people with reported food intolerances. The researchers gave all the subjects blood tests for 14 food-specific IgG antibodies using ELISA – the enzyme-linked immunosorbent assay.

The foods tested for IgGs included wheat, mushrooms, eggs, fish, chicken, beef, soybeans, rice, tomato and others.

From the 21,306 subjects tested, 5,394 of them were randomly selected to complete surveys on their diets and their food tolerance-related symptoms.

The researchers first calculated the results of the testing without the surveys, and mapped these test results by region and population. Then they compared the surveys with the IgG testing to determine if there was a correlation between the intolerant foods reported by the patients with the food-specific IgGs gained from the test results. *No correlation found between higher IgG levels and food intolerances was found.*

Instead of finding the IgG test results closely matching those food intolerances reported, the researchers found that higher IgG test results often related to foods they were eating without intolerance symptoms. They also found just as often, lower IgG results among those foods subjects reported as producing intolerance symptoms.

In fact, the results were so varied that the researchers could not find any correlation between the IgG results and the reported food intolerances. They found that higher IgG levels were found among women. They also found that older people had more food-related spikes in IgG levels.

More revealing was that higher IgG levels were also distinctly related to where the subjects lived and that region's general diet. For example, in areas where more corn was consumed, more people had higher IgGs related to corn – regardless of whether they reported any intolerance to corn or not.

In other words, the IgG testing revealed nothing about food intolerances among the population.

And healthy people can have similar levels of heightened IgGs as those who have food intolerances. The researchers concluded:

> *"In summary, the present study demonstrates for the first time that food-specific IgG serum concentrations are variable in both healthy and symptomatic Chinese adults."*

Again, when a test result that is being promoted to indicate a particular condition shows a positive result for a person who does not have that condition, the result is called a false-positive.

And the so-many cases in this study that showed positive IgG test results for foods without any sensitivity to that food are, by definition, false-positives.

This also explains the scenario of a patient receiving a IgG positive test result for a food they are sensitive to. Because there is a past history of eating that food and an attempt by the immune system at tolerance, there is a positive IgG result.

But when an IgG ELISA assay comes back with 10-150 foods with positive IgG results for foods that do not produce intolerance signs, there is good reason to question those positive results.

As the above study's scientists indicated in their discussions, this and other studies have indicated the probability that by eating more of a food, our immune system creates a greater tolerance to it, and this tolerance mechanism produces a greater likelihood of positive IgG results. As to whether this IgG-related tolerance produces some protection against allergies was not able to be answered by this study:

> *"Finally, the study does not provide an answer to the question of whether food-specific IgGs play a protective role or an allergic role in adults."*

This also explains why a particular test result can be positive for a person who has an intolerance to that particular food. If a patient reports food intolerance to a particular food or foods, this typically means they have been eating that food with at least a measure of frequency. And their immune system is also working to develop a tolerance to the food.

Further questioning of IgG testing for food sensitivities

While the above study is the largest and first of its kind to objectively test such a large population of both healthy and food-intolerant individuals, previous studies on IgG testing have concluded similar results. In a review of the data from a number of studies, the Task Force from the European Academy of Allergy and Clinical Immunology (EAACI) found:

> *"Testing for blood IgG4 against different foods is performed with large-scale screening for hundreds of food items by enzyme-linked immunosorbent assay-type and radioallergosor-*

bent-type assays in young children, adolescents and adults. However, many serum samples show positive IgG4 results without corresponding clinical symptoms. These findings, combined with the lack of convincing evidence for histamine-releasing properties of IgG4 in humans, and lack of any controlled studies on the diagnostic value of IgG4 testing in food allergy, do not provide any basis for the hypothesis that food-specific IgG4 should be attributed with an effector role in food hypersensitivity."

Other allergy associations from around the globe have stated similar findings and guidelines against utilizing IgG testing to diagnose food intolerances. These include:

- American Academy of Allergy, Asthma and Immunology & American College of Allergy, Asthma and Immunology
- American Academy of Allergy, Asthma and Immunology (AAAAI)
- Australasian Society of Clinical Immunology and Allergy (ASCIA)
- Allergy Society of South Africa
- The Food Allergy Initiative

Here is a statement from the ASCIA:

"Inappropriate use of Conventional Testing: Food specific IgG, IgG4; Use: Diagnosis of food sensitivity / allergy.
Method: Antibodies to food are measured using standard laboratory techniques.
Evidence: Level II
Comment: IgG antibodies to food are commonly detectable in healthy adult patients and children, independent of the presence of absence of food-related symptoms. There is no credible evidence that measuring IgG antibodies is useful for diagnosing food allergy or intolerance, nor that IgG antibodies cause symptoms. In fact, IgG antibodies reflect exposure to allergen but not the presence of disease. The exception is that gliadin IgG antibodies are sometimes useful in monitoring adherence to a gluten-free diet patients with histologically confirmed coeliac disease. Otherwise, inappropriate use of food allergy testing (or misinterpretation of results) in patients with inhalant allergy, for example, may lead to inappropriate and unnecessary dietary restrictions, with particular nutritional implications in children. Despite studies showing the uselessness of this technique,

it continues to be promoted in the community, even for diagnosing disorders for which no evidence of immune system involvement exists."

Here is a position statement from the Allergy Society of South Africa:

Position Statement: ALCAT and IgG Allergy & Intolerance Tests, "Diagnostic tests for food allergy: Sixth Report on Allergy":
"We are concerned both that the results of allergy self testing kits available to the public are being interpreted without the advice of appropriately trained healthcare personnel, and that the IgG food antibody test is being used to diagnose food intolerance in the absence of stringent scientific evidence. We recommend further research into the relevance of IgG antibodies in food intolerance, and with the establishment of more allergy centres, the necessary controlled clinical trials should be conducted. We urge general practitioners, pharmacists and charities not to endorse the use of these products until conclusive proof of their efficacy has been established."

From the Food Allergy Initiative:

"IgG Testing: This test checks your blood for the presence of food-specific immunoglobulin G (IgG) antibodies. Unlike IgE antibodies, which occur in abnormally large quantities in people with allergies, IgG antibodies are found in both allergic and non-allergic people. Experts believe that the production of IgG antibodies is a normal response to eating food and that this test is not helpful in diagnosing a food allergy."

Other Diagnostic Tests used for Food Sensitivity

There are a variety of other diagnostic tests that health care practitioners may subscribe to. These include sublingual testing, immune-complex tests, cytotoxic tests, provocative tests, the Mediator Release Test, galvanometer skin testing and others. While some of these may have value in some instances, most have not been met with the rigor of definitive scientific study (Boyce *et al.* 2010).

Researchers from the Ospedale Civile Maggiore hospital in Varona, Italy (Senna *et al.* 2002) conducted a study of alternative food allergy tests, including the cytotoxic test, the sublingual provocation test, the subcutaneous test, the heart-ear reflex test, kinesiology, electro-acupuncture, the ELISA IgG test, and hair analysis. They concluded that none of these tests were reliable diagnostic tests for food sensitivities.

Some of these tests, such as applied kinesiology, have been met with success by some practitioners. While the author is not condemning any of these, they should still nevertheless be approached with caution, and possibly not trusted without some inclusion of a double-blind placebo-controlled food challenge.

We can quote from a few diagnostic guidelines to help the reader orient themselves. Here is the guideline from the From the European Academy of Allergy and Clinical Immunology (Stapel *et al.* 2008):

4.2.2.9. Nonstandardized and Unproven Procedures; Guideline 12:

The (Expert Panel) recommends not using any of the following nonstandardized tests for the routine evaluation of IgE-mediated (food allergy):

- *Basophil histamine release/activation*
- *Lymphocyte stimulation*
- *Facial thermography*
- *Gastric juice analysis*
- *Endoscopic allergen provocation*
- *Hair analysis*
- *Applied kinesiology*
- *Provocation neutralization*
- *Allergen-specific IgG*
- *Cytotoxicity assays*
- *Electrodermal test (Vega)*
- *Mediator release assay (LEAP)*

Researchers from the UK consumer group *Which?* (2008) trialed alternative tests that claim to diagnose food intolerances through analysis of blood samples or strands of hair, changes in electric current, or resistance to pressure applied to their legs or arms. Here is an excerpt from their findings:

> ***Results***
> *We found that:*
> *- the tests diagnosed 183 intolerances – although the researchers actually had just one medically confirmed allergy and one food intolerance between them*
> *- identical blood and hair samples sent under different names to the same company produced different test results*
> *- there was little or no overlap between test results from different companies*

- the testers felt the practitioners applied more pressure when measuring resistance for certain foods – which they were then told to avoid
- the tests recommended excluding up to 39 foods – which could make it difficult to eat a balanced diet and lead to nutritional problems.

The study found the IgG tests ranged from £45 and £275 (about $76 to $467) each. The investigation's medical experts felt that none of the tests had any value for diagnosing allergies or intolerances. The author adds that these were the results of actual tests – up to 39 foods tested positive. The author has seen tests in the U.S. document well over a 100 foods. The number of foods tested depends largely upon the size of the scan – typically related to the cost of the assay.

The Food Elimination Study

Some of the more recognized tests discussed above are no more reliable than a simple food elimination study. Furthermore, the food elimination study can be conducted at home by oneself if the symptoms are not severe. If the symptoms are severe, the elimination program should be supervised by a health professional or observed by someone prepared for anaphylaxis if there are serious symptoms involved in the sensitivity response. This said, the only expense is time, patience, and careful record-keeping.

Here the person simply begins to eliminate suspect foods, one at a time, from the diet. If symptoms subside after the food is withdrawn, one can be fairly certain of a sensitivity. The period of elimination should be enough to confirm the test, however. A good period is seven days without a symptom, but the longer the better. The results should also probably be confirmed by returning to the inclusion diet and then eliminating the food again, assuming the symptoms are manageable and not severe or assuming there is supervision as mentioned above when the food is added back.

Elimination testing can also be conducted using foods from similar food groups to pinpoint whether there is a common protein sensitivity or otherwise.

To confirm the sensitivity, the food or group can also be tested with a double-blind, placebo-controlled food challenge test. If symptoms are severe, this should be performed or supervised by a health professional trained in anaphylactic response.

But if we are talking about an intolerance, this test will likely not achieve any diagnostic results. Why?

Before we dig into the mechanisms related to this, let's get to know the proposed and actual effects of gluten and gluten-containing foods.

Chapter Two

Are Gluten and Wheat Toxins?

Correlation versus Causation

This is a key element we will discuss throughout this book as we investigate the current thesis regarding gluten intolerance – that gluten is the cause of the problematic symptoms being attributed to gluten sensitivity, which would make gluten essentially a toxin.

This comparison – correlation versus causation – should pop up first for any scientist seeking to solve any problem. And certainly for anyone looking to find the real cause of a physical condition needs to distinguish between the potential cause of that physical condition and a sign or symptom of that condition.

The issue is association. When a scientific study associates – or links – two things – be they conditions, signs of a condition, foods or otherwise – that association is called a *correlation*.

In a correlation, one occurrence will be found existing more frequently with another occurrence – more frequently than the occurrence will exist otherwise. This is also called a link or association.

Furthermore, is the issue of causation. When is an event a cause?

Let's use an example regarding causation. Let's say our car is leaking oil. Is the oil leak the cause of the problem? No, the oil leak is a sign of a problem – some might also consider it a symptom. How can we say this? Because there has to be a reason for the oil to leak. It is not a problem in itself because oil is typically tightly contained within and circulated within an enclosed engine block. So if it began leaking oil, there is a cause for the leak outside of the leak itself.

Let's try another example – this of a correlation. Let's say that in addition to our engine oil leak, our transmission is making noise. As soon as we shift into a new gear we hear a grinding noise.

What do we assume from these two occurrences? We can correlate that the two are occurring at the same time. But can we say that either one is causing the other?

Could either occurrence be the cause of the other? Is the noise related to the oil leak? Could the oil leak be causing the noise? Or could the noise be causing the oil leak – perhaps the vibration from the noise or something?

There are four logical possibilities:

1) We could assume the transmission noise is being caused by the oil leak.
2) We could assume the oil leak is caused by the transmission noise.

3) We could assume the oil leak is completely unrelated to the transmission noise outside of the fact that they happen to be occurring at the same time.
4) We could assume they are related by an underlying problem that is affecting both the transmission and the crankcase.

Which of the assumptions above is a correlation? And which is a causation?

Number one and two assumptions above are proposing causation: That one occurrence is causing the other.

And number four is assuming correlation without causation – assuming there is a common but different cause of both.

Meanwhile, number three assumes neither causation nor correlation – except for the correlation of coincidence – their unrelated occurrence at the same time.

Thus number three would essentially assume the noise is a separate problem from the oil leak, and each is a sign of two distinct problems with the transmission.

In the realm of possibilities, it would be hard not to correlate the events since two things typically don't go wrong with a car at the same time. At least as far as we know.

But this would be an unscientific approach. There is no observational reason for a related occurrence assumption. The two events would just as likely be unrelated as they would be related. In fact, if we were to statistically analyze it, the possibility of unrelated occurrence would probably overwhelm any possibility otherwise. This is because of the number of moving parts within a car. If we were to multiply the probabilities of any moving part to have an independent problem together and compare this with the multiplied probabilities that one problem is related to another, unrelated occurrence would prevail.

Unless of course there is an underlying reason for their mutual occurrence. This would increase the probability of a related occurrence dramatically.

In fact, the joining of those two as signs of one underlying problem would essentially be saying they are related. They are linked – somehow. But to make this assumption, we would also need to observe an underlying cause.

Otherwise it would be an unscientific assumption.

Now what if we were told by someone at work that they read on the internet that transmission noises are often related to being low on engine oil. The person at work may admittedly know nothing about cars. But we might immediately correlate the two events based upon the statement of the person at work.

Would it then be more scientific for us to correlate the two problems? Well, that depends upon the basis for the information found on the internet.

Whether it was from a reliable source – perhaps an automobile mechanic. If so, the basis for correlation may be sound.

But if the information passed on by our co-worker was also gained in passing, say from a person who wrote an article after reading another article in passing – and perhaps none of them knew much about cars – well, that would not be a scientifically valid reason to correlate the two occurrences.

But let's consider our assumption of the two problems if the leak was transmission oil instead of engine oil. Would it be more scientific for us to assume the two occurrences were connected?

Certainly it would – assuming the underlying relationship between the transmission oil and the transmission – confirmed by a mechanic or auto manufacturer – that because transmission oil lubricates the transmission, a lack of lubrication offered by the oil can cause the transmission to make noise.

In other words, there is an observable underlying reason – a mechanical connection between transmission oil and transmission noises – that would allow us to make the assumption of correlation.

In fact, the same scenario might allow us to make a reasonably scientific causation as well. We could make a reasonable assumption that the transmission noise was caused by the lack of lubrication, because of the oil leak.

And this could be considered a scientifically valid assumption, but with one great limitation: The possibility that in our particular case, the transmission noise is being caused by something unrelated to the transmission oil leak.

Yes, a transmission oil leak might cause transmission noises. But the only way we can make such a conclusion is if we had a mechanic open up the transmission and investigate the problem further. Then the assumption of causation would depend upon the reliability of the mechanic's diagnosis – and whether the noise stopped when the transmission was refilled with oil.

Disease Associations with Gluten Sensitivity

As we step through this subject of whether gluten or wheat in general are toxins or not, we should take a minute to review some of the disorders that have been associated with gluten. These are perfect candidates for utilizing our understanding of the difference between causation and correlation.

Intestinal Issues

Starting from studies done in the 1950s and 1960s, there has been significant research that associates gluten with intestinal problems such as irritable bowels, bloating and cramping, headaches and fatigue. However, most of these early studies investigated those with the emerging disease called celiac sprue. As such, in celiac patients, gluten was found to negatively affect cells of the intestinal wall.

This research has matured over the decades, and now it is well-accepted that celiac patients and those who are pre-celiac will have increased anti-tissue transglutaminase2 (anti-TG2) antibodies, which relate to an immune response to eating gluten among the intestinal cells – specifically of the small intestine.

For example, in a study of 129 celiac or pre-celiac patients from Italy's University Federico II (Tosco *et al.* 2014), most patients showed anti-TG2 antibodies. And anti-TG2 antibodies directly related to worsened symptoms. Those celiac patients on gluten-free diets the longest had fewer anti-TG2 antibodies than those who recently went gluten-free or who not gluten-free.

Other research has found that unhydrolyzed gliadin proteins will stimulate something called epidermal growth factor (EGF) among celiac intestinal cells. This has been shown to be part of the mechanisms for gluten sensitivity among celiac sufferers (Barone *et al.* 2007).

Furthermore, other research has found that among celiac patients, gluten stimulates an increase in intestinal permeability. One study found that zonulin levels were spiked among celiac intestinal cells in the presence of gluten (Fasano *et al.* 2000). As we'll discuss further, the zonulin protein is associated with increased intestinal permeability.

Indeed, further research indicates that the undigested gliadin protein may also produce increased zonulin levels and thus potentially disturb intestinal permeability among the cells of some non-celiac patients.

This fact was discovered in laboratory testing from the University of Maryland School of Medicine (Drago *et al.* 2006). The researchers biopsied both celiac patients and non-celiac persons to obtain their IEC6 and Caco2 cells from their intestines.

Within the environment of the laboratory, they exposed these cells to complete gliadin proteins. The proteins increased zonulin levels among both the celiac and the non-celiac patients. But the zonulin increase among the non-celiac patients was "limited" and "transient" according to the researchers.

While this research certainly establishes a correlation between the production of zonulin and intestinal cells – and possibly increased intestinal permeability – we would point out two issues with this study:

1) The intestinal cells were removed from their normal mucosal membrane-covered environment within the digestive tract, and were directly exposed to the gliadin proteins.
2) The gliadin proteins were isolated and thus not exposed to the normal digestive processes which should – in a healthy person as we will show – break down the gliadin proteins into their respective amino acids and small peptide chains.

Certainly these studies do illustrate a link between non-digested gliadin protein and intestinal cells.

But other undigested proteins can also cause these sorts of issues. For example, casein – a central protein in milk – also produces intestinal permeability issues, and an inflammatory response when exposed to intestinal cells without being broken down (Miller *et al.* 1991 and others).

And as was found by researchers from Hiroshima University (Yasumatsu and Tanabe 2010) when the casein macromolecule is broken down into smaller peptides, these can actually help strengthen the intestinal barrier. This study found that the peptide chain, Asn-Pro-Trp-Asp-Gln (NPWDQ) – from positions 107 to 111 of a casein protein – stimulated occludin (known to decrease permeability) but not zonulin. The researchers noted:

> *"Therefore, it is suggested that NPWDQ up-regulated the expression of occludin in particular and enforced the tight junction barrier."*

As we will show evidence for later, many macromolecule food proteins that can produce an allergy – if they are not broken down by enzymes in the digestive tract – including proteins from fish, nuts and others – can produce intestinal permeability issues when exposed to intestinal cells. But once they are broken down properly by the digestive tract, they become nutrients that can nourish our bodies. This issue was discussed at length in the author's book, *Natural Solutions for Food Allergies and Food Sensitivities.*

The bottom line among these studies on gluten's impact upon intestinal cells is: Yes, there is a correlation between undigested gluten proteins – particularly gliadins – and negative impact on intestinal cells.

But as we will show within this text, this is correlation and not causation. It is an isolated correlation without taking into account the other elements at play within the anatomy of the mucosal membranes and the intestinal cells they protect – and the mechanisms that relate to the physiology of digestion along with the strength of the immune system.

With this in mind, let's look more closely at some of the specific disorders gluten has been associated with.

Gluten and Irritable Bowel Syndrome/Inflammatory Bowel Disease

Research has found that from seven to twenty percent of U.S. adults suffer from irritable bowel syndrome (IBS) (Chey *et al.* 2002, Longstreth *et al.* 2006).

And sometimes – despite the anecdotal discussions, only sometimes – IBS is correlated with some form of gluten sensitivity. In fact, sometimes IBS is correlated with other food sensitivities. Illustrating this, Italian researchers (Carroccio *et al.* 2010) tested 120 patients diagnosed with IBS. Of the 120, 24 patients showed sensitivities to cow's milk and/or wheat. While they didn't test for other food sensitivities – this research indicated that 75% of the IBS patients did not have a sensitivity to either wheat or milk.

Furthermore, many who had a sensitivity or intolerance to gluten also had a sensitivity or intolerance to dairy.

Many celiac disease patients also often have IBS (Ford *et al.* 2009).

But the converse is not true. In a study from the National Naval Medical Center (Cash *et al.* 2011) of 492 IBS patients, only 0.41% of them had celiac disease. This was compared to 458 healthy control patients with no symptoms – of which 0.44% were confirmed with celiac disease. By the way, both of these results are less than the estimated 0.75% celiac rate according to Fasano and associates (2003).

The Navy study also found that more of the IBS patients – though a mere 7.3% compared to 4.8% in the control group – showed antibodies to gliadin and tissue transglutaminase. While this is a small correlation, it does pose the possibility of a small (2.5%) correlation between gluten sensitivity and some IBS sufferers.

But noting that nearly 5% of those without IBS also showed these antibodies, a little over 7% is not so convincing. It surely doesn't indicate that IBS is caused by gluten sensitivity – or even that gluten sensitivity necessarily results in IBS.

Much of the research correlating gluten with irritable bowel syndrome and inflammatory bowel disease has been made through exclusion: That a gluten-free diet has helped many of these patients.

For example, a study from the University of North Carolina (Herfarth *et al.* 2014) gave questionnaires to 1,647 patients with inflammatory bowel diseases. From this study population, 10 subjects had been diagnosed with celiac disease and 81 (about 5%) had been diagnosed with non-celiac gluten sensitivity.

Meanwhile, 19% of the respondents (314) had at some point tried a gluten-free diet, and less than half of those – 8% (135) – were on a gluten-free diet at the time of the survey.

Of these, 66% of those who had tried a gluten-free diet said the diet led to some improvement in their intestinal symptoms, while 38% reported fewer or less severe flare-ups.

And in those who were currently on a strict gluten-free diet, many reported less fatigue. The researchers wrote in their conclusion:

> *"Testing a gluten-free diet in clinical practice in patients with significant intestinal symptoms, which are not solely explained by the degree of intestinal inflammation, has the potential to be a safe and highly efficient therapeutic approach."*

This sums up the current situation with regard to the association between gluten sensitivity with respect to IBS:

1) There is an association between gluten and intestinal wall health among celiac patients.
2) Many of those who are not celiac patients who have intestinal bowel disorders – in the study above about two-thirds – who try a gluten-free diet find some improvement in their symptoms.
3) A portion of those with inflammatory bowel disease, also sometimes called irritable bowel syndrome – 38% according to the above study – report fewer or less severe flare-ups.

So these are pretty clear associations. They should be taken seriously, and indeed, many doctors do, as many are now recommending a gluten-free diet for those patients who report IBS or IBD.

But we must be clear that these are correlations not causations.

For example, from the UNC study above, a third of those IBD patients who went gluten-free did not report any improvement of symptoms. And about two-thirds of those who went gluten-free did not report any reduction in the severity or number of flare-ups from going gluten-free.

These points break down the assumption that gluten is the cause of IBS or IBD disorders.

And furthermore, if gluten was the cause of even those patients that reported some improvement in symptoms or some reduction in flare-ups, then going gluten-free should have completely removed all of their symptoms and all of their flare-ups – right?

Yes, that is right. If a person was having headaches because they were banging their head against the wall, if they stopped banging their head against the wall the headaches would go away, right? If the headaches did not go away – and even if they only partly went away – we would know there is another cause of those headaches – right?

As we will be discussing further on this issue, this is indeed the trick of the gluten-free issue – as it is in so many other *panacea*-related issues. As more and more people begin to believe in a *panacea*, the more real that *panacea's* ability to heal appears. It doesn't mean that the *panacea* is having the healing effect, however. It just means there is a surge in the belief that the *panacea* is helping.

And while the author is not discounting the 66% who reported a reduction of symptoms, or the 38% who reported fewer flare-ups; self-reported notions of reductions or "fewer" symptoms is not a compelling case for causation, especially when considering the surge of websites, books and articles that pledge the benefits of a gluten-free diet.

This is specifically why studies are conducted with double-blind, placebo-controlled protocols. Because if a person knows he/she is partaking in a therapeutic protocol, there is a strong likelihood the person will report benefits from that protocol.

This effect of knowing the person is undertaking a therapeutic protocol is so strong that acceptable peer-reviewed studies not only require the patient not know they are being treated – but the doctor must also not know who is being treated. This is called double-blindedness.

But in the UNC study above – as has been the case in most of the other recent studies associating a gluten-free diet with some improvement in intestinal symptoms – each of the patients knew they were on the gluten-free diet. And most of them were on the diet because either they were told the diet should help their symptoms or they read somewhere that the gluten-free diet will help their symptoms.

Therefore, while we can certainly accept there may be a correlation between gluten and intestinal symptoms *in some cases,* we cannot accept that outside of allergies, gluten causes intestinal disorders such as IBS or IBD.

But we cannot draw such a conclusion from just one study. Other studies have made the same correlations.

For example, in a study from Germany's University Hospital Ernst Moritz Arndt and the University of Greifswald (Wahnschaffe *et al.* 2007) tested 145 patients who had diarrhea-dominant irritable bowel syndrome along with 74 celiac patients and 57 other irritable bowel patients.

More of the patients with diarrhea IBS showed antibody and genetic tests similar to the celiac disease patients than in the other irritable bowel patients. And of those with antibody and genetic tests similar to the celiac disease patients, 60% had improved symptoms after six months on a gluten-free diet.

But again this is a correlation. About 40% of the diarrhea IBS patients showed genetic testing similar to celiac patients, and of those, 60% improved with a gluten-free diet. Only 12% of those diarrhea IBS patients without celiac-like test results showed any improvement with a gluten-free diet. Not so much.

A lack of blindedness and placebo control makes the conclusion that a gluten-free diet actually helped suspect. Even among the few studies that tried to employ blindedness, correlation is confirmed but causation is not.

In one of the few blinded studies, researchers from Australia's Monash University (Biesiekierski *et al.* 2011) studied 34 patients with IBS gastrointestinal symptoms. The patients were given either a gluten-free diet or a gluten diet for six weeks. Theoretically, the patients were blinded as to whether they were eating the gluten foods. While hiding gluten within a food with regard to mouthfeel or taste may be somewhat difficult, we can accept it from a scientific assumption.

At the end of the six weeks, 68% of the gluten-eating group saw no improvement in IBS symptoms while 40% of the gluten-free group reported no improvement in IBS symptoms after the six weeks.

This illustrates both sides of the equation once again. A full 32% of the group that ate gluten during the six weeks reported improved ("controlled") symptoms. And six out of the 15 patients (40%) who were gluten-free saw no improvement in symptoms.

The researchers also noted there were no changes in physiological markers between the gluten-free and gluten-eating IBS subjects:

> *"Anti-gliadin antibodies were not induced. There were no significant changes in fecal lactoferrin, levels of celiac antibodies, highly sensitive C-reactive protein, or intestinal permeability. There were no differences in any end point in individuals with or without DQ2/DQ8."*

And in the conclusion, the researchers wrote:

> *"Non-celiac gluten intolerance" may exist, but no clues to the mechanism were elucidated."*

Again this means that some but not all of IBS patients may have a gluten sensitivity. And some but not all IBS patients may benefit from a gluten-free diet.

But again in this study and among others, we find the gluten-free diet does not lead to a reversal of IBS symptoms in suspected gluten-intolerant people. Among celiac sufferers, yes: In many cases, going gluten-free lessens and sometimes resolves their IBS symptoms. But this has not been proven among non-celiac IBS or IBD sufferers, as the evidence illustrates.

So again, is IBS caused by gluten sensitivity in a non-celiac? No, because abstaining from gluten does not remove IBS symptoms. It might lessen the symptoms in some cases. And therefore, it might be a good option to try for IBS patients to help relieve some symptoms.

But this is because IBS is typically so mysterious to conventional medicine that there is typically no better choice of therapy.

If we were to return to our analogy using the leaking engine oil and the transmission noise, let's say that fixing the oil leak decreased the transmission noise in more cases than it didn't – say in 60% of cases as in the Biesiekierski university study. Does this mean the oil leak causes the transmission noise?

No, first because the transmission noise was not eliminated – it only was not as loud. And second, because it didn't work in all cases. This means there may be some sort of relationship between the oil and the transmission noise. But it isn't causational.

Stated in terms of IBS and gluten sensitivity, we will illustrate as we go that there is a common element between many IBS cases and cases of gluten sensitivity. Something that can cause both.

Gluten and schizophrenia

An observation of some schizophrenia patients having celiac disease was made as far back as 1953 (Bender) and in 1961 with five case histories. (Graff and Handford). This led to a proposal that schizophrenia was possibly caused by celiac disease but this was later disproved by the sheer volume of schizophrenia cases that did not present with celiac disease or even a gluten sensitivity.

For example, a 1977 study (Stevens *et al.* 1977) performed blood testing on 380 schizophrenia patients from two mental hospitals. They found that 26 had antibodies to reticulin – a test that indicates celiac disease in about 60% of positive tests. It also indicates Crohn's disease in about 20% of positive tests.

While this study illustrated a possible association, it is clear that not everyone with schizophrenia has celiac disease.

The research investigating a potential link between schizophrenia and celiac disease has persisted over the years. And some have proposed that wheat gluten produces an effect similar to opiates (Heubner *et al.* 1984). However, the ability of gluten to produce a serum opiate response was also disproven in other research (Morley *et al.* 1983).

In a study (Lambert et al 1989) of 24 schizophrenia patients, researchers from St Mary's Hospital Medical School in London stated:

> *"It is concluded that schizophrenia is, at least in the majority of cases, unrelated to coeliac disease."*

But then another study (Perisic *et al.* 1990) found a possible genetic link between celiac disease and schizophrenia. Because celiac disease has been considered a genetic disorder, the proposal wasn't that gluten sensitivity produced schizophrenia. Rather, the possibility – which has never been proven out – that the two genetic markers may co-exist in some people.

In terms of an increased risk of schizophrenia among those with celiac disease, this was studied by a Danish (Eaton *et al.* 2004) study of 7,997 people admitted to a psychiatric facility and diagnosed with schizophrenia. They compared the rates of celiac disease among the schizophrenia patients with the rates of celiac disease among people without schizophrenia.

While the study concluded increased occurrence of celiac disease among schizophrenia patients, the association was not direct. The true results of the study are revealed in the case numbers. There were 7,337 cases of schizophrenia studied, and there were only four patients who had celiac disease, which calculates to less than one half of one half percent. This is far less than the

0.73% found in the general population. And even when the researchers included family members – five mothers of patients and three fathers of patients who didn't have schizophrenia – this still equated to only 1.5 per 1,000 schizophrenia patients.

The calculation that determined an increased risk of schizophrenia among celiac patients (3.2) utilized a conditional logistic regression taken from an increased risk of celiac disease among children of parents with the disorder (Mortensen *et al.* 1999). Since their children had not been diagnosed with celiac disease, the researchers utilized regression statistics to calculate a risk based upon research indicating a potential increased risk.

The fact that so few of the schizophrenia patients were celiac was illustrated in the researchers' discussion:

> *"The risk relation is strong but reflects a small proportion of cases of either disorder, since both disorders are rare."*

This point of rarity is critical. Noting that 1 out of 133 people or so have tested positive for celiac disease in the most accepted research, 1.5 out of 1,000 among schizophrenia patients would hardly indicate any kind of causation relationship, at least on the part of celiac disease.

A better designed study from the UK's University of the Highlands and Islands (Law *et al.* 2011) studied celiac disease and schizophrenia among 223 families. They found no association between celiac disease and schizophrenia. They concluded:

> *"This synthesis, in light of our review of previous reports, suggests a differing developmental trajectory for schizophrenia and coeliac disease. It is possible that these two conditions do not share any functional overlap."*

However, the possibility of an association was found in another study (Cascella *et al.* 2011) of 1,401 schizophrenia patients. The patients were given blood antibody tests and these were compared to a group of 900 healthy control subjects – though we should note they were not matched controls.

Nonetheless, this research found the schizophrenia group had an increased prevalence of tTG antibodies and anti-gliadin antibodies. Twenty-three percent of the schizophrenia group had higher levels of AGA-IgA while 3% of the healthy group did. And 5.4% of the schizophrenia group had tTG antibodies compared to only 0.8% of the healthy group.

This should indicate a clear association except there was no association between these antibodies and the severity of the patients' schizophrenia. PANSS (Positive and Negative Syndrome Scale) scores were compared to the AGA and tTG antibody levels, and there was no association.

In a causation scenario, severity would be related. For example, a person who swallows more poison will have more severe poisoning symptoms than a person who swallows less. This indicates a causation relationship between the poison and the symptoms.

Furthermore, there was no association between anti-endomysial antibodies (EMA) and schizophrenia. This presents a glaring problem with a thesis that schizophrenia is associated with celiac disease because EMA is one of the most common markers of celiac or pre-celiac disease.

In their discussion, the researchers identified that gluten was likely not the culprit, but rather, schizophrenia might increase the risk of some minor intestinal tissue issues, giving rise to increased sensitivity to gluten:

> *"We believe that the most likely explanation is that patients with schizophrenia suffer from mild intestinal tissue damage that might also be consistent with the extremely low number of EMA-positive cases found in this study."*

We should note that the vagus nerve – and the vagal system in general – connects brain and nervous system issues with intestinal health and digestion. For example, the vagus nerve stimulates peristalsis, the motions of digestion. The relationship between ones mental condition and intestinal upset has been observed for thousands of years. People who are anxious will often have intestinal upset, for example.

Mental issues have often been associated with other intestinal disorders – as we'll illustrate below – along with metabolic diseases and other conditions.

Illustrating this, a study from the University of Wyoming (Lee *et al.* 2013) confirmed other research that schizophrenia patients have a higher risk of diabetes. Does this mean diabetes, or even glucose, causes schizophrenia?

Further to the point of association, a study (Wu *et al.* 2014) from Taiwan's National Yang-Ming University studied 337 patients with schizophrenia and compared them with healthy individuals. They found that the schizophrenia patients had a greater incidence of skin diseases such as dermatitis and others.

Does this mean that skin problems cause schizophrenia? Certainly not.

We should note that other studies have associated mental disorders with markers for gluten sensitivity. A review of 12 research studies from the University of Toronto (Lachance and McKenzie 2014) found (as measured from the different studies) that anti-gliadin IgG, anti-gliadin IgA, anti-tTG2 IgA, anti-wheat and anti-gliadin antibodies were higher among those with psychosis.

However, several other important biomarkers for gluten sensitivity – anti-EMA IgA (important for a connection with celiac disease), anti-TTG2 IgG, anti-DGP IgG and anti-gluten antibodies – were not found to be higher among schizophrenia patients. These would be critical to an association with celiac disease. The researchers concluded:

> *"Not all serum biomarkers of gluten sensitivity are elevated in patients with schizophrenia. However, the specific immune response to gluten in this population differs from that found in patients with Celiac disease."*

In other words, as the Cascella study and others found, there may be an association between schizophrenia and celiac disease but the evidence is thin. There appears to be a stronger association between schizophrenia and potential sensitivity to gluten based upon antibodies, but the type of antibodies appear related to intestinal deficiencies rather than gluten itself.

This notion is supported by research that has correlated irritable bowel syndrome with schizophrenia and other psychiatric disorders. This association was confirmed by researchers from Mt. Sinai School of Medicine (Garakani *et al.* 2003). The medical scientists conducted a review of multiple studies relating IBS and psychiatric disorders, and found among the studies that 19% of schizophrenia patients were diagnosed with IBS. In addition, 29% of those with major depression were diagnosed with IBS and 46% of those with panic disorder were diagnosed with IBS.

They also found that as many as 70% to 90% of IBS patients will also have some sort of psychiatric disorder.

Thus we can conclude that psychiatric disorders such as schizophrenia are significantly associated with IBS, whereas their link with gluten sensitivity is weaker and only teased out using antibody tests and heredity regression calculations. This contrasts the stronger relationship between IBS and other neurological or psychiatric disorders.

In other words, there is no evidence that gluten causes schizophrenia. Rather, there is strong evidence that schizophrenia and other psychiatric disorders are associated with intestinal deficiencies, which indicates a potential link between gluten sensitivity and an underlying intestinal issue.

ADHD, Autism and Gluten Sensitivity

This is a similar case, where the associations have been sketchy, and indicative of another underlying issue. In the most quoted study (Niederhofer *et al.* 2011) among 67 ADHD patients, ten were found to be celiac, and among those ten, a gluten-free diet helped reduce their symptoms.

But then a study from Turkey's Inönü University (Gungor *et al.* 2013) tested 362 children diagnosed with ADHD and compared them with 390 healthy controls of the same age. They gave them tissue transglutaminase (tTg) tests for both IgA (immunoglobulin A) and IgG (immunoglobulin G) and compared the results among the group.

Out of the entire population of ADHD children, the researchers found only four instances of tTg-IgA positive results. Among the healthy children, the researchers found three cases of tTg-IgA positive results.

The researchers concluded that gluten sensitivity is unrelated to ADHD.

Just as other physical conditions have been linked with schizophrenia with diabetes and other metabolic disorders. ADHD is also linked to a number of other metabolic conditions such as diabetes, thyroiditis, and even neurological diseases such as epilepsy. ADHD is also significantly linked to major depression – which is also linked to a higher risk of intestinal issues such as IBS as evidenced in research mentioned earlier.

Autism is a disorder that often exists with ADHD. And autism has been correlated with increased IgG antibodies to gliadin (Lau *et al.* 2013). But autistic children have also been reported to have significantly increased IgG levels to other macromolecules, including casein (de Magistris *et al.* 2013).

At the same time, other research has found autism is linked with abnormal intestinal permeability – often referred to as leaky gut syndrome. The researchers found that 37% of autism patients had abnormal lactulose/mannitol ratios, and 21% of their relatives had abnormal intestinal permeability. This compared to only 5% of healthy matched control subjects having abnormal intestinal permeability.

This research also established that gastrointestinal symptoms affected nearly 47% of the autism sufferers. This further authenticates the associations between intestinal issues and neurological conditions evidenced earlier.

Researchers from Italy's Marche Polytechnic University (Catassi *et al.* 2013) reviewed this and other research and reported concerns about the efficacy of a gluten-free diet for autism:

> *"Despite its popularity, the efficacy of the gluten-free casein-free diet in improving autistic behavior remains not conclusively proven."*

Indeed, there appears to be an association between the lack of digestion of casein and gluten components with the developmental disorders. Researchers from Brazil's São Paulo University (Souza *et al.* 2012) tested seven children with developmental childhood disorders, and found greater intestinal permeability among them. They also found higher intake of dairy products and wheat products. But then again, they also found all of the seven children were overweight.

So while there appeared to be a correlation between the consumption of dairy and wheat among these disorders, most will agree that a person who is overweight from eating a Western diet will certainly consume more dairy and wheat products than others. This is also a correlation.

We will discuss the link between food sensitivities and intestinal permeability later on.

Gluten sensitivity and bipolar disorder

Some of these same associations have been seen with bipolar disorder – a shifting between manic and depressive moods. Researchers from the Stanley Research Program (Dickerson *et al.* 2011) tested 102 persons with bipolar disorder along with 173 control subjects. They gave all the subjects antibody tests for IgG and IgA to gliadin and tTG using ELISA.

The bipolar subjects indeed showed higher IgG antibodies to gliadin and deamidated gliadin compared to the healthy controls. But there was no difference between the two groups' levels of IgA to gliadin or tTG.

The researchers concluded the lack of allergic or celiac association:

> *"Individuals with bipolar disorder have increased levels of IgG antibodies to gliadin. However, such antibody increase is not accompanied by an elevation in IgA antibodies to gliadin or the celiac disease-associated antibodies against deamidated gliadin and tTG."*

We illustrated in the last chapter the lack of clear evidence that IgG testing using ELISA indicates a sensitivity to gluten. There is good reason to believe it reveals exposure and likely a lack of protein hydrolyzation within the gut – which can produce the exposure to the gluten macromolecule. We'll discuss more of the evidence for this later.

This relates back to the previous discussions regarding the link between neurological issues and IBS.

This is supported by a large study from the Norwegian Institute of Public Health (Mykletun *et al.* 2010). The researchers found that mood and/or anxiety disorders occurred more than twice (2.62) as often among IBS patients, and half of those with IBS at some point in their life also had a mood or anxiety disorder at some point in their lives.

Furthermore, a study from Canada's University of Manitoba (Walker *et al.* 2008) found in a study of 351 people matched with 779 controls that depression and "possibly other anxiety disorders" were significantly greater among those with an intestinal bowel disease condition at some point.

They also found that 27% of IBD patients suffered from major depression.

But as to why those with bipolar disorder have higher levels of IgG – once again, the co-existence of two metabolic signs or conditions does not mean one condition caused the other. Assuming the IgG testing even indicates a sensitivity to gluten, there may be another underlying metabolic issue that produces both – along with the other conditions common among the two. And certainly bipolar disorder – along with ADHD are both associated with a myriad of other conditions, such as diabetes, intestinal issues as well as others.

This myriad of relationships with bipolar disease was illustrated by a study from Johns Hopkins University School of Medicine (Severance *et al.* 2014). The researchers tested 264 bipolar patients together with 207 healthy controls. They tested the patients' blood for antibodies to casein, gluten, herpes simplex 1, Epstein-Barr virus, influenza A, influenza B, measles, and *Toxoplasma gondii*.

They found that more bipolar patients had antibodies to both casein and gluten. They also found higher antibodies to measles and Toxoplasma.

Just as the ADHD research found, there is a relationship between neurological disorders and the health of the intestines. Intestinal health relates directly with digesting complex proteins found in our foods, including casein (from milk) and gluten. When the digestive system is not doing a good job, there is increased exposure to unhydrolyzed protein molecules.

Gluten sensitivity and other reported symptoms

Yes, there is a great deal of documentation that has connected gluten sensitivities – celiac disease and wheat allergies – to the specific symptoms we listed in the previous chapter.

And these have been confirmed over the decades by numerous studies. In these cases, there is repeated correlation between these symptoms and the allergic response.

But there is also a mechanism that links these symptoms with those allergies. This is related to the inflammatory processes that occur when the body's immunological (antibody) system recognizes an invader and works to remove that invader from relative tissues – along with warning the owner to otherwise avoid the allergen with other symptoms.

We will discuss these mechanisms at length later.

But what about symptoms reported from a non-celiac, non-wheat allergy intolerance to gluten?

For these, the relationships are completely fuzzy. There may be correlation but even the correlations are suspect because there is no diagnostic confirmation of a non-celiac, non-wheat allergy gluten intolerance – as we illustrated in the first chapter.

In fact, the evidence given in many of the studies that have shown a relationship between these types of symptoms (primarily bloating, irritable bowels, headaches and fatigue) and gluten intolerance has relied upon the subjective reports of symptoms from the patients themselves.

In other words, as was illustrated in the Biesiekierski study, there has been little or no physiological marker or mechanism that has directly linked gluten intolerance to these symptoms.

Thus the only evidence given in most studies – that the symptoms are related to gluten intolerance – has been questionnaire-obtained reports that a gluten-free diet has lessened some symptoms among those who reported them initially.

Thus most of these patient report studies have a lack of placebo control.

In other words, not eating a certain type of food is extremely difficult to mask with a placebo. In the rare (short) study – such as in the Biesiekierski two-week study – one group could be given breads made with other grains while another group might be given breads with gluten grains.

But outside the confines of such a short, well-planned study, gluten elimination is very difficult to mask for any serious length of time. The study subjects have to locked within a treatment facility where their meals can be tightly controlled. Even then, gluten has a specific flavor profile and mouth feel that would be hard to match.

And it is for this reason that self-reported results of gluten-free diets are not very reliable.

In fact, most studies that utilize self-reported gluten-free diets as a basis for diagnostic information rely completely upon the patient's reporting. This means the patient knows he or she has been on a gluten-free diet.

Therefore, the results of these studies are difficult to rely upon.

But gluten-free studies have confirmed that celiac patients will become free of symptoms. In these cases, however, the symptoms of allergic response are clear. They are observable. And their antibody tests are also clear.

An allergic symptom – such as a hive or anaphylaxis, is completely observable. But the feelings of fatigue, bloating and even headaches – are quite subjective. Indeed, these types of symptoms – such as bloating and fatigue – can also occur naturally in healthy persons for reasons unrelated to any disease condition let alone the specific condition of gluten sensitivity.

Remember for example, the Carroccio 2012 study discussed in the first chapter. Here wheat-sensitive patients were found to have eosinophil infiltration. This is associated with intestinal damage and when full-blown, a condition known as eosinophilic gastroenteritis. This condition is symptomized by many of the same symptoms reported for gluten sensitivities.

And the researchers found higher eosinophil infiltration amongst practically every wheat-sensitive patient.

In other words, the symptoms being reported may be real, but gluten might not be the cause of those symptoms. Those symptoms may not only be unrelated to gluten: They may be unrelated to themselves. Each symptom may well have a different cause, or one unrelated underlying cause.

But certainly, if gluten was removed from the diet and the symptoms went away, it might seem to be a scientific assumption that gluten caused those symptoms.

But this would be equivalent to saying that if we didn't put any oil in the car – causing the car to not leak oil anymore – the oil caused the oil leak.

Certainly the same logic is being used. That if we take away a component and the symptoms of the problems stop, then the component was the problem. But that is actually an unscientific conclusion. Why?

If you don't put oil in the car, right: You will not have any more oil leaks. Because there is no more oil to leak out.

This, however, doesn't solve the problem because oil is necessary to keep the car running.

While this analogy isn't perfect, we can say that if a certain otherwise nutritious food is withheld from the body's digestive system, the damaged digestive system will no longer produce the symptoms it produced before.

Yes, certainly we can survive without eating wheat: Those who can afford the higher costs of a gluten-free diet. But we cannot survive for long without the fiber of grains, because this fiber is critical to our artery health and our colon health.

And remember that in many of the conditions mentioned above casein was also problematic – in that there were more casein antibodies or signs of possible casein sensitivity.

So now we have to eliminate two otherwise nutritious foods from the diet. How many other nutritious foods will have to be eliminated before we begin to suspect that the digestive system is the problem and not these foods?

It is the same with oil in the car. Certainly we can put synthetic oil in the car or regular oil – both will supply the lubrication necessary to keep the car running. But if the synthetic oil also leaks – and we blame the problem on the oil – guess what? There won't be many other options to keep the car running.

In the same way, we will quickly run out of foods to eat if we continue to blame the foods. This is in fact evidenced by the many IgG food sensitivity tests that will show sensitivity to dozens – even hundreds – of nutritious and healthy foods.

Canaries in the Coal Mine

This is not saying there isn't a good reason to believe that gluten and casein might be involved in the symptoms when a person goes on a gluten-free and/or dairy-free diet reports feeling better. Certainly gluten and casein may be involved.

But this still doesn't mean these are the culprits. In fact, as we've shown in some of the research, many gluten and/or casein intolerances occur in those with multiple food sensitivities. For these, eliminating all the sensitive foods will bring some relief.

Rather that blaming these foods, however, we might also consider these foods as canaries in the coal mine.

This expression comes from the mining industry, where canaries were taken into the mines. Because canaries are more sensitive to carbon monoxide or methane, when the canary fell over and died, the workers knew there was a problem.

In the same way, because gluten and casein are some of the more difficult proteins to break down for the digestive system, a sensitivity to one or both of these indicates a problem with the digestive system.

And then sensitivity to multiple foods reveals the deficiencies that were revealed by the gluten or casein sensitivity have become worse.

This might be compared to the miners staying in the mine after the canary died. The result would be their own demise.

In other words, instead of 'killing the messenger' so to speak and blaming a food or foods that have nourished billions of people for hundreds of thousands of years; as we will show with the evidence, the issue relates to the health of the digestive tract and its various components.

This might be like stating that the oil leak and the transmission noise are both related to a car with several worn out engine and transmission components. Instead of blaming the engine oil or the noise, they are simply symptoms that those worn out parts need to be repaired.

So why is gluten a problem and not other foods?

This is an over-generalization without a scientific basis. In fact, it is wholly inaccurate. We mentioned casein, but many other proteins from foods can cause far worse responses when the body's intestinal and internal tissues are exposed to not properly broken-down proteins. In fact, sensitivities to some of these can be significantly more dangerous than gluten or casein. In such exposures, such reactions to other foods outside of these two can even be fatal – as we discussed earlier in the section on anaphylaxis.

Examples include peanut proteins, fish proteins, tree nut proteins and many others, any of which can spark dangerous inflammatory processes when they are presented to intestinal tissues.

And as far as food allergies go, celiac disease and wheat allergies are one of the least occurring conditions when compared to peanut allergies, seafood allergies, tree nut allergies and others. More information on these is available in the author's book, *"Natural Solutions for Food Allergies and Food Intolerances."*

We will discuss this with more detail later, but this relates to the fact that these various food proteins are each complex. This complexity creates a more demanding enzymatic process to break down these large proteins before they can be presented to intestinal tissues.

And it is specifically for this reason that many who have symptoms such as bloating, irritable bowels, headaches and fatigue report reduced symptoms when they go on a gluten-free diet. They have eliminated the offending protein from the equation, so they feel better.

But because gluten was not the central culprit, many of these people will continue to have some of the same symptoms after going gluten-free. They might report these symptoms as being reduced, but they will still have them.

This is because the problems of a lack of protein breakdown and intestinal wall protection are still there after the gluten is taken out of the diet.

Just as the problem that caused the oil leak still exists when the oil is no longer put in the car.

But what about the improvements reported on gluten-free diets?

There are many reports of people who have gone on a gluten-free diet having better sleep, increased mental clarity and more energy. What is going on here?

First we should consider the general effects of digestion in general. Digestion requires a significant burden for the body's resources. The body must dedicate much of its blood flow, cellular energy and nervous energy into the process of digesting and absorbing the nutrients within foods. Then there is the necessity of eliminating those parts of our foods that our bodies don't require.

In addition is the energy required to eliminate those toxins that come with the foods we eat.

Yes, it is true that fasting will produce many positive results due to this reality. Fasting will help clear the mind and improve sleep for a while. Fasting will increase one's energy and even one's brain activity.

But there is a clear reason for this. By fasting, we are removing the work the body must do in order to digest the food. This frees up the body's energy to be used for other things.

And when we fast, we are eliminating some of the potential toxins that come within foods – toxins that might be in the foods or hitchhiked with the foods, including pesticides, plasticizers and others. This elimination relieves the liver of some of its burden relating to clearing toxins out of the body.

But there is a big problem with fasting. We are also eliminating carbohydrates, vitamins, minerals, proteins and so many other nutrients the body needs in order to continue to survive.

As a result, in any fast there are typically several stages. In the beginning there may be increased energy, better sleep, more mental clarity and so forth. But after awhile the body goes into acidosis and/or ketosis – as the body has to utilize fat and proteins for energy and begins breaking down and throwing off toxins store in fat cells and other tissues.

While a gluten-free diet is not the same as fasting, it is removing a component from the diet that typically requires significant digestive energy. We may still eat the same amount of calories even. But if we eliminate a portion of the body's digestive requirements, there will be a reduced burden upon the body.

We might accomplish a similar result by eating only vegetables. If we were to eat only vegetables, we would relieve those parts of our digestive capacity that are used to digest many other components of the diet. As a result, a person who has eliminated practically any part of a diet will find some increase in energy as the body has less of a digestive burden.

In the same way, a gluten-free diet might well result in more energy and psychological effects. This can be the result of the body not having to deal with as much proteins, fiber and carbohydrates coming into the body – at least of certain types.

But to take such a report and conclude that gluten is a toxin because of the effects of a gluten-free period is an extreme reach with no scientific validity.

The increased energy produced in a gluten-free diet may come not only from the lack of gluten protein: It may also come from the elimination of toxins that are in many grain-based foods such as breads, muffins, cakes and so forth. These include refined sugars, aluminum-based baking powders, certain yeasts (for those without probiotic balance), and many other ingredients that are typically mixed with grain-based foods. We'll review these shortly.

And this doesn't include the most suspect of all – the use of white refined flours that have had most of the nutritious and fibrous elements of the grain removed while leaving an unnatural balance of simple carbohydrates shown to spike insulin levels and push the cells towards insulin resistance.

Removing these foods from our diet would certainly produce positive health effects – including benefits to our sleep, energy levels and other less obvious effects.

To this we can add the placebo effect. Most of the reports showing benefits of a gluten-free diet are not only subjective: Many of the symptoms themselves are psychological symptoms. Psychological symptoms are frequently traced to the placebo effect: In fact, when someone believes a certain change will produce a psychological effect, that psychological effect becomes an almost certainty. This is because of a *double-entende*: The expectation is psychological and the effect is psychological.

This placebo effect is a long-standing observation in scientific research, and it is the reason why every bonafide research study engages in not only a placebo, and not only in blindedness, but also double-blindedness.

Blindedness is when the patient doesn't know whether he/she is being treated or being given a placebo. And double-blindedness refers to the doctor or treatment-provider also not being aware of whether the subject is being given the treatment or not.

But in the case of a gluten-free diet, everyone knows the patient is receiving the treatment. There is no blindedness. In addition, the effect of feeling better, whether it is cognitive-based or observation-based – gives such a report of feeling better a psychological element. This is because medical science has found that if a person thinks they will feel better with a certain therapy, they most likely will feel better.

This is the placebo effect in a nutshell. If a person believes the treatment will heal his or her ailment, in many cases it actually does even if the treatment was a sham – be it a sugar pill or otherwise.

In fact, the standard placebo effect assumed in most scientific studies is about a third. This is based upon previous scientific study that showed that about a third of all subjects will respond physically from just being given a pill even though that pill is not therapeutic.

This is certainly a huge number – a third of everyone. But the number becomes even greater when the benefit is not physical but psychological. Because a subjective report of increased cognition, mental clarity or better sleep is a subjective psychological report, there is a double placebo effect if you will.

The big proof of this is the so-many positive-thinking prognosticators that have taught over the decades that we will feel better about the world around us if we simply think optimistically. If we think things will turn out good then they have a greater likelihood of turning out good according to the teaching.

This optimism will not just affect the result, but will also affect the view of the result. For example, if we think we will get a positive result out of something, we can create a positive spin from practically any result. We can see the positive in practically anything.

And many of us will sometimes do this: We will say there is some benefit to practically anything: A lesson at least. And certainly this is not necessarily a false statement. But the notion of it reduces the likelihood we will ever see any result otherwise.

Yet this has no sense of objectivity or science. Once the belief is there, the science will be practically impossible to ascertain.

And while one might say they didn't expect some of the positive results resulting from a gluten-free diet, simply the fact that they gave up gluten expecting some kind of positive result means they had a psychological expectation. Thus, some kind of positive result is practically a certainty.

Noting these realities, let's look at some other potential issues regarding gluten and wheat-based foods.

Is Wheat Genetically Modified?

Let's clear the air on this question.

This is an often-stated argument for the reason to give up eating wheat. But sorry, commercial wheat is not currently a GMO – a genetically modified organism.

Genetically modified wheat is not being grown and sold commercially. This is the fortunate result of wheat traders and farmers coming to understand that Japan, Europe and other markets would reject their wheat exports if the wheat was grown from genetically modified seeds. In 2005, as a result of pressure from these groups, Monsanto abandoned its testing program for developing genetically modified wheat.

The genetically modified wheat variety called glyphosate tolerant wheat – or Roundup Ready Wheat – was being field tested at the time. Monsanto applied to the U.S. Department of Agriculture for a license to sell the seed commercially. The permit was on hold when Monsanto abandoned the program.

Monsanto had field-tested the crop between 1998 and 2005 in Oregon.

However, another variety of wheat that is commercially available has been the subject of controversy. This variety is called Imazamox-tolerant Clearfield winter wheat. This wheat variety has not been genetically modified. Let's get clearer on Clearfield wheat, without attempting to defend it:

Clearfield wheat was developed – hybridized – to tolerate the application of an increased amount of herbicide Imazamox – now trademarked as Beyond. It was licensed to be sold in 2001. The Clearfield system marketed by the company combines the seed with the use of the herbicide to control weed growth among the wheat fields.

However, as stated clearly by the BASF company and researchers who helped develop the technology:

> *"No foreign DNA was inserted into the wheat plant at any time during the development of Clearfield wheat."*

Rather, what the developers did was expose certain varieties of wheat to the herbicide and the plant naturally developed resistance to the herbicide.

Certainly, this doesn't mean that wheat from herbicide-sprayed wheat fields is what nature intended. While Imazamox is considered one of the less toxic – more short-lived – herbicide, herbicide use is prevalent in growing practically every non-organic food.

And it is not as if Clearfield wheat is that popular. It is an expensive program that requires the farmer to buy new seed from BASF every year – rather than use some of the harvested wheat berries for seed. It also requires the farmer to rotate crops much as organic growers do because of the fear that the weeds will become resistant to the BASF herbicide.

And this is what plants naturally do. They learn to become tolerant and resistant to what is sprayed on to them generation after generation.

As such, while Clearfield wheat is not toxic because of its hybridization process, the sustainable solution to bypass this technology completely is to simply consume organic wheat and wheat flours whenever possible.

This is because certified organic growers will not utilize Clearfield wheat seeds.

But we can state with confidence that commercial wheat in today's marketplace – even if it is Clearfield wheat – is currently not genetically modified.

Rather, the wheat on the commercial market has been hybridized – over thousands of years. Hybridization occurs either when plants are cross-pollinated, cross-grafted, or challenged by environmental conditions. In any of these cases, the plant naturally responds through resistance. This will typically result in a slight DNA change, which will then be passed on to the next generation.

This natural process of tolerating and responding to our environment occurs constantly in every organism. Even humans. Every body's DNA is changing from generation to generation in a process called evolution.

In fact, every food we eat from plants comes from hybridized plants. Every plant is a hybrid of those species and varieties that were growing before it hybridized.

Most plants are hybridized by cross pollination. This means planting two different varieties of the same species of plants nearby each other. When the plants begin to send out their pollen, pollen from one variety will pollinate with another variety. This produces a natural hybrid that combines the DNA from one plant with that of another. Typically, cross-pollination does not occur between two different species, but it has been known to occur with two species that are otherwise related.

Many have stated that hybridization is somehow wrong or unhealthy. But this is a mistake. Hybridization utilizes nature's own evolutionary processes – including natural selection and adaptation.

For example, if the weather in an area begins to change over time, the plants will adapt to the new weather. The plants will produce genetic changes to adapt to that new weather system.

This is a survival mechanism that not only continues the species, but also allows the plants to evolve with the environment – which continues the health of the planet.

In the same way, when a plant receives pollen from another variety, it invokes its natural environmental adaptation processes to incorporate some of the new variety's strengths. This typically creates a stronger plant. Plants will typically not assume the weaknesses of another, simply because the plant wants to survive.

And a stronger plant is often more nutritious, because strength – immunity – within a plant translates to its antioxidant properties.

This process was utilized by Dr. Norman Borlaug, who received the Nobel Peace Prize for his plant-breeding work in developing high-yield, nutrition-rich semi-dwarf wheat varieties that were bred to be resistant to many diseases that often effect wheat farming in different areas.

Dr. Borlaug's wheat varieties, developed between 1965 and 1970, allowed wheat yields to nearly double in places such as Mexico, Pakistan and India – places where hunger and starvation have weighed heavy.

But many will say that modern wheat is unhealthy because it has undergone hybridization – not just recently, but over the past 10,000 years or more.

This is a short-sighted view. Humans have been employing nature's natural hybridization processes in order to sustain ourselves in every food we grow.

Early on, we found that planting nutritious grains nearby others produced new varieties that combined the best of both. Later humans found that when they challenged plant seeds in certain ways, the plant itself made changes to prevent its seeds from being damaged in the future.

Why is this natural? Because the plants are naturally choosing their new genetic arrangement as they procreate. They are adapting to the environment around them – which is a completely natural process.

Even if that environment utilizes a chemical.

In other words, if a plant is exposed to a chemical and the plant adapts to the chemical – this is still a natural process. The plant isn't incorporating the chemical into its DNA. It is setting up a facility that will resist the damage that chemical will cause. It is not as if the new DNA now contains that chemical. The plant is simply becoming tolerant to the chemical by becoming stronger. This would be the same type of mutation a plant might make if the weather got hotter over a period of time.

Those new gene sequences produced during such natural mutations – even if the seed is exposed to chemicals – are still plant genes. It is still plant material.

Yes, a living plant may absorb a chemical that is applied to the plant. This is called bioaccumulation. The chemical may bioaccumulate among the plant's cells as the plant absorbs nutrients that stimulate its growth. If there are chemicals in the environment, the plant may absorb some of those chemicals.

But this is not occurring in the hybridization process, and this did not occur in the case of Clearfield wheat. In the case of Clearfield wheat, seeds were exposed to the chemical, and this exposure stimulated the plant's natural selection processes to resist and tolerate the chemical in the future.

The application of chemicals onto seeds before they are germinated is not a new technology. Many of the foods we eat are hybrids that have been developed using ethanol (alcohol), ethyl methane sulphonate, sodium azide and others. These are called mutagens because they can encourage the plant to rearrange its own DNA to adapt to the next substance it is exposed to.

Natural mutagens include superoxides, hydrogen peroxide, nitrous acids, lipid peroxides, nitrosamines, and a variety of other compounds qualified as plant alkaloids.

In fact, many of our medicinal herbs stimulate a process of mutagenesis. Mushrooms are one of the most powerful.

And radiation from the sun is a mutagen. The UVB, UVA, gamma rays and other waves within sunlight can stimulate mutation. In a healthy system, the mutation will produce a stronger, more resilient species in the future – one able to counteract such challenges. And in many hybrid projects, gamma rays will be applied to the seeds prior to their being exposed to other elements that produces the hybrid.

While the author is not defending the process used to produce the Clearfield hybrid, the process simply stimulated the plants' own defense systems. The resulting DNA was not an unnatural arrangement – as occurs with many GMO projects. The plant naturally re-arranged its own DNA to become more resistant to a particular chemical.

Let's review the method that the American Cyanamid Company utilized to produce the first Imidazolinone-tolerant wheat back in the late 1980s (Newhouse *et al.* 1992):

The scientists took 5,000 seeds of French winter wheat. They soaked the seeds in water for 18 hours. They bubbled air through the seed bath for six hours. Then they soaked the seeds in a 1 millimolar (very tiny) solution of sodium azide – the chemical used in airbags – for two hours. After drying and cleaning the seeds, they planted the seeds into the ground.

They took the seeds that these plants produced, and they soaked the seeds in sodium hypochlorite (to disinfect them). Then they soaked the seeds in a one molar solution of imazethapyr – an imidazolinone – for three days. After cleaning and drying the seeds, they planted them into the ground.

The plants grown from these seeds were found to be more tolerant to imidazolinone herbicides. They could better resist the damage normally occurring from the application of the herbicide. They had become stronger in this respect.

The subsequent wheat did not contain either sodium azide or imidazolinone. They simply learned – naturally as they sprouted – to become tolerant to the imidazolinone. They were still nutritious wheat seeds. The wheat plant still took the same nutrients from the soil and produced the same nutrients as the wheat they were originally taken from.

In other words, becoming more resistant to the imidazolinone was no different than a plant becoming tolerant to hotter weather. It is not as if a plant that has become tolerant to heat now produces hotter wheat berries.

There are billions of chemicals in nature – including natural versions of sodium azide. Plants develop genes to become tolerant to so many chemicals. It is a natural process.

Genetic modification, on the other hand – also called transgenics – works outside of the organism's natural selection process. Genetic modification synthetically manipulates the genes outside of nature. The process synthesizes the new genetic sequencing by inserting genes from one species into another species. It is not a natural selection process, where plants adapt to exposures or incorporate new pollen within their own genetic mechanisms.

Sometimes genetic modification will utilize a virus in order to effect the transfer of the gene(s). Or the lab can simply combine the various genes independently of the organism and then insert the DNA into the organism to effect the genetic change.

Because these genetic modifications work outside of nature's processes of procreation and natural selection they can produce unexpected results. Risky results.

This is completely different from cross-pollination or natural selection through environmental challenge.

Does Gluten Cause Weight Gain?

Some would have us believe this, but the science just isn't there.

Consider a study that has been used to prove a gluten-free diet results in weight loss. In this Mayo Clinic study (Murray *et al.* 2004) 215 people (160 female and 55 male) who were diagnosed with celiac disease went on a gluten-free diet. While it has been purported that the gluten-free diet resulted in weight loss, the numbers do not indicate this. The researchers stated with regard to their results:

> *"The same proportions of males and females gained or lost weight after the institution of a gluten-free diet (for the males,*

31% gained and 41% lost; for the females, 36% gained and 35% lost)."

They also stated that 91 of the patients gained weight within six months of going on the gluten-free diet.

While this study showed that those with celiac disease have reduced celiac disease symptoms after going gluten-free, this study does not indicate that a gluten-free diet produces weight loss.

In fairness, however, we should note that in 2013, researchers from Brazil's Federal University of Minas Gerais (Soares *et al.*) published a study that tested C57BL/6 mice by giving them either a high-fat diet with gluten or a gluten-free diet.

The researchers found that the gluten-free diet resulted in reduced weight compared with the high-fat gluten diet.

This sounds super encouraging, except that mice are not humans, and there are differences between glycemic processing between rats and humans. Furthermore, different species of mice will process fat and carbohydrates differently from one another.

For example, researchers from Duke University Medical Center (Parekh *et al.* 1998) studied two strains of mice. One of the strains – the C57BL/6J strain – was found to develop diabetes on a high-fat diet. And when the mouse diet was changed to a low-fat diet for eight months, their diabetes disappeared.

Duke University excitedly announced that only a high-fat diet – not a high glycemic diet – causes diabetes. This of course contradicted the now-understood effects of high-glycemic foods on diabetes. One of the researchers – Dr. Mark Feinglos even stated in a 1998 Duke University press release:

"The only thing sugar has ever been shown to do is cause dental cavities. It's the fat that appears to be most detrimental."

Of course, this theory was refuted in short-order by a number of human studies over the next decade – both epidemiological and clinical – that proved that high-sugar diets indeed produce type 2 diabetes (Lustig *et al.* 2012).

Furthermore, the type of fat is the bigger issue than the fat itself with respect with insulin sensitivity, it has been found.

And the research has also clearly identified that diets high in sugar also produce obesity, again negating the Duke mice study. We can present the headline of a review from Harvard University (Hu 2013):

"Resolved: there is sufficient scientific evidence that decreasing sugar-sweetened beverage consumption will reduce the prevalence of obesity and obesity-related diseases."

With respect to sugar and type 2 diabetes, Harvard researchers (Hu and Malik), published a large review of evidence through 2010. There were 13 large human studies up until 2006 that showed the relationship, and more between 2006 and 2010. Then additional human studies between 2010 and 2013 resulted in the study headline above.

These studies repeatedly showed the relationship between sugar and obesity, and sugar and type 2 diabetes. Meanwhile, diets high in saturated fats have been linked with obesity, but a link with diabetes is not clear.

So what about the C57BL/6J mice showing the link between diabetes and high fat diets?

Well first know that the link between the high-fat diets and diabetes in the C57BL/6J mice did not occur in the other strain of mice tested at that time at Duke. The A/J mice fed the same high-fat diet did not develop diabetes. Why not?

In 2003, researchers from Louisiana State University studied the C57BL/6J mice along with AKR/J mice. They fed both groups of mice a high-fat diet for eight weeks. The C57BL/6J mice ended up way fatter (three times more adipose tissue) than the AKR/J mice. They also found that the C57BL/6J mice were more insulin sensitive than the AKR/J mice and produced far less insulin.

Furthermore, the C57BL/6J mice tissue contained three times more GLUT4 protein than the AKR/J mice. They also expressed more PDPCK in the liver, which prompted the researchers to state the C57BL/6J mice quite simply processed carbohydrates differently than the other mice – producing *"elevated glycemia."*

Now in the 2013 Brazilian gluten study mentioned above, the researchers chose to test these highly glycemic C57BL/6J mice. And interestingly, they also found that the elevated GLUT4 protein was one of the main reasons for the increased weight among the gluten-eating mice. The researchers found:

> *"The overexpression of PPAR is related to the increase of adiponectin and GLUT-4."*

The bottom line of this review of some mice research with respect to gluten, obesity and diabetes is that the reason why the Duke University researchers erroneously concluded that diabetes was related only to a high-fat diet was because they found this effect upon one particular strain of mice – and curiously, not the other strain.

Furthermore, later research from Florida State University found the same strain of mice – the C57BL/6J – had a tendency for greater weight gain and diabetes because it processed carbohydrates and fats differently.

In other words, the two other mice strains tested did not display this intense glycemia found in the C57BL/6J mice.

And this is the mice that the Brazilian researchers used in their gluten-free study. Can we with good conscience apply this research to humans?

No.

This is especially in the face of a clinical *human* study (Murray *et al.* 2004) that showed a gluten-free diet did not result in more weight loss.

And finally, we present more evidence: A lot more evidence:

We can leave this topic by looking at the other side of the coin, with *human* research. An extensive review of research by Pennsylvania State University scientists (Harris and Kriss Etherton 2010) found that whole grain intake – consisting primarily of wheat-containing foods – significantly reduces body mass index. In a meta-analysis of 20 studies – many large-scale – the researchers found those who eat one or more servings a day of whole grain foods had a body mass index of nearly two BMI points lower (27.1 versus 29) and a waist circumference of more than three centimeters lower (90.3 versus 93.9) than those who ate less whole grains.

Certainly if gluten causes weight gain, that would be determined by these extensive human studies – some of which followed tens of thousands of people for more than a decade. We'll discuss some of this research later.

As far as the anecdotal evidence given by many that their gluten-free diet has produced weight-loss, there is a very reasonable explanation:

Many of the fattiest foods – such as cookies, donuts, cakes and others – also happen to contain gluten. If a person is avoiding gluten, then these foods will suddenly be off limits.

Unless of course similar fatty foods are purchased or cooked as gluten-free. But in most public venues – such as a party, work event or family event – the cookies, cakes and crackers will typically all be standard wheat foods containing gluten. Thus you have a situation of forced calorie reduction.

Furthermore, gluten-free replacement foods are typically available primarily in health food markets and/or by healthier food brands. Thus these may also likely have less sugary, fatty ingredients compared with the donuts, cakes and other gluten-containing *junk foods.*

At the same time, one of the problems with a wheat-free diet is that commercial gluten-free foods often require some unhealthier ingredients in order to match the mouthfeel of a gluten-based food.

This means in order to accomplish the doughy texture or chewiness that consumers want in a food, a gluten-free food might contain more refined sweeteners and refined carbohydrates than a matching gluten-containing food would require.

The bottom line is there is not only no real evidence that healthy diets with gluten-containing whole wheats will produce weight gain: there is significant evidence that diets high in whole wheats actually lead to weight loss and decreased body fat.

Amylopectin

Some have stated that the dwarf hybrid of the wheat family contains excessive amounts of amylopectin – and this is responsible for straining our glucose levels and producing insulin resistance.

The reality is that amylopectin is actually a complex carbohydrate that provides more than half of the carbohydrates that humans and most other plant-eating animals ingest. About 60% of our entire diet is composed of amylopectin.

While most plants contain about 75% to 80% amylopectin – with the rest being mostly amylose – some plants contain higher levels of amylopectin. These include potatoes, rice, corn, cassava and wheat.

And the simpler carbohydrates produced as amylopectin is broken down initially are maltose and isomaltose. These are still more complex than simple sugars such as glucose and fructose. They will still break down into glucose, but this will typically take place in the small intestines through the enzyme process of pancreatic amylase as opposed to the amylase produced in the oral cavity.

And the potatoes, rice, corn, cassava, wheat and other higher-amylopectin-containing foods are all healthy foods to eat in their whole forms. Yes, depending upon whether they are whole or refined, they may contain more amylopectin and might provide more complex carbohydrates per serving. But along with those amylopectins, these whole foods also contain a significant amount of nutrition.

But certainly, if the amylopectins are isolated from the rest of the plant's compounds in refining they may present some metabolic challenges, unless they are blended sensibly with other whole foods. These refined versions include potato starch, cassava starch, white rice and white flour. In these cases, the ratio between amylopectin and other nutrients – including protein, lipids, minerals, vitamins and other phytocompounds such as sterols, alkylresorcinols, beta glucans and others – increases significantly.

If consumed exorbitantly, these refined versions of real foods could then become a challenge to our metabolism because as they are broken down by amylase within our mouth and digestive tracts, they can be more quickly absorbed into the bloodstream.

This hastened glycemic response produces more pressure on our pancreas to produce more insulin to escort the glucose to the cells.

This in turn – over time – can produce an increased resistance to insulin – called reduced insulin sensitivity because the cells become less sensitive or ready to receive insulin on its cellular receptors in order to guide glucose into the cell.

This lack of insulin sensitivity leaves the body in a state of heightened glucose in the bloodstream. This can result in blood vessel wall damage as the extra glucose produces greater levels of oxidized lipids – called lipid peroxidation – along with higher levels of oxylipins. The lipid peroxides are known to directly damage the blood vessel walls, and oxylipins are involved as signaling systems for inflammation according to recent research.

So yes – should we eat an abundance of white rice, refined potato starch or a lot of foods made with white flour, we are possibly burdening our metabolism with a faster absorption of glucose being converted from these refined versions of real foods.

But worse than these are refined simple sweeteners such as white sugar, high-fructose corn syrup, dextrose and others that require little or no amylase to break them into their assimilated forms of glucose. These push our metabolism far worse than even refined carbohydrates will. These refined sweeteners have no nutrients to offer outside of their simple sucrose, glucose and fructose molecules, and thus they are almost immediately absorbed into the bloodstream.

But interestingly, molasses, maple syrup and honey do not have these same metabolic effects as the refined sweeteners do, even though they also contain extreme amounts of simple sugars. Why not?

In fact, honey is actually antimicrobial, proven to kill numerous pathogens including MRSA (*Methicillin-resistant Staphylococcus aureus*) (Anthimidou *et al.* 2013) – while the refined sweeteners like white sugar actually feed MRSA and other pathogenic microorganisms.

It is because these natural sweeteners such as honey and maple syrup contain numerous other components. These include phytonutrients that will slow the absorption of the glucose (see more information about sweeteners in the author's book, *The Ancestors Diet*.)

And for this reason, these natural sweeteners are not considered causes for pre-diabetes as refined sugary foods are.

Whole wheats are like these natural sweeteners in that they contain numerous phytonutrients – as we'll discuss in the next chapter. But even better, wheats also contain dietary fibers and sterols that further slow the absorption of their complex carbohydrates.

This is illustrated by the glycemic index. The glycemic index measures how fast a food will increase blood sugar. The scale is based on glucose – the purest form of sugar the body utilizes – which is given a standard measure of 100. All other foods, then are based upon that 100 standard of glucose.

The glycemic index does not alone indicate the blood sugar effects of a food, however. There is also the glycemic load – which multiples the glycemic index by the amount of carbohydrates in a serving. This is further complicated by the production of insulin from a particular food. Different foods produce different levels of insulin, and thus put more pressure upon the insulin-glucose relationship within the bloodstream.

That said, both glycemic index and load have been shown to relate to metabolic syndrome, obesity and weight loss in different studies. They are well-accepted measures among the scientific community.

In general, whole grains are considered low glycemic, and refined flour foods – even whole wheat bread which typically contains 50% white flour – is in the mid-range of glycemic levels. Let's look at this more specifically.

Cooked whole wheat pasta has a glycemic index from 43 to 58, and pumpernickel bread will have a GI of about 41 with a glycemic load of 5. And cracked wheat breads, and course wheat kernel breads will also range from 48-58 GI with glycemic loads ranging from 10 to 12.

Whole wheat breads can have GI's that range from 43 to 75, depending upon their content of white flour – often about 50% as mentioned. Many whole wheat breads also contain many other ingredients added to sweeten up the bread such as sugar.

In general, the more whole the wheat is – more whole wheat flour and more whole kernels (cracked for example) – the lower the GI will be, as indicated above.

White bread is another case altogether. White wheat breads will have a GI of 70-77 with a glycemic load of around 10-15. White bagels are also in this category of 70+ in many cases on the GI scale. But Bagels will typically have much higher glycemic loads, ranging around 25.

Baguettes, however, will often have incredibly high GIs, some around 95, with glycemic loads that can range from 25 to 48.

In other words, we cannot make a sweeping judgment of whole wheat bread one way or another. There are good whole wheat breads and not so good ones in terms of their glycemic index and load.

And yes, a white bread that is enriched with vitamins such as folic acid may indeed not have much greater a glycemic load than whole wheat bread. But the issue is not just blood sugar. It is also the effect of the bread upon the intestines. In other words, its fiber content and whole-grain nutrient availability are also key considerations as we'll discuss shortly.

In comparison to the above numbers on wheat products, rice has far higher glycemic numbers than wheat foods do. A medium grain white rice will have as much as an 89 GI. And just as the cooked pasta has much lower GI levels, brown rice has much lower GIs, ranging from 48 to 62 – the latter being Japonica short-grain brown rice.

But a sponge cake – made from white flour – can have a GI that approaches white rice, of 87.

Meanwhile, blackstrap molasses has a glycemic index of 55, and maple syrup, 54. And honey, 50. And barley malt syrup, 42 – indicating the lower glycemic burden of those first-stage amylopectin derivatives – maltose.

And it is not as if gluten-free bread is any better. In fact, most gluten-free breads have significantly higher glycemic indices than wheat breads.

Here is a listing of gluten free breads (Revised International Table of Glycemic Index and Glycemic Load 2002):

- Gluten-free multigrain bread: Glycemic Index: 79±13 Glycemic Load: 10
- Gluten-free white bread, unsliced: GI: 71 GL: 11
- Gluten-free white bread, sliced: GI: 80 GL: 12
- Gluten-free fiber-enriched, unsliced: GI: 69 GL: 9
- Gluten-free fiber-enriched, sliced GI: 76 GL: 10

Compare this to:

- Wholemeal flour bread: GI range: 52-73 GL: 6-10
- White flour bread: GI range: 69-73 GL: 9-11

This means that most whole wheat breads and white breads have better glycemic index and load numbers than gluten-free breads do.

So certainly we can't accuse gluten or amylopectin as being distinctively bad for blood sugar.

In addition, research has found that wheat's amylopectins are very similar to rice's amylopectins – which has also been a mainstay of human nutrition for billions of people for thousands of years. And repeated studies of populations that eat generous portions of rice have continually showed lower rates of obesity, diabetes, heart disease and other metabolic-related disorders.

Furthermore, wheat's amylopectins have been found to be more complex and harder to break down than those in potatoes and sweet potatoes (Want *et al.* 2014). So wheat has less of an effect upon our blood sugar than these nutritious foods. Do we have to give up sweet potatoes too?

Wheat Germ Agglutinins

This is somewhat of a misnomer. Because the word agglutinin contains the root "glut" it is presumed that an agglutinin is a gluten and/or grain-related element.

The word agglutination comes from the Latin word *agglutinare*, which means 'to glue.' In chemistry and biology it refers to a clumping of cells or particles. The cells can be bacteria, immune cells or even red blood cells. In particles it can mean the clumping together of molecules into a precipitate.

In medicine, this word agglutinin refers to something that will produce a clumping of antibodies or even red blood cells within the bloodstream. The latter is often referred to as hemagglutination.

Agglutination can also occur during an allergic response, when cells clump together to prevent the admission of a foreigner.

Proteins called lectins can also form a clumping – in this case often to polysaccharides or carbohydrates.

And as far as the agglutinin in wheat germ – yes, a particular type of protein called wheat germ agglutinin will bind to a glucose derivative called N-Acetylglucosamine. And note that wheat germ agglutinin – or WGA – is unrelated to gliadin and glutenin proteins termed 'gluten.'

The investigation into WGA's effect upon the intestines has provided some grist for gluten-free advocates. But what must be examined with the science is the context and rationale for studying WGA lectins. Many food plants produce lectins as a natural part of their immunity, so it is important for food scientists to understand the effects of these lectins from an isolated viewpoint – out of the context of normal dietary use of the foods they are contained within.

So is WGA a toxin or not?

Some lab research (Pellegrina *et al.* 2009) found that WGA, at certain doses, can provoke an inflammatory response, specifically upon intestinal Caco2 cells. However, in this study, the immune system also appeared to balance these effects with cytokines.

But did the research duplicate the intestinal tract? Actually, no. The research utilized divided intestinal cells within a laboratory environment that did not duplicate all of the elements involved in human digestion – namely the various probiotics and enzymes, as well as the mucin layer that in a healthy intestinal tract protects the intestinal cells from such exposures.

Rather, the researchers simply exposed the isolated intestinal cells to purified WGA and watched the immune response within the laboratory.

At the same time, however, other research has illustrated in animal research that a vast range of WGA doses are safe and non-inflammatory in a healthy intestinal tract. But when doses that dramatically exceed any normal human diet – the equivalent to over 600 grams for an adult male (over a pound of not just wheat germ but a pound of purified WGA lectin in one sitting) – can cause small intestinal issues and if crossed into the internal tissues.

Not only was the quantity far greater than any realm of realism, but the WGA was not within its natural matrix of the plant nutrients around it. This also relates to the enzyme availability of the rats' digestive tracts to break down the WGA. As we will discuss later, our bodies produce particular proteases which break apart proteins such as WGA.

Furthermore, research has indicated that much of wheat germ agglutinin is neutralized by cooking. A study by researchers from Italy's University of Verona (Matucci *et al.* 2004) determined that WGA is largely deactivated at cooking temperatures of 65 degrees Celsius (about 149 degrees Fahrenheit). The researchers stated:

> *"Detectable amounts of WGA were found in raw foodstuffs and wheat flours, whilst variable amounts of agglutinin were found in wholemeal pasta probably as a consequence of thermal inactivation during food processing."*

The "variable amounts" would refer to significantly reduced levels

This means, of course that baked breads and most uses of whole wheat (which contain wheat germ) will have, to the degree the bread was fermented with yeast and cooked, largely inactivated wheat germ agglutinin.

But should a lab isolate and purify a huge dose of practically any protein – especially a protein that is a known lectin – there certainly will be intestinal consequences relating to the fact that the protein was not properly broken down in the intestinal tract.

Lectins in general – when isolated and purified as they were in these studies – are not normal foods. It is similar to isolating and purifying sugar from beets. Beets are healthy foods that provide significant nourishment. But when refined sugar is isolated and purified from beets (and cane) – as has been done over the past century – that sugar becomes a cause of diabetes, metabolic disease, heart disease and other conditions. Should we stop eating beets because of the sugar that has been extracted from them?

Furthermore, even within the doses considered healthy, WGA has been shown to be *selectively* cytotoxic to human colon cancer cells (Pusztai *et al.* 1993 and others). The WGA was able to select, bind to and destroy colon cancer cells while leaving the healthy intestinal cells alone. So WGA is actually – as many lectins are – pretty smart. And beneficial to humans.

This simply means that within a healthy diet and healthy intestinal tract, WGA is not only safe for human consumption, but helps protect against colon cancer.

In fact, N-acetylgalactosamine is a typical element of living cells – and binding to them can serve to stimulate better intercellular communication.

And wheat germ is known to effect the translation between amino acids and mRNA – which produces enzymes and other proteins necessary for life.

Yet wheat germ extract contains little of its own mRNA, indicating its sustainable contribution to the health of the reproduction within the grain seed – the wheat berry.

But in some wheat allergies, people have been found to become sensitive to – form antibodies against – wheat germ agglutinin. But this is the same as other proteins of many other foods that are otherwise considered nutrients. So while an allergy to wheat germ agglutinin might not be a good thing, it doesn't mean that WGA in itself is bad.

So is wheat germ agglutinin unhealthy or not? Agglutinated N-Acetylglucosamine, for example, is found throughout the body, for example in cartilage and eye tissue.

Lectins bind with innumerable biomolecules in millions of life-sustaining biological processes. Some of them are particularly healthy in fact. For example, lectins from *Wisteria japonica* bind with cancer cells but not normal cells, just as lectins from wheat germ do.

And some lectins are known to bind to bacteria and viruses and other foreign elements – helping to protect cells from their intrusion.

In fact, this is one of the reasons for these important proteins. They help protect the plants that produce them from being harmed by bacteria and viruses. They do this through molecular affinity, and the binding-reception process that takes place on the surface of most cells.

In other words, lectins are found throughout nature. They conduct so many processes that it is unreasonable to define them as toxins in general, because many are health-promoting. Lectins are in bananas, coconuts, potatoes, beans nuts, seeds and so many other health-promoting foods. To define them as anything but health-promoting is to look at health through a very narrow bandwidth indeed.

This is not to say that all lectins are healthy. Ricin, for example, is a lectin. It is a lectin found within castor beans of the castor plant (*Ricinus communis*).

But just as beans, nuts, seeds, potatoes, coconut and many other foods are healthy, wheats and wheat germ are also healthy, as we will prove in the next chapter.

Wheat germ, for example, has been shown in several human clinical studies to reduce intestinal inflammation, boost liver health, stimulate immunity and help normalize cholesterol levels. In a study from France's INSERM (National Institute of Health and Medical Research) (Cara *et al.* 1992) researchers found that WGA-containing wheat germ reduced triglycerides, improving cardiovascular health.

The Mayo Clinic had this to say about wheat germ in a slideshow of *"10 great health foods:"*

"Wheat germ is the part of the grain that's responsible for the development and growth of the new plant sprout. Although only a small part, the germ contains many nutrients. It's an excellent source of thiamin and a good source of folate, magnesium, phosphorus and zinc. The germ also contains protein, fiber and some fat. Try sprinkling some on your hot or cold cereal."

Phytic Acid

Gluten-containing grains contain phytic acid. Is this harmful?

Yes, it is true that wheat does contain a significant amount of phytic acid. Raw wheat and uncooked wheat flour can contain no more than about 1.4% by weight.

Yet grains are not the only foods containing considerable amounts of phytic acid. Nor do they have the most phytic acid compared to other foods.

In fact, phytic acid is found in a large range of foods. Practically any food with a shell or a husk will contain phytic acid. In fact, some of the highest amounts of phytic acid are contained among some of the healthiest nuts such as Brazil nuts and almonds, as well as sesame seeds and other healthful foods. These mentioned nuts and seeds can have as much as twice the phytate levels as many gluten-containing grains.

To be clearer, many foods have higher phytic acid levels than wheat by weight: Sesame seeds have 5.4%, Brazil nuts contain up to 6.3%, oat meal contains up to 2.4%, pinto beans contain up to 2.4%, corn contains up to 2.2% and peanuts contain up to 1.8%. This is compared to whole wheat, which as mentioned can contain up to about 1.35% by weight – not much more than raw walnuts and rice, both of which come in at about 1% (Reddy *et al.* 2001; Phillippy *et al.* 2002; Macfarlane *et al.* 1988, Gordan *et al.* 1984).

Yes, research has found that many unprocessed nuts, beans and grains contain phytic acid. And phytic acid has been shown in multiple laboratory studies to potentially decrease the absorption of certain minerals, including calcium, iron and zinc, through the wall of the intestines.

However, it is not as simple as that. Phytic acid – also called inositol hexakisphosphate as well as phytate – is broken down into its soluble components (hydrolyzed) during soaking, cooking, fermentation and germination processes.

Phytates are also hydrolyzed by enzymes called phytases – which become available during the processes just mentioned. In the presence of a phytase, phytates are converted to inositolphosphates such as myo-inositol triphosphate, which do not block mineral absorption.

Phytases are available throughout nature. Upon germination, most grains will produce phytases to neutralize phytates. (Yes, nature is intelligent.)

And many bacteria also produce phytase – including intestinal bifidobacteria such as *Bifidobacterium infantis* – a bifidobacterium passed from mother to infant during birth and within breast milk – and lactobacilli such as *L. acidophilus, L. plantarum* and *L. paracasei* – which are present in the guts of healthy persons. These and many other probiotic strains produce phytase, which in turn hydrolyze any remaining phytic acids not hydrolyzed during soaking, cooking, fermentation and/or germination (Sandberg 1991; Famularo *et al.* 2005).

Multiple studies have successfully tested the ability of these and other probiotic strains to hydrolyze phytic acid by producing phytase. Other probiotics that have been found to produce phytase include *Bifidobacterium bifidum* (Nalepa *et al.* 2012); *Bifidobacterium pseudocatenulatum, Bifidobacterium longum* (Tamayo-Ramos *et al.* 2012); and other bifidobacteria (Sanz-Penella *et al.* 2012). This adds to other Lactobacillus strains that have also been shown to produce the phytase enzymes (Tang *et al.* 2010; Lavilla-Lerma *et al.* 2013).

Even before wheat is cooked and eaten – both of which can remove most if not all phytates – the process of yeast fermentation will reduce much of its phytate content. A study from France (Leenhardt *et al.* 2005) found that sourdough fermentation of dough can reduce phytate content by up to 70% – depending upon its pH. A pH of 5.5 found the highest removal of phytate.

The ancient Ayurvedic formula for consuming grains with meals is to include yogurt with the meal. Though the soaking and longer cooking style of Ayurvedic rice and wheat chapattis and so forth naturally reduce its phytic acid content, the accompanying yogurt helps immediately jump start the body's fermentation process.

This is followed up by the phytase produced by the intestine's probiotics – leaving little if any phytic acid not hydrolyzed.

The bottom line: If we cook our grains and maintain a healthy microbiome – our gut's probiotic populations – phytic acid is not a concern.

Wheat Amylase Trypsin Inhibitors

What is a wheat amylase trypsin inhibitor? Trypsin is an enzyme produced in the pancreas that breaks down proteins. It is a protease – an enzyme that breaks down protein.

So a trypsin inhibitor is also a protease inhibitor. In a nutshell, a trypsin inhibitor is a substance that slows or blocks the enzyme functions of trypsin.

So what is the problem? Recent research has suspected that trypsin inhibitors from wheat are involved in mechanisms related to celiac disease. A study from Harvard (Junker *et al.* 2012) found that amylase trypsin inhibitors may be involved in the inflammatory processes related to celiac disease – and possibly other immune sensitive persons.

This effect was found in mice that were deficient in a particular toll receptor gene called TLR4. And interestingly, the toll-like receptor 4 is set up to sense liposaccharides – which are the waste products from pathogenic bacteria. Thus it is interesting that the connection between sensitivity to amylase trypsin inhibitors in wheat lies within the TLR4 gene. More on this in a bit.

Like phytic acid, there are many trypsin inhibitors in nature. Many exist among plants because the plant is trying to protect its proteins against being broken down or hydrolyzed by other elements in nature. As such, many seeds, beans and other types of eggs contain trypsin inhibitors to help protect the precious embryo. Hen's eggs, for example contain more than their weight in trypsin inhibition potency.

And a lima bean contains more than two times its weight in trypsin inhibiting power. And our own bloodstream contains trypsin inhibitors.

Other foods with notable trypsin inhibitors include squash, peas, legumes, potatoes, sweet potatoes, tomatoes and so many others. While there has not been enough research to arrive at this conclusion, it is safe to say that practically every plant produces trypsin inhibitors to help protect themselves.

So far a cataloging of proteins and their inhibitors called the MEROPS database (Rawlings *et al.* 2011) has cataloged 192,053 proteases (enzymes that digest proteins) and 17,451 different protease inhibitors among plants.

For example, McGill University researchers (Waglay *et al.* 2014) juiced potatoes, and found 53.3% trypsin inhibitors from their extraction.

Plants produce trypsin inhibitors in their leaves to help deter animals from eating those leaves.

Fermentation and cooking will break down most of these plant-based trypsin inhibitors. A Brazilian study (Trugo *et al.* 2000) for example, showed that cooking completely neutralized trypsin inhibitors among germinated soybeans, lupins and black beans. Another study (Cabral *et al.* 1005) found cooking hulled soybeans inactivated 99% of their trypsin inhibitors, and storage decreased the remaining levels.

A study at the University of Agriculture in Krakow (Pysz *et al.* 2012) found that microwaving reduced trypsin inhibitor levels among legumes by 70-75%. Another study (Yuan *et al.* 2008) found that blanching and UHT processing inactivated trypsin inhibitors in soymilk manufacturing. Other research has found that cooking and flour-making reduces most of the trypsin inhibitors of these foods. It is for this reason that cooking some of these foods is important.

However, trypsin inhibitors are also neutralized during the gut fermentation among those animals – including humans – that eat leaves, seeds and vegetables.

Yes, probiotic bacteria resolve not only phytic acid, but trypsin inhibitors. Why? Because like us, our intestinal bacteria need to eat. Like us, they also need to break down proteins for their own consumption. This is called symbiosis.

Researchers from India's Haryana Agricultural University (Sindhu and Khetarpaul 2002) tested a mixture of barley flour, dhal flour, milk powder and tomato pulp for phytic acid and trypsin inhibitor content among other elements. They fermented multiple mixtures with *Lactobacillus casei, L. plantarum* and *S. boulardii,* and found that the fermentation significantly decreased the phytic acid levels and trypsin inhibitor levels. They noted:

> *"All the fermentations drastically reduced the contents of phytic acid, polyphenols and trypsin inhibitor activity while significantly improving the in vitro digestibilities of starch and protein."*

This study was repeated (Binita and Khetarpaul 2007) with just *Lactobacillus acidophilus,* whereupon the same results were found – a significant reduction in both phytase and trypsin inhibitor.

Indeed, many of the studies that showed intestinal probiotics reduced phytic acid levels among grain foods also found reduced trypsin content.

What this means is that trypsin inhibitors from so many plant foods – just as phytates – will not be problematic for a healthy digestive tract that houses good colonies of intestinal bacteria.

As this text will reveal, the smoking gun in gluten sensitivity is not necessarily simple, but there is clear evidence that it relates to the relative health of our intestinal bacteria.

But there is more to it than just that.

A Case of Mistaken Identity?

To these various points we should add that once the hypothesis that gluten is a toxin was put forth and hit the mainstream – since around 2010 – researchers from different institutions have doubled-down their attempts to objectively establish if this is truly the case.

One of the main problems is that outside of the subjective reports of symptom relief after trying a gluten-free diet; the research linking the consumption of gluten with gastrointestinal and other symptoms outside of those caused by wheat allergies or celiac disease (non-celiac gluten sensitivity) has been hazy. There has been correlation, but no causation.

Illustrating this, researchers from the Department of Gastroenterology of Monash University along with The Alfred Hospital in Melbourne (Biesiekierski *et al.* 2013) conducted an extensive review of gluten research that included 59 studies and research papers. Here is the abstract of their findings:

> *"The avoidance of wheat- and gluten-containing products is a worldwide phenomenon. While celiac disease is a well-established entity, the evidence base for gluten as a trigger of symptoms in patients without celiac disease (so-called 'non-celiac gluten sensitivity' or NCGS) is limited. The problems lie in the complexity of wheat and the ability of its carbohydrate as well as protein components to trigger gastrointestinal symptoms, the potentially false assumption that response to a gluten-free diet equates to an effect of gluten withdrawal, and diagnostic criteria for coeliac disease. Recent randomized controlled re-challenge trials have suggested that gluten may worsen gastrointestinal symptoms, but failed to confirm patients with self-perceived NCGS have specific gluten sensitivity. Furthermore, mechanisms by which gluten triggers symptoms have yet to be identified."*

In the conservative language of research, the word *"limited"* means basically, a lack of clear evidence. The *"potentially false assumption"* mentioned here being discussed is the misleading inclusion of celiac disease research as evidence that gluten is a toxin for those who are not allergic to gluten.

And this is certainly what is seen in much of the consumer literature that promotes the gluten-free diet for those without wheat allergies or celiac disease: It will quote research done on celiac disease patients.

Who can argue that a gluten-free diet will benefit a person who is allergic to gluten? Certainly, many if not most symptoms of celiac disease will be reduced by a gluten-free diet. There is no question here, because there is the definite element of causation.

Furthermore, it is a theoretical presumption to utilize any research that tests celiac patients to promote a theory of gluten being a toxin.

Just consider the ramifications of such a strategy. Just think of all the other foods that some people become allergic to. A considerable proportion of the population is allergic to fish, milk, eggs, nuts, beans, shellfish and others. Some of the allergic responses of these are life-threatening as we have discussed. Does this mean these foods are toxins for the rest of us?

Such an assumption would lead to mass starvation.

University of Oslo researchers (Lundin and Alaedini 2012) stated the following after their scientific review of the research on non-celiac gluten sensitivities:

> *"Gluten sensitivity has been best recognized and understood in the context of two conditions, celiac disease and wheat allergy. However, some individuals complain of symptoms in response*

to ingestion of "gluten," without histologic or serologic evidence of celiac disease or wheat allergy. The term non-celiac gluten sensitivity (NCGS) has been suggested for this condition, although a role for gluten proteins as the sole trigger of the associated symptoms remains to be established."

Let's consider some of the clinical evidence.

Monash University researchers (Biesiekirski *et al.* 2013) conducted a trial that came with the initial observation from other research:

"Patients with non-celiac gluten sensitivity (NCGS) do not have celiac disease but their symptoms improve when they are placed on gluten-free diets."

The researchers tested 37 people in a double-blind cross-over study. Of the group, 31 were women and 6 were men. All the patients complained of gluten sensitivity and did not have celiac disease or a wheat allergy.

The patients were randomly divided into groups and each underwent a high-gluten diet or a low-gluten diet or a whey-protein diet for a week. The high-gluten diet contained 16 grams of gluten per day and the low-gluten diet contained 2 grams of gluten per day. Another group ate a control diet with 16 grams of whey protein per day.

Now before the diets began, all the groups were subjected to two-week period where other foods were eliminated. These included what is termed FODMAPs – "fermentable, poorly absorbed, short-chain carbohydrates," including fermentable, oligo-, di-, monosaccharides, and polyols.

After the one-week diets, the subjects had wash-out periods, and then each crossed over into the other groups for three days after finishing their testing period. This eliminated odd metabolic differences between the subjects.

The results of the study were clear. All the subjects reported significantly improved gastrointestinal symptoms during the initial two-week period where the processed ingredients were removed from their diet.

But only 8% of the subjects reported any improved symptoms during a low-gluten or gluten-free period. And even those who went gluten-free reported worse symptoms than the two-weeks of FODMAPs elimination.

This clear result questions gluten's role as being the culprit. And it was confirmed during a three-day re-challenge. Here gastrointestinal symptoms increased among the gluten-free subjects again. The researchers concluded:

"In a placebo-controlled, cross-over rechallenge study, we found no evidence of specific or dose-dependent effects of gluten in patients with NCGS placed diets low in FODMAPs."

This is not the only study finding this conclusion. Another study, published in 2014 (Halmos *et al.*), studied 30 IBS patients along with 8 healthy control persons. This study also found that while gluten-foods did not reduce symptoms of IBS, reducing FODMAPs – again foods including fermentable oligosaccharides, disaccharides, monosaccharides, and polyols – resulted in significantly fewer IBS symptoms.

The researchers concluded:

> *"In a controlled, cross-over study of patients with IBS, a diet low in FODMAPs effectively reduced functional gastrointestinal symptoms. This high-quality evidence supports its use as a first-line therapy."*

As such, we can offer that the latest research suggests that for some, a gluten-free diet may offer some relief from intestinal difficulties such as bloating, gas and indigestion. However, for most others, this relief of symptoms is accomplished by the discontinuance of many other foods and food ingredients that are producing GI symptoms.

This of course indicates a much deeper gastrointestinal problem occurring rather than simply a case of gluten being a toxin. The fact that discontinuing all of these FODMAPs was therapeutic while a gluten-free diet alone was not indicates simply that the problems being attributed to gluten are misplaced: *A case of mistaken identity.*

Interestingly enough, many foods classified as FODMAPs are broken down by probiotics – including foods containing lactose, casein, fructans, vinegar and others. They also include oligosaccharides – which are the prebiotics that our probiotics utilize for food. This is of course why they are called *fermentable* oligosaccharides, disaccharides, monosaccharides, and polyols (FODMAPs).

What does "fermentable" mean? It means they are consumed – broken down – by gut probiotics during the fermentation process.

Yes, our guts are fermenters. We, like most other plant-eating mammals, ferment plant-based foods within our digestive tract using probiotics.

That is, if our guts are healthy.

Unhealthy guts can also ferment, via yeasts like *Candida* species and pathogenic bacteria such as *E. coli* and *Bacteroides fragilis.* When these microorganisms ferment in our guts, the results aren't as pretty.

As the researchers have expanded and tested the notion of certain foods causing more digestive issues than others, many, many foods have now been classified as FODMAPs. This is an exhaustive venture however, as nearly every plant-based food requires fermentation in order to digest it.

Some very wholesome foods are also categorized as FODMAPs. These include apples, pears, asparagus, artichokes, garlic, beets, cabbage, beans, pulses, legumes, peaches, snap peas, watermelon, nectarines, peaches, plums, cashews, pistachios, sweet corn and many others.

Some dairy foods are also considered FODMAPs, including cow's milk, cheese, ice cream and even yogurt are considered FODMAPs.

In addition, rye and wheat-containing foods are also considered FODMAPs.

Higher fructan levels are often defined as determinants of FODMAPs. Monash University researchers (Biesiekierski *et al.* 2011) tested a number of foods and found fructan levels range from 1.12 grams per 100 grams in cous-cous to 0.6 grams in rye, and 0.07 grams in spelt bread. They also found 0.11 grams in oats, 1 gram in wheat-free muesli, and 0.81 grams in a muesli fruit bar.

They also found that many FODMAPs contain important prebiotics such as GOS and FOS. As such, the elimination of FODMAPs will also necessarily eliminate a lot of healthy foods in general – foods necessary for feeding our intestinal bacteria.

There are also some processed food FODMAPs because they become acidic, either through processing with lactic acid or other preservation/acidification processes. This makes them difficult to digest for many. FODMAPs also include many junk foods – including those with refined sugars and refined carbohydrates, and sugar-alcohols such as sorbitol and others – often ingredients of many breads and other wheat products.

FODMAPs in general are not unhealthy foods and do not cause any problems for those with healthy digestive systems (read: healthy microbiomes). This was shown in a Monash study (Ong *et al.* 2010) of 15 healthy people and 15 IBS patients. During a two-day testing period, the researchers found that FODMAPs did not affect healthy persons outside of producing slightly different gas levels – which relate directly to increased fermentation. And increased intestinal fermentation relates to probiotic populations in a healthy gut. But in the IBS patients, FODMAP consumption produced significant IBS symptoms.

And isn't it interesting that FODMAPs, like the TLR4 factor and the enzyme factor, all seem to relate to our intestinal bacteria? Is this a coincidence? The reality is that our intestinal bacteria and their various workings within our digestive tract are still somewhat mysterious.

Yes, researchers have been investigating our intestinal bacteria for the past five decades. But there is still a lot that conventional science still doesn't understand about the various processes of our microbiota.

And the understanding of how yeasts like *Candida* species and pathogenic bacteria like *E. coli* and *B. fragilis* can build up within our guts and destroy the health of our intestines is also emerging. Later we will show just how important these are in the gluten equation later.

Later on we will discuss the underlying issues related to these cases. Certainly, we can accept that all those healthy foods mentioned above that are defined as FODMAPs – including many, many others – are not toxic in themselves. There is something in common among them, and there is an underlying reason the digestive tracts of these food sensitivity sufferers cannot handle these types of foods, when many of these foods have been eaten for millions of years by humans.

Junk Food Gluten

With regard to gluten in particular, we should also consider that many junk foods that contain gluten are lumped in with healthy gluten-containing foods. Is that fair? Certainly not, because junk foods containing gluten are not in the same nutritional classification as whole wheat foods – which will be discussed shortly. Rather, junk foods are, well, fake foods – unhealthy foods.

Consider all the gluten-containing foods with junky food ingredients:

- ✓ high-fructose corn syrup, white sugar and other refined sugars
- ✓ synthetic sweeteners
- ✓ refined salts
- ✓ refined flour
- ✓ bleaching agents
- ✓ dough conditioners
- ✓ ammonium sulfates and chlorides
- ✓ emulsifiers
- ✓ preservatives
- ✓ nitrites
- ✓ hydrogenated oils (and trans fats)
- ✓ glutamates
- ✓ synthetic food dyes
- ✓ aluminum-containing baking powders
- ✓ thinning and thickening agents
- ✓ acidification ingredients
- ✓ so many other ingredients that help make processed grain products sweet, fluffy and lip-smacking tasty.

These ingredients create foods that are basically junk foods.

Deceptively, many of these foods might say NATURAL or MADE WITH NATURAL INGREDIENTS on the label.

And this doesn't even include the fact that the wheat flour itself used to create most of these junk foods is often refined bleached flour – flour after the germ and the bran have been stripped away.

Just consider for a moment, the ingredient panel for the leading bread in the U.S. We won't mention the brand of this soft white bread but it is one of the oldest, most trusted U.S. bread brands:

> WHEAT FLOUR, WATER, HIGH FRUCTOSE CORN SYRUP OR SUGAR, YEAST. CONTAINS 2% OF LESS OF SOYBEAN OIL, BARLEY MALT, WHEAT GLUTEN, SALT, CALCIUM CARBONATE, SODIUM STEAROYL, LACTYLATE, VITAMIN D3, VINEGAR, MONO- AND DIGLYCERIDES, CALCIUM SULFATE, MONOCALCIUM PHOSPHATE, YEAST NUTRIENTS (AMMONIUM CHLORIDE, AMMONIUM SULFATE), ENZYMES, YEAST EXTRACT, WHEAT STARCH, CALCIUM DIOXIDE, FERROUS SULFATE (IRON), B VITAMINS (NIACIN, THIAMINE, MONONITRATE (B1), RIBOFLAVIN (B2), FOLIC ACID, SOY LECITHIN, AZODICARBONAMIDE, SOY FLOUR, WHEY, CALCIUM PROPOINATE (TO RETAIN FRESHNESS), DATEM, SORBIC ACID.

First, the WHEAT FLOUR is refined, and bleached, with little or no bran and germ within the flour – only the endosperm-originated flour. And remember, the endosperm contains the gluten and the amylopectin, while the bran and the germ contain most of the nutrients and fiber.

The second ingredient after water is HIGH FRUCTOSE CORN SYRUP OR SUGAR. Then the 2% listing means that none of those ingredients make up more than 2% of the contents, but 2% is quite a bit when some of these junky ingredients, such as AZODICARBONAMIDE and AMMONIUM CHLORIDE are added together. Yummy? *Junky* is more like it.

Or consider an ingredient the author found in some commercial shortcakes: PROPYLENE GLYCOL. This is the chemical used as radiator coolant.

Some junk foods will say they are made with WHOLE WHEAT. And many breads labeled as WHOLE WHEAT BREAD don't even have WHOLE WHEAT FLOUR as the primary flour ingredient. Many will have ENRICHED FLOUR (bleached refined flour enriched) or UNBLEACHED ENRICHED FLOUR as the main ingredient. While it is generally understood from the USDA that the primary flour should be whole wheat, there is an allowance for fiber enhancement that brings the bread up to the standard of being considered WHOLE WHEAT, even if WHOLE WHEAT FLOUR runs second or third on the list.

One of the takeaways here is that most bread labels will not list that the flour it is made with is refined with the bran and germ removed. It will only be listed as WHEAT FLOUR or ENRICHED WHEAT FLOUR. But they will list WHOLE WHEAT FLOUR if the bran and germ have been added back. And if the FLOUR is BLEACHED, it also will not be listed as such, but if it is UNBLEACHED, you betcha *that* will be listed.

In other words, a whole wheat bread might be almost as junky as the white bread, with the addition of a little more fiber. We'll discuss healthier options later on.

Junk Food Gluten Toppings

We cannot forget the *junk food* often put between and on top of gluten-containing foods. Just consider a few junky things commonly put in or on top of gluten-containing foods:

- ✓ Frostings
- ✓ Icings
- ✓ Sugary jellies
- ✓ Mayonnaise
- ✓ Imitation butter spreads
- ✓ Polyunsaturated oil spreads
- ✓ Processed meats
- ✓ Imitation cheese
- ✓ Sugary, hydrogenated oil peanut butters

These and many other toppings contain ingredients that are also damaging to our intestines, not to mention the harm they can have upon our physiology. Some of their ingredients include nitrites, preservatives, color dyes, high-fructose corn syrup, trans fats and others.

As such, these foods can help stimulate the overgrowth of yeasts like Candida, spike blood glucose, reduce insulin sensitivity, produce lipid free radicals that damage blood vessel walls and produce inflammatory responses. These physiological responses in turn can cause headaches, bloating, diarrhea, indigestion, fatigue and other symptoms often attributed to gluten intolerance.

In other words, some of the same symptoms observed by those who have been eating junk gluten foods may actually be related to a pre-diabetic condition, driven by the consumption of an overload of refined and bleached flour, too much refined sweeteners, too much hydrogenated and polyunsaturated oils, too little fiber and too many chemicals.

And to the contrary, once all these junky foods are removed from the diet, a person might indeed feel quite a bit better.

This is a point to consider carefully because a person may be able to eat junky foods for years, and suddenly, seemingly out of the blue, become pre-diabetic or type 2 diabetic. This is in fact a common syndrome among adults today. This is because sugary, refined foods will slowly stress the metabolism of our intestines, pancreas, liver, cells and blood vessels. In addition to damaging our intestinal tracts and liver, over time the blood sugar spikes and the lack of fiber from these junky foods produce insulin resistance among our cells. This pushes our blood into high glucose levels, leading to blood vessel damage and a host of metabolic issues.

We might compare this to stacking building blocks without mortar. At some point there are too many blocks stacked up too high and the whole stack collapses.

As we'll discuss later, these foods and ingredients can also irritate intestinal cells, stimulating zonulin (reducing the intestinal barrier), and increasing the colonization of pathogenic yeasts and bacteria. As the research we will examine proves, these can produce intestinal cramping, bloating and other symptoms being attributed to gluten.

Certainly if going gluten-free means bypassing all these junk foods and junk food ingredients and toppings, gluten-free is certainly a good strategy. There is no doubt that gluten-free diets will typically reduce these junk foods and junky food ingredients. Why? Because these have been built into the corporate food machine that has risen to the top of the food chain among Western countries.

But it doesn't mean that gluten proteins are the culprit.

Ironically, some of these junk foods and junky ingredients also create the intestinal environment allowing a person to become sensitive to gluten.

Later on, we will review the science that further supports this case of mistaken identity.

For now, let's flip the coin and look at the other side of gluten-containing grains.

Chapter Three

Health Benefits of Whole Wheat

The perplexing issue to those who would claim gluten is a toxin is that gluten-containing grains have been found to lower the risk of heart disease, diabetes and other metabolic conditions. Could a toxin do this?

Gluten-containing foods also dominate one of the most health-providing food categories – a category that forms the largest tier of the food pyramid introduced by nutritionists and government agencies over the past century. Yes, whole wheat cereals and grains provide the foundation for a healthy diet according to nutritional experts – with the consensus arriving at five servings a day of these foods in order to maintain a nutritious and health-giving diet.

There have been hundreds of studies that provide the foundation and evidence for this consensus.

We could list and document the dozens of studies that have found these effects here, but these would fill a thick book. While we will discuss a few of these in this chapter, in the interest of science we'll rely upon an extensive scientific review of the research:

Penn State University researchers (Harris and Kriss Etherton 2010) reviewed the multitude of studies that have connected whole grains – consisting primarily of gluten-containing grains with several important health benefits. They found:

- Persons with a diet high in whole grains have a reduced risk of obesity.
- Persons with a diet high in whole grains have a reduced risk of cardiovascular diseases.
- Whole grains such as barley decrease low-density lipoprotein cholesterol (LDL-c).
- Whole grain barley also lowers blood pressure.
- Whole grain barley and whole grain wheat improves glucose control and reduces insulin sensitivity.
- Whole grain wheats increase intestinal probiotics.

Here are some highlights of some of the studies that helped the researchers arrive at these conclusions:

- ➢ A 14-year study of 42,850 adult men that found diets high in whole grains reduced coronary heart disease by 18%
- ➢ A 12-year study of 75,521 adult women that found diets high in whole grains reduced ischemic stroke by 36%
- ➢ This study also found that diets high in whole grains reduced type 2 diabetes incidence by 27%

- A 9-year study of 38,470 women that found diets high in whole grains reduced cardiovascular disease deaths by 18% and coronary heart disease was reduced by 18%
- A 9-year study of 34,491 adult women that found diets high in whole grains reduced ischemic heart disease by 30%
- This study also found diets high in whole grains reduced type 2 diabetes incidence by 21%
- A study of 535 elderly men and women that found diets high in whole grains reduced mortality from cardiovascular disease by 52%
- This study also found that diets high in whole grain foods reduced incidence of metabolic syndrome
- A 11-year study of 15,972 adult men and women that found diets high in whole grains reduced deaths from all causes by 23% and reduced coronary artery disease incidence by 28%
- An 18-year study of nearly 350,000 men that found those who ate more whole grain foods had the least incidence of hypertension – high blood pressure
- Studies that showed whole grain wheat reduced cholesterol
- Studies that showed whole grain intake was associated with lower body mass index (weight) and lower average waist circumference
- A meta analysis of 11 studies showed diets high in whole grain foods reduced colorectal cancer incidence
- A five-year study of 291,988 men and 197,623 women found that diets high in whole grain foods reduced colon cancer incidence by 14% and rectal cancer by 36%
- This study also found a 41% reduction in small intestinal cancer incidence
- A study of 61,433 women over the age of 40 found a diet high in whole grains reduced colon cancer incidence by 33%

The Penn State meta-analysis found that most of these results were achieved with three servings a day or more of whole grain foods. And the predominant form of whole grain foods – by far – was whole grain wheat foods such as bread, rolls, pasta and other wheat flour products.

The relationship between grains and heart disease relates directly to mortality. Because greater consumption of whole wheat reduces our risk of cardiovascular disease, there is a direct link between whole grains and mortality.

One of the reasons for the link between lower risk of heart disease and gluten-containing grains is aleurone. Aleurone is located at the outer shell of the grain endosperm, and it is known to have therapeutic health effects.

Illustrating this, a study from Ireland's University of Ulster (Price *et al.* 2010) tested 79 healthy adults. For four weeks, the subjects were given either a diet high in aleurone-rich grain foods or a control diet with the same amount of fiber and nutrients. Those eating the grain foods high higher levels of plasma betaine (helps blood vessel walls) and lower levels of homocysteine (lower inflammation).

Other heart-healthy compounds in gluten-containing grains include arabinoxylans, beta-glucans, alkylresorcinols, tocols and phytosterols, as well as lignans and B-vitamins. Phytosterols have been associated with lower LDL-cholesterol levels, better hormone levels and other health benefits. We will discuss some of the benefits of all these in a bit.

Metabolic Syndrome and Diabetes

Metabolic syndrome is one or a combination of obesity, glucose metabolism issues such as pre-diabetes or diabetes, and cardiovascular inflammation. Rounding out the metabolic syndrome is often coronary artery disease – which typically affects those with glucose metabolism issues and higher inflammation among the blood vessels.

The research illustrates that metabolic disorder conditions can be at least partly mitigated by a diet rich in whole gluten grains.

For example, in a study of 166 people from Swedish and Finnish researchers (Magnusdottir *et al.* 2014), whole rye grain consumption was found to significantly increase insulin sensitivity. This is a significant therapeutic benefit because diabetes and pre-diabetes are linked with insulin resistance. The element of rye found by the research to have this effect is alkylresorcinol. We'll discuss this in a bit.

A review of the research from scientists from the Norwegian University of Science and Technology (Aune *et al.* 2013) conducted a systematic meta-analysis of the research to date – a total of 16 studies – relating to grain intake and type 2 diabetes. The researchers found that a diet containing three servings per day of whole grains including wheats, rye and barley lowered the risk of type 2 diabetes by 32%. Among the grain sub-types, whole grain bread and wheat bran were both associated with a reduced risk of diabetes.

The researchers concluded:

> *"Our results support public health recommendations to replace refined grains with whole grains and suggest that at least two servings of whole grains per day should be consumed to reduce type 2 diabetes risk."*

A 32% drop in diabetes incidence is significant. This certainly illustrates that gluten-containing grains do not produce the high-glycemic metabolism that is associated with *both* diabetes and obesity.

Another study, from the Boston University School of Medicine (Newby *et al.* 2007) studied 1,572 people within the Baltimore Longitudinal Study of Aging. They found those who ate the highest levels of whole grains in their diets had significantly lower body mass index (BMI) than those who ate less whole grain.

They also found those who ate whole grains had significantly less total cholesterol, less LDL-cholesterol (the "bad" cholesterol), and lower two-hour glucose levels – a test for diabetes risk.

A study from Tufts University (McKeown *et al.* 2002) tested 2,941 people and found those who ate the highest levels of whole grains also had the lowest body mass index levels, the lowest waist-to-hip ratios, the lowest levels of total cholesterol and LDL-cholesterol, and the lowest levels of fasting insulin – indicating a lower risk of diabetes.

A study from the University of Maryland (Sahyoun *et al.* 2006), followed 585 elderly people for three years. They found those who ate the most whole grains had the least indications of metabolic syndrome. They found fasting glucose levels lower and lower mortality among those who ate the most whole grains in their diet.

A study from the University of Minnesota School of Public Health (Murtaugh *et al.* 2003) found among 160,000 people that those who ate the most whole grains had 30-36% lower incidence of type 2 diabetes.

Other studies have tested people with diabetes or pre-diabetes, and found that a diet high in whole grains increased insulin sensitivity and lowered blood glucose levels (Pereira *et al.* 2002; Rave *et al.* 2007; Nisson *et al.* 2008).

This is just a small sampling of the many studies done over the years that have substantiated the ability of gluten-containing whole grains to prevent metabolic syndrome.

As we'll discuss, whole wheat grains contain phytocompounds within the pericarp, aleurone and germ – removed from refined flours. Because refined flour comes from primarily the endosperm, this means white breads, cookies, cakes and other gluten-containing (junk) foods will not contain many of these phytocompounds, and thus not provide the metabolic syndrome protection that whole wheat provides.

This was evidenced in a study (Nilsson *et al.* 2008) of 15 healthy people who were fed, at different meals, either barley kernel bread or white wheat bread. The barley kernel bread produced better glucose response the day following the meal. The researchers concluded:

> *"In conclusion, the composition of indigestible carbohydrates of the evening meal may affect glycemic excursions and related*

metabolic risk variables at breakfast through a mechanism involving colonic fermentation. The results provide evidence for a link between gut microbial metabolism and key factors associated with insulin resistance."

Inflammation is a big part of metabolic syndrome – specifically among the blood vessels, which can become inflamed as a result of high blood sugar and poor lipid (cholesterol) quality. This sort of inflammation is typically measured with a blood test for C-reactive protein.

A study from Pennsylvania State University (Katcher *et al.* 2008) followed 50 overweight adult men and women with metabolic syndrome for three months. The researchers split the subjects into two groups. Both groups ate a reduced calorie diet (500 less calories), and three servings of grain foods per day (mostly wheat-based) for the three months. But one group ate whole grain foods and the other group ate only refined grain foods.

Both groups experienced significant body weight reductions by the end of the three months, ranging from 3 to 5 kilograms – or up to about 11 pounds. However, the group eating whole wheats had greater reductions in percentage body fat and abdominal fat – by more than double the refined grain group.

More importantly, the whole grain group also had significantly reduced C-reactive protein levels – by an amazing 38%. CRP levels were not reduced in the other refined grain group. Triglyceride levels and LDL-c levels also went down considerably in the whole grain group.

Greater abdominal and body fat loss among the whole grain group reveals an interesting point: As gluten-containing foods are sometimes accused of producing more abdominal fat. While the refined grain group also saw body fat and abdominal fat reductions, whole grains provided significantly more.

As a result of some of this evidence discussed above, health organizations focused on metabolic syndrome such as the American Heart Association, the American Diabetes Association, Healthy People, the World Health Organization and the U.S. Department of Agriculture (among others) recommend three or more servings of whole grain foods daily, inclusive of whole wheats.

Whole Wheats and Colon Cancer

Research from the Danish Cancer Society Research Center in Copenhagen (Kyrø *et al.* 2014) has confirmed what some previous studies also indicated: That whole grain foods made from wheat and rye significantly reduce the risk of colon cancer.

The researchers followed 1,372 colorectal cancer patients together with 1,372 matched healthy persons as part of the European Prospective Investigation into Cancer and Nutrition study.

To confirm whole grain wheat and rye consumption, the researchers measured blood levels of alkylresorcinols – phenolic lipids from the bran of cereal grasses wheat and rye.

The researchers found those with higher levels of alkylresorcinols in their bloodstream had between 52% and 72% lower incidence of distal colon cancer.

Furthermore, among Scandinavians, higher levels of alkylresorcinols had a 27% reduced incidence of all types of colon cancer.

Their research also found that populations that ate greater amounts of alkylresorcinols – notably Central Europe and Scandinavian countries – there was a significantly lower incidence of colon cancer. This means it isn't about eating a few whole wheat and rye foods here and there: It is about consistently including whole grains in the diet.

The researchers stated this clearly:

> *"Plasma alkylresorcinols concentrations were associated with colon and distal colon cancer only in Central Europe and Scandinavia (i.e., areas where alkylresorcinol levels were higher)."*

Those areas where *"alkylresorcinol levels were higher"* relate to regions where more whole-grain wheats are consumed. In other regions of Europe and among many other Western countries, common wheat foods are primarily made from refined flours, which contain little alkylresorcinol content.

Again this is not the first study to correlate reduced colon cancer incidence with the consumption of whole-grain wheat. A larger study from the Danish Cancer Society Research Center (Kyrø *et al.* 2013) followed 108,000 Danish, Swedish, and Norwegian persons for eleven years. From this population 1,123 were diagnosed with colorectal cancer during the 11 years.

As the researchers analyzed diets across the board, they found the consistent (daily) consumption of whole-grain foods, including whole-grain breads and cereals, resulted in a 44% lower incidence of colorectal cancer among the population studied.

The research has shown that alkylresorcinols have numerous biological effects, including curbing mutagenic activity and inhibiting carcinogenic enzymes in the gut. They also have been shown to have antifungal activities. We'll discuss alkylresorcinols in a moment.

But another component of whole-grain wheat is something we have investigated before – that of supplying a certain prebiotic called arabinoxylan oligosaccharide that promotes the growth of probiotic bacteria. Several studies have shown certain gut probiotics reduce levels of colon-cancer related enzymes such as beta-glucosidase and beta-glucuronidase. We will also cover this topic in more depth later.

Whole Wheat Nutrition

Wheat contains a considerable amount of health-giving nutrients – nutrients that have sustained billions of people for millions of years on the planet.

One of the greatest benefits of wheat is its superior protein content: One hundred grams of whole wheat flour will contain over 16 grams of protein – that's 16% protein by weight. Furthermore, wheat is a complete protein. Common wheat varieties will contain up to 21 amino acids, including all nine of the essential amino acids.

According to USDA research (Krull and Wall 1969) common whole wheat contains the following amino acids:

Alanine	Leucine*
Arginine	Lysine*
Asparagine	Methionine*
Aspartic acid	Phenylalanine*
Cysteine	Proline
Cystine	Serine
Glutamic acid,	Threonine*
Glutamine	Tryptophan*
Glycine	Tyrosine
Histidine*	Valine*
Isoleucine*	

*Essential amino acid

Note that amino acids that are often deficient because they either aren't contained in all foods or they aren't properly cleaved include methionine and cystine – critical to the formation of methyl donating and detoxification elements.

For this reason, wheat supplies more protein on a global basis than any other food. Other mass-fed foods such as rice and corn have significantly less protein content.

As you can see from the table below, wheat is also rich in folate, thiamin, riboflavin, pantothenic acid, niacin and vitamin B6. Wheat also contains significant vitamin E and vitamin K. In terms of minerals, wheat is rich in magnesium, selenium, manganese, phosphorus, and is also a good source of iron, copper, potassium and zinc. Wheat also contains calcium. Consider the table on the next page:

Whole Wheat Flour Nutrients Per One Cup (120 grams)

Nutrient	Measure	% Daily Value (US)
Calories	407	20%
From Carbohydrate	329	
From Fat	18.8	
From Protein	59	
Carbohydrates		
Total Carbohydrate	87.1 grams	29%
Dietary Fiber	14.6 grams	59%
Sugars	0.5 grams	
Fats & Fatty Acids		
Total Fat	2.2 grams	3%
Saturated Fat	0.4 grams	2%
Monounsaturated Fat	0.3 grams	
Polyunsaturated Fat	0.9 grams	
Total trans fatty acids	0	
Total Omega-3 fatty acids	45.6 milligrams	
Total Omega-6 fatty acids	886 milligrams	
Protein & Amino Acids		
Protein	16.4 grams	33%
Vitamins		
Vitamin A	10.8 IU	
Vitamin E (Alpha Tocopherol)	1 milligram	5%
Vitamin K	2.3 micrograms	3%
Thiamin	0.5 milligrams	36%
Riboflavin	0.3 milligrams	15%
Niacin	7.6 milligrams	38%
Vitamin B6	0.4 milligrams	20%
Folate	52.8 micrograms	13%
Pantothenic Acid	1.2 milligrams	12%
Choline	37.4 milligrams	
Betaine	87.4 milligrams	
Minerals		
Calcium	49.8 milligrams	4%
Iron	4.7 milligrams	26%
Magnesium	166 milligrams	41%
Phosphorus	415 milligrams	42%
Potassium	486 milligrams	14%
Zinc	3.5 milligram	23%
Copper	0.5 milligrams	23%
Manganese	4.6 milligrams	228%
Selenium	84.8 milligrams	121%

Wheat is an extraordinary food. Consider wheat's superior selenium, manganese, copper and zinc levels. These are critical macrominerals utilized amongst the many enzymes of the body. These include the body's detoxification systems as well as brain processes. For this reason, foods with higher levels of selenium and zinc have been associated with increased immunity and lower levels of inflammation, cancer and heart disease.

Magnesium is also associated with lower levels of heart disease. This relates to the artery walls becoming more flexible.

Potassium is critical to the health of the cells' kidneys and to blood pressure, as potassium balances the sodium levels within the blood and urinary systems. Research from the University of Naples Medical School (D'Elia *et al.* 2014) found, after conducting a meta-analysis that included 333,250 participants among 14 large studies, that diets high in potassium significantly reduce the risk of stroke.

With regard to wheat's generous supply of choline and betaine, these two elements help promote healthy brain cells and neuron activity. They are also instrumental in blood vessel health, and have been linked with lower risk of cardiovascular diseases. Research from Spain's University of Murcia (Vidal *et al.* 2014) has found that betalains (betaine is a betalain) inhibit the enzymes lipoxygenase and cyclooxygenase – both of which are enzymes involved in pain and inflammation (e.g., COX and LOX inhibitors).

The nutrient table above used common wheat varieties. Other wheats such as rye, spelt, Kamut and barley, contain different nutrient levels – sometimes higher. Let's review barley's.

Whole Barley Nutrition

As mentioned, barley contains similar yet slightly different nutrient levels. Oats and barley are very similar in their phytonutrient content, and are often eaten together in oatmeal and other applications. But oats do not contain gliadin proteins – whereas barley does.

Like whole wheat flour, barley flour also contains considerable nutrients. A cup of flour will supply 15.5 grams of protein – a very high quality protein with a balance of amino acids. In fact, barley is a complete protein food. Here is a list of its amino acids according to laboratory analysis of multiple varieties (Folkes and Yemm 1956):

Alanine
Arginine
Asparagine
Aspartic acid
Cysteine
Cystine
Glutamic acid,
Glutamine
Glycine
Histidine*
Isoleucine*
Leucine*
Lysine*
Methionine*
Phenylalanine*
Proline
Serine
Threonine*
Tryptophan*
Tyrosine
Valine*

*Essential amino acid

That is 21 amino acids – including all of the nine essential amino acids.

Barley flour also contains a number of important vitamins and minerals. These include it being a good source of thiamin (37% DV), niacin (46% DV), vitamin B6 (29% DV) and riboflavin (10% DV). Barley flour also contains 47 milligrams of calcium (5% DV), 142 milligrams of magnesium (36% DV), 457 milligrams of potassium (13% DV), zinc (20% DV), copper (25% DV), manganese (77% DV) and selenium (80% DV), along with 56 milligrams of choline and 97 milligrams of betaine.

Barley is also a good source for healthy fats. A serving of barley can contain 173 milligrams of omega-3 alpha-linolenic acids (ALA), and 3,781 mg of omega-6 fatty acids. The fat content of barley – higher than most other grains – is also well balanced between monounsaturated and polyunsaturated fats.

Barley also contains glycolipids, diacylglycerols, alkylresorcinols and estolides. These unique fatty acids distinguish barley from other grains.

Alkylresorcinols

Wheat, barley and rye contain unique alkaloid polyphenols called alkylresorcinols. What are alkylresorcinols?

Alkylresorcinols are lipids classified as resorcinolics. They have extremely long phenolic rings that are contained in the bran layer of wheats, and not as much in the inner endosperm.

In fact, alkylresorcinol content tends to be highest in the outer layers of the bran and endosperm, and decreases towards the middle of the endosperm.

Alkylresorcinols are transported throughout the body within lipoproteins – important for transporting cholesterol. Alkylresorcinols will thus build up in fat cells and other cells – contributing to better fatty acid metabolism and a reduction of artery damage.

Recent research indicates that alkylresorcinols reduce incidence and complications of atherosclerosis – the scarring and inflammation of the artery walls. Alkylresorcinols have also shown significant antioxidant capacity.

Recent research is now measuring the amount of whole grain intake of people by the presence of alkylresorcinols in the bloodstream and urine. And higher levels of these are being linked with health benefits.

Wheats produce alkylresorcinols as a defense mechanism. During 2004 field testing by scientists from the Agricultural University in Poland (Zarnowski and Suzuki 2004), winter barley varieties grown in different regions showed higher alkylresorcinol content in regions with greater environmental stressors – notably harsher weather. This means alkylresorcinols are produced as part of the plant's immunity.

This converts to health benefits. Multiple studies have found that higher alkylresorcinol levels are associated with lower cancer rates and lower rates of heart disease, as indicated in some of the research mentioned earlier.

Some of the highest alkylresorcinol levels among Europe, for example, exist among the Swedes – which also have lower levels of heart disease and cancer than countries such as the United Kingdom and the U.S.

Remember the Magnusdottir study (*et al.* 2014), mentioned earlier. The research that tested 166 people with metabolic syndrome found higher levels of alkylresorcinols in the blood was associated with better glucose control and specifically, insulin sensitivity. The subjects ate either a control diet or a diet rich in whole grain wheats for up to six months.

A study from Tufts University (Ma *et al.* 2012) found higher plasma alkylresorcinols levels was associated with lower body mass index scores. Those in the higher quartile of alkylresorcinols levels had an average of nearly 1 kg/m2 lower BMI, effectively lowering the average of the subjects from 27.6 to 26.7.

Remember also the Danish Cancer Society Research Center study (Kyrø *et al.* 2014) that found higher levels of alkylresorcinols in the diet reduce the risk of colon cancer.

Another study, from researchers at the North Carolina Agricultural and Technical State University (Zhu *et al.* 2012) found, in a study of 15 different alkylresorcinols, that alkylresorcinols inhibited colon cancer cells from growing and replicating. This study concluded that wheat's alkylresorcinol content drives much of its anti-cancer effects.

In 2011, researchers from Canada's Carleton University (Gliwa *et al.*) found that alkylresorcinols protect our cells from free radical damage. The researchers tested alkylresorcinols in the laboratory, which included testing their oxygen radical absorbance capacity (ORAC) and gas chromatography-mass spectrometry. They also tested the alkylresorcinols with cells, and found the alkylresorcinols helped protect the cell from damage.

Another study from Sweden's Lund University (Andersson *et al.* 2011) found that alkylresorcinols from rye bran significantly inhibited lipolysis among fat cells – which leads to higher levels of triglycerides and fatty acid-derived free radicals.

An analysis of the research from University of Helsinki (Adlercreutz 2010) indicated that the combined effects of the lignans and alkylresorcinols within wheats result in lowering plasma estrogen concentrations. This, indicated the research, produces protection against breast cancer.

This was confirmed in another University of Helsinki study (Aubertin-Leheudre *et al.* 2010). This study of 56 people including 16 women with breast cancer found that lower alkylresorcinol levels were associated with higher incidence of breast cancer.

Multiple studies have shown that alkylresorcinols will build up in fat cells, improving the nature of their production of fatty acid metabolites.

University of Helsinki researchers (Parikka *et al.* 2006) measured alkylresorcinol activity and found they were able to inhibit oxidation of low-density lipoprotein – a common cause of artery damage. They also found alkylresorcinols inhibited genetic damage from oxidation.

Research from the Swedish University of Agricultural Sciences (Frank 2005) conducted studies on vitamin E utilization in the body and found that alkylresorcinols increase the availability of natural vitamin E within the body. The research found several mechanisms for this, along with reducing the amount of vitamin E excreted through the urine.

Because vitamin E is an antioxidant with many benefits, its increased utilization as offered by whole wheat provides a significant advantage.

Beta Glucans

Beta-glucans – referred more scientifically as beta-D-glucans or better, (1,3),(1,4)-beta-D-glucans – are contained within the fibrous cell walls of cereal grains and wheats. For this reason, the fibers from whole wheat and barley are rich in beta-D-glucans. This is one of the reasons fiber has been shown in university research to maintain healthy cholesterol levels.

More specifically, beta-glucans are found in the plant family *Gramineae* – including rye, oats, wheat and barley. While wheat contains less than 1% beta-D-glucans content, barley appears to contain the highest levels, with typical varieties containing from 5-7% beta-D-glucans. Meanwhile rye provides about 2% beta-D-glucans content by weight.

A number of studies have linked beta-D-glucans with less cardiovascular disease risk. Researchers from The Netherlands' Maastricht University (Theuwissen and Mensink 2008) calculated from many of these studies that LDL-c levels were decreased by .52 mmol/L for each gram of beta-glucan-rich water-soluble fiber added to the daily diet.

Beta-D-glucans reside in cell walls throughout the bran and endosperm of the wheat berry. In 2002, the U.S. Food and Drug Administration, after reviewing scientific evidence from a number of studies, announced that beta-D-glucans soluble fiber is proven to have significant cardiovascular benefits.

In a six-week study from University of Minnesota's Medical School (Keenan *et al.* 2007) 155 volunteers were divided into four treatment groups, with or without beta-D-glucans. The beta-D-glucans groups were given either high or low molecular weight barley beta-D-glucans in either five gram or three gram per day doses. The five gram high molecular weight beta-D-glucan group experienced a 15% reduction of LDL-c, while the low molecular weight five gram beta-D-glucan group had a 13% reduction of LDL-c. The three gram groups both experienced 9% LDL-c reduction. This illustrates the gold standard of dose-relationship between beta-D-glucans consumption and LDL-cholesterol levels.

Beta-D-glucans can also increase high-density lipoprotein (HDL-c) levels. In a study at Venezuela's University of Zulia (Reyna-Villasmil *et al.* 2007), 38 volunteers with mild hypercholesterolemia were given either the American Heart Association Step II diet alone or the AHA Step II diet plus 6 grams of beta-D-glucans per day for eight weeks. HDL-c levels among the beta-D-glucans group increased by an average of 28% – from 39.4 to 49.5. The beta-D-glucans group also experienced significant decreases in LDL-c and total cholesterol – along with smaller decreases in VLDL-c and triglycerides.

Sterols

Plant sterols, also called phytosterols, are compounds found in most plant foods, including fruits, vegetables, seeds and nuts. There are a variety of different types of sterols, including avenasterol, campesterol and beta sitosterol. These are the lipids that make up the cells membranes of plants. A healthy plant cell membrane made of these phytosterols helps protect the plant's cells from becoming vulnerable to free radicals.

They also help reduce oxidized radicals in human nutrition because they attach and neutralize unstable lipids within the intestines.

Foods notably high in sterols include fresh corn with 952 milligrams per 100 grams; rice bran with 1055 milligrams per 100 grams; and flax seed with 338 milligrams per 100 grams. Nuts also have good sterol content. Cashews have 146 milligrams per 100 grams and peanuts have 206 milligrams per 100 grams.

But wheats are also high in phytosterols. Wheat germ, for example, has been found to contain a lofty 553 milligrams per 100 grams – higher than flax and nuts.

Furthermore, German and French researchers (Nurmi *et al.* 2012) found that wheat's phytosterol content was greatest within the bran. Sitosterol and campestanyl ferulate were the primary sterols found.

These results confirmed an earlier study from Finland (Nystrom *et al.* 2006) that found as much as 17% of wheat and rye phytosterols were steryl ferulate and less than 10% was steryl glycosides.

Researchers from Canada's University of Toronto and St Michael's Hospital (Jenkins *et al.* 2011) found that people who ate diets rich in plant-based foods rich in plant sterols experienced reductions in LDL-cholesterol by 13% after six months. The study, published in the *Journal of the American Medical Association*, found the average reduction in LDL-cholesterol went from 171 mg/dL down 25 mg/dL to 156 mg/dL. That is quite significant for this critical and difficult-to-lower element of our cardiovascular health.

The study followed 345 volunteers who were either instructed to eat a low-saturated fat diet or were given specific dietary advice to eat certain foods known to lower cholesterol during clinic visits. Those who ate the low-saturated fat diet showed a 3% reduction in LDL-cholesterol levels during the same period. Their levels reduced from the average of 171 mg/dL to 168 mg/dL.

This illustrates the significantly increased benefit of increasing whole wheat foods compared to reducing saturated fats – a typical recommendation of many physicians for those patients with high LDL-c levels.

Higher LDL-cholesterol levels have been associated with higher incidence of heart disease, atherosclerosis (hardening of the arteries), strokes and other cardiovascular issues. This is because LDL-cholesterol is less stable, and readily oxidizes. This oxidation produces free radicals that damage the walls of the blood vessels. This causes scaring, which tends to harden the arteries, as well as releases scar tissue into the blood. This release is what causes thrombosis.

The Canadian researchers concluded that:

> *"Use of a dietary portfolio compared with the low-saturated fat dietary advice resulted in greater LDL-C lowering during 6 months of follow-up."*

One sterol from wheat is octacosanol. Octacosanol is primarily contained within the germ of the wheat berry – although for supplements it is often derived from the leaves of some plants such as Eucalyptus. Clinical research (Stüsser *et al.* 1998) has illustrated that long-term supplementation with policosanol – formed from octacosanol – has cardiovascular and cholesterol-lowering benefits.

Another sterol-type element in wheat germ is lecithin. While lecithin is often used to describe several types of phospholipids, lecithin from wheat is phosphatidylcholine. It also often accompanies an enzyme called phosphatidylcholine-sterol O-acyltransferase. This enzyme converts cholesterol to cholesterol esters, which are able to be captured by lipoproteins.

Meanwhile, phosphatidylcholine is known as being beneficial for nerve and brain cells as it donates choline. It has also been shown in clinical research to increase memory (Ladd *et al.* 1993). Other research (Tovey *et al.* 2013) has shown phosphatidylcholine may help protect against ulcers, notably because of its ability to promote healthy mucosal membrane lining.

In fact, there is some indication (Tovey 2009) that the phospholipid and sterol content gained from eating staple whole foods (including whole wheat) may provide one of the explanations for the significantly lower rates of ulcers among second and third world countries.

Aleurone Antioxidants

Few realize that wheat contains significant antioxidant content. This is primarily because most wheat is eaten in the form of refined flour – made after separating the more antioxidant-containing parts of the grain.

Plants typically produce antioxidants to protect themselves from the environment, pests, bacteria and fungi. These same antioxidants also help protect our arteries, our hearts, our livers and other organs from the ravages of free radicals within our foods and our environment.

This is the reason why much of wheat's antioxidants are contained in the outer bran. Because this is where most of the protection against invaders takes place.

In general, the antioxidants in wheat include carotenoids, tocopherols, tocotrienols and polyphenols including flavonoids and lignans, phenolic acids and phytosterols.

We discussed some of the sterols such as sitosterol, campestanyl ferulate, steryl ferulate and steryl glycosides. Other antioxidants in wheats include beta-glucans as also discussed.

Phenolic acids within wheats include ferulic acid – the major phenol – along with valillic acid, coumaric acid, protocatechuic acid, syringic acid, hydrooxybenzoic acid, caffeic acid, gentistic acid and chlorogenic acids.

One of the major effects of phenolic acids is their ability to inhibit lipid peroxidation. Lipid peroxidation is the oxidation of fat molecules – notably those fatty acids that carry cholesterol – such as low density lipoproteins. Low-density lipid-protein combinations can be oxidized more easily. When they do, they become lipid peroxide radicals that can damage our artery walls – producing atherosclerosis, also called hardening of the arteries. Phenolic acids protect fatty acids from being oxidized by neutralizing free radicals.

Experiments specifically testing lipid peroxidation of LDL-c have found that wheat bran provides the most protection – along with those flours that include the wheat bran (Yu 2007).

Ferulic acid and cinnamic acid in particular have also been found to help protect brain cells and other tissues of the body even more than ascorbic acid and tocopherols.

All of these antioxidants mentioned above are significant free radical scavengers and provide other preventive health benefits. They are no slouches. In fact, many of these compounds are the reasons why some medicinal herbs have such therapeutic effects.

Aleurone

Aleurone is a key component of the bran – lying within the pericarp and epicarp covering over the wheat berry. Aleurone is responsible for the release of many of the antioxidants mentioned above. Aleurone-released antioxidants help protect the rest of the wheat berry.

And aleurone itself is considered an antioxidant.

Two of the central enzymes that stimulate the production of antioxidants from aleurone are xylanase and feruloyl esterase. Two others are cytokinin and abscisic acid. As the seed germinates, these convert nutrients for the emerging plant.

But aleurone's co-factors also protect the wheat berry in the form of free radical scavenging. They neutralize free radicals before they can damage cells, just as they neutralize lipid peroxides before they can damage cell walls. This same antioxidant affect carries through to our physiology as we eat wheat foods – assuming we consume the bran and the germ.

Research from France (Rosa *et al.* 2013) found that aleurone's antioxidant productive capacity was maintained through digestion – meaning that its free radical scavenging abilities benefit us when we eat whole grains that include the pericarp and epicarp. This means eating breads made with cracked wheat and other complete whole grain products such as whole wheat flour.

Aleurone is also complicit in storing and then releasing antioxidants such as ferulic acid, zinc and others. A good 50% of miller's bran contains live aleurone cells (Lilloja *et al.* 2013). This means removing and separating the bran in flour making does more than reduce the flour's fiber content – or even nutrient content: It also reduces its antioxidant capacity.

Illustrating the practical capacity of aleurone antioxidants, researchers from Ireland's University of Ulster (Price *et al.* 2014; Price *et al.* 2010) tested 79 healthy older volunteers, half of whom ate aleurone-rich meals each day. The other half of the group – the control group – ate grain meals with no aleurone content.

After the month, the aleurone-consuming group had significantly lower levels of C-reactive protein – a marker for inflammation and particularly for cardiovascular disease. The aleurone-consuming group also had significantly lower levels of LDL-cholesterol and lower homocysteine levels – two other markers for cardiovascular disease.

In terms of antioxidant capacity, milled wheat germ has the highest at 8400 uM TE/100g followed by whole grain flour at 7400, then red dog flour at 4300 and course wheat bran at 3500. Refined white flour contains 1450 (Yu 2007).

Lignans

The bran of the wheat kernel also contains lignans. These are tough molecules called biopolymers and more technically termed phenylpropanoids. Lignans help protect the stability of plant cell walls while in the wheat berry. But within our digestive tracts, lignans are polyphenolic, which means they help protect and defend our own cells from free radical damage. They are also anti-inflammatory and selectively antimicrobial (Korkina 2007).

The lignans in wheat and rye brans include pinoresinol, lariciresinol, secoisolariciresinol, syringaresinol, matairesinol and hydroxymatairesinol. Rye contains higher amounts of syringaresinol while wheat contains higher amounts of hydroxymatairesinol.

Lignans also have a unique ability to weakly attach to estrogen receptors, making them phytoestrogens. Phytoestrogens have been known to help menopausal symptoms because they help buffer the dramatic decrease in estrogen production that occurs during menopause.

Illustrating this, researchers from Sweden's University of Zurich (Richard *et al.* 2014) followed 193 perimenopausal women between 45 and 55 years old. They found that higher levels of urinary lignans – indicating greater consumption of lignans – reduced the incidence of perimenopausal depression by 34%.

Other studies have found that increased consumption of phytoestrogens significantly reduces the incidence of other conditions, including lung cancer. A study from University of Texas (Schabath *et al.* 2005) compared the diets of 1,674 lung cancer cases together with 1,735 healthy matched control volunteers. They found that the higher phytoestrogen consumption reduced the risk of lung cancer.

More specifically, those consuming higher amounts of phytoestrogens in their diets had a 46% reduced incidence of lung cancer. This was added to a 21% reduced risk of lung cancer among those consuming greater amounts of phytosterols.

Whole wheats contain phytoestrogens in the form of lignans as well as phytosterols.

One of the reasons why whole wheat reduces the risk of colorectal cancers may lie in the phytoestrogen lignan content of wheat. Research from Italy's University of Bari (Principi *et al.* 2010) found that supplementing phytoestrogens with insoluble fibers increased estrogen receptor-beta protein levels among 60 colonic adenoma patients. ER-beta protein has been linked with a decreased risk of colon cancer.

Isoflavones

Isoflavones act similarly, but more powerfully than lignans with respect to estrogen and other hormone receptors, and are thus more powerful phytoestrogens. They also help balance hormone levels.

This means that the research mentioned above regarding phytoestrogens doubly applies to wheat because wheat is a source of isoflavones as well as lignans.

More specifically, isoflavones daidzein and genistein are components of other healthy foods as well, including asparagus; many types of beans including soybeans, fava beans, lupins, mung beans and lentils; seeds such as sesame, linseed and flax; and yams, apples, pomegranates and some others. Isoflavone-rich herbs include black cohosh, licorice root, fennel, anise, hops and chaste berry.

A study by researchers from (Liggins *et al.* 2002) found that whole wheat flour, brown flour, pasta and other whole wheat foods contain both daidzein and genistein, up to 279 micrograms per kilogram of daidzein in the case of self-rising brown bread flour and 255 micrograms per kilogram of genistein in the case of bread-making brown flour.

They also found both diadzein and genestein in several other wheat foods including pasta and whole wheat flour.

However, white (bleached and refined) wheat flour had no detectible diadzein or genistein content.

Whole wheat breads contained considerably more of both genistein and daidzein – but this was likely the result of soy flour being added in to the breads – as do many bakers.

In other words, while the levels of genistein and daidzein in wheat are not as high as soy or rice, they are higher than oats and many other gluten-free foods such as tapioca, which has no genistein or daidzein content.

The broad swath of research on isoflavones has found that isoflavone consumption reduces the risk of heart disease, diabetes, several cancers, osteoporosis, menopausal issues and mortality in general. They also appear to increase learning and other cognitive abilities, particularly in women (Wang *et al.* 2013).

An analysis of multiple studies by researchers from Sichuan University's Hainan Medical College (Wei *et al.* 2012) confirmed that isoflavones also effectively increase bone density and reduce bone loss.

The study analyzed multiple published international clinical studies on the application of soy isoflavones to prevent osteoporosis, the central cause of hip fractures and other bone fractures around the world.

In their meta-analysis of the various studies, the researchers found that soy isoflavones increased bone density by 54% while reducing bone loss by 23% as measured by a bone loss marker called deoxypyridinoline. Deoxypyridinoline is typically measured from urine, and is often at higher levels among menopausal women.

The research found that doses above 75 milligrams a day of soy isoflavones had the most effect among the menopausal women.

Osteoporosis is the leading cause of disability among the elderly. Nearly half of women over 60 will have a hip fracture among industrialized nations.

And not coincidentally, foods that contain the active phytoestrogens such as genistein and daidzein are also consumed significantly less among industrialized nations, primarily because of the increased consumption of refined foods.

S-equol and Menopause

Some of these effects come from an isoflavone metabolite called S-equol, which is produced by probiotic bacteria in the presence of isoflavone-containing foods.

Higher circulating levels of S-equol have been linked to decreases in bone loss, reduced prostate cancer and reduced menopausal symptoms, including hot flashes, night sweats and irritability. Some research has also indicated that S-equol reduces the risk of breast cancer and endometrial cancer.

One clinical study (Bicíková *et al.* 2012) tested 28 menopausal women. They were given 80 milligrams of phytoestrogens daily while being tested for S-equol within their urine and bloodstream. Prior to the study, the researchers identified the "S-equol producers" versus "S-equol non-producers."

Among the S-equol producers, their S-equol urine levels went from 0.34 to 10.67 ng/ml after the isoflavone supplementation, while the non-producers' levels went from 0.29 to a scant 0.34.

Meanwhile, Kupperman index ratings decreased substantially, but only for the S-equol producers. In the producers, Kupperman index values went from 23.44 to 14.44, while there was little change among the non-producers.

The Kupperman index measures hot flashes, insomnia, nervousness, melancholia, vertigo, weakness, arthralgia or myalgia (muscle pain), headache, paresthesia (tingling sensations), palpitations (quickening heart beats), and formication (skin sensations). A reduction in the index indicates reduced menopausal symptoms.

Actually, S-equol (4,7-isoflavandiol) – also called 5-hydroxy-equol – is actually produced by intestinal probiotics after they consume the isoflavones daidzein and genistein we eat. Some have proposed that S-equol only comes from daidzein but recent research clearly indicates that certain probiotics will produce S-equol from genistein.

Many other studies have shown lower menopausal symptoms among those consuming isoflavones. In one (Jou *et al.* 2008), 96 menopausal Taiwanese women were given 135 milligrams of isoflavones daily for six months. The isoflavone group reported significantly decreased menopausal symptoms. But again, this effect was only among those who were S-equol producers.

This of course points to the health of our intestinal probiotics.

Revealing this relationship, a study from Italy (Benvenuti *et al.* 2011) with twelve menopausal women found *Lactobacillus sporogenes* supplementation produced a 24% increase in genistein-related equol.

Another study (Tamura *et al.* 2011) indicated that *Lactobacillus rhamnosus* increased daidzein S-equol production.

This research indicates the mechanisms related to isoflavones are a bit more complex than simply eating more grains and beans. We also have to consider the health of our gut's probiotics, as we'll discuss in more detail later.

Arabinoxylans

Arabinoxylans are another component of the bran of wheats. They are long-chain polysaccharides in the format of arabinose.

More specifically, gluten grains – and wheat in particular – contain arabino-xylan-oligosaccharides. These are, quite simply, prebiotics: food components that feed our intestinal probiotics. This has now been established in a number of laboratory and human clinical studies over recent years.

For example, in research led by Dr. Glenn Gibson, Professor of Food Microbial Sciences at the UK's University of Reading (Maki *et al.* 2012) 55 healthy men and women were given different doses of a wheat bran for three weeks. Those eating more wheat bran showed an increase in healthy probiotic bifidobacteria in their intestines and colons.

Another study conducted by some of the same researchers (Walton *et al.* 2012) tested 40 adults and arrived at the same conclusion: The long-chain polysaccharide arabino-xylan-oligosaccharides were found to be prebiotic, feeding and increasing lactobacilli probiotic populations within the gut.

Dr. Gibson's research has also tested a multitude of probiotic species and their response to prebiotic fibers. Dr. Gibson explained:

> *"Currently the main prebiotic targets are bifidobacteria and lactobacilli, however more genera may be soon included, such as roseburia, eubacteria faecalibacteria."*

Other research has confirmed these findings. In a double-blind study (Maki *et al.* 2012) published in the journal *Nutrition* – researchers gave 55 healthy men and women no arabinoxylans, or 2.2 grams or 4.8 grams of arabinoxylan oligosaccharides with their cereal every day for three weeks.

The researchers tested the subjects' levels of bifidobacteria using laboratory analysis of stool samples. This by the way is a standard means of establishing levels of probiotics within the gut – and it allows researchers to track the growth or lack of growth of probiotic colonies.

The researchers measured stool samples throughout the study, and they also measured the subjects' serum ferulic acid concentrations along with other metabolic factors.

They found that bifidobacteria colonization was significantly higher in the subjects who consumed the arabinoxylan-rich cereals. Furthermore, this improvement was found to be dose-dependent, which means the higher dose of 4.8 grams per day produced more bifidobacteria colonies than the 2.2 grams per day dose produced. And both of these produced significantly more probiotics than the no arabinoxylan cereal produced.

A dose-dependent result is the gold standard in clinical research as it establishes not only effect, but direct effect.

How did they produce more probiotics? Because the probiotics had more food to eat, and their colony sizes grew as a result.

The arabinoxylan-rich cereals also produced higher levels of antioxidant ferulic acid within the bloodstream.

The researchers concluded:

> *"These results indicate that arabinoxylan oligosaccharide has prebiotic properties, selectively increasing fecal bifidobacteria, and increases postprandial ferulic acid concentrations in a dose-dependent manner in healthy men and women."*

In a study from Belgium's Catholic University of Leuven (François *et al.* 2012) researchers gave wheat bran extract containing arabinoxylans (or not) to 63 healthy adults. The volunteers were divided into three groups and each group consumed three grams, ten grams or zero grams of the wheat extract for three week periods in succession with two-week washout periods in between.

Before and after each three-week session, the subjects were tested with stool sampling, as well as urine samples for p-cresol content. Higher p-cresol levels indicate greater pathogenic bacteria and fewer probiotic colonies in the gut.

The researchers found that consuming the greater amounts of the arabinoxylan-rich wheat extract significantly increased bifidobacteria counts. The 10 grams per day consumption produced the highest probiotic counts – again creating a dose-dependent result.

In addition, consuming greater amounts of the wheat extract significantly decreased levels of urinary p-cresol, while increasing short chain fatty acids – which have been shown to be linked with colon cancer prevention. The wheat extract also reduced pH, which is connected with greater probiotic fermentation in the gut.

The researchers concluded:

> *"Wheat bran extract is well tolerated at doses up to 10 g/d in healthy adult volunteers. Intake of 10 grams wheat bran extract per day exerts beneficial effects on gut health parameters."*

This effect also occurs in children. A study from the University of Groningen and the Leuven Food Science and Nutrition Research Center (François *et al.* 2013) tested 29 healthy children for three weeks in a placebo-controlled cross-over clinical study.

The researchers fed the children five grams of a similar wheat bran extract or placebo for three weeks. This study found the wheat bran extract increased probiotic bacteria in the gut and also reduced gastrointestinal issues such as flatulence, cramping and abdominal pain among those children consuming the wheat bran extract with arabinoxylans.

The wheat bran extract group also had lower levels of isobutyric acid and isovaleric acid. Like p-cresol, these are pathogenic bacteria byproducts (also called endotoxins) seen in greater amounts in dysbiosis. The researchers concluded:

> *"Wheat bran extract is well tolerated at doses up 5g/day in healthy children. In addition, intake of 5grams per day exerts beneficial effects on gut parameters, in particular increase of faecal bifidobacteria levels relative to total faecal microbiota, and reduction of colonic protein fermentation."*

Other studies have confirmed similar results. A study from the University of Reading (Walton *et al.* 2012) gave 30 healthy adults subjects breads enriched with arabinoxylan oligosaccharides or placebo. The researchers found that levels of both bifidobacteria and lactobacilli (healthy intestinal probiotics) were significantly increased in the subjects given the breads enriched with bran arabinoxylans.

Another university study (Damien *et al.* 2012) of 27 healthy adults utilized wheat bread with or without arabinoxylans from the bran. The subjects given the arabinoxylan had significantly higher levels of bifidobacteria. The researchers wrote:

> *"In conclusion, consumption of breads with in situ-produced arabinoxylan oligosaccharide may favorably modulate intestinal fermentation and overall gastrointestinal properties in healthy humans."*

As for the meaning of *in situ* from this conclusion, this means the arabinoxylan oligosaccharides are being produced naturally by the wheat plant. It is a natural part of the wheat bran.

A study by researchers from the University Hospital Gasthuisberg in Belgium (Cloetens *et al.* 2010) gave wheat fiber rich in arabinoxylans or placebo to 20 healthy adults. The subjects given the arabinoxylan wheat fiber had significantly higher levels of bifidobacteria.

All of these studies utilized double-blind placebo-controlled protocols, all were published in peer-reviewed medical journals – such as the *British Journal of Nutrition* and the journal *Nutrition* – and each study resulted in the same finding:

Consuming wheat products with arabinoxylan oligosaccharides increases probiotic colonies within the gut and decreases gastrointestinal issues.

Other earlier studies (Pyle *et al.* 2005; Stenman *et al.* 2009; Smecuol *et al.* 2013; Grant *et al.* 2001; Farkas 2005; Ostlund 2003; Cara *et al.* 1992; Demidov *et al.* 2008) demonstrated that arabinoxylans are critical for the health of our intestinal probiotics. The more recent research confirmed their clinical efficacy for gastrointestinal problems.

An applicable and fascinating finding of these studies is (drum roll please): *Many of the same probiotic species fed by arabinoxylans actually produce the enzymes that break down gliadin and glutenin proteins.*

This underscores the need for eating whole wheat foods, and at least one of the reasons why eating refined wheat foods can cause gluten issues: Because these important probiotic species are not being fed, there are fewer colonies to produce the enzymes that break down gluten proteins – before they have a chance to be exposed to intestinal cells.

We will discuss the importance of prebiotics and probiotics to the topic of gluten sensitivity later.

Wheat Bran and Cancer

This prebiotic potential of wheat leads to a discussion regarding the fermentation that takes place within our gut. Gut fermentation is what takes place to our foods before they are digested. Fermentation is the process whereby bacteria begin decomposing something because they are ingesting it as their food. In the gut, this process is performed by probiotics in health, and pathogenic bacteria in disease.

In other words, our digestive tracts are basically fermentation chambers.

When whole wheat is eaten by a person with a healthy gut, the wheat will initially be fermented in the small intestines. That's where the magic takes place, including disease prevention and the delivery of other health benefits from whole grains.

We can reference some of these effects specifically from research studying the effects of fermented wheat germ.

Fermented wheat germ – especially using sourdough fermentation methods which use bacteria typically found in healthy guts – has been shown to halt the growth of cancer cells.

Research from Italy's University of Bari and Germany's Martin Luther University (Rizzello *et al.* 2013) screened over 40 fermenting bacteria types and tested wheat germ fermented using traditional sourdough methods against raw wheat germ.

The laboratory researchers then tested these against multiple human cancer cell lines. They found that while the raw wheat germ had no anticancer potential, the fermented wheat germs showed significant inhibition of cancer cell growth.

The researchers commented that:

> *"These results are comparable to those found for other well-known pharmaceutical preparations…"*

There was a variance between the extent of cancer inhibition among the types of cancer tested, which included ovarian cancer, colon cancer and germ cell tumors. The researchers found that the fermented wheat germs inhibited ovarian cancer cells the most between the three, but all three were significantly inhibited by the fermented line.

The research also found that two of the bacteria used in fermentation – bacteria normally found among fermented wheat germ – were especially productive because they produced an enzyme called beta-glucosidase. The two highest beta-glucosidase producing fermentation processes utilized the bacteria species *Lactobacillus plantarum* and *Lactobacillus rossiae.*

Beta-glucosidase is an enzyme that breaks down glucose and other plant matter, releasing their beneficial phytonutrients.

Two of the beneficial phytonutrients released by the fermentation process of wheat germ are methoxybenzoquinone and dimethoxybenzoquinone. These are also referred to by biochemists as quinones. Quinones of different types are used in the body for metabolic purposes. One of the most famous of these is ubiquinone, also known as Coenzyme Q10 – or CoQ10.

But these quinones are also benzoquinones, as they have a benzene ring. This means they can be toxic in some cases, but in the case of fermented wheat germ they are *selectively* toxic against cancer cells.

This was described by the researchers:

> *"Quinones consist of a class of bioactive compounds with promising potential as components for anticancer chemotherapy drugs."*

Fermented wheat germ has been progressively studied for many years. For example, researchers from Florida's Lee Moffitt Cancer Center and Research Institute (Judson *et al.* 2012) also found that fermented wheat germ extract significantly inhibited ovarian cancer cell lines. The researchers tested the fermented wheat germ against no less than 12 ovarian cell lines.

Clinical testing has also been done on fermented wheat germ. A phase II clinical trial of fermented wheat germ was done by researchers from Russia's N.N. Blokhin Cancer Research Center (Demidov *et al.* 2008) in conjunction with the Russian Academy of Medical Sciences.

The researchers gave a fermented wheat germ extract product (Avemar) together with conventional therapy to patients with melanoma – a type of skin cancer. The patients were classified as *"high-risk"* in terms of survival rates.

The patients were given the fermented wheat germ extract for one year, and all the patients were followed for seven years after the treatment. The researchers found that the average survival period was 66 months among those who took the fermented wheat germ extract, while the average survival period was nearly 45 months among the control group – who were given conventional treatment without the wheat germ product.

The researchers also found that the fermented wheat germ patients had significantly less progression of their cancers. They had an average of nearly 56 months of no progression of their cancers, while the conventional treatment group had an average of 30 progression-free months.

Besides the cancer cytotoxic effects of benzoquinones produced by the fermentation process, one of the potential mechanisms of fermented wheat germ relates to its ability to block the cancer cell's energy source – a process called glycolysis (Comin-Anduix *et al.* 2002).

Glycolysis is a critical part of the process of converting glucose and oxygen into energy. To block this process among cancer cells means to smartly cut off their food source.

It should be noted that the bacteria used to ferment wheat germ – especially *Lactobacillus plantarum* – are often normal inhabitants of healthy intestines. *Lactobacillus plantarum* and other species have also been used to ferment various other cultured foods over the centuries.

Fiber

We've been dancing around this topic so far because most of the healthy components of wheat are contained within its fiber content.

This obscures the fact that one of the most important aspects of wheat is its fiber content.

Most of the fiber from wheats comes from the bran layer and the germ of the grain. The bran layer surrounds the endosperm. It is not to be confused with the grain's chaff – the husk that surrounds the grain. It is the outer layer that surrounds the endosperm. See the illustration in the first chapter.

The American Diabetes Association recommends 40 grams of fiber per day to prevent adult-onset diabetes. Others, such as the Mayo Clinic, recommend up to 25 grams per day for women, and up to 38 grams of fiber for men.

Fiber is composed of a number of polysaccharides and oligosaccharides – beta-D-glucans, arabinoxylans, alkylresorcinols, lignans among others – as discussed in this chapter. These are utilized by the wheat plant for stability and protection against the elements, pests and microorganisms.

Plants also use dextrins, inulins, lignans, pectins, chitins and waxy substances to create their root, leaf and stem cell structures. These give plants stability and flexibility – giving the plant the ability to stand tall against the elements yet sway with the wind and weather as needed.

The beauty of this feature of plants is symbolic to how fibers from plant foods assist our bodies. When we consume plant fibers, they stimulate our immunity but also render greater tolerance for toxins.

How so? In our intestines plant fibers will bind to toxins and lower low-density lipoproteins. Then they will escort these unneeded elements out of the intestines. This combined action reduces the burden of toxicity on our livers and reduces the risk of atherosclerosis on our blood vessels.

The health of the colon is a critical part of the health of the entire body. The colon might be compared to the exhaust of an engine. Certainly we cannot utilize all of the food we consume. Those unused parts and toxins within our foods must be escorted out through the colon.

These are combined with numerous waste elements input into the intestines from the liver. This includes bilirubin byproducts – from the breakdown of red blood cells. These waste products from the liver travel with the bile through the gallbladder.

These are added to the various endotoxins produced during the process of fermentation – by both probiotic and pathobiotic microorganisms. All of this has to be escorted out of the intestines, through the colon and out with our bowel movements.

What will escort them out through the colon?

Plant fibers. Plant fibers will bind to most of these waste products and bring them though the colon.

The binding of toxins by plant fiber has a double effect. The toxins are removed from the intestines. But while they are being removed, they are unable to damage the intestinal walls: Because they are bound to the fiber molecules. Their free radical nature – and their ability to damage intestinal cells – is neutralized because they become bound within the fiber molecules.

Healthy elimination of waste products through the colon is critical to the health of the body because if these waste products are not bound and not eliminated – they can become resorbed through the colon wall into the bloodstream.

In other words, without good elimination, waste products will putrefy, possibly finding their way back into the bloodstream.

In healthy intestines, there is a layer of protection to protect the intestinal wall against this mix of acidic endotoxins and waste matter. This will extend into the colon.

But in an unhealthy colon, there is a self-defensive, inflammatory build up of mucous that will occur. This self-defensive layer is referred to as a *mucoid plaque layer*. This layer will build around the inside of the colon, clogging much of the passageway for food and waste to pass. Bacteria and endotoxins will assimilate into the layer, thickening it much as tar might build up.

This mucoid plaque layer will sometimes be so thick and hard a pencil can hardly fit through the colon space. Because pathogenic microorganisms can grow inside the mucoid layer, outside the reach of probiotics, their populations can expand with little hindrance.

There are a number of ailments associated with this build up of mucoid plaque within the intestines and colon. This includes constipation, polyps and colon cancer.

This mucoid plaque layer and resulting constipation is a result of a diet with minimal fiber intake, as the intestinal gap (or *lumen*) becomes constricted.

But these are not the only conditions resulting from this increased mucoid plaque layer. Because the waste products that build up in the mucoid plaque layer can become resorbed into the bloodstream, these endotoxins are involved in numerous inflammatory conditions, as evidenced by significant research linking constipation and inflammation around the body.

Some of these inflammatory conditions include:

- ✓ Sinusitis
- ✓ Allergies

- ✓ Asthma
- ✓ Bronchitis
- ✓ Back pain
- ✓ Liver toxicity
- ✓ Gall bladder problems
- ✓ Skin issues like psoriasis and eczema
- ✓ Chronic fatigue
- ✓ Food sensitivities

Other disorders are worsened by or connected to this build up of mucoid plaque in the colon. Recent clinical evidence has indicated that endotoxin build up – in the form of lipopolysaccharides – can infect joints, causing rheumatoid arthritis (Lorenz *et al.* 2013).

Fiber is either soluble or insoluble. Neither soluble nor insoluble fiber is digested. This is referring to water-soluble or water-insoluble – a laboratory term. Both types of fiber move through our intestinal tract, escorting waste, facilitating digestion, and balancing nutrient absorption. As many know by experience, they also help facilitate our bowel movements.

While soluble fiber becomes gelatinous in the presence of liquids, insoluble fiber passes through our small and large intestines without much change. Soluble fiber will bind with fats in the stomach, slowing down the process of absorption. This delays glucose absorption into the bloodstream, which means that it provides an evenly balanced stream of energy to the cells. Some might call this a *timed release.*

For this reason, soluble fiber is good for regulating blood sugar in those who have blood sugar issues – both hyperglycemic (high) and hypoglycemic (low) problems. Soluble fiber also lowers levels of the "bad" forms of LDL cholesterol by rendering LDL particle size at more optimal levels.

Soluble fiber is plentiful in wheat, barley, flax, vegetables, psyllium husk, and various nuts and beans.

Insoluble fiber facilitates the easier movement of food and waste through our intestines. This means that insoluble fiber helps prevent constipation and helps eliminate toxicity in the colon due to its aiding regular, rhythmic bowel movements. It is like an escort service. Insoluble fiber also helps balance the pH of the intestinal tract.

This of course assists the survival and viability of the important probiotic colonies so important to the immune system.

The general agreement among nutrition experts – as confirmed by the American Diabetes Association recommendation – is that a typical adult should have at least 25-40 grams of total fiber in the diet, with about 75% of that fiber being insoluble. Yes, it is possible to get this amount of fiber without eating gluten-containing grains. But it will be quite difficult.

Wheat contains both types of fiber, but its fiber content is mostly insoluble. Whole wheat breads and flour will contain about 75-80% insoluble fiber, while whole rye can contain more like 55-60% insoluble fiber.

If we have constipation, irritable bowels, or just a lack of regular bowel movements, a lack of insoluble fiber is often the key contributing factor.

The Million Year Old Food

This discussion of real grain foods verses fake grain foods bears another regarding humanity's history of eating grains. One of the basic questions rarely being asked and certainly not being answered well is the history of gluten-containing foods in the human diet.

Recent findings indicate that common varieties of wheat were cultivated in the Holocene period – some 12,000 years ago. This, however, is a limited view – one tracking agriculture from the end of the last ice age.

The look back in agriculture thus tends to focus upon the diet of those Northern European and Northern American survivors of the last ice age. They have assumed grain-based agriculture developed shortly after the ice age receded. Does this mean humans only began to eat wheat at that time?

This is rather short-sighted, because the history of the human race extends a lot further back than 12,000 years. Way further back. Millions of years in fact.

As peer-reviewed archeological science has revealed, humanity arose between two and three million years ago in Africa.

But wait, aren't we descendants of the cavemen?

Actually, no.

The early human species of *Homo heidelbergensis* and the *Homo erectus* species, migrated to Europe from Africa, evidently during a period where the climate was more hospitable than it became during the ice age. *Homo heidelbergensis* evidently evolved into the Neanderthals (*Homo neanderthalis*), the archetype caveman. And unfortunately, or perhaps fortunately, *Homo neanderthalis, Homo heidelbergensis* and *Homo erectus* all went extinct.

In other words, we did not evolve from the cavemen.

The assumption is that previous to this era, the ancestors of the Neolithic humans were primarily nomadic. This is based upon a variety of archeological evidence, finding early tribal man moving from one region to another in periodic fashion.

What does this remind us of? Most certainly, the migration habits of animals. Many animals are also nomadic in the sense that they travel with the seasons to regions with better weather and food to their liking.

For this reason, birds and many other critters will migrate south in the winter and north in the summers (in the northern hemisphere, opposite for southern hemisphere), because their favorite foods are more plentiful in these regions during these seasons. And with this migration will come seasonal mating and birthing habits, which are passed down to the next generation.

Modern humans genetically retain this seasonality to this day, as spring months and summer months bring increased outdoor activities such as gardening, traveling and vacationing.

The evidence shows that early humanoids traveled between the warmer comfortable climates of Africa, Asia and the Mediterranean primarily, and less frequently into Southern Europe during summers when foraging food was plentiful. Excursions into Northern Europe during the winters were more rare, requiring an arduous journey over the Swiss Alps.

This history has been documented by archeologists:

> *"Ethnographically, human forager densities were particularly low in high latitudes, a pattern attributed to low plant and mammal species diversity and high fluctuations in ungulate productivity. Human densities generally were higher in more temperate environments..."* (Morin 2007)

To this effect we can examine the migrating habits of any number of species of migrating animals – such as the antelope. These and other grass-eating creatures migrate to those areas where the grasses are more plentiful, so they can eat what their bodies were designed to eat. Would they migrate into an icy snow-bound northern location without a compelling reason? Be serious.

This is supported by archaeological finds that illustrate the early nomadic *Homo erectus* and *Homo neanderthalensis* went extinct because they were unable to survive harsh winter conditions. Some recent archeological finds have indicated some got locked in a territory struggle. Other digs have found what looks to be a combination of hunger and struggles for territory.

So we know the Neanderthals weren't our ancestors. Let's focus on our real ancestors.

Archaeology has determined that our real ancestors, the *Homo sapiens,* eventually did migrate out of Africa into Southern Europe and Asia – and on to Indonesia, Polynesia and the Americas.

Research also finds the presence of fire among hominids from about 300,000 to 400,000 years ago. This means that humans did not have fire from their ascent at about two million years ago to 400,000 years ago. This means that our ancestors had no fire for over 75% of their existence – at least 1.6 million years.

What did our ancestors eat then? The evidence indicates early humans were nomadic foragers who subsisted primarily on a diet of nuts, fruits, berries, roots, barks, vegetables, seeds and grains.

The evidence also shows that the majority of early humans maintained their ancestral diets and logical migration patterns, just as we see among other migrating animals today.

The clearest evidence the archaeology presents is that our ancestors, the early *Homo sapiens,* did ascend from and eventually migrate from Eastern Africa, where the lush forests provided plentiful fruits, berries, barks, roots and other gathered foods.

But research also finds they also ate grains as the weather warmed and the savannah lands increased.

In fact, ice core readings taken over the past two decades have revealed that there were 10 or 11 ice ages over just the past million years, and the temperatures modern man has dealt with over the past 10,000 years are *colder* than the average temperatures of the past million years.

This means that humanity existed in warmer temperatures more often than in colder temperatures, and even in northern regions there was far less snow and ice during the winters, yielding more vegetation – grasses and sedges – for our ancestors to eat along with fruits, roots and nuts.

With this we can also reference some of the archaeological evidence of the oldest humanoids, living in Africa 2-3 million years ago. These are the earliest humanoids, and they contended with no ice or snow in their first two million years of existence.

The archaeological evidence indicates that humans first arose from the taxonomy of the Family of Hominidae – which included orangutans (Pongo), gorillas (Gorilla) chimpanzees (Pan) – eventually evolving to modern humans – *Homo sapiens sapiens.*

And the direct ancestors of *Homo sapiens* evolved from their last common ancestors, the australopithecines, about four to five million years ago in eastern Africa.

Eventually one of these australopithecine species evolved to become *Homo habilis* and *Homo ergaster.* Then eventually to *Homo cepranensis, Homo erectus, Homo heidelbergensis* and *Homo neanderthalensis* (the theoretical "caveman") and other species. But it was only the *Homo cepranensis* branch that eventually evolved to become *Homo sapiens sapiens. Homo heidelbergensis* and *Homo neanderthalensis* went extinct as mentioned.

This means in order to understand our ancestral diet we need to look back at the earliest humanoid ancestors – our real ancestors – the australopithecines.

The australopithecines – which include *Australopithecus afarensis, A. africanus, A. bahrelghazali, Paranthropus robustus, Ardipithecus ramidus* and others – are our true ancestors. They stood up and walked on two feet (bipedalism) and had larger brains than their ape predecessors. They marked the distinction between the human race and its animal origins (Ruff 2010).

Recent research has discovered clear archaeological evidence of the diet of these ancestors. The technologies developed over the past decade by archaeological experts have included advanced scientific instrumentation and analysis, revealing our early diets.

By analyzing fossil teeth enamel, modern researchers have determined the primary diet of our earliest ancestors. The data has been unlocked from their teeth enamel. Basically, the teeth enamel retain carbon isotopes that identify the composition of what they were putting in their mouths to chew, digest and assimilate.

Much of these enamel carbon isotope techniques were originally developed by Dr. Thure Cerling, a professor of Geology and Geophysics at the University of Utah. Dr. Cerling developed a process that analyzes a process in nature called carbon photosynthesis – where plants essentially convert carbon dioxide plus water to glucose and oxygen with some leftover water.

The teeth data are determined by comparing the two stable carbon isotopes – carbon-12 and carbon-13. This is because most carbon is carbon-12 (six protons and six electrons), and many plants – especially those of grasses and sedges – fix carbon-13 more heavily.

Thus by analyzing the ratio of carbon-12 to carbon-13, scientists have been able to determine the nature of the diet of the australopithecines.

One type of carbon conversion is crassulacean acid metabolism. This is a carbon fixation process found among certain plants as they adapt to a lack of water and an increasingly arid environment – analyzed by measuring carbon 13 (C-13) levels. In other words, greater C-13 levels indicate the adaptation of an arid climate by these plant species.

The research of Dr. Cerling and his many colleagues has generally found three types of carbon photosynthesis – picked up by carbon isotope analysis from the teeth enamel of our earliest ancestors. Two in particular relate to early grain diets.

These isotopes reveal our earliest ancestors were eating a diet that included the warm-season grasses among the savannas. These take part in C4 photosynthesis, utilizing both C-12 and C-13 carbons. The gluten-containing grasses like wheat, rye and barley utilize C-12 over C-13 photosynthesis, but also use both. The later type is referred to as C3 photosynthesis.

Carbon analyses of our ancestors' teeth enamel have found that our earliest humanoid ancestors, the australopithecines, ate primarily a plant-based diet taken from bushes, trees and grains – from both C3 and C4 plants. Carbon-wise, the ratios of their diets ranged from 75% C4 with 25% C3; to 65% C4 with 35% C3 plant foods. (Cerling *et al.* 2013).

This research indicates that gliadin proteins – which come from the C3 photosynthesis – were part of humanity's earliest diet, millions of years ago.

The researchers have also been able to verify these early diets though a combination of their surroundings, teeth shape and other identifying features of their habitats, including the soils, which have a carbon footprint of their own.

But just to be sure, the data from these early teeth fossils is typically confirmed by analysis of teeth abrasion patterns, along with soil analysis around the digs to confirm the composition of their surrounding food availability. The analyses of abrasion is called dental "microwear."

Research by Dr. Cerling and his associates have concluded that the diet of australopithecines such as *Paranthropus boisei* was dominated by a diet in grasses and sedges.

As for the bulk of early man's diet, the researchers also stated:

> *"the evidence indicates that the remarkable craniodental morphology of this taxon represents an adaptation for processing large quantities of low-quality vegetation rather than hard objects."*

What is *"low-quality vegetation?" "Low quality"* relates to foods from the primary plant. This includes the raw grains and stems of the plant.

While this doesn't necessarily mean early man was out grazing – and certainly our digestive tracts can ferment greens so such a diet would be nutritious – the finding of ancient tools reveals additional technology for grinding plants. The early stone tools of *Homo habilis* around three million years ago reveals plant grinding and chopping tools – which were inherited by *Homo erectus* a million years later, and carried to such distant places as Java.

This and other research finds that these and other early ancestors such as *Australopithecus afarensis* and *A. anamensis* and related species primarily consumed diets consisting of fruit, roots, leaves, grains and nuts of different varieties. (Ungar *et al.* 2008; Peters and Vogel 2005; Grine *et al.* 2006; Ungar *et al.* 2010; Ungar *et al.* 2011)

And more recent fossil discoveries have indicated that the australopithecines species were met with a warming trend that forced some to migrate from forests to savannah grasslands. This was determined by identifying Crassulacean acid metabolism among the plant-based carbon isotopes within their teeth enamel.

In other words, the research indicates that our ancestors began to increasingly consume diets of grasses and sedges nearly 2 million years ago.

Grasses and sedges? What are grasses and sedges? Grains. We're talking about early grains here, along with the nutritious stalks of such grains.

This is consistent with other determinations that have found the consumption of seeds to be prevalent among early hominids (Jolly 1970).

As the australopithecines developed into *Homo sapiens* humans, their intelligence increased, and they figured out how to utilize the seeds of those sedges and grasses to cultivate more. They also learned new ways to grind and consume those grain seeds as food.

Yes, a few *Homo sapiens* migrated north and got themselves trapped in deserts or icy regions may have been forced to scavenge animals for survival. When the snow covered the ground for several months, those not smart enough to migrate south for the winter were forced to hunt for food. Or die.

Which many did.

But the vast majority of our ancestor *Homo sapiens* in the Paleolithic era settled throughout Africa, Asia, Indonesia, the Mediterranean and other more hospitable environments where they continued to eat grains along with other plant-based foods.

We cannot ignore the fact that those early societies rising from the late Paleolithic era among the world's more hospitable climes were also the most advanced human societies of those periods.

We evidence the early societies of the Indus Valley, China, Northern Africa, the Middle East, North and South America and Polynesia: These were known for their incredible leisure time, as they became adept at survival using well-organized plant-based food gathering and cultivation strategies. Whole some also foraged for animal and sea foods when survival necessitated, their fundamental diets included nuts, grains, fruits, vegetables, roots, seeds, kelps and a variety of fermented foods derived from dairy and grains. And it is from this core diet we find the most intelligent culinary invention – baked breads and later fermented breads – began to flourish.

And yes, humans are industrious and creative. Certainly those of our ancestors who landed on hard times in the wintertime in colder regions of Europe and North America, or in the desert, eventually had to figure out how to eat without plant-based foods.

But this period didn't last long. Soon we figured out how to store grains in cold-weather climates, retrieving them in the dark of winter from bushel storage. And it wasn't long before Northern humans resumed eating grains without having to migrate to warmer climates.

Is this Northern grain different from the C3 grains eaten by the australopithecines? Surely grains have evolved just as man has evolved over the millions of years. But the gliadin protein – this is an ancient protein that traveled the span of time.

Even evidence from the 'Old World' Europe – dating back to 5,000-10,000 years ago, indicates a human population that was primarily agricultural-based, with grains as a primary element of the diet (Flandrin 1999). Did this penchant for eating grains happen all of a sudden? Certainly not. Humans had been eating wild grains for millions of years.

Wheat is actually one of the oldest cultivated foods – currently thought to have been domesticated about 10,000 years ago as a hybrid of *Aegilops squarrosa* and early wheat from the Poaceae family.

One of the earliest domesticated wheats is Einkorn, or *Triticum monococcum*. This variety grows in the wild as well as among farms. This plant will also grow amongst salt-ridden, poorly-nourished soils.

Among the more populated and more ancient regions of the Middle East, Asia Minor and Africa, grain consumption played an even greater role in the diet.

Even among ancient Biblical times and among desert regions where there was seemingly little vegetation, clear passages indicate that grains were an important part of the diet, as indicated by this statement by Isaac to Esau:

> *"May God give you heaven's dew and earth's richness – an abundance of grain..." (Genesis 27:28)*

The grain-based diet was pervasive among the Etruscans who were the ancestors of the Romans and the Greeks, and prior to these civilizations, the Bronze Age populaces of the Anatolians and Aegeans, the Minoans, the Mycenaeans, the ancient Egyptians, the Punts of ancient Somalia, the Norte Carals, Olmecs and Zapotecs of the South Americas, the North American Indians, and two of the oldest advanced societies, the ancient Chinese and Indus Valley civilizations of ancient Asia along with the Kush and Nok civilizations of the Afrikaans, along with other tribal civilizations around the world.

Each of these ancient societies treasured grains as part of their essential diet. Whether they hunted or not, they included grains that contained gluten. Why? Because these grains made them strong. And healthy.

And intelligent. The ancient Asian and Indus Valley civilizations, which included the civilization of the Aryans, were the first civilizations to have organized math and science, advanced architecture, an advanced alphabet with lengthy writings, advanced medicines with Materia Medica and other advancements that eventually spread to other cultures via trade and cultural exchange. Other ancient societies that created languages and complex science were also grain eaters.

All this was possible because gluten-containing grains nourished our ancestors, rendering the most intelligent species to inhabit our planet.

And gluten-containing foods have the potential to keep feeding our planet when other means may fall short. We mentioned earlier the University of Minnesota Institute on the Environment (Foley 2014) research. They found that if humans continue our shift from traditional plant-based foods such as wheat, by 2050 we will have to double the food we grow just to feed the animals we are eating.

In other words, wheat is one of the most efficient forms of protein we can grow. In cost per pound of protein at 1989 prices, the cost to produce a pound of protein from wheat was $1.50 while the cost of a pound of protein from beefsteak was $15.40 – a good ten times the cost. These costs have skyrocketed just as the price of meat has over the past 25 years.

And this does not include costs related to the increased environmental costs of water and water purification and so on. A pound of wheat requires about 25 gallons of water, while a pound of meat requires about 2,500 gallons (EarthSave 1989).

Food scarcity is real and it will become a greater problem over the next decades. Will we survive? Today, millions of people around the world are hungry, and many of these are being fed by food brought in by charity organizations from the U.S. and other regions. How are so many people preventing starvation? By eating wheat. Because wheat contains significant protein and nutrient content, as we've laid out in this chapter.

Conclusion: Gluten/Toxin Thesis

To make an informed decision regarding the thesis proposed in the previous chapter, the evidence provided in both of these last two chapters should be reviewed objectively. Yet even this information will be lacking without considering the evidence to be offered through the next two chapters, which prove the underlying causes for gluten sensitivity and intolerance.

The evidence presented so far illustrates that without a varied diet of fibrous whole foods, including grains produced by Mother Nature, we will be robbing the body of some of nature's best resources for health. While seeds are intended for the procreation of plants, the wheat seed also provides essential nutrients that benefit every cell, organ and metabolism within our bodies.

These include an array of vitamins, minerals, essential oils, and complex phytocompounds – some of which are only available in grains.

The thesis that gluten or wheat is a toxin certainly comes with circumstantial evidence. And those who have arrived at this conclusion scientifically are no slouches. And certainly some of the evidence is solid. Undigested gluten proteins can damage the intestinal walls of those who are either genetically or immunologically susceptible.

However, we will provide clear evidence as we proceed that this susceptibility is not irreversible. We will also illustrate that such susceptibilities are abnormal. In other words, a healthy gut should have no susceptibility to gluten.

This includes celiac disease and wheat allergies along with gluten intolerances.

And this also happens to be supported by thousands of years of traditional diets that included wheat – eaten by billions of people around the world.

The gluten-toxin postulation also opposes decades of scientific research showing precisely the opposite: Whole grain plant foods contain important nutrients, fibers and phyto-chemicals that extend our lives and prevent metabolic diseases and oncological diseases (cancers).

Unfortunately, those who have bought into the gluten-toxin postulation end up turning their diets upside down as they seek alternatives to healthy whole grains. They also find themselves on the wrong side of the fiber equation, because many grains that supply important soluble and insoluble fibers also happen to contain gluten.

Further to the thesis, wheat contains lectins that can cause inflammation, and phytic acid from grains can block mineral absorption. The theory also proposes that wheat germ – a healthy food rich source of B-vitamins and other nutrients – is a cause for "leaky gut syndrome" because it contains wheat germ agglutinin (WGA).

But the evidence for these postulations – like the theory that gluten is a toxin – is weak, and largely inconclusive. We showed how phytic acid is contained in so many foods such as beans, nuts, rice and many others. We also illustrated that phytic acid is largely neutralized during the cooking and storage processes. And what may be left over is neutralized by healthy intestinal probiotics.

On the lectin issue – WGA – we illustrated that lectins are produced throughout nature and they have many protective and health-giving properties. The assertion that WGA is a toxin holds to the notion that some become allergic to WGA and this produces inflammatory symptoms.

But sensitivities to any food component – any protein – can also produce inflammatory symptoms. Some proteins, such as those in cow's milk, fish, peanuts and others, can produce fatal inflammatory symptoms – known as anaphylaxis.

Meanwhile the research showing whole wheat foods as nutritious and health-giving is solid and substantial. Studies have followed hundreds of thousands of people among the different populations. Diets have been compared and diseases have been calculated.

The evidence is in: Gluten-containing wheat is not a toxin.

Furthermore, this conclusion is sustained by the fact that humanity has been eating gluten-containing grains for not just thousands, but for millions of years.

Now let's uncover the real causes for gluten sensitivities, starting with the physiology of food hypersensitivity.

Chapter Four

Hypersensitivity and Gluten

Before we go much further, a discussion of the mechanisms of gluten sensitivity, and food sensitivity in general is in order. In this chapter the mechanisms will be laid out with respect to how the immune system works, how foods become allergens and how the body marks and remembers allergens.

Intelligent Recognition

In general, the immune system is an intelligent scanning and defense mechanism, combined with an efficient toxin removal process. There are, however, numerous systems in place to achieve these objectives.

The immune system has a number of intelligent abilities. The first is recognition, as mentioned. The immune system has the facility to memorize and then recognize threats previously memorized. The immune system focuses on the distinguishing features that identify a threatening molecule or pathogen.

In the case of a pathogen, the immune system may remember proteins or peptides on the invader's cell membrane, or even the invader's waste products.

The immune system is set up to recognize and later retrieve whether a particular molecule, cell or organism is healthy for the body. This requires a complex biochemical identification system and a process of memorization. It also means the immune system must monitor the health of the body's cells and tissue systems.

We might compare the recognition system to a criminal fingerprint search system. The computer maintains a database of fingerprints, and the program searches for matches by breaking down elements of the fingerprints into a mapping system that classifies their type and position. When enough of these elements are found, the fingerprint is declared a match.

Utilizing a database of information, the immune system also scans and checks molecular structures against its database of threat memory. If the molecular structure matches with the elements of something that threatened the body previously, the immune system begins to mobilize the appropriate mechanisms to block entry to the threat.

But if the threat has already entered the tissues and gained access to cells, the immune system will be forced to launch an inflammatory response to attack the foreigner and those cells the threat has invaded.

When it comes to a food molecule, the immune system scans and remembers distinctive molecular sequences or combinations – these may be polypeptides, individual peptides or a portion of a peptide. These molecular sequences are called *epitopes*.

Epitopes are antigens that are often referred to as allergens because they stimulate an allergic inflammatory response. They stimulate the inflammatory response because their epitopes are recognized by the immune system as threatening.

But this doesn't mean that all epitopes are allergens. Epitopes are often segments of proteins. Remember from our discussion on proteins that in theory the digestive tract should break apart most proteins – and their epitopes – into their fundamental amino acid parts and small combinations of amino acids called peptide chains.

For example, gliadins and glutenins will contain parts of their protein configurations that might – if they are seen as threatening – become identified by the immune system as an allergen or otherwise as a foreigner.

But as we'll discuss later, they don't have to be and typically they are not – as evidenced by the extremely low rate of wheat allergies and celiac disease (in the range of 1%) found in scientific research.

But this ability to be marked as an allergen matches the ability of many other food proteins – those from nuts, dairy, seafoods and other foods. In these cases as well, there are very few cases of allergies against the proteins in those foods, even though a heck of a lot of people are eating them.

Even larger macromolecules – food proteins – that end up passing through the intestinal wall into the bloodstream can still present no danger to the body. Why? Because the liver and other tissues produce free radical scavengers such as superoxide dismutase that can break down these uninvited molecules.

In fact, this is how the body typically handles many types of toxins, including pharmaceutical toxins: The liver churns out enzymes that will break these down – upon which they will quickly escorted out of the body – assuming a healthy liver and metabolism.

When the immune system first records a foreign epitope, it also develops a special receptor for that epitope. This receptor might be compared to a lock, while the allergen epitope is a particular type of key that will only open that lock. These 'locks' are the antibodies or immunoglobulins. The lock-and-key system of immunoglobulins provides a switch for the immune system to recognize an allergen and activate the immune system to remove it.

The immune system is located throughout the body. We find immune cells on the skin, in the blood, in the lungs, in the bones and in every organ system. We also find the immune system within trillions of probiotic bacteria scattered around the body.

As we'll discuss, the body's probiotic bacteria are integral within the immune system. They also help the immune system recognize foreign entities or toxins. This information is invaluable to the rest of the immune system. Probiotic bacteria also have the ability to remember invaders and toxins. They can thus assist the body in the breakdown and ejection of foreign molecules and pathogens, and often do this before the rest of the immune system even has to get involved.

We might compare such a system to a castle from the middle ages. The castle typically has very tall walls and a moat surrounding it. It would most likely have a very large and heavy gate system. These together prevent attacking enemies from easily gaining access to the castle.

But the moat and gate systems would be easy to get through were it not for defending marksmen and spear-chucking warriors who stand guard in the towers and castle walls. These guards prevent enemies from climbing the walls, jumping over the moat, or setting fire to the gate. Without these living guards, the defense systems of the castle would be quite useless to any enemy with some conviction.

This is where the body's intelligent recognition systems come into play. Just as the castle guards are able to recognize who is an invader versus their own citizens as they try to get into the castle, the body employs several layers of intelligence to identify and record for the future those threats to its future survival.

This intelligence of the immune system is incredible in its ability to identify and recognize molecular specificity and diversity. These characteristics allow the immune system to respond to literally millions, if not billions of different antigens. Moreover, each particular antigen and epitope will require a distinct type of response to get rid of it. The immune system also remembers this particular response.

This issue of recognition brings up an important question to discuss in relation to food sensitivities: How does the body distinguish between "good" food molecules and "bad" (or threatening) food molecules?

Remember that the immune system recognition process is based upon memorization. The immune system accesses a variety of databases, including antibodies (immunoglobulins), MHC memory, T-cell, B-cell and probiotic memory systems.

Like branches of a large but centralized database system, these memory systems interact and confirm the threat levels of particular antigens. This confirming process, of course, relies upon a balanced and strong immune system. If the system is overloaded or in emergency mode; its responses may not be balanced. We'll be discussing this in more detail later.

One of the databases the immune system utilizes comes from the body's DNA. DNA sequences code the foods that our ancestors ate, and even those foods our ancestors' bodies didn't like. This DNA coding is quite complex, but is generally an accumulated record of not just our parents, but many generations back.

For example, researchers from the Johns Hopkins Bloomberg School of Public Health (Liu *et al.* 2004) found that nucleotide polymorphisms among genes were associated with specific allergies. They found that a gene variant labeled C-1055T was associated with food or environmental allergies. They found that the variant Gln551Arg was associated with cat allergies. They found that the variant C-590T was associated with dust mite allergies.

The immune system also 'remembers' the foods our mother ate during pregnancy. Here we are sensitized to whatever nutrients managed to get through to our umbilical cord blood – which provided us with nutrition for the first nine months of our physical lives.

The next recognition process takes place through our own food consumption. This also can get complicated, as this relates to our body's initial immunoglobulin response to the food, how well the food was digested, how easily it accessed our bloodstream and many other factors, including even our state of mind when we began eating the food. All of these can cause the immune system to 'mark' a food in a particular way.

Once this identification takes place, the immune system will memorize the body's interaction with the food. If the body's interaction with the food was negative, the immune system may remember the food as being potentially threatening to the body, and launch an immune response to rid the body of the pertinent food molecule(s).

In food sensitivities, molecules identified as foreign or harmful will initially access the body via the mouth and digestive tract, and sometimes the nose, skin and/or eyes through dust or processing exposure.

To keep up with these different vehicles of exposure, there are four general facilities – or strategies – the immune system utilizes to keep foreigners out. Let's dig into each strategy a bit further:

Non-specific Immunity

The first layer of defense against the invasion of foreigners into our body is called non-specific because it provides a barrier that doesn't differentiate between the bad guys This general defense utilizes a network of physical and biochemical barriers that work synergistically to block just about anything potentially threatening from getting into the body.

The barrier structures include the ability of our body to shut down its orifices. We can close our eyes, mouths, noses and ears to prevent foreigners from entering the body. Our skin is also a barrier. Within and around these lie further defenses: Nose hairs, eyelashes, tongue, tonsils, ear hair, pubic hair and hair in general are all designed to help screen out and filter invaders within and around the body's entry areas.

These barriers utilize the body's programmed autonomic systems, which automatically respond to even the slightest indication that there may be a threat to the body. For example, if there is a little smoke in the room, the eyes will become more watery to protect the eyes from the smoke.

Nearly every one of the body's passageways is also equipped with tiny cilia, which block but also assist the body in evacuating invaders by brushing them out. These cilia move rhythmically, sweeping back and forth, working caught pathogens outward with their undulations.

The surfaces of most of the body's orifices are also covered with mucous membranes. These thin liquid membrane films contain a combination of biochemicals (also called *mucin*) and cells that prevent invaders from penetrating any further. These special biochemicals include mucoproteins, glycoproteins, glycosaminoglycans, glycolipids, and various enzymes. These are designed to stick to, alter and break down large molecules that the body is not used to consuming. These mucus films lining our passageways also contain a combination of immune cells, immunoglobulins and colonies of probiotics.

The digestive tract is equipped with another type of sophisticated defense technology. Should any foreigners get through the lips, teeth, tongue, hairs, mucous membranes and cilia, and sneak down the esophagus and through the sphincter, they must then contend with the digestive fire of the stomach. The gastrin, peptic acid and hydrochloric acid within a healthy stomach keep a pH of around two. This is typically enough acidity to kill or significantly damage or neutralize many toxins and pathogenic bacteria.

Unfortunately, many of us mistakenly weaken this protective stomach acid by taking antacids or acid-blockers. In this case, the stomach's ability to neutralize pathogens will be handicapped.

Another critical part of the body's non-specific immune system – especially as it relates to food sensitivities – is the intestinal barrier. The walls of the intestines are also lined with a special mucosal membrane chock full of the elements described above: immunoglobulins, acids, enzymes, glycoproteins, mucopolysaccharides, probiotics and more.

There is also an intricate barrier system installed between the intestinal cells called the *brush barrier.* The brush barrier screens and filters larger molecules and toxins so that only certain molecules – nutrients the body can use – can gain entry into the intestinal tissues and bloodstream.

This latter type of non-specific defense system relates specifically to gluten foods because these intestinal barriers – when they are healthy – are designed to prevent the intrusion of and undigested proteins such as gluten, as well as lectins such as WGA from affecting our intestinal cells and those tissues and blood lying within the intestinal wall.

As we'll discuss further, if this defense system is corrupted, undigested macromolecules like uncleaved proteins and lectins from various foods have the ability to produce inflammatory responses. Later we'll also dig into the technology of the intestinal cells and their barrier elements.

Humoral Immunity

The second layer of immune defense takes place when foreign entities (toxins, food molecules or pathogens) gain access to these intestinal cells, tissues or bloodstream beyond the intestinal wall.

The word *humoral* originates from *"the body's humours,"* which Hippocrates and other Greek physicians used to describe the body's different physiological regions and tissue mechanisms. Allergies and food sensitivity responses are most often humoral responses.

The humoral immune system involves a highly technical strategic attack that first identifies the invader's weaknesses, followed by a precise and immediate offensive attack to exploit those weaknesses.

The body can draw from more than a billion different types of antibodies, macrophages and other immune cells to execute specific attack plans. As an immune cell scans a particular invader, it may recognize a particular biomolecular or behavioral weakness within the toxin or pathogen. Upon recognizing this weakness, the immune system will devise a unique plan to exploit this weakness. It may launch a variety of possible attacks, using a combination of specialized B-cells (or *B-lymphocytes*) in conjunction with specialized antibodies – the immunoglobulins mentioned earlier.

Cruising through the blood and lymph systems, the humoral system's antibodies and/or B-cells can quickly sense and size up foreigners. Often this will mean the antibody will lock onto or bind to the foreigner to extract and confirm critical molecular information. This process will often draw upon the identity databases held within certain helper B-cells that recognize and memorize molecular vulnerabilities. In other words, the immune system will either devise or draw from a memorized strategy for breaking down and ridding the body of the invader.

As mentioned, the specific vulnerability of the foreigner is typically revealed by its molecular structures or cell membrane structures. Each pathogen will be identified by these unique structures, called antigens. The B-cell then reproduces a specific antibody designed to record and communicate that information to other B-cells through biochemical signaling. This allows for a constant tracking of the location and development of pathogenic antigens – or in the case of food allergies, allergens – allowing B-cells to manage and constantly assess the response.

Meanwhile, the B-cell's antibodies will lock on to the epitope of the antigen. This "locking on" is also called *binding*. When the antibody binds or locks on to a foreign molecule, inflammatory mediators such as histamine, prostaglandins and leukotrienes are released. This stimulates a systemic inflammation response, which is often symptomized as an allergy.

For this reason, antibodies – immunoglobulins – are tested. Those antibodies that have locked on to certain proteins or molecules will remember those. And for this reason, antibodies in the blood that respond to a particular food or protein will be considered active to that food or protein.

But that doesn't mean there is an allergy or other sensitivity. It just means there is a history of the antibody having responded to that protein or food sometime in the past for some reason.

Cell-Mediated Immunity

The third defense process used by the immune system is the cell-mediated immune response. The cell-mediated response occurs when cells are damaged or invaded by foreigners. With respect to gluten sensitivities, this can occur when gluten macromolecules or lectins gain access to intestinal cells and damage those intestinal cells.

Cell-mediated immunity can also be provoked should food macromolecules gain access to the bloodstream and damage tissue and blood cells.

Our cell-mediated immune system incorporates a collection of smart white blood cells called T-cells. T-cells and their surrogates wander the body scanning the body's own cells. They are seeking cells that have become infected or otherwise have been damaged by foreigners. Infected cells are typically identified by special marker molecules (also called antigens) that typically sit atop infected cell membranes. These cell antigens have particular molecular arrangements that signal to the roving T-cells that damage has occurred within the cell, or the cell is otherwise compromised.

Once a damaged cell has been recognized by the T-cell system, the cell-mediated immune system will launch an inflammatory response against the cell and its tissue system. This response will typically utilize a variety of cytotoxic (cell-killing) cells and helper T-cells. These types of immune cells will often directly kill the damaged cell by inserting toxic chemicals into it. Alternatively, the T-cell might send signals into the damaged cell, switching on a self-destruct mechanism within the cell.

The reader may wonder why this would be important to a food sensitivity. We must remember that T-cells also carefully scan the body's intestinal cells. If the T-cells pick up that cells within the intestinal system have been compromised somehow, they will stimulate an immune response against these intestinal cells. This immune response results in an inflammatory response within the intestines. The type of inflammatory response is directly related to the T-cell helpers, also called Th-cells, as we'll discuss further.

An inflammatory response of T-cells and T-cell helpers can greatly damage the tissues of that region. In other areas, inflammation can cause arthritis, heart disease and a variety of other problems. In the intestines, this T-cell inflammatory response can compromise the barrier function that keeps certain food molecules from gaining access to the blood.

In celiac disease, for example, T-cells are activated through a complex enzymatic process that involves transglutaminase type II (TG2) and T-cells. When this enzyme binds with gliadin proteins, the immune system launches T-cells that will provoke an inflammatory response among the intestinal cells. This inflammatory response among celiac patients will in turn damage the intestinal barrier function – as we'll discuss in a bit.

This TG2/T-cell mechanism among celiac patients is typically referred to as an autoimmune process because gliadin proteins should theoretically not provoke this antibody response in a healthy person. However, as we've seen in some of the research, there are healthy people with no intestinal issues and no issues to gluten that can test positive to TG2. So it isn't bullet-proof.

However, the TG2/T-cell mechanism has also been seen during Crohn's disease flare-ups and irritable bowel syndrome, polyps and a variety of other conditions. As we'll discuss in greater detail, damage to the intestinal barrier function allows food macromolecules such as gliadins and glutenins into the intestinal tissues and bloodstream. When that happens, the T-cell immune system may launch an inflammatory response.

Probiotic Immunity

The fourth and most powerful part of the immune system takes place among the body's colonies of probiotics. The human body can house more than 32 billion beneficial and harmful bacteria and fungi at any particular time. When beneficial bacteria are in the majority, they constitute up to 70-80% of the body's immune response, as mentioned earlier. This takes place both in an isolated manner and in conjunction with the rest of the body's immunity and digestive systems.

About one hundred trillion bacteria live in the body's digestive system – about 3.5 pounds worth. The digestive tract contains about 400-500 different bacteria species. About twenty species make up about 75% of the population, however. Many of these are our resident strains, which attach to our intestinal walls. Many others are transient. These transient strains will typically stay for no more than about two weeks.

The majority of our probiotics live in the colon, although billions also live in the mouth and small intestines. Other populations of bacteria and yeast can also live within joints, under the armpits, under the toenails, in the vagina; between the toes; and among the body's various other nooks and body cavities.

First, probiotics are critical to the body's recognition of foreign molecules. Remember the DNA memory system mentioned earlier? Well, probiotics also contain DNA, and their memory systems also catalog the various foods we eat. They also have a stored history of the foods our ancestors consumed and worked around.

This is significant as we discuss the relationship between grains and human metabolism. As we illustrated in the previous chapter, wheat grains contain prebiotics that actually feed our probiotic species. This means that our probiotics have been recognizing these foods for thousands – even millions – of years.

If a particular food is recognized by a probiotic as being typical of its historical food or working environment, there is no problem. But if the molecules are foreign, the probiotic system can signal the immune system to launch a response, as well as launch its own response to get rid of the foreigner.

In other words, probiotic colonies work alongside as well as cooperatively with the body's immune system to organize strategies to prevent toxins and pathogenic microorganisms from harming the body.

Probiotics communicate and cooperate with the immune system through complex signaling systems. Probiotics utilize complex cytokine and immunoglobulin communication processes. They will stimulate T-cells, B-cells, macrophages and NK-cells with smart messages that promote and coordinate specific immune responses. They can also activate phagocytic cells directly to mobilize an intelligent toxin-removal response.

Using this communication, probiotics can activate cell-mediated responses and humoral responses. Probiotics also organize and police the body's mucosal barrier mechanisms.

Probiotics can also quickly identify harmful bacteria or fungal overgrowths and work directly to eradicate them. This process may not directly involve the rest of the immune system. In an infection, the immune system may act in a supportive manner, by breaking up and escorting dead pathogens out of the body.

Probiotics produce chemical substances that break down some food molecules into digestible form. They also release biochemicals and nutrients that are healthy for the body.

Lactic acid produced by *Lactobacillus* and *Bifidobacteria* species sets up the ultimate pH control in the gut to repel antagonistic organisms and aid the breakdown of food.

The environment that probiotics contribute to within the mucosal membrane include a number of complex acids. These include a hydrogen peroxide complex called *lactoperoxidase*. They also include acetic acids, formic acids lipopolysaccharides, peptidoglycans, superantigens and heat shock proteins. These inhibit challengers to ultimately benefit the intestinal environment.

Probiotics also secrete a number of key nutrients crucial to their hosts' (our body) immune system and metabolism, including B vitamins pantothenic acid, pyridoxine, niacin, folic acid, cobalamin and biotin, and crucial antioxidants such as vitamin K. Research is increasingly finding that these critical nutrients are often lacking in modern society. The reason, of course, is the destruction of these important probiotic species within our intestines.

Probiotics also help the break down (or police the break down) of food molecules into useable nutrients. This is the case for the lactose in milk. Probiotics produce lactase, an enzyme that breaks down lactose into smaller, digestible sugars. The lack of this enzyme (and those probiotics) is the primary reason many people become lactose intolerant.

Probiotics also produce antimicrobial molecules called *bacteriocins*. *Lactobacillus plantarum* produces lactolin. *Lactobacillus bulgaricus* secretes bulgarican. *Lactobacillus acidophilus* can produce acidophilin, acidolin, bacterlocin and lactocidin. These and other antimicrobial substances equip probiotic species with territorial mechanisms to combat and reduce pathologies related to *Shigella, Coliform, Pseudomonas, Klebsiella, Staphylococcus, Clostridium, Escherichia* and other infective genera.

Furthermore, antifungal biochemicals from the likes of *L. acidophilus, B. bifidum, E. faecium* and others also significantly reduce yeast outbreaks caused by the overgrowths of *Candida albicans* (Shahani *et al.* 2005).

Furthermore, probiotics will specifically stimulate the body's own immune system to attack pathogens. Probiotics will simulate T-cells by initiating cytokines and other intelligent components.

The research confirming the role that probiotics play with the immune system is impeccable, consistent and undeniable. We will cover some of this research in this text, but for a more complete review of the research and practical application of probiotics, see the author's book, *Probiotics: Protection Against Infection*.

In the case of gluten and WGA sensitivities, probiotics exert three types of defense: The first is that they line the mucosal membrane of the intestines, helping to provide a barrier. Second, probiotics secrete enzymes that break down these macromolecules before they can be exposed to the intestinal cells. And third, our intestinal probiotics provide anti-inflammatory chemicals and signals that communicate with the body's immune system – providing a fail-safe mechanism.

But this protection factor provided by our probiotics – including their ability to break down gluten proteins discussed earlier – is completely lost by those things that kill our colonies of probiotics. These include antibiotics, alcohol, pharmaceuticals and a variety of *junk foods* among others.

Let's discuss the specific players among the body's immune system, and their interaction with food sensitivities.

The Immune Cells

Remember when we discussed the lack of mechanism encountered by researchers as they investigated non-celiac gluten sensitivities? Part of those mechanisms not found were the lack of immune cell flare-ups among those reporting gluten sensitivities. When an inflammatory event takes place, it can be traced to immune cells that have organized to combat or remove the foreigner. But if there is no organization to take out the foreigner, how could we profess there is a foreigner?

The immune system is composed of a number of different cells, and most are referred to as white blood cells or leukocytes. There are at least five different types of white blood cells. Each is designed to identify and target specific types of antigens (or allergens).

Once an antigen/allergen is identified, these immune cells will initiate an attack specific to the condition of the body and the weakness of the antigen. Generally, the weaker the condition of the body's immunity, the more systemic the response. The stronger the body's immune system is relative to the threat of the antigen, the more efficient (and less systemic) the response will be. This is the reason why a high white blood cell count in a blood test will indicate that the body is fighting a big infection or toxin relative to its strength.

We might compare this to getting bit badly by red ants as we walk by an ant hill. The only reason the ants began to bite is because they felt threatened. The size of the foot was very large relative to the proximity of the ant hill. If we were walking by a few of the same ants further away from the ant hill, we probably would not get bit. They didn't feel that we threatened their ant colony and queen from that distance.

In the same way, the immune system kicks into high gear when it is most vulnerable. In the face of a less-threatening food molecule, a strong immune system would not need to launch a full scale attack. It could easily take care of the invasion by less drastic means, and with fewer white blood cells. If the attack was a lethal virus, on the other hand, then even the strong immune system will kick into high gear and launch a systemic immune response.

The main types of white blood cells are lymphocytes, neutrophils, basophils, monocytes and macrophages. Each WBC plays an important role in the antigen/allergen-identification and inflammatory process. WBCs are the body's immune response soldiers. They tackle invaders head on. Here are the specific types of immune cells along with some examples of how they organize in response to food allergens:

Monocytes

Monocytes are like the Neolithic ancestors of the attack soldiers. After being produced in the marrow, monocytes differentiate into either macrophages or dendrite cells. The macrophages are particularly good at engulfing and breaking apart pathogens. Dendritic cells are interactive cells that stimulate certain responses. They may, for example, isolate and present antigens to B-cells or T-cells. Dendritic cells also stimulate the production of those special communication proteins called cytokines.

Lymphocytes (T-cells and B-cells)

Lymphocytes are identification cells that code and target specific invaders. The primary lymphocytes are the T-cells (thymus cells) or B-cells (bone marrow cells). These cells and their specialized communication proteins work together to strategically attack and remove invaders. Then special memory helper cells memorize the strategy in preparation for a future invasion.

All white blood cells are initially produced by stem cells within the bone marrow. Following their release, T-cells undergo further differentiation and programming within the thymus gland. B-cells undergo a similar process of maturity before release from the spleen. Both T-cells and B-cells circulate via lymph, bloodstream and intercellular tissue fluids. Both T-cells and B-cells have a number of special types, including memory cells and helper cells to identify and memorize invaders.

As mentioned earlier, B-cells look for foreign or potentially harmful antigens moving freely. These might include allergens, toxins or microbes. Once identified, B-cells will stimulate the production of a particular type of antibody, designed to bind to and neutralize the foreigner.

Most B-cells are monoclonal, which means they will adjust to a specific type of invader. Once they set up for a particular type of invader, they can make "clones" or copies that will launch an attack and bind to the foreigners.

Most B-cells are investigative and surveillance oriented. Once activated, they launch a variety of inflammatory responses through the release of mediators such as histamine and leukotrienes. This process allows them to interrupt antigen penetration. B-cells that circulate and scan the bloodstream are often called plasma B-cells. Others – like memory B-cells – record and communicate previous invasions for future attacks.

B-cells typically work through legions of antibodies called immunoglobulins. We'll discuss immunoglobulins further in a bit. B-cells may also attach to or bind directly to antigens. In this case, their immunoglobulins are attached to their cell membrane. Once this binding takes place, the inflammatory mediators are released.

T-cells, on the other hand, are oriented toward the body's own cells, and those foreigners who get mixed up with the cells' metabolism. This means T-cells are focused upon internal cellular and tissue systems. In other words, when antigens are absorbed by or invade cells, the cell becomes damaged. T-cells look for these damaged cells. Once found, the damaged cells will be destroyed or crippled by the T-cells.

There are different types of T-cells. Each is programmed in the thymus to look for a different type of problems that may occur inside cells, such as infection or toxin contamination. This is programmed in the thymus by the major histocompatibility complex, or MHC (see the Thymus section on pages 50-51 for more on MHC programming).

Many T-cells simply respond to a pathogen that has invaded the cell by destroying the cell itself – this is the *killer* T-cell. It does this by inserting deadly (cytotoxic) chemicals into the cell or by submitting instructions into the cell to kill itself. Cell death is called *apoptosis*, and those T-cells capable of killing our cells are called cytotoxic T-cells (*cyto* refers to cells) and natural killer T-cells.

T-cells work through the communication cytokines to relay instructions and information amongst the various T-cells. Prominent cytokine communications thus take place between helper T-cells, natural killer cells and cytotoxic T-cells.

The initial screening of an infected cell by a helper T-cell utilizes an electromagnetic scanning system not unlike the scanning systems airports use to screen passengers before they get on a plane.

The T-cell's scanning system includes delta-gamma T-cells. Delta-gamma T-cells are sensitive to specific receptors on intestinal cell membranes. Thus, delta-gamma T-cells are considered key to the body's tolerance to foods, as food molecules make contact with intestinal cells.

Helper T-cells record and communicate database information on previous invaders. They also communicate previous immune responses, memorize current ones, and pass on strategic information regarding the progress of pending attack plans.

The helper T-cell scan initially surveys the cell's membrane for indications of either microbial infection or some sort of genetic mutation due to a virus or toxin. This antigen scan might reveal invasions of chemical toxins or allergens that may have intruded or deranged the cell. The scanning helper T-cell immediately communicates the information by releasing their tiny coded protein cytokines. These disseminate the information needed to coordinate macrophages, NK-cells and cytotoxic T-cells.

B-cells and T-cells often coordinate their strategies through what is called *T-cell-dependent responses.* In other words, the B-cell is activated through cytokines after a T-cell recognizes the antigen.

Most healthy cells contain tumor necrosis factor or TNF – a self-destruct switch of sorts. When signaled from the outside by a cytotoxic T-cell, TNF will initiate a self-destruct and the cell will die. These "death-switch" communications sometimes also utilize intermediary cytokines.

Under some circumstances, entire groups of cells or tissue systems may become damaged. Macrophages may be signaled to cut off the blood supply to these deranged or infected cells.

The two primary helper T-cell types are the Th1 and the Th2. The Th1 T-cell focuses on the elimination of bacteria, fungi, parasites, viruses, and similar types of invaders. The Th2 cells stimulate more B-cell activity. This focuses the immune response toward antibody and allergic responses. The Th2 cells are thus explicitly involved in the inflammatory responses of allergic reactions. The Th2 response coordinates with the B-cell-antibody system to stimulate allergic symptoms.

This is important to note on a number of levels. Research has revealed that stress, chemical toxins, poor dietary habits and a lack of sleep tend to suppress Th1 immune responses and elevate Th2 levels. With an overabundance of Th2 cells in the system compared to Th1, the body is prone to respond more strongly to allergens and toxins, causing more pronounced reactions like hay fever and food sensitivities. This is also why we sometimes see people who are under physical or emotional stress overreacting with hives, psoriasis and other allergic-type responses.

Probiotics modulate the balance between the Th1 and Th2 response. This was illustrated by Japanese researchers (Odamaki *et al.* 2007). Yogurt with *Bifidobacterium longum* BB536 or plain yogurt was given to 40 patients with allergies to Japanese cedar pollen. After 14 weeks, the peripheral blood mononuclear cell counts of the patients indicated that the probiotics reduced the body's Th2 counts and activity.

Mast Cells, Neutrophils and Basophils

Mast cells, neutrophils and basophils are granulocyte white blood cells that release inflammatory mediators. They circulate within the bloodstream and lymph, looking for abnormal behavior or toxins. Once they identify a problem or are stimulated by B-cells and immunoglobulins, they will initiate a process to clean up the area. This invokes inflammation and allergic symptoms, as they work to remove toxins.

This cleaning process is conducted by their release of inflammatory mediators such as histamines and leukotrienes. The release of these mediators in the case of an allergen is provoked by signals following the binding between immunoglobulins and allergen epitopes. Upon being signaled, the granulocyte releases mediators through its cell membrane.

While histamine is famously released by mast cells, recent research has confirmed that both basophils and neutrophils also release histamine. Neutrophils have been associated with infective microorganisms, while basophils and mast cells have been associated with allergens. Furthermore, neutrophils have been found to release histamine within the lungs in allergic lung responses related to both allergic asthma and food allergies (Xu *et al.* 2006).

The Communicators

When there is a foreign invader, the various immune cells need to communicate strategies to allow them to organize appropriately.

Cytokines are the communication systems that allow different immune cells to signal each other. Probiotics also utilize cytokines to communicate between the immune system's cells.

Cytokines come with complex names like interleukin (IL), transforming growth factor (TGF), leukemia inhibitory factor (LIF), and tumor necrosis factor (TNF).

There are five basic types of cell communication, driven by these cytokines: intracrine, autocrine, endocrine, juxtacrine and paracrine.

Autocrine communication takes place between two different types of cells. This message can be a biochemical exchange or an electromagnetic signal. The other cell in turn may respond automatically by producing a particular biochemical or electromagnetic message. We might compare this to leaving a voicemail on someone's message machine. Once we leave the message, the machine signals that the message has been received and will be delivered. Later the machine will replay the message. The immune system uses this type of autocrine message recording process to activate T-cells. Once the message is relayed, the T-cell will respond specifically with the instructed activity.

Paracrine communication takes place between neighboring cells of the same type, to pass on a message that comes from outside of the tissue system. Tiny protein antennas will sit on cell membranes, allowing one cell to communicate with another. This allows cells within the same tissue system to respond in a coordinated manner.

Juxtacrine communications take place via smart biomolecular structures. We might call these structures relay stations. They absorb messages and pass them on. An example of this is the passing of inflammatory messages via immune cell cytokines.

Intracrine communication takes place within the cell. First, an external message may be communicated into the cell through an antenna sitting on the cell's membrane. Once inside the cell, the message will be communicated around cell's organelles to initiate internal metabolic responses.

Endocrine communication takes place between endocrine glands and individual cells. The endocrine glands include the pineal gland, the pituitary gland, the pancreas, adrenals, thyroid, ovary and testes. These glands produce endocrine biochemicals, which relay messages directly to cells.

Endocrine communications stimulate a variety of metabolic functions within the body. These include growth, temperature, sexual behavior, sleep, glucose utilization, stress response and so many others. One of the functions of the endocrine glands relevant to food sensitivity is the production of inflammatory co-factors such as cortisol, adrenaline and norepinephrine. These coordinate and initiate instructions that help regulate inflammatory processes. Cortisol, for example, shunts or slows the inflammatory cascade, as we'll discuss more later. This is critical to the body's ability to control or balance the allergic immune response.

Cytokines Associated with Food Sensitivities

T-cell cytokines: Allergic T-cell-dependent responses utilize specific cytokines to develop and communicate response strategies. Also their cell membrane CDs are influenced by cytokines.

For example, microbiology researchers from the Academy of Sciences of the Czech Republic (Tuckova *et al.* 2002) found that when the intestinal cells of celiac patients are exposed to gliadin proteins, the cytokines TNF-alpha and IL-10 are produced. These were found to stimulate the activity of T-cells that initiate inflammatory activity.

Other research (Anderson *et al.* 2000) found that among celiac patients, gliadin stimulated a particular type of T-cell – a gliadin-specific CD4 T-cell initiated through a modification of tissue transglutaminase.

Another study (Sapone *et al.* 2009) found that IL-17A was significantly increased among intestinal cells in celiac disease patients but not among non-celiac gluten sensitive subjects.

INSERM research (Hüe *et al.* 2004) found CD8 T-cells were involved in the damage of intestinal cells in celiac disease, which was relayed through IL-15.

National Institutes of Health researchers (Prussin *et al.* 2009) have found that anaphylactic food allergy and eosinophil-related digestive disorders are both linked with Th2 and food-specific IgE responses, even though the two produce different symptoms. When they tested peanut allergy patients with allergic gastroenteritis patients together with control subjects, they found that cytokines such as interleukin-5 (IL-5) for Th2 cells were specific to the allergen.

They both had IL-5 Th2 responses but with different binding. Th1s were similarly active, but dominated by the Th2 response.

Finnish medical researchers (Rautava and Isolauri 2004) found that cow's milk allergy was accompanied by increased levels of the cytokine interleukin-4 (IL-4).

With regard to gliadin interleukin responses, Second University of Naples researchers (Sapone *et al.* 2009) determined that gluten allergies such as celiac disease are related to an interleukin-17 (IL-17) response. They found that IL-17A was expressed among mucosal cells during the inflammatory response.

This identification of interleukin (IL)-17 – found among CD4+ T helper cells, has allowed researchers to understand the celiac disease immune and inflammatory response – which is more complex than the more generalized balance of Th1 to Th2.

University of Helsinki researchers (Westerholm-Ormio *et al.* 2010) found that particular T-regulative cells and toll-like receptors (TLR) increased within the intestines of allergic subjects. These T-reg cells play a key role in the inflammation process with regard to allergies. Foxp3- and TLR4- driven cytokines were greater among food allergy patients. The Foxp3 cells stimulated primarily CD4, CTLA-4, or CD25. The researchers also found that Foxp3 mRNA cell ratios were lower among food allergy and celiac patients. Foxp3 T-cells were increased within the duodenum.

B-cell cytokines: Food allergic responses tend to utilize the CD19+CD5+ related cytokines to stimulate B-cells. Allergen-oriented B-cells tend to stimulate the further allergic response utilizing the IL-10 cytokine (Noh *et al.* 2010).

B-cells regulate immune responses with antigens in late atopic skin reactions. When eight milk allergy patients and thirteen milk-tolerant (no allergy) subjects were challenged with casein and tested for B cell subsets, researchers found that CD19+ B-cells were lower in the milk tolerant group, and apoptotic B-cells were lower in the allergy group. IL-10 producing CD19+CD5+ regulatory B-cells were also lower in the milk allergy group, compared with the no-allergy group.

The Inflammatory Mediators

Our body's immune system launches inflammatory cells and factors to rid toxins, heal injury sites and prevent bleed-outs. This means there is a smoking gun behind the mediator. This is important because many confuse the cause of the condition with the mediator, as though the mediator caused the inflammation. When these inflammatory mediators are increased, it indicates an invasion and subsequent tissue damage from that invasion.

Leukotrienes

Leukotrienes are molecules that identify problems and stimulate the immune system. They pinpoint and isolate areas of the body that require repair. Once they pinpoint the site of repair, one type of leukotriene will initiate inflammation, and others will assist in maintaining the process. Once the repair process proceeds to a point of maturity, another type of leukotriene will begin slowing down the process of inflammation.

This smart signalling process takes place through the biochemical bonding formations of these molecules. Leukotrienes are paracrines and autocrines. They are paracrine in that they initiate messages that travel from one cell to another. They are autocrine in that they initiate messages that encourage an automatic and immediate response – notably among T-cells, engaging them to remove bad cells. They also help transmit messages that initiate the process of repair through the clotting of blood and the patching of damaged tissues.

Leukotrienes are produced from the conversion of essential fatty acids (EFAs) by an enzyme produced by the body called arachidonate-5-lipoxygenase (sometimes called LOX). The central fatty acids involved of this process are arachidonic acid (AA), gamma-linolenic acid (GLA), and eicosapentaenoic acid (EPA). These are obtained from the diet. Lipoxygenase enzymes produce different types of leukotrienes, depending upon the initial fatty acid.

The key considerations with regard to fatty acids and leukotrienes is that the leukotrienes produced by arachidonic acid stimulate inflammation, while the leukotrienes produced by EPA halt inflammation. The leukotrienes produced by GLA, on the other hand, block the conversion process of polyunsaturated fatty acids to arachidonic acid. This means that GLA also reduces the inflammatory (and allergic) response.

Prostaglandins

Prostaglandins are also produced through an enzyme conversion from fatty acids. Like leukotrienes and mast cells, prostaglandins are mediators that transmit inflammatory messages to immune cells. Their messaging is either paracrine or autocrine. Prostaglandins, especially PGE2, are critical parts of the allergic process. They also initiate a number of protective sequences in the body, including the transmission of irritation and pain, and some swelling from inflammation.

Prostaglandins are produced by the oxidation of fatty acids by an enzyme produced in the body called cyclooxygenase – also called prostaglandin-endoperoxide synthase (PTGS) or COX. There are three types of COX, and each converts fatty acids to different types of prostaglandins. The central fatty acid that causes inflammation is arachidonic acid. COX-1 converts AA to the PGE2 type of prostaglandin. COX-2, on the other hand, converts AA into the PGI2 type of prostaglandin.

The central messages that prostaglandins transmit depend upon the type of prostaglandin. Prostaglandin I2 (also PGI2) stimulates the widening of blood vessels and bronchial passages, and pain sensation within the nervous system. In other words, along with stimulating blood clotting, PGI2 signals a range of responses to assist the body's wound healing at the site of injury.

Prostaglandin E2, or PGE2, is altogether different from PGI2. PGE2 stimulates the secretion of mucus within the stomach, intestines, mouth and esophagus. It also decreases the production of gastric acid in the stomach. This combination of increasing mucus and lowering acid production keeps healthy stomach cells from being damaged by our gastric acids and the acidic content of our foods. This is one of the central reasons NSAID pharmaceuticals cause gastrointestinal problems: They interrupt the secretion of this protective mucus in the stomach.

This means that the COX-1 enzyme instigates the process of protecting the stomach, while the COX-2 enzyme instigates the process of inflammation and repair within the body. In the case of allergies, the COX-2 process often lies at the root of allergic wheezing.

Cyclooxygenase also converts ALA/DHA and GLA to prostaglandins. Just as lipoxygenase converts ALA/DHA and GLA to anti-inflammation leukotrienes, the conversion of ALA/DHA and GLA by cyclooxygenase produces prostaglandins that either block the inflammatory process or reverse it.

The arachidonic acid conversion process that produces prostaglandins also produces thromboxanes. Thromboxanes stimulate platelets in the blood to aggregate. They work in concert with platelet-activating factor or PAF. Together, these biomolecules drive the process of clotting the blood and restricting blood flow. This is good during injury healing, but the inflammatory process must also be slowed down as the injury heals. We'll discuss the role of fatty acids in the inflammatory process in more detail later on.

Histamine

Histamine is produced by mast cells, basophils and neutrophils as mentioned earlier. Histamine is a key mediator in the allergic response because it serves to increase the permeability of blood vessels. This in turn allows white blood cells to spread out among the various tissues of the body. As the WBCs spread, they attack any kind of foreign molecule.

As blood vessel permeability increases, the mucous membranes become fuller with fluid. This takes place concurrent with the destruction of antigens by white blood cells, producing phlegm. This also produces the watery eyes, sinus congestion and lung congestion known in allergic responses.

When histamine is released, it will bind with specific receptors located around the body. Depending upon the type of receptor, histamine will elicit a particular response.

For example, the H1 histamine receptor located within the tissues of the lungs, muscles, nerves, sinuses, and other tissues stimulates the allergic responses of congestion, watery eyes, sinusitis, skin rashes and so on. H2 receptors lie in the digestive tract and control the release of stomach acids and intestinal mucous membrane. H3 receptors stimulate the nervous system and the flow of neurotransmitters. H4 receptors involve the directional function of immune cells and intestinal cells in function.

While histamine in general might be considered a "bad guy" in the process of food sensitivity, histamine is critical for maintaining equilibrium around the body. Histamine helps establish homeostasis among cells and tissue systems. Without histamine to communicate balance and imbalance, the body would have little reference to respond to threats. When histamine is released in abundance, this will often stimulate all four receptor systems, putting the body into hyper-vigilance mode. In this mode, the body is responds on a hair-trigger.

The bottom line is that none of these inflammatory mediators are the bad guys. This type of isolation approach is what causes medications that target mediators to have so many side effects. The body is a 'smart' organism, and it operates through a series of checks and balances that intermix with information and communications. Thus, the attempt to try to shut off one process or another (such as histamines with antihistamines) with a single chemical can temporarily halt a few symptoms, but they cannot reverse or heal the basic issue of imbalance. They also come with side effects, because they can further imbalance other parts of the body's natural homeostasis.

The Immunoglobulins

This topic is of particular concern to gluten sensitivities, but it is important to understand that immunoglobulins are not independent entities. They are role-players within the macrocosm of the immune system as a whole.

Immunoglobulins are proteins that attach to the epitopes (peptide sequences typically on the surface) of antigens. They are either released into the blood or lymph by B-cells, or they remain on the surface of B-cells, enabling B-cells to attach to antigens. The immunoglobulins that are secreted and released into the blood and lymph are called antibodies. Those that stay attached to the B-cells are called surface immunoglobulins (sIg) or membrane immunoglobulins (mIg).

Secretory IgA (SIgA) immunoglobulins typically line the mouth, nose, ears, tears and digestive tract. Here they scan for pathogens or toxins that might harm the body. Serum IgAs look for initial tissue entry antigens. Most IgAs are SIgAs, however.

IgDs sense early microbial infections and activate macrophages. IgEs attach to early entry foreign substances (such as food molecules they do not recognize) and stimulate the release of inflammatory mediators – associated with most allergic responses. IgGs cross through membranes, responding to growing and maturing antigens within the body. IgMs are focused on earlier (but not new) intrusions into cells and body fluids that have yet to grow enough to garner the attention of IgGs.

Type	Where located	Targets
IgA	Mucus membranes, intestines, saliva, tears, breast milk (SIg), also blood/lymph (serum IgA)	Prevent initial entry of antigens or early entry into bloodstream; May also indicate a tolerance
IgD	Blood/lymph/B-cells	Detect initial microbial infections
IgE	Blood/lymph/B-cells	Detect early toxins and allergens in blood and tissues
IgM	Blood/lymph/B-cells	Detect infections and toxins that begin to damage cells
IgG	Blood/lymph/placenta	Detect mature infections that have damaged cells and invaded tissues; May also indicate a tolerance

Each of these general immunoglobulin categories contain numerous subtypes geared to different types of pathogens and responses. Other immunoglobulin proteins also exist. Some of these aid macrophages and lymphocytes in identifying specific pathogens.

The science of immunoglobulins is deep and still being uncovered, as we illustrated with the IgG research earlier.

We might try to generalize and say the status of the body's immunoglobulins indicates the immune system's strength and health – but again this depends upon which ones are active. An immune system with a large number of IgAs (SIgAs and serum IgAs) for example, will often be more tolerant of all foods, toxins and pathogens; because antigens will typically be identified and removed before they can access the body's bloodstream and tissue systems.

On the other hand, high IgE counts indicate a hypersensitivity mode for allergens and/or other toxins, and possibly a weaker immune system.

For example, a Swiss allergy study (Bell and Potter 1988) found that following the consumption of milk and whey, children allergic to milk produced more milk-specific IgE antibodies.

Likewise, high IgM and IgG levels indicate a past infection or toxicity that is being increasingly managed or tolerated. And this correlates with the research we discussed earlier: That large studies have indicated that IgGs associated with certain foods occur quite often with those without sensitivities to that food. This and other research in this area – as we've discussed – has indicated that past consumption of that food – and the possibility of being able to tolerate that food – creates the relationship between high IgGs and a particular food.

Higher levels of protein-specific immunoglobulins can also mean different things in different situations. For example, a food protein-specific IgE will typically mean an allergic response to that protein. But a food-protein specific IgG – as the first chapter research indicated – may simply mean the body has been exposed to that protein in the past and the body has become tolerant to it.

A protein-specific IgA may indicate a sensitivity or a tolerance, depending upon the situation. Because IgAs are typically focused towards mucosal contact, food protein-IgAs will often be heightened in a situation where the mucosal membranes are thinner and not as well protective – as we will discuss further.

For this reason, irritable bowel syndrome has been linked with higher IgA's to food proteins. For example, a Singapore study (Lu *et al.* 2014) found among 186 IBS patients that 18% were positive for IgA to gliadin (deamidated gliadin).

Italian researchers (Catassi *et al.* 2013) found while some have proposed IgAs in non-celiac gluten sensitivity patients might trend towards celiac disease, there was no evidence for this. The researchers stated:

> *"So far no specific biomarker of non-celiac gluten sensitivity has been identified. Recently, Volta and colleagues reported on the pattern of CD serology found in 78 untreated patients affected with NCGS. Many patients displayed an elevated prevalence of high titer, "first-generation" IgG AGA [anti-gliadin antibody] directed against native gliadin (56.4%). The prevalence of IgG AGA detected in NCGS, although lower than that found in CD (81.2%), was much higher than other pathologic conditions such as connective tissue disorders (9%) and autoimmune liver diseases (21.5%) as well as in the general population and healthy blood donors (2%–8%). On the other hand, the prevalence of IgA AGA in NCGS patients was very low (7.7%)."*

As we've mentioned earlier, other studies have found that another IgA type of antibody response to tissue transglutaminase exists alongside the IgA sensitivity to deamidated gliadin. We'll discuss this relationship in more detail later.

With regard to IgG, in the first chapter we discussed research illustrating uncertainty that a positive ELISA IgG test to a food necessarily means sensitivity to that food.

Remember that the immune system utilizes immunoglobulins to identify and recognize incoming elements that might endanger the body. If the element is indeed a danger to the body, the immune system is signaled to initiate the process of inflammation, which produces atopic responses, headaches, intestinal difficulty and other symptoms.

This relates of course to how the tissues are exposed, when they were/are exposed and how ago the exposure was.

But – and this is a big *but* – if the foreign element is *not* seen as a danger to the body, the immune system's job is to develop a tolerance to that element. This tolerance may or may not include the mechanism to remove that foreigner without inflammation.

This tolerance requires the immune system to store the molecular *fingerprint* for this element, which utilizes the immunoglobulins. A *tolerant fingerprint* allows the immune system to recognize it upon future exposures without responding – because it is not a danger to the body. Perhaps the body knows how to use or even remove the foreigner without utilizing an inflammatory response. Or perhaps the molecule poses no threat at all.

Furthermore, in the case of a food molecule, there is another element to consider as we ponder the reality that many have positive IgGs to commonly eaten foods they are not sensitive to. That is, food molecules are typically not considered foreign to the body after they are properly broken down to their respective nutrients and amino acids within the digestive tract.

If they are not properly broken down – from proteins into amino acids and small peptides – there is a different situation at hand. The food molecules will be considered foreign because they are macromolecules – they are not properly broken down.

But they still may not pose much of a danger to the body, as the body may be able to utilize liver processes such as superoxide dismutase and other enzymes to break them down within the blood or tissues. This of course depends upon the complexity of the macromolecule and the strength of the liver.

So the immune system may form an IgG antibody to a macromolecule as it develops tools to otherwise break it down or otherwise remove it. This will result in developing a tolerance to a tissue/blood exposure of that protein or proteins in the future.

At the same time, if the immune system is weakened, the intestinal cells are on a hair trigger, and/or the proteins are not properly broken down, gliadin proteins may be marked as threats that require an inflammatory response – regardless of whether the response is necessary. This, as we'll discuss, has been described as an autoimmune mechanism.

When the immune system is weakened, either from a bombardment of various toxins or otherwise, this is called immunosuppression. In such a condition, unhydrolyzed macromolecule proteins may invoke an inflammatory response simply because the body's other detoxification systems – its probiotic systems, immune cells, liver, lymphatic system and digestive tract – are overworked or under-equipped. If these important systems are weakened or overloaded, the body may switch into inflammatory response for something that a healthy body would ordinarily be or become tolerant to.

Somewhere in between this response and a tolerant response lies the intolerant response – resulting in other metabolic changes, which may directly or indirectly cause intestinal difficulties, brain fog, headaches, fatigue and other symptoms attributed to gluten.

The evidence discussed in the first chapter regarding IgG testing illustrated a positive IgG test to gluten may not even correlate with a food sensitivity, but may well simply indicate repeated exposure and a resulting tolerance to that food – or not.

This makes sense, as certainly most people with an intolerance to a food also have a history of eating the food. Otherwise how would they have known they were intolerant?

Even in the case of positive IgG correlation, remember that correlation – relating a symptom to eating of a food – is not the same as causation, as we discussed in the second chapter.

Clusters of differentiation

An important element of immunoglobulins is the CD glycogen-protein complex. CD stands for *cluster of differentiation*. CDs are molecules that sit on top of immune cells to navigate and steer their behavior. They will sit atop T-cells, B-cells, NK-cells, granulocytes and monocytes, identifying threats and infected cells. They will also sometimes negotiate with and bind directly to pathogens. This allows the lymphocytes to proceed to strategically attack the threat.

Clusters of differentiation are identified by their bindable molecular structure: This is also referred to as a ligand. The specific molecular arrangement (or CD number) will also match a specific type of receptor at the membrane of the cell or pathogen. Each CD number maintains a bonding relationship with a certain receptor structure on the cell to allow the accompanying immunoglobulin or lymphocyte to have interactivity with the pathogen. This gives the immunoglobulin or lymphocyte an access point from which to attack the perceived threat, and a coding vehicle to remember the invader later on.

Immunoglobulins and CDs are also tools probiotics utilize to define or influence appropriate responses for the immune system. Probiotics stimulate IgAs through CDs, for example, when they discover a pathogen has invaded the body's mucous membranes.

CDs are also utilized by probiotics to alert the immune system to intestinal cells and tissues that have been damaged by toxins, bacteria, or viruses. Probiotics signal back and forth with the immune system to maintain a check and balance system among the intestines. This signaling process can stimulate particular immune responses as needed.

Different CD types are found among different food sensitivities. For example, University of Helsinki researchers (Savilahti *et al.* 2010) studied T-cell cytokine markers for CD4, CD25, CD127 and FoxP3 after they were stimulated by beta-lactoglobulin among milk allergy children. They also found that constant levels of these related cytokines were higher among milk-allergic children as compared with non-allergic children. These cytokines directly affected the profiles of the Th2 response.

The Thymus

One of the most important players in the immune system is the thymus gland. The thymus gland is located in the center of the chest, behind the sternum. The thymus is one of the more critical organs of the lymphatic system. Some have compared the thymus gland of the lymphatic system to the heart of the bloodstream.

The thymus gland is not a pump, however. The thymus activates T-cells and various hormones that modulate and stimulate the immune and autoimmune processes. The thymus converts lymphocytes called thymocytes into T-cells. These activated T-cells are released into the lymph and bloodstream ready to protect and serve. Within the thymus, the T-cells are infused with CD surface markers – which identify particular types of problematic cells or invading organisms. Their CD markers define the mission of the T-cells.

In other words, the thymus codes the T-cells with receptors that will bind to and damage particular cells or toxins. The types of cells or toxins they bind to or identify are determined by the *major histocompatibility complex,* or MHC determinant. During the process of converting thymocytes to T-cells, their CD receptors are programmed with MHC combinations. This allows them to tolerate particular frailties within the body while attacking what the body considers to be true invaders (Kazansky 2008).

Therefore, it is the MHC that gives the T-cell the ability to identify the difference between the "self" and "non-self" parts of the body. A non-self identification will produce an immunogen – a factor that stimulates an immune response. Once the immunogen is processed, it stimulates the inflammatory cascade.

The thymus gland develops and enlarges from birth. It is most productive and at its largest during puberty. From that point on, depending upon our diet, stress and lifestyle, our thymus gland will shrink over the years. By forty, an immunosuppressed person will often have a tiny thymus gland. In elderly persons, the thymus gland is often barely recognizable. For many people today, the thymus is practically non-functional.

Throughout its productive life, the thymus gland processes T-cells with the appropriate MHC programming. If the thymus gland is functioning, it will continue to produce T-cells with MHC programming that reflects the body's current status. Its constantly updated programming will accommodate the various genetic changes that can happen to different cells around the body as we age and adapt to our changing environment. With a shrunken and non-functioning thymus, however, its ability to re-program T-cells with a new MHC – enabling them to identify the body's cells that have adapted – is damaged. The T-cells will have to keep working from the old MHC programming. This means the T-cells will not be able to properly identify "self" versus "non-self" within the body's cells.

With this progression of thymus weakness and the resulting lack of updated MHC determinants, T-cells begin attacking the body's own tissues instead of becoming tolerant to their new conditions.

The Liver

The liver is the key organ involved in detoxification and the production of a variety of enzymes and biochemicals. The liver produces over a thousand biochemicals the body requires for healthy functioning.

The liver is also a critical component in celiac disease. A study from the Cleveland Clinic (Wakim-Fleming *et al.* 2014) found that a person with liver cirrhosis has twice the risk of celiac disease compared with the general population. This means that celiac disease is somehow linked with liver disease.

Does this mean that one causes the other? Nope. But it does illustrate the importance of a healthy liver with regard to food sensitivities.

The liver has many functions, but an important one relates to blood glucose control. The liver maintains blood sugar balance by monitoring glucose levels and producing glucose metabolites. It manufactures albumin to maintain plasma pressure. It produces cholesterol, urea, inflammatory biochemicals, blood-clotting molecules, and many others.

These functions are major reasons for the liver's involvement in food sensitivities. When the liver is overwhelmed with removing a heavy burden of toxins, its capacity to produce enough enzymes to break down larger macromolecules shrinks. This means that those macromolecules that slip through the intestinal wall – including gluten proteins and other large food proteins like casein – are more likely to provoke antibody and immune cell responses. This then turns a relatively docile invasion of protein into the bloodstream into a major inflammatory event.

The liver sits just below the lungs on the right side under the diaphragm. Partially protected by the ribs, it attaches to the abdominal wall with the falciform ligament. The *ligamentum teres* within the falciform is the remnant of the umbilical cord that once brought us blood from mama's placenta. As the body develops, the liver continues to filter, purify and enrich our blood. Should the liver shut down, the body can die within hours.

Interspersed within the liver are functional fat factories called stellates. These cells store and process lipids, fat-soluble vitamins such as vitamin A, and secrete structural biomolecules like collagen, laminin and glycans. These are used to build some of the body's toughest tissue systems.

Into the liver drains nutrition-rich venous blood through the hepatic portal vein, together with some oxygenated blood through the hepatic artery. A healthy liver will process almost a half-gallon of blood per minute. The blood is commingled within cavities called sinusoids, where blood is staged through stacked sheets of the liver's primary cells – called hepatocytes. Here blood is also met by interspersed immune cells called kupffers.

These kupffer cells attack and break apart bacteria and toxins. Nutrients coming in from the digestive tract are filtered and converted to molecules the body's cells can utilize. The liver also converts old red blood cells to bilirubin to be shipped out of the body. Filtered and purified blood is jettisoned through hepatic veins out the inferior vena cava and back into circulation.

The liver's filtration/purification mechanisms protect our body from various infectious diseases and chemical toxins. After hepatocytes and kuppfer cells break down toxins, the waste is disposed through the gall bladder and kidneys. The gall bladder channels bile from the liver to the intestines. Recycled bile acids combine with bilirubin, phospholipids, calcium and cholesterol to make bile. Bile is concentrated and pumped through the bile duct to the intestines. Here bile acids help digest fats, and broken-down toxins are (hopefully) excreted through our feces. This is assuming that we have healthy intestines containing healthy mucous membranes, barrier mechanisms and probiotic colonies.

The liver's filtration and breakdown process is critical to food sensitivities. If an allergen gets through the intestinal IgA process of removal, the liver gets a crack at removing it. If the liver is not able to metabolize and neutralize the molecule, the body must rely upon the inflammatory immune response to rid the body of the molecule. Often this process is concurrent, but a strong liver will reduce the body's dependence upon the inflammatory processes for removing macromolecules.

If the hepatocytes and kuppfer cells are abundant and resilient, they can remove many toxins. Should those cells be damaged or overwhelmed by too many toxins at once, their ability to break down and remove problematic macromolecules becomes diminished.

Research and a wealth of clinical evidence tells us that the liver is damaged by chemical and food-based toxins. This is the very reason that alcohol (ethanol) causes liver disease: ethanol damages the liver's hepatocytes and kuppfers.

Today our diets, water and air are full of many other chemicals that produce the same result. These include plasticizers, formaldehyde, heavy metals, hydrocarbons, DDT, dioxin, VOCs, asbestos, preservatives, artificial flavors, food dyes, propellants, synthetic fragrances and more. With every additional chemical comes a requirement for the liver to work harder to break down these synthesized chemicals.

Frankly, most modern livers – especially those in urban areas of industrialized countries – are now overloaded and beyond their natural capacity. What happens then? Generally, two things. First, the hepatocytes collapse from toxicity, causing an overactive immune system due to the additional burdens placed upon it. Second, liver exhaustion leads to increased susceptibility to infectious diseases such as viral hepatitis. The combined result is a downward spiraling of hypersensitivity.

Liver disease – where one or more lobes begin to malfunction due to the death or dysfunction of hepatocytes – can result in a life-threatening emergency. Cirrhosis is a common diagnosis for liver disease, often caused by years of drinking alcohol or taking prescription medications combined with other toxin exposure. During this progression towards cirrhosis the sub-functioning liver can also produce symptoms such as jaundice, high cholesterol, gallstones, encephalopathy, kidney disease, clotting problems, heart conditions, hormone imbalances and many others. As cirrhosis proceeds, it results in the massive die-off of liver cells, and the subsequent scarring of remaining tissues, causing the liver to begin to shutdown.

While most of us have heard about the damage alcohol can have on the liver, many do not realize that pharmaceuticals and so many other synthetic chemicals can also be extremely toxic to the liver. The liver must find a way to break down these foreign chemicals. The liver's various purification processes can become overwhelmed by these synthetic molecules. As liver cells weaken and die, their enzymes leak into the bloodstream. Blood tests for two particular enzymes, ALT (alanine transaminase) and AST (aspartate transaminase) reveal this weakening of the liver.

We must therefore closely monitor the quantity and types of chemicals we put into our body. Eliminating preservatives, food dyes and pesticides in our foods can be done easily by eating whole organic foods. We can eliminate exposures to many environmental toxins mentioned above by simply replacing them with natural alternatives.

A number of herbs help strengthen liver function. These include goldenseal, dandelion, milk thistle and others.

Probiotics also play a large role in liver disease. When pathogenic bacteria get out of control in the intestines, they can overload the liver with endotoxins – their waste products. This bombardment of endotoxins onto the liver produces a result similar to alcohol or pharmaceuticals: During the putrefaction of pathogenic bacteria such as *Clostridium* spp., for example, one of the endotoxins is ammonia. Like ethanol, ammonia is toxic to the liver (Shawcross *et al.* 2007). Ammonia from pathogenic bacteria in the gut damages the liver, in other words.

Because probiotics reduce pathogenic bacteria, probiotics prevent these metabolites and endotoxins from affecting the liver. For example, researchers from the G.B. Pant Hospital in New Delhi (Sharma *et al.* 2008) gave 190 cirrhosis patients a combination of probiotics or placebo for one month. The probiotic group experienced a 52% improvement in cirrhosis symptoms and significantly lower blood ammonia levels.

Intestinal Permeability

This topic is of critical importance to any food sensitivity. This is because the intestines not only provide a barrier between the digestive tract and the rest of the body: The intestine is made up of cells that can become damaged.

In order to police the health of the intestinal cells, the immune system must be on guard to prevent if possible, and repair damage should it occur. And believe it, our diets today contain a lot of compounds that can seriously damage our intestinal cells.

The intestines utilize non-specific, humoral, cell-mediated and probiotic immunity to protect intestinal tissues from larger peptides, toxins and invading microorganisms. In a healthy body, these are primarily packaged nicely into the mucosal membrane that lines the intestines – also referred to as the intestinal brush barrier.

The intestinal brush barrier is a complex mucosal layer of mucin, enzymes, probiotics and ionic fluid. It forms a protective surface medium over the intestinal epithelium. It also provides an active nutrient transport mechanism. This mucosal layer is stabilized by the grooves of the intestinal microvilli.

It contains glycoproteins, mucopolysaccharides and other ionic transporters, which attach to amino acids, minerals, vitamins, glucose and fatty acids – carrying them across intestinal membranes. Meanwhile the transport medium requires a delicately pH-balanced mix of ionic chemistry able to facilitate this transport of useable nutrient.

The mucosal layer is also policed by billions of probiotic colonies, which help process incoming food molecules, excrete various nutrients, and control pathogens.

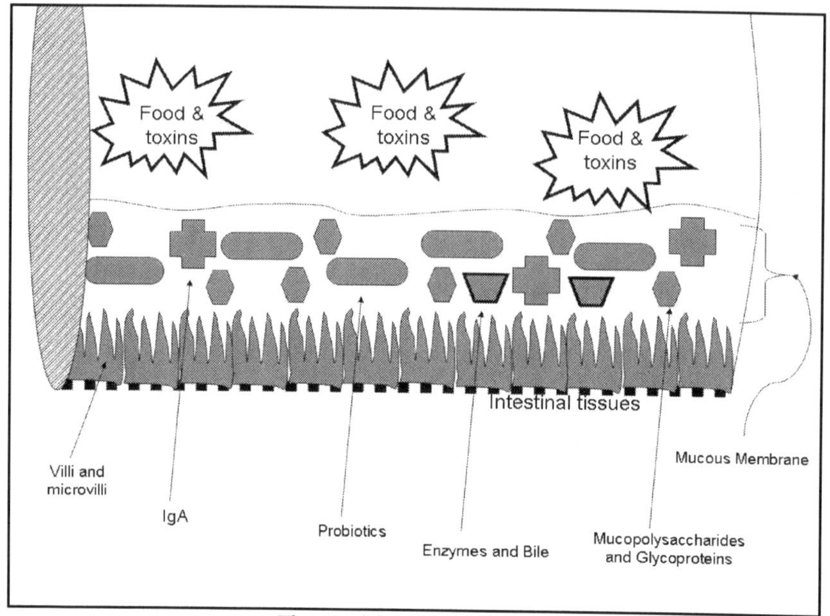

The Healthy Intestinal Wall

The brush barrier is a triple-filter that screens for molecule size, ionic nature and nutrition quality. Much of this is performed via four mechanisms existing between the intestinal microvilli: tight junctions, adherens junctions, desmosomes, and colonies of probiotics.

The tight functions form a bilayer interface between cells, controlling permeability. Desmosomes are points of interface between the tight junctions, and adherens junctions keep the cell membranes adhesive enough to stabilize the junctions. These junction mechanisms together regulate permeability at the intestinal wall.

This mucosal brush barrier creates the boundary between intestinal contents and our bloodstream. Should the mucosal layer chemistry become altered, its protective and ionic transport mechanisms become weakened, allowing toxic or larger molecules to be presented to the microvilli junctions. This contact can irritate the intestinal cells and their microvilli, causing a subsequent inflammatory response. This is now considered associated (appearing concurrently) with many cases of IBS, type 1 diabetes, Crohn's disease, celiac disease, multiple sclerosis and others.

The intestinal wall is not simply one layer of cells. While our drawings show just the inner layer of cells, there are inner layers. These cell layers are not accustomed to interacting with large macromolecules such as food proteins.

The breakdown of the mucosal membrane causes it to thin. This depletes the protection rendered by the mucopolysaccharides and glycoproteins, probiotics, immune IgA cells, enzymes and bile. This thinning allows toxins and macromolecules that would have been screened out by the mucosal membrane to be presented to the intestinal cells.

The tight junctions are also equipped with some organizing factors, which keep them healthy and, well, tight.

These include communication systems that allow the intestinal cells to regulate the permeability – the space – between them. While the precise mechanisms are still largely a mystery, research has indicated that intestinal cells utilize a protein called zonulin to help regulate their permeability.

When intestinal cells become stressed or damaged, they tend to produce increased amounts of this protein called zonulin. Thus zonulin has now been found to be a biomarker for increased intestinal permeability – also referred to as leaky gut syndrome (Fasano 2011; 2013).

Zonulin is apparently involved in an increase of another molecule called haptoglobin. Haptoglobin is made within the intestinal cells – within the endoplasmic reticulum – a site where increased zonulin has been found among damaged intestinal cells.

High zonulin levels and subsequent haptoglobin increases have been linked with increased gaps between intestinal cells.

Can gluten provoke intestinal permeability? In one study (Lammers *et al.* 2008) gliadin proteins were shown to increase zonulin levels among laboratory cells biopsied from intestines. In this study, gliadin proteins attached to CXCR3 receptors in the laboratory analysis. CXCR3 receptors are typically elevated among celiac disease sufferers during gluten consumption.

One issue of this and similar studies is that cells are extracted and tested outside of the real environment of the intestines – where intestinal cells are covered by a layer of mucous membrane, which includes probiotics that should hydrolyze (break down) gliadin proteins before they come into contact with the intestinal cells.

This was illustrated in a study from the University of Bari (De Angelis *et al.* 2006) where the researchers treated wheat flour with a combination of probiotics. First they found the gliadins were practically completely hydrolyzed by the probiotics. Then they exposed *human* intestinal cells from celiac disease patients to both unhydrolyzed gliadins and hydrolyzed gliadins from the probiotic dough. They found the hydrolyzed gliadins did not provoke the same zonulin response. All intestinal permeability markers including zonulin were reduced by the probiotic-hydrolyzed dough.

Further on this relationship with hydrolyzed food proteins and intestinal permeability, some clarity on the subject is revealed by research (Courtois *et al.*

2005) finding a hydrolyzed casein diet decreases zonulin secretion and signs of intestinal permeability. Hydrolyzed casein feeding and other hydrolyzed foods have also been shown helpful for milk allergies and others among infants, as we'll show later.

But what is interesting with regard to the rat research and intestinal permeability is that the casein must be hydrolyzed in order to have this effect of reducing zonulin levels and intestinal permeability.

This means that while unhydrolyzed casein (in pasteurized milk) can cause allergies, irritate and even inflame intestines in some – thereby increasing zonulin – hydrolyzed casein – casein protein that has been broken down into amino acids and small peptides – is therapeutic for intestinal permeability.

What does this say? Quite certainly, it says that casein needs to be hydrolyzed – broken down – by casein-hydrolyzing enzymes – which are produced by probiotics – in order to be a healthy protein.

This is a natural mechanism. Cow's milk and human milk are both breastfed milks. Healthy mothers and healthy cows naturally secrete probiotics with their breast milk. These probiotics produce enzymes that hydrolyze – break down – much of the casein within those products during the digestive process. Assuming, of course, the milk is not pasteurized first – killing those probiotic colonies.

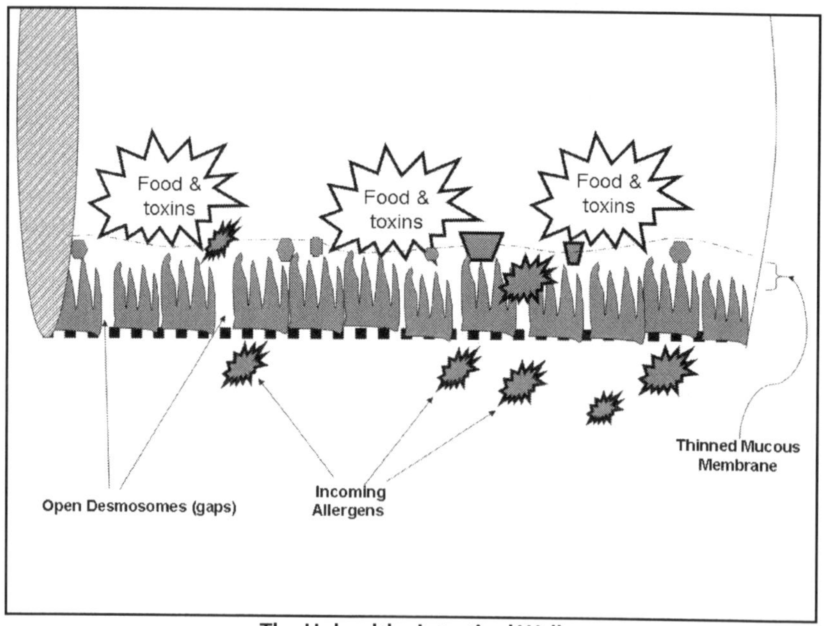

The Unhealthy Intestinal Wall

Furthermore, the other studies we will discuss in the early diet section later have shown that other feeding formulas such as hydrolyzed soy – also help children recover from allergies. This means what – the children do not have the enzymes – produced by probiotics – to properly digest those proteins before the intestinal cells are exposed to them.

But let's not get off track. Zonulin's precise role is still mostly at large. The bottom line is that mucous membrane thinning, intestinal cell irritation and a combined inflammatory immune response cause desmosomes and tight junctions to open. These gaps allow food macromolecules to further damage intestinal cells, and enter the tissues.

But increased intestinal permeability may just be one dimension of this picture. As we discussed earlier, a condition called eosinophilic gastroenteritis leads to the development of both food sensitivities and increased intestinal permeability. In this condition, there is a build up of inflammation-related white blood cells – eosinophils – within the intestinal wall tissues.

Eosinophilic gastroenteritis comes with many of the same symptoms as reported in gluten sensitivities. And the researchers found higher eosinophil infiltration. Does one cause the other? For the time being we can state it is only a correlation – although we will dig into the science regarding the link between intestinal wall damage and food sensitivities in the next chapter.

The Inflammatory Process

Most people think of inflammation as bad. Especially when they hear that allergies involve inflammation.

Inflammation simply coordinates the various immune players into a frenzy of healing response. This is a good thing. Imagine for a moment cutting your finger pretty badly. First you would feel pain – letting you know the body is hurt. Second, you will probably notice that the area has become swollen and red. Blood starts to clot around the area. Soon the cut stops bleeding. The blood dries and a scab forms. It remains red, maybe a little hot, and hurts for a while. After the healing proceeds, soon the cut is closed up and there is a scab left with a little redness around it. The pain soon stops. The scab falls off and the finger returns to normal – almost like new and ready for action.

Without this inflammatory process, we might not even know we cut our finger in the first place. We might keep working, only to find out that we had bled out a quart of blood on the floor. Without clotting, it would be hard to stop the bleeding. And without some continuing pain, we would be more likely to keep injuring the same spot, preventing it from healing.

Were it not for our immune system and inflammatory process slowing blood flow, clotting the blood, scabbing and cleaning up the site, our bodies would simply be full of holes and wounds. Our bodies simply could not survive injury.

The probiotic system and immunoglobulin immune system work together to deter and kill particular invaders – hopefully before they gain access to the body's tissues. Should these defenses fail, they can stimulate the humoral immune system in a strategic attack that includes identifying antigens and recognizing their weaknesses. B-cells and probiotics coordinate through the stimulation of immunoglobulins and CDs.

This progression also stimulates an activation of neutrophils, phagocytes, immunoglobulins, leukotrienes and prostaglandins. Should cells become infected, they will signal the immune system from paracrines located on their cell membranes. Once the intrusion and strategy is determined, B-cells will surround the pathogens while T-cells attack any infected cells. Natural killer T-cells may secrete chemicals into infected cells, initiating the death of the cell.

Leukotrienes immediately gather in the region of injury or infection, and signal to T-cells to coordinate efforts in the process of repair. Prostaglandins initiate the widening of blood vessels to bring more T-cells and other repair factors (such as plasminogen and fibrin) to the infected or injured site. Histamine opens the blood vessel walls to allow all these healing agents access to the injury site to clean it up.

Prostaglandins also stimulate substance P within the nerve cells, initiating the sensation of pain. At the same time, thromboxanes, along with fibrin, drive the process of clotting and coagulation in the blood, while constricting certain blood vessels to decrease the risk of bleeding.

In the case where the pathogen is an allergen, the inflammation response will also accompany an H1-histamine response. As mentioned earlier, histamine is primarily produced by the mast cells, basophils and neutrophils after being stimulated by IgE antibodies. This opens blood vessels to tissues, which stimulates the processes of sneezing, watering of the eyes and coughing. These measures, though sometimes considered irritating, are all stimulated in an effort to remove the toxin and prevent its re-entry into the body. As histamine binds with receptors, one of the resulting physiological responses is alertness (also why antihistamines cause drowsiness). These are natural responses to help the body and mind remain vigilant in order to avoid further toxin intake.

At the height of the repair process, swelling, redness and pain are at their peak. The T-cells, macrophages, neutrophils, fibrin and plasmin all work together to purge the allergen from the body and repair the damage.

As macrophages continue the clean up, the other immune cells begin to retreat. Antioxidants like glutathione will attach to and transport the byproducts – broken down toxins and cell parts – out of the body. As this proceeds, prostaglandins, histamines and leukotrienes begin to signal a reversal of the inflammation and pain process.

One of the central features of the normalization process is the production of bradykinin. Bradykinin slows clotting and opens blood vessels, allowing the cleanup process to accelerate. A key signalling factor is the production of nitric oxide (NO). NO slows inflammation by promoting the detachment of lymphocytes to the site of infection or toxification, and reduces tissue swelling. NO also accelerates the clearing out of debris with its interaction with the superoxide anion. NO was originally described as endothelium-derived relaxing factor (or EDRF) – because of its role in relaxing blood vessel walls.

The body produces more nitric oxide in the presence of good nutrition and lower stress. Probiotics also play a big role in nitric oxide production in a healthy body. Lactobacilli such as *L. plantarum* have in fact been shown to remove the harmful nitrate molecule and use it to produce nitric oxide (Bengmark *et al.* 1998). This is beneficial to not only reducing inflammation: NO production also creates a balanced environment for increased tolerance.

Low nitric oxide levels also happen to be associated with a plethora of diseases, including diabetes, heart failure, high cholesterol, ulcerative colitis, premature aging, cancers and many others. Low or abnormal NO production is also seen among lifestyle habits such as smoking, obesity, and living around air pollution.

There is more to the food sensitivity process than simply an allergen being met by immunoglobulins and releasing histamine (as simplified by many health writers). The intestinal cells are often damaged first by other toxins, resulting in an inflammatory cascade. Once the intestine's cells are damaged, macromolecules/allergens can enter the system through the damaged intestinal wall.

Thus a food sensitivity is usually the result of two events: The first being an inflammatory process responding to an injury to the cells of the intestinal wall. These cells can be damaged by an assortment of toxins, poor dietary choices, microorganism pathogens, stress, smoking, alcohol, pharmaceuticals and toxins. Food macromolecules or allergens can also produce this damage to the cells of the intestinal walls.

Once the cells of the intestinal wall are damaged, the immune system will launch an inflammatory injury response through the T-cell system as described earlier. The T-cells will "repair" the problem by killing off these intestinal cells. This is often described as an autoimmune issue, but in reality, the T-cells are responding to real damage of toxins to these cells. They are not confusing "self" with "non-self."

While this damage and response is active, the intestinal cell wall barrier is altered. This alteration creates a problem called *increased intestinal permeability* as we just described.

The Hypersensitivity Responses

There are four kinds of hypersensitivity responses within the body once an intruder gains access to the body: Type I, Type II, Type III and Type IV. These might sound very similar but they are actually quite different. Let's review these:

Type I: Immediate Hypersensitivity

This response occurs when IgE antibodies bind to food antigens. Food antigens include proteins, fatty acids, and polysaccharides among others. They may also be combined subparts of any food. When this binding between an antigen and IgE takes place, the bound IgE will typically set off the release of inflammatory mediators from mast/basophil/neutrophil white blood cells. These mediators include histamine, prostaglandins and leukotrienes. Depending upon the location and type of mast/basophil/ neutrophil cells, these mediators will spark an allergic response within the airways, sinuses, skin, joints and other locations. This kind of response will typically be immediate, within about two hours of ingestion of the offending food.

Type II: Cytotoxic Response

In this type of immune response, food antigens have penetrated the tissues, and the body responds to kill these cells. This typically takes place through an antigen binding to IgG or IgM immunoglobulins in a delayed immune response. This response can happen concurrently to other allergic responses; though it is still most often a delayed response.

Should the red blood cells be involved in the antigen absorption, hemolysis (the destruction of red blood cells) and anemia (a lack of red blood cells) may result.

Type III: Immune-Complex Response

Here the allergen-bound antibody complex actually penetrates cell tissues and injures them. This can occur within the intestinal cells, liver, or virtually anywhere around the body. In some instances these immune complexes can increase vascular permeability or intestinal permeability, as we've discussed.

This type of response is also often a delayed response, occurring hours or even a day or two after eating the offending food.

Sometimes the immune complexes will stimulate mast cell degranulation of histamine, prostaglandins and leukotrienes, and stimulate inflammation within the tissue system. This can result in a variety of conditions, which are sometimes attributed to autoimmunity.

Type IV: T-Cell Responses

This type of response is independent of other types of sensitivity. For example, the Type III may generate a T-cell response once the cell and tissue damage begins. But this Type IV occurs without the binding of an antigen by an antibody. In this response, a cell is directly affected by the allergen or food constituent. Conditions of colitis are typical of this type of response, because the antigen directly stimulates toxicity within the intestinal cells. Once the intestinal cells are damaged, T-cells launch an immune response to clear out the invaded cells. As mentioned, this response is also often attributed to autoimmunity. Rather it is an immune response to cellular toxicity.

This type of response will typically take from two to four days from exposure to response.

Food Allergy Responses

There are multiple immune responses to food that result in food sensitivity. A food may spark an inflammatory response by stimulating any number of inflammatory mediators, including prostaglandins, serotonin, platelet-aggregating factor, kinins and others. In these instances, any number of conditions may result.

To this we can add that some foods actually contain histamine, as we'll discuss later. These can sometimes stimulate an inflammatory response, especially among immunosuppressed people with hair-trigger immune systems.

While most of these different types of responses might relate to the body's immune system, most of them are not often referred to as a food allergy by physicians and researchers. Many refer only to the IgE form of allergen-antibody response (Type I) as a pure food allergy. The others sometimes are present in food allergies, but some are often simply food intolerances that have involved the immune system.

Furthermore, the **Type I** allergic response can be broken down into two stages: sensitization and elicitation.

Sensitization

The food molecule sensitization process takes place when a potential protein antigen happens to come into contact with a type of immune cell called a progenitor B-cell. As part of their immune system responsibilities, these B-cells will break apart the protein into smaller peptides. These will be attached to hystocompatibility complex class II complex molecules.

The T-cell hystocompatibility complex is transferred onto the surface of the B-cell, which binds to a particular allergen. Once upon the B-cell surface, T-helper cells take notice of this foreign particle stuck to the B-cell. The T-helper cell cytokine CD4 receptors trigger a response, and this stimulates the production of the IgE immunoglobulins. These particular IgE immunoglobulins are now sensitized to the particular epitope of the antigen in the future.

The below diagram illustrates sensitization:

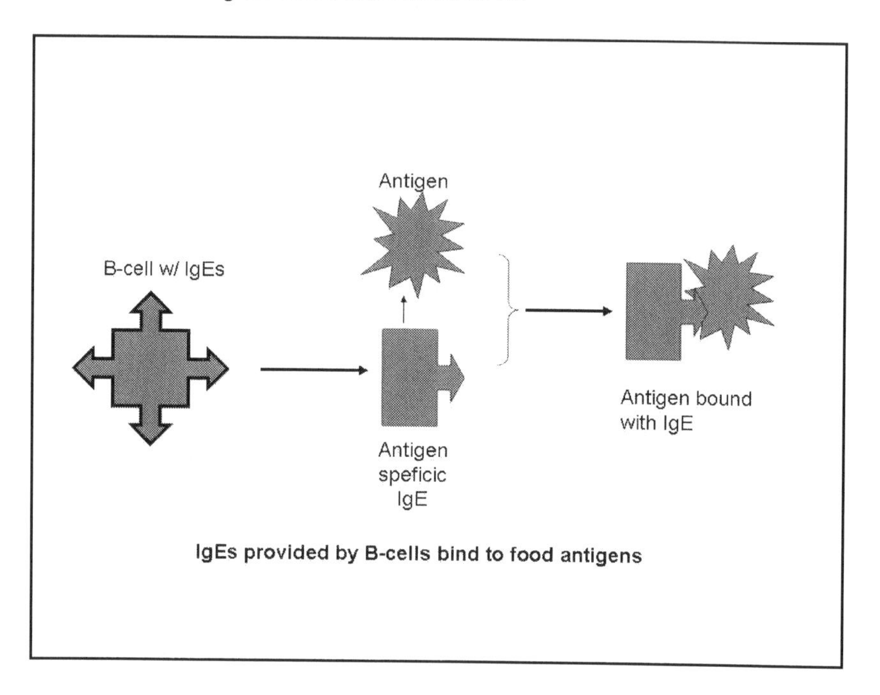

IgEs provided by B-cells bind to food antigens

Elicitation

Once sensitized, the IgE associates with the specific IgE receptors that lie on the surface of the neutrophil, basophil or mast cells. Within these cells are packages called granules.

The granules are stock full of a variety of inflammatory mediators. The most notorious of these in food allergies is histamine as we've been discussing. As the allergen-specific IgEs connect with the IgE receptors on these immune cells, the immune cells will release the inflammatory mediators such as histamine and leukotrienes into the bloodstream and lymph. This is what drives much of the symptoms of an allergic attack, including but not limited to hives, asthma, uritica, sinusitis and others.

The next diagram illustrates elicitation:

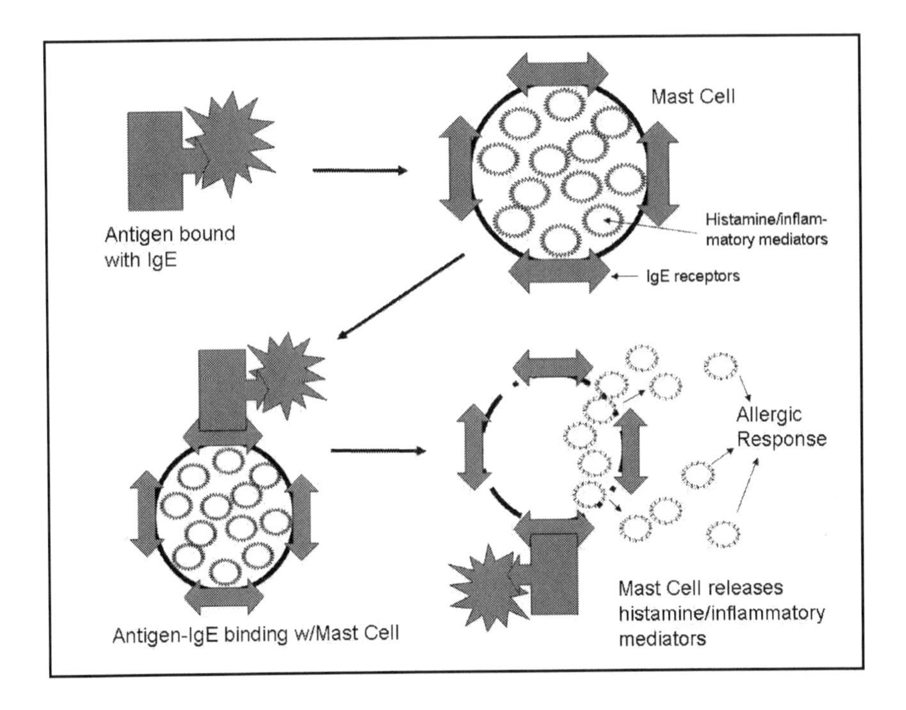

The Role of Probiotics in Immune Responses

Outside of producing enzymes that hydrolyze or break down certain foods, probiotics also play a critical role in many of the processes of the immune system as it relates to food sensitivities. Probiotics also temper and balance the immune response so that the body responds with less hypersensitivity. Let's discuss some of the science that illustrates the important role probiotics play in the immune system:

Probiotics tend to increase IgA responses within the intestines and reduce the IgE allergic response. Finnish scientists (Ouwehand *et al.* 2009) gave healthy elderly volunteers *Lactobacillus acidophilus* or a placebo. Immune factors were tested, and the probiotics had modulated their IgA and PGE2 levels. They also observed improved spermidine levels – an enzyme involved in DNA synthesis. The researchers concluded that these improvements suggested increased mucosal and intestinal immunity among the probiotic group.

Researchers from the Teikyo University School of Medicine in Japan (Araki *et al.* 1999) gave *Bifidobacterium breve* YIT4064 or placebo to 19 infants for 28 days. IgA levels significantly increased among the probiotic group.

In a study of 105 pregnant women, University of Western Australia scientists (Prescott *et al.* 2008) found that *Lactobacillus rhamnosus* and *Bifidobacterium lactis* stimulated higher levels of cytokine IFN-gamma, higher levels of TGF-beta1, and higher levels of breast milk IgA. Plasma of their babies had lower CD14 levels, and greater CB IFN-gamma levels. These indicated that the probiotics strengthened immunity and moderated hypersensitivity.

Researchers from the Turku University Central Hospital in Finland (Rinne *et al.* 2005) gave 96 mothers either a placebo or *Lactobacillus rhamnosus* GG before delivery and continued the supplementation in their infants after delivery. At three months of age, immunoglobulin IgG-secreting cells among breastfed infants supplemented with probiotics were significantly higher than the breastfed infants who received the placebo. In addition, the non-hypersensitivity IgM-, IgA-, and IgG-secreting cell counts at 12 months were significantly higher among the breastfed infants who supplemented with probiotics, compared to the breastfed infants receiving the placebo.

Probiotics help modulate the inflammatory processes. In research from Poland's Pomeranian Academy of Medicine (Naruszewicz *et al.* 2002), scientists found that giving *Lactobacillus plantarum* 299v to 36 volunteers resulted in a 37% decrease in inflammatory F2-isoprostanes. Isoprostanes are similar to prostaglandins, formed outside of the COX process.

Probiotics also stimulate a healthy thymus gland. Illustrating this, medical researchers from the University of Bari (Indrio *et al.* 2007) gave a placebo or a probiotic combination of *Bifidobacterium breve* C50 and *Streptococcus thermophilus* 065 to 60 newborns. The thymus glands of the probiotic group was significantly larger compared to babies that consumed the standard (placebo) formula.

Scientists from the Nagoya University Graduate School of Medicine (Sugawara *et al.* 2006) found in a study of 101 patients that supplementation with probiotics increased NK activity and lymphocyte counts. Pro-inflammatory IL-6 cytokines also decreased significantly among the probiotic group. Serum IL-6, white blood cell counts, and C-reactive protein also significantly decreased among the probiotic group.

Furthermore, probiotics have the ability to *uniquely* modify cytokines depending upon the condition and disease of the person. Illustrating this, a probiotic drink with either placebo or a probiotic combination of *Lactobacillus paracasei* Lpc-37, *Lactobacillus acidophilus* 74-2 and *Bifidobacterium animalis* subsp. *lactis* DGCC 420 (*B. lactis* 420) was given to 15 healthy adults and 15 adults with atopic dermatitis.

After eight weeks, CD57(+) cytokines levels increased significantly among the healthy group taking probiotics, while CD4(+)CD54(+) cytokines decreased significantly among the atopic patients who were taking the probiotics, compared with the placebo group and compared to the levels at the beginning of the trial (Roessler *et al.* 2008).

In another study, researchers from Poland's Pomeranian Academy of Medicine (Naruszewicz *et al.* 2002) gave *Lactobacillus plantarum* 299v or placebo to 36 healthy volunteers for six weeks. Monocytes isolated from probiotic subjects had significantly reduced adhesion to endothelial cells, and the probiotic group had a 42% reduction in pro-inflammatory cytokine interleukin-6. No changes were observed among the placebo group.

Probiotics are often involved in the production of intermediary fatty acids used for LOX and COX enzyme conversions, producing anti-inflammatory effects. To illustrate this, scientists from the University of Helsinki (Kekkonen *et al.* 2008) measured lipids and inflammation markers before and after giving probiotic *Lactobacillus rhamnosus* GG to 26 healthy adults. After three weeks of probiotic supplementation, the subjects had decreased levels of intermediary inflammatory fatty acids such as lysophosphatidylcholines, sphingomyelins, and several glycerophosphatidylcholines. Probiotics also reduced hyper-inflammatory markers TNF-alpha and CRP in this study.

The bottom line is that our body's probiotics and our immune system are interconnected. They are inseparable. At least 70% of the immune system *is* probiotic. Consider this carefully: If the intestine's probiotics were decimated by either a lethal bacteria infection or a course of antibiotics, *we would lose nearly three quarters of our gut's immune system.*

Remember our discussion about how wheats contain prebiotic fibers (arabinoxylans) that feed certain types of probiotic colonies. And as we'll show further evidence of later, some of these same species also produce the enzymes that break down gliadin and glutenin proteins.

There is a lot more involved within our immune system when it comes to food sensitivities as we've discussed in this chapter, but probiotics are fundamental in gluten sensitivities.

Chapter Five

The Causes for Gluten Sensitivities

As we will illustrate in this chapter, gluten sensitivities can have a myriad of causes. Knowing this is critical for understanding what causes gluten allergies and wheat allergies: Many of these are also related to non-allergic intolerances to gluten, WGA or other components of gluten-based foods.

Thus the task is complex. We are covering several overlapping conditions that may or may not relate to each other. In some cases, we will show that the physiological elements at play in food intolerance may also eventually produce an allergy to the food.

But in other instances, we'll illustrate that intolerance and allergy are two different conditions, and not necessarily linked when it comes to causational aspects.

To achieve this, this chapter will list many *contributing factors*. In other words, a single factor is not likely to be solely at the root of a food sensitivity. A myriad of factors – a combination of these discussed – will come into play to create the conditions by which the sensitivity may arise.

Or it may not arise. Depending upon the strength of our immune system and our ability to process foreigners, some of the factors may put a dent in our digestive system yet not produce a food sensitivity.

In some cases, this chapter will illustrate the connection between the element discussed and gluten sensitivity by showing research connecting the factor with a food sensitivity other than wheat or gluten. Admittedly some of the research is limited with respect to wheat or gluten. But the evidence with respect to food sensitivities in general – also large proteins comparable to gliadins and glutenins – is strong.

In a few cases this chapter will illustrate that the cause of the sensitivity is actually the condition. Remember the oil leak analogy discussed earlier, and the difference between correlation and causation. The food, like the oil, isn't causing the problem of sensitivity.

If it were, most of us would be starving.

But a condition might also create a digestive weakness that predisposes us to gluten sensitivity.

The bottom line here is that food sensitivities are better seen as symptoms rather than diseases in themselves. Food sensitivities may be medically diagnosable, but there is an undercurrent of physiology that lies at the root of these conditions.

Therefore, in terms of our general physiology, food sensitivities are not a disease: They are symptoms of disease.

Breaking Down Glutenins and Gliadins

Remember that proteins are typically composed of very long chains of amino acids. Gluten proteins are good-sized, but not gigantic. They can contain between 275 and 360 amino acids linked together. But some proteins contain thousands of amino acids.

The body typically breaks apart these chains through an enzyme reaction called hydrolysis – also referred to as proteolysis.

Proteolysis breaks down proteins using hydrolysis into amino acids and small groups of amino acids called polypeptides. This is also called *cleaving.* As enzymes break off these polypeptides or individual amino acids from proteins, they replace the protein chain linkages with water molecules to stabilize the peptide or amino acid. This process is called *enzymatic hydrolysis*. We've discussed this process earlier. Breaking away the peptides or amino acids allows the body to utilize the amino acid or polypeptide to make new proteins within the body.

The body then assembles its own proteins from these amino acids and polypeptides. The body's protein assemblies are programmed by DNA and RNA. For this reason, the body must recognize the polypeptide combinations. Strange polypeptide combinations can burden the body, especially if the body does not have the enzymes to break those peptides apart. While some enzymes can break apart multiple proteins and polypeptides, some proteins, such as gliadins, require special enzymes to be properly broken down into body-friendly peptides and aminos. Protein-cleaving enzymes are called *proteases.*

In a study that analyzed treatment alternatives for celiac disease from George Washington University School of Medicine (Bakshi *et al.* 2012), researchers found that probiotics provide a viable solution for gluten digestion and intestinal health – and likely their absence provides at least one smoking gun for the cause of gluten sensitivities.

As we discussed, celiac disease – an inflammatory immune response to primarily the gliadin protein – has been increasing over the past few years, and research is illustrating that celiac disease is more prevalent than previously considered.

Significant research focus and several teams of investigators including the George Washington University researchers mentioned above have confirmed that the inflammatory response to gliadin – initiated with an interleukin-15 mediated response – is inhibited by healthy intestinal probiotics.

In fact, intestinal probiotics break down gliadin into healthy, non-inflammatory amino acid nutrients.

A 2012 paper by three medical school professors studied the various means by which the effects of celiac disease may be mitigated – by inhibiting the inflammatory response. The paper's authors include two doctors who are gastroenterology professors at George Washington University School of Medicine, Anita Bakshi, M.D. and Sindu Stephen, M.D. Two other clinical M.D.s co-authored the research.

The researchers focused first upon the mechanisms of wheat gliadin protein upon the intestinal cells – which produce inflammation and intestinal permeability. These include the activation of a CD4+ T-cell response among the intestinal cells – which induces the secretion of a protein called zonulin. Zonulin then stimulates an increase in the spaces in the tight junctions between the intestinal cells, creating gut permeability.

This opening between intestinal cells is accompanied by an even greater inflammatory response as the immune system responds to larger proteins having potential contact with the bloodstream.

While there are a number of studies that have shown these effects, the researchers singled out a few studies that clearly and specifically illustrated how intestinal probiotics in a healthy body will inhibit this process by breaking down gluten through protease (enzyme) activity.

In one of these, Irish researchers found that two enzymes produced from probiotic bacteria – prolyl endopeptidase and endoprotease B – were able to break down gluten into non-reactive elements, completely sidestepping the possible intestinal response.

This research was confirmed in a clinical setting by scientists at the Celiac Sprue Research Foundation in Palo Alto, California. Here 20 celiac patients were given small doses of gluten with and without being pretreated with one of these probiotic-produced enzymes – prolyl endopeptidase. The cross-over study utilized two 14-day treatment periods in total, in a staged format.

The pretreatment with the enzyme allowed a majority of the celiac patients to avoid malabsorption of carbohydrates and fats – a typical symptom of celiac sprue response.

The researchers concluded that:

> *"Pretreatment of gluten with prolyl endopeptidase avoided the development of fat or carbohydrate malabsorption in the majority of those patients who developed fat or carbohydrate malabsorption after a 2-week gluten challenge."*

In a series of studies from Finland's University of Tampere Medical School, researchers (Lindfors *et al.* 2008) tested the probiotics strains *Lactobacillus fermentum* and *Bifidobacterium lactis* with gluten digestion and the inflammatory effects of gliadin.

They found these live probiotics were both able to inhibit the inflammation response among sensitive intestinal (Caco-2) cells. In both instances the probiotics prevented the inflammatory response as well as prevented the formation of *"membrane ruffles."*

The researchers stated:

> *"B. lactis inhibited the gliadin-induced increase dose-dependently in epithelial permeability, higher concentrations completely abolishing the gliadin-induced decrease in transepithelial resistance."*

This of course means the probiotics reduced the amount of intestinal damage caused by the inflammatory response related to the gluten ingestion.

In their discussion, the researchers stated:

> *"In the present study we have shown for the first time that B. lactis probiotic bacteria are able to protect epithelial cells from cellular damage induced by gliadin administration."*

And in their conclusion, the researchers stated:

> *"We conclude thus that live B. lactis bacteria can counteract directly the harmful effects exerted by coeliac-toxic gliadin and would clearly warrant further studies of its potential as a novel dietary supplement in the treatment of coeliac disease."*

While the inflammatory response in celiac sprue is typically described as being the result of a genetic abnormality, intestinal irritation and indigestion to gluten in non-celiac people provokes similar mechanisms of inflammation – though not as vigorous – and not linked with genetic abnormality.

The UGW researchers concluded after reviewing the research that:

> *"Inclusion of probiotics appears to be able to reduce the damage caused by eating gluten-contaminated foods and may even accelerate mucosal healing after the initiation of a gluten-free diet."*

These results have been confirmed by other research. A study from Argentina's University of Buenos Aires (Smecuol *et al.* 2013) tested a probiotic supplement with 22 adults with celiac disease. The patients were given either capsules with the probiotic *Bifidobacterium infantis* or a placebo for 3 weeks.

Those taking the probiotic supplement had significantly lower levels of indigestion, constipation and other intestinal symptoms as gauged by the Gastrointestinal Symptom Rating Scale. Levels of IgA antibodies to gluten were also lower among the probiotic group.

The researchers stated:

> *"The study suggests that B. infantis may alleviate symptoms in untreated celiac disease."*

Another study illustrated that probiotics can provide safety for gluten foods even for celiac disease patients. Researchers from Italy's University of Bari (Di Cagno *et al.* 2004) made a sourdough bread with 30% wheat flour together with four strains of probiotic bacteria (*Lactobacillus alimentarius, L. brevis L. sanfranciscensis and L. hilgardii*) combined with baker's yeast. Of the 17 celiac patients given the bread, all of them tolerated the bread without signs of allergic reaction. We'll elaborate on the formula in the last chapter.

In addition, Argentina researchers (Rollan *et al.* 2005) tested two strains of *Lactobaccillus plantarum* in the laboratory. They found that both were able to break down gliadin proteins within sourdough bread.

The University of Bari researchers (Rizzello *et al.* 2007) conducted a similar study using 12 celiac patients. Their bread fermented with probiotics and sourdough yeast completely hydrolyzed (broke down) all of the gliadins, all the albumins, and all the globulin proteins within the flour. And the fermentation also hydrolyzed 80% of the glutenin proteins – which are typically inconsequential in most gluten-sensitive people.

As most celiac patients react to gliadin proteins and not glutenins, the bread was tolerated by the celiac patients without *"immunoreactivity."* This of course means they had no allergic response. The researchers stated:

> *"Food processing by selected sourdough lactobacilli and fungal proteases may be considered an efficient approach to eliminate gluten toxicity."*

We might take a moment to comment on the use of *"toxicity"* here. This should not be taken out of context. The researchers were not stating the gluten in itself is toxic. The aspect of *"toxicity"* discussed relates specifically to celiac disease – where gluten proteins (gliadin proteins in particular) that are not broken down into their components by our intestinal bacteria or otherwise, can be toxic to a celiac patient allergic to those unhydrolyzed proteins.

This also indicates an interesting paradigm. Because probiotic bacteria are colonizing healthy intestinal tracts – as we'll discuss in detail later – the smoking gun behind the proclivity of celiac disease may very well be misplaced. Instead of it being a genome disorder, it may very well be a disorder related to a lack of microbiome.

How is this related to the hereditary link in celiac disease then? Again as we'll discuss in detail later, our resident probiotic colonies are typically passed down from mother to child during birth. This means a lack of particular probiotic stains in the mother will typically be passed down to the child.

The basis for the understanding that probiotics break down gliadin and glutenin proteins is solid. Let's look at a few other studies.

We previously discussed a study from the University of Bari (De Angelis *et al.* 2006) earlier. Here the researchers tested a probiotic combination called VSL#3 with wheat flour and tested the ability of the gliadins to interact with intestinal cells in celiac disease patients. The researchers found the flour fermented with the probiotics produced an almost complete hydrolysis (break down) of the gliadin proteins in the flour.

They also found the probiotic combination reduced by agglutinating activity (lectin/WGA related) by 100 times.

In their intestinal cell testing, the researchers found the probiotic dough resulted in lower intestinal permeability markers all around, including CD3+ intraepithelial lymphocytes – an autoimmune response.

A study from Argentina's Centro de Referencia para Lactobacilos (Gerez *et al.* 2006) tested 42 strains of bacteria with gluten. They found that 13 lactic acid bacteria including nine lactobacillus species used gluten as food. This resulted in an increase in amino acids – meaning the bacteria were breaking down the gluten proteins into their amino acid components.

One of these components, for example, was lysine – an essential amino acid found in wheat. This illustrates the ability of our intestinal bacteria – assuming we are colonizing them – to break down gluten proteins and turn them into those healthy amino acids our body requires for nutrition.

Some of the same University of Bari researchers discussed above (Di Cagno *et al.* 2002) tested a number of strains of probiotic bacteria as they fermented some sourdough breads. This is one of the precursor studies that resulted in the formulation of the bread and the clinical testing with celiac patients.

While the researchers found the bacteria produced hydrolysis among the gliadin proteins as the later studies determined, they also found the resulting fermented flour prevented agglutination among the intestinal cells of celiac patients.

This means these probiotic bacteria – *Lactobacillus alimentarius, Lactobacillus brevis, Lactobacillus sanfranciscensis* and *Lactobacillus hilgardii* – also broke down those wheat germ agglutinins, and prevented any agglutination effects upon the intestinal cells. This of course was confirmed by the 2006 study on VSL#3.

The research clearly identifies the true smoking gun for the growth of intestinal irritability and gluten insensitivity in our society: The steady and growing destruction of healthy probiotics within our intestines through an unbridled use of antibiotics and antiseptics. This lack of probiotics exposes the intestines to large unbroken gliadin molecules the intestines are not intended to contend with. Healthy probiotic colonies would otherwise break these gliadins down into components our intestines were designed to deal with.

When we examine the evidence: The fact that gluten sensitivities have been growing during the same period the use of antibiotics and antiseptics has exploded; together with the findings that enzymes produced by probiotics break down gluten and gliadin into non-toxic constituents, we can only arrive at the conclusion that our gut microflora has everything to do with wheat and other gluten sensitivities.

And with this conclusion, avoiding all forms of gluten in our diets can not only be an arduous and close to impossible task – but it may become unnecessary when we learn how to promote and maintain healthy intestinal flora.

Remember the research discussed in the second chapter regarding FODMAPs. These are foods that have been found to reduce – if they are eliminated from the diet – symptoms of bloating, intestinal irritability, cramping and indigestion. Research has found that many complaining of gluten intolerance are in fact intolerant to multiple foods.

And remember some of the foods defined as FODMAPs:

> Prebiotic foods, acidic processed foods, dairy foods, apples, pears, asparagus, artichokes, garlic, beets, cabbage, wheat, beans, pulses, legumes, peaches, snap peas, watermelon, nectarines, peaches, plums, cashews, pistachios, sweet corn, and many others, including processed foods containing sugar-alcohols and refined sugars and carbohydrates.

What do most of these foods have in common?

They require particular enzymes to break them down. Many of which are produced by intestinal probiotics.

The Role of Oral Bacteria in Gluten Hydrolysis

The probiotics that live within healthy digestive tracts are not the only probiotics that produce the enzymes that break down gluten proteins. Actually, there are several bacteria that live within a healthy oral cavity that also hydrolyze gliadins and other gluten proteins.

This was illustrated by a study from Boston University's Henry M. Goldman School of Dental Medicine (Helmerhorst *et al.* 2010). The researchers tested oral bacteria residing in dental plaque and found that several produced glutamine endoproteases, which break down gliadin proteins.

They stated clearly about their findings:

> *"Plaque bacteria efficiently hydrolyzed Z-YPQ-pNA, Z-QQP-pNA, Z-PPF-pNA and Z-PFP-pNA, with Z-YPQ-pNA being most rapidly cleaved. Gliadin immunogenic domains were extensively degraded in the presence of oral bacteria."*

To *"cleave"* means to break apart, and those combinations such as *Z-YPQ-pNA* describe different gliadin protein types – types described here as *"immunogenic." Immunogenic* relates to something that produces an immune response (*"genic"* relates to *genesis*).

Furthermore, the medical scientists established other food components that require bacteria-produced enzymes to break them down outside of gluten and other food proteins:

> *"Complex carbohydrates that cannot be degraded by the arsenal of human digestive enzymes can in most cases be hydrolyzed by bacterial glycosidases."*

This and other research has clearly confirmed the reality that gliadin and other gluten proteins are not the only complex molecules that our bodies do not produce enzymes for without bacteria. There are many – as the FODMAPs listing of foods indicates.

As such, without these important bacteria – living within our digestive tracts and our oral cavity – our intestinal cells must be exposed to the macromolecules being identified as "complex carbohydrates" here, in addition to proteins coming from gluten, milk, fish, nuts, and others that cause food sensitivity if not properly hydrolyzed.

The researchers used state-of-the-art technology to analyze the hydrolyzation process of the gliadin proteins. They utilized mass spectrometry using capillary nano-flow liquid chromatography and electrospray ionization tandem mass spectrometer analysis. These allowed the medical scientists to pinpoint the precise molecular compositions and the particular amino acids that were cleaved – broken down – from the gluten proteins by the enzymes produced by the bacteria. Here is a description of the hydrolyzation of two of the gliadin peptides considered "superantigens"– 33-mer in alpha2-gliadin and 26-mer in omega-gliadin:

> *"We confirmed that both peptides are resistant to digestion by the major human digestive enzymes trypsin, chymotrypsin and pepsin after 24 hours of incubation. In a suspension of plaque bacteria, however, the 33-mer completely degraded after 5 hours of incubation, as evidenced by disappearance of the peak at 66 minutes and appearance of degradation fragments eluting between 60–66 minutes and between 25 and 30 minutes. The 26-mer was also cleaved by dental plaque bacteria, yielding fragments eluting between 25 and 30 minutes and between 35 minutes and 52 minutes. No degradation of the 33-mer and the 26-mer was observed when incubations were carried out in saliva ion buffer alone, indicating that the peptides*

were stable unless oral bacterial enzymes were present in the incubation mixture."

"Stable" here means not broken down. The *"saliva ion buffer alone"* means human saliva without oral bacteria.

So what were these bacteria that were found to cleave and hydrolyze the immunogenic gliadin molecules? There are some-600 species of bacteria residing in our oral cavity (oral bacteria – see the authors book, *Oral Probiotics*).

The researchers did not focus upon the microorganism species identification in this study. However, the same researchers conducted another study (Zamakhchari *et al.* 2011) shortly after in order to identify these species. They identified a number, but found the bacteria species able to hydrolyze gliadin proteins the most were *Rothia mucilaginosa* and *Rothia aeria*.

These two microorganisms were found to more completely hydrolyze gliadin proteins within a shorter time period. The researchers stated:

"Gliadins were however rapidly cleaved in a suspension of R. aeria, as evidenced from the finding that within 2 hours of incubation the added amount of gliadin (250 micrograms in a 1 milliliter volume) was completely degraded. The precise time course for gliadin degradation by R. aeria was established in a separate experiment in which sampling was carried out at shorter time intervals within the 2 hour incubation time period."

The researchers found that at least half of the gliadin protein was completely hydrolyzed within 30 minutes, and completely within two hours.

A more recent study from Boston University's dental school (Fernandez-Feo *et al.* 2013) found the "highly immunogenic" alpha-gliadin-derived 33-mer peptide showed hydrolysis in multiple assays by the two Rothia species mentioned above, along with:

Actinomyces odontolyticus
Streptococcus mitis
Streptococcus sp.
Neisseria mucosa
Capnocytophaga sputigena

The Rothia species were the most active, as the Zamakhchari found. This study being active in all four assays. Notice that some of these bacteria species are also known to produce plaque on the teeth, and some – like *S. mitis* – have been known to be involved in periodontal disease.

But as shown conclusively in the author's book, *Oral Probiotics,* these and other bacteria can be controlled and thus inconsequential when they are colonized in balance with other (probiotic) species. In other words, it is the balance of bacteria that helps prevent disease, and even bacteria otherwise known to be probiotic can produce ill health if they are allowed to over-colonize.

So does this mean that we'd have to chew bread for two hours to completely break down the gliadin proteins – assuming we have healthy colonies of oral bacteria?

Nope. First, these bacteria and others produce the enzymes, which mix with the bolus of our food. The bolus – the mixture of food, saliva, enzymes and bacteria – then travels down our esophagus where it enters the stomach. The stomach may produce some die-off of a portion of the oral bacteria, but the enzymes will continue with the food, eventually helping to hydrolyze the remainder – which can be finished off by enzymes produced by intestinal probiotics.

We should note also that *R. mucilaginosa* also inhabit the upper intestinal tract in a healthy gut. We should note that Rothia species in general have been found in celiac patients as well as healthy patients within the duodenum.

However, as we will illustrate in the next chapter, the intestines of celiac disease children also tend to contain pathogenic rod shaped bacteria – such as Clostridium and Actinomyces.

What this illustrates as we'll discuss later in more detail is dominance – territorial control. When part of our intestines is dominated by certain bacteria or yeast – the ability of other bacteria to do their thing becomes limited. This goes for the ability to produce enzymes. If the dominant bacteria are controlling the territory, other bacteria find themselves controlled as to their major activities.

This is done by creating certain chemical and pH environments. Colonies of dominant bacteria species will control the chemical nature of a certain region. They will also produce their own antimicrobials, acids and chemicals to counteract or even prevent the production activity of those bacteria they dominate.

The rub here is that just as our so-many antibacterial strategies such as antibiotics have killed off many of our intestinal probiotics, the many antibacterial mouth washes and toothpastes have destroyed many of those bacteria that produce not only these enzymes but others helpful in digesting the foods we eat.

The researchers stated the importance of maintaining the balance of healthy microorganisms within intestinal bacteria as well as oral bacteria:

> *"Such microorganisms may play a hitherto unappreciated role in the digestion of dietary gluten and thus protection from celiac disease in subjects at risk."*

But we cannot conclude that only probiotics are involved in causing gluten sensitivities. Let's keep going.

Enzyme Deficiencies

So proteins must be broken down in the gut in a process called proteolysis using hydrolysis as we've discussed. This is the result of the food's exposure to proteolytic enzymes.

Okay, so we've already discussed much of this, and how certain probiotics provide the enzymes that break down gliadins and glutenins.

But we may not realize that our body's own production of enzymes is also critical to food sensitivities, including wheat allergies and gluten intolerance.

In other words, sensitivities to wheat may or may not be related to the gluten proteins only broken down by probiotic-produced proteases. Some may even be related to some of the polysaccharides or even lectins not being properly broken down.

This is because our body produces general proteases and peptidases that break down different parts of different proteins. And if these are not properly broken down, protein and even carbohydrate macromolecules can be presented to intestinal cells, producing immune responses that can turn into multiple food sensitivities.

Trypsin, for example, is produced in the pancreas and secreted into the small intestine through the pancreatic duct as trypsinogen. Trypsinogen then partners with enteropeptidase to activate trypsin.

Trypsin breaks apart the bonds between many amino acid and peptide sequences – called polypeptide bonds – producing smaller peptides and amino acids. As we've discussed, these can readily be absorbed into the blood and utilized by the body.

The importance of trypsin to gluten sensitivity is that it is often used in flour-making. Why? To make the dough softer and easier to use. This dough-softening takes place as the trypsin enzymes break down the stiffer proteins in wheat – many of which are gluten-type proteins.

We might also consider that wheat allergies and other food allergies often accompany a metabolic process called enzyme inhibition. For example, trypsin-inhibiting foods can block trypsin activity, producing a reduction in protein assimilation.

If we are deficient in a particular enzyme, the food that enzyme breaks down will not be properly broken down. This can create a macromolecule that may be exposed to the cells and tissues of the intestines.

If the intestinal barrier is weakened, the immunoglobulins within the intestines can mark the macromolecule as an invader. Worse, the macromolecule can get into the internal tissues and bloodstream – where the immune system can launch an immune attack against it – often resulting in allergies.

The body has a very exacting way it breaks down proteins. This requires specific protease enzymes and the process of natural enzymatic hydrolysis. This of course means that the body also needs to have plenty of water on hand as well.

Food allergies are directly related to our digestive enzymes. Researchers from the Medical University of Vienna (Untersmayr *et al.* 2007) studied the effects that incomplete digestion of fish proteins have on fish allergies. Healthy volunteers and those with diagnosed codfish allergies were challenged with codfish. They were also tested with fish proteins incubated with varying degrees of digestive enzymes. The subjects were tested for histamine release from fish allergen sensitivity with each type.

The researchers found that the inadequate breakdown of fish proteins produced more allergic responses, while a more complete breakdown by enzymes produced fewer allergic responses among both groups. Inadequate digestion produced allergens that the body sensitized to.

Our body requires numerous enzymes to digest our foods. Here is a short list of the major digestive enzymes and the foods they break down. Note this includes enzymes produced by probiotics, and some supplied by foods:

Major Digestive Enzymes

Enzyme	Foods it Breaks Down
Amylase	Starches
Bromelain	Proteins
Carboxypeptidase	Proteins (terminal)
Cellulase	Plant fiber (cellulose)
Chymotrypsin	Proteins
Elastase	Proteins and elastins
Endoprotease B	Gluten proteins
Glucoamylase	Starches
Glutamine endoproteases	Gliadins
Isomaltase	Isomaltose and Maltose
Lactase	Lactose
Lipase	Fats
Maltase	Maltose
Nuclease	Protein nucleotides
Pepsin	Proteins
Peptidase	Proteins
Prolyl endopeptidase	Gluten proteins
Rennin	Milk
Steapsin	Triglycerides
Sucrase	Sucrose
Tributyrase	Butter Fat
Trypsin	Proteins
Xylanase	Hemicellulose (plant fiber)

We can see from this list there are many different protein enzymes. This is because there are so many different types of proteins to break down. There are numerous enzyme sub-types and others that break down specific food constituents and particular foods.

Exposure to Glyphosate

Multiple studies have found that food sensitivities aren't necessarily the results of sensitivities to the food itself: Sometimes there are additives that produce the sensitivity.

There is now good evidence that in fact glyphosate – or more specifically the herbicide RoundUp® – may be a contributing factor for wheat sensitivities and even allergies including celiac disease.

The implication comes in the form of what is referred to by many wheat farmers as *desiccation*. This is the spraying of the herbicide RoundUp® onto a commercial crop of wheat just prior to harvest. According to Monsanto and many farm advisors, this kills the wheat plant and stimulates heavier wheat berries in order to yield a greater harvest.

It also makes the harvest easier, since the wheat plants are dried out – or better, killed – after being sprayed with the herbicide.

According to data provided by the USDA, the application of glyphosate onto wheat crops in the U.S. has significantly increased over the past few decades. In 1998, 91% of spring wheat, 88% of durum wheat and 47% of winter wheat was sprayed with glyphosate herbicides. In 2012, the percentages were 97%, 99% and 61%, respectively.

This means that most of the conventionally grown U.S. wheat is sprayed with glyphosate herbicide at some point. This doesn't mean that all this percentage underwent desiccation prior to harvest, however.

In fact, farmers are realizing that desiccation will produce seed abnormalities, making it difficult for the farmers to replant the seed harvested with this method. According to a release from Steve Sebesta, the Deputy Commissioner North Dakota State Seed Department regarding planting wheat:

> *"Don't use grain harvested from fields treated with glyphosate as a harvest aid for seed. It's grain, not seed."*

Mr. Sebesta indicated that testing showed 98% of desiccated seed was not productive. The first question this brings up is why would such a practice be horrible for planting seed yet be okay for humans to eat? The concept is absurd at the least.

The fact is, glyphosate and the other chemicals including surfactants utilized in RoundUp® are implicated in inhibiting gut bacteria from producing enzymes that are critical to our health. And by inhibiting these bacteria, we are essentially setting up the means for intestinal abnormalities.

Research has confirmed that glyphosate specifically reduces gut bacteria populations. Among other studies, research from Germany's Leipzig University (Shehata *et al.* 2013) found the glyphosate significantly reduces probiotic bacteria including *Enterococcus* species, *Bifidobacterium* species and *Lactobacillus* species, while promoting the growth of pathogenic bacteria such as *Salmonella* species and *Clostridium* species.

The reason for this? Glyphosate interferes with the shikimic acid pathway, a crucial part of cell metabolism among plants and bacteria. In other words, the same destructive effects that glyphosate has upon plants also produces a die off of probiotic gut bacteria. This leaves the less vulnerable pathogenic bacteria such as *Clostridium difficile* to thrive in the gut, producing chaos within the digestive system along with an inability to break down wheat proteins.

That's because, as shown in the last section, it is our gut probiotics that produce the enzymes that break down gluten proteins.

Furthermore, a study by MIT scientists (Samsel and Seneff 2013), reveals that the rise in celiac disease incidence in the U.S. is directly proportionate with increases in glyphosate spraying to wheat crops since 1990.

And because celiac disease is linked with decreased populations of probiotic gut bacteria such as lactobacilli, bifidobacteria and enterococci, we can thus associate farmers' increased use of glyphosate – not only among wheat crops but also many other crops – with the dramatic increase of celiac disease among Western populations including the U.S. and the U.K.

Note that glyphosate is not sprayed onto organic food crops.

Increased Intestinal Permeability

Increased intestinal permeability is the scientific name for the less credible name of *leaky gut syndrome.* This is stated as *less credible* because we are not talking about the gut "leaking" as a balloon with a hole might leak.

As we've discussed the intestines were designed to absorb nutrients – through tiny gaps in the intestinal walls – normal intestinal permeability.

But in some of us, the intestines have increased permeability: They allow larger molecules through their gaps. Some of these larger molecules include complex, unbroken proteins from foods. In this case, we are speaking of gluten and gliadin proteins, which in healthy guts are broken down before they have contact with the intestinal wall.

So how do we know that gluten sensitivity is related to increased intestinal permeability? Numerous studies have connected the two.

In one of the earliest, researchers from Italy's University of Naples (Greco *et al.* 1991) tested 27 celiac patients who had been on a gluten-free diet for two years. They also tested 19 healthy control subjects. They tested lactulose/rhamnose ratios (see below) on the subjects before and after eating biscuits containing 50 grams of gluten each.

The researchers found that the gluten significantly changed the urinary excretion ratio of lactulose/rhamnose among the celiac patients – indicating increased intestinal permeability.

But in the healthy control group, there was no change in the lactulose/rhamnose ratio after eating the gluten-containing muffins.

This study result has been repeated over and over by researchers testing celiac patients and wheat allergy patients over the years. And over the years, the specific mechanisms of increased permeability have been discovered.

Fast forward to 2014, researchers from Spain's University of the Basque (Jauregi-Miguel *et al.*) discovered, in a study of 16 celiac patients and 16 healthy control subjects that there are genetic differences related to the tight junctions that regulate intestinal permeability between celiac patients and healthy persons. In particular, they found 23 genes related to the tight junctions that were different between the celiac patients and their healthy counterparts. These genetic differences confirmed the relationship between increased intestinal permeability and celiac gluten sensitivity.

The consensus of the research is that the gastrointestinal tract, from the mouth to the anus, is the primary defense mechanism against antigens as they enter the body. The mucous membrane integrity, the probiotic system, digestive enzymes, and the various immune cells and their mediators work together to orchestrate a "total defense" structure within the mucosal membrane. However, should this barrier be weakened or become imbalanced, hypersensitivity can result. The weaknesses in the barrier can be influenced by a number of factors, including pharmaceuticals, toxins, diet, genetics, and environmental factors (Chahine and Bahna 2010).

In other words, poor dietary choices, toxin exposures and environmental forces related to lifestyle and living conditions can wear down and thin this mucosal membrane. Once the membrane is damaged, the intestinal cells become exposed to the foods and toxins we consume.

The intestines also have a microscopic barrier function. The tiny spaces between the intestinal epithelial cells – composed of villi and microvilli – are sealed from the general intestinal contents with what are called tight junctions. As we discussed earlier, should the tight junctions open up, this barrier or seal will be broken.

When tight junctions are open – as they are normally open in the bladder or the colon – the wrong molecules can cross the epithelium through a transcellular pathway. Researchers have found more than 50-odd protein species among the tight junction. Should any of these proteins fail due to exposure to toxins, the barrier can break down, giving access to what are called macromolecules – molecules that are larger than nutrients that the intestinal cells, liver and bloodstream are accustomed to. Once these macromolecules access the intestinal tissues, they can stimulate an immune response: an inflammatory reaction.

The epithelial mucosal immune system has two anti-inflammatory strategies: The first is to block invaders using antibodies, probiotics and acids. This controls microorganism colonies and inhibits new invasions. The body's immune response counteracts local and peripheral hypersensitivity by attempting to remove them before a full inflammation attack is launched. This is referred to as oral tolerance when it is stimulated in the intestines.

The biochemical constituents of the mucosal membrane (glycoproteins, mucopolysaccharides and so on) also attach and escort nutrients across the intestinal barrier, while resisting the penetration of unrecognized and potentially harmful agents. Intestinal permeability allows molecules that are normally not able to cross the intestines' epithelial barrier access to the bloodstream.

When the intricate balance between the intestinal epithelial layer is destroyed by exposure and inflammation, abnormal protein antigens gain access to the intestinal subepithelial compartment. Here they stimulate the release of immune cells and degranulation (Yu 2009).

Let's examine the research supporting these conclusions:

Medical researchers at Norway's University of Bergen (Lillestøl *et al.* 2010) found that self-reported food hypersensitivity was highly associated with irritable bowel syndrome and intestinal permeability. Of the 71 adult subjects, 93% had irritable bowel syndrome and increased intestinal permeability, while 61% had atopic disease – primarily rhinoconjunctivitis. All the atopic sufferers had respiratory allergies, and 41% had food allergens.

Louisiana State University researchers (Chahine and Bahna 2010) found that the intestinal wall uses specific immunologic factors to defend the body against antigens. They showed that integrity of the mucous membrane lining of the intestine is critical. A defective lining, on the other hand, leads to allergic responses and hypersensitivity reactions, according to their research. They named the cause of these *"defects in the gut barrier."*

French researchers (Vivinus-Nébot *et al.* 2012) tested 34 IBS patients and 15 healthy volunteers. After collecting and testing biopsies of intestinal cells, they found that the severity of IBS symptoms correlated with the severity of intestinal permeability.

Medical researchers (Jackson *et al.* 1982) gave polyethylene glycol to eight eczema patients with food allergies and 10 patients with supposed non-allergic eczema in order to investigate intestinal permeability. Both groups absorbed macromolecules in excess of the normal subjects. They concluded that eczema with and without food allergy was associated with *"intestinal mucosal defects"* (increased intestinal permeability).

Hungarian researchers (Kovács *et al.* 1996) tested intestinal permeability among 35 food allergic patients and 20 healthy controls. Intestinal permeability was determined using EDTA. Of the 35, increased intestinal permeability was determined in 29 of the food allergy patients. Of these 29, 21 volunteers were tested for intestinal permeability five years later. IgA antibody titers were increased, among wheat, soy and oat antigens. Significant correlations between intestinal permeability and IgA antibody titers was found, especially against soy and oat proteins.

French researchers (Bodinier *et al.* 2007) studied wheat proteins with patients with intestinal permeability syndrome. They compared the translocation of native wheat proteins with those in a pepsin-hydrolyzed state. They found that the native wheat proteins were crossing the intestinal cell layer, and were able to associate this with their allergic responses.

Hospital Saint Vincent de Paul researchers (Dupont *et al.* 1991) pointed out in their research that the extent of intestinal permeability depends upon the molecule size and the state of the intestinal mucosa. Some intestinal *"porosity,"* as the researchers put it, is normal. However, when macromolecules that were normally not allowed to enter the bloodstream gained entry – primarily protein macromolecules – this stimulated the immune system, according to their research.

The Intestinal Permeability Index

So how do scientists and physicians test for increased intestinal permeability? Intestinal permeability is typically measured by giving the patient molecules that do not break down in the intestines. For example, alcohol-sugar combinations such as lactulose and mannitol are often used. These indicate intestinal permeability because of their different molecular sizes. After ingestion, the patient's urine is tested to measure the quantities that these two molecules were absorbed through the intestinal walls.

Because lactulose is a larger molecule than mannitol, it will thus be more present in the urine compared to mannitol when there is greater permeability of the intestinal wall. Intestines with normal permeability will have little lactulose absorption. This creates a ratio between lactulose and mannitol, which scientists call the L/M ratio. This L/M ratio is used to quantify intestinal permeability. When the lactulose-to-mannitol ratio is higher, more permeability exists. When it is lower, less (and normal) intestinal permeability exists. Higher levels are graduated using what many researchers call the *Intestinal Permeability Index.*

Other large molecule markers are also sometimes used to detect intestinal permeability using the same protocol of measuring recovery in the urine over a period of time (typically 5-6 hours). Substances used include polyethylene glycols of various molecular weights, horseradish peroxidase, EDTA (ethylenediaminetetraacetic acid), rhamnose, lactulose and cellobiose. Because these substances are not readily metabolized in the intestine or blood, and they also happen to have distinct molecular sizes – larger and smaller – they can also give accurate readings on the level of intestinal permeability. Let's see how researchers have used the Intestinal Permeability Index to discover how food sensitivities are related to intestinal permeability:

Researchers from Italy's University of Bari Medical School (Ventura *et al.* 2006) studied intestinal permeability among 21 patients with food allergies, and 20 patients with food intolerances who were on an allergen-free diet. They measured intestinal permeability using the L/M ratio from urinary excretion. Their results found a progressive state of intestinal permeability among all the allergy and food sensitive subjects. They also found that clinical symptoms were increased among those with higher scores on the Intestinal Permeability Index. In other words, intestinal permeability was greater among those with IgE food allergies with worse symptoms. This was also the case to a lesser degree among those with food intolerances.

Researchers from the Charité University Medical School in Berlin (Buhner *et al.* 2004) studied 55 patients with non-IgE allergic (food intolerant) chronic urticaria (hives). The researchers used a triple-sugar-test to determine duodenal permeability, and the lactulose/mannitol ratio to measure intestinal permeability. Gastroduodenal and intestinal permeability levels were both significantly higher among urticaria patients as compared to controls. After the 55 patients were given an allergen-free diet, 29 of the patients displayed reduced or eliminated skin eruptions. These 29 "responders" had significantly greater levels of intestinal permeability than those who did not respond to the diet.

Researchers from the Department of Pediatrics of the Cochin St Vincent de Paul Hospital in Paris (Kalach *et al.* 2001) studied intestinal permeability and cow's milk allergy among children as they aged. The research included 200 children who exhibited symptoms of cow's milk allergies. Of this 200, 95 were determined as allergic using challenge testing. This left 105 children as control subjects. The researchers measured intestinal permeability using the L/M ratio. They found that the L/M ratio was significantly greater among the milk-allergic children. Abnormal intestinal permeability levels were present among 80% of the milk-allergic children who had digestive symptoms, and 40% of children who exhibited anaphylactic symptoms. Furthermore, L/M ratios improved among older children who became more tolerant to milk.

Researchers from the French national research institute, INSERM (Andre *et al.* 1987) compared intestinal permeability between 90 healthy persons and 60 food allergy patients using the mannitol-lactulose test. In healthy subjects, the average urinary excretion of mannitol was 14.11% and of lactulose 0.26%. The food allergy patients had levels of 11.57% and 1.04% after eating a meal that included the allergen – a considerable difference from the healthy controls.

Researchers (Fälth-Magnusson *et al.* 1984) utilized sodium cromoglycate (a similar test to L/M) to determine intestinal permeability among 22 children between eight and ten years of age. Half of the children were previously diagnosed as allergic using history and laboratory tests. Half of the children were healthy. The sodium cromoglycate test revealed that the allergic children had significantly greater levels of intestinal permeability.

Researchers (Ukabam *et al.* 1984) used the lactulose-mannitol ratio to test 11 allergic eczema patients plus control subjects. Lactulose absorption was significantly greater among eczema patients, and their excretion ratios were significantly higher than control subjects. The researchers concluded that small intestinal permeability was greater among the patients with atopic eczema.

Medical researchers from Kuwait University (Hijazi *et al.* 2004) studied 32 asthmatic children together with 32 matched controls. The lactulose/mannitol test was performed to determine intestinal permeability. The asthmatic children had significantly higher levels of intestinal permeability.

Medical researchers from Italy's University of Naples (Troncone *et al.* 1994) tested intestinal permeability among 32 children aged from three months old to 84 months old. They utilized a ratio related to L/M called the cellobiose/mannitol (C/M) ratio. Of those who had allergy symptoms after a challenge with milk, 90% had significantly increased C/M ratios, indicating increased intestinal permeability.

INSERM scientists from the Lyon-Sud Center Hospital in France (Andre *et al.* 1991) compared 15 healthy volunteers with 20 food allergy patients using the L/M ratio. When both groups were fasting, there was little difference between their L/M indices. However, when the allergic group ingested food containing their allergen, the absorption of lactulose doubled among this group.

Researchers (Fälth-Magnusson *et al.* 1986) gave 16 children with milk allergies different-sized polyethyleneglycolsy molecules (approx. 400 and 1000 Daltons – the same principle as the L/M ratio), and then measured their urinary recovery over six hours. The children with the most severe allergic symptoms also had the greatest levels of permeability. The molecule and milk challenge among healthy children produced only minor permeability symptoms. In other words, the allergic subjects had significantly greater changes in the absorption of large molecules.

Researchers from France's St. Vincent de Paul Hospital (Dupont *et al.* 1989) measured intestinal permeability using mannitol and lactulose among 12 children with milk allergy, 28 children with atopic dermatitis and 39 healthy children. They found that while the allergy sufferers' L/M ratio was similar to the healthy group while fasting, intestinal permeability was three times higher than the healthy group when the allergic group drank milk.

Researchers (Pike *et al.* 1986) tested permeability among 26 children with food-sensitive atopic eczema together with 29 non-allergic children. This time they used urinary excretion rates of di- and monosaccharides lactulose and rhamnose after eating. The average absorption ratio was significantly higher among the 26 allergic children as compared with the control group of 29 children. The researchers concluded that:

> *"This increased permeability may be a primary abnormality of the gut or may reflect intestinal mucosal damage caused by local hypersensitivity reactions to food antigens."*

Intestinal Permeability and Other Disorders

French researchers (Heyman and Desjeux 2000) found that not only can intestinal permeability cause various disorders, disorders can worsen intestinal permeability. They pointed out that as undigested food antigens are transported through the intestinal wall, the immune system launches an inflammatory response. Intact proteins and large peptides, they pointed out, stimulate inflammation among the mucosa of the intestinal wall. IFN gamma and TNF alpha are cytokines that are often part of this inflammatory response. These two – IFN gamma and TNF alpha – also so happen to increase the further opening of the tight junctions.

Researchers from Ohio State University's Medical School (Zhou *et al.* 2009) studied 54 patients with irritable bowel syndrome along with 22 controls. They found those patients with higher pain intensity and higher levels of diarrhea also had greater levels of increased intestinal permeability.

Researchers from Brazil's Federal Fluminense Medical School (Soares *et al.* 2004) studied the associations between IBS and food intolerance. The researchers used 43 volunteers divided into three groups: an IBS group, a dyspepsia group, and a group without gastrointestinal difficulties. All test subjects were given skin prick tests for nine food allergens. The IBS group presented the highest level of positive allergen responses. The researchers concluded that:

> *"The higher reactivity to food antigens in group I compared to groups II and III suggests that intestinal permeability may be increased in patients with IBS."*

This link was also found at Nottingham University Hospital (Dunlop *et al.* 2006) when researchers tested 87 IBS sufferers and healthy controls. They found that 84% of diarrhea-predominant IBS patients had increased intestinal permeability.

Researchers (Forget *et al.* 1985) tested intestinal permeability using EDTA in ten normal adults, eleven healthy children, seven children with acute gastroenteritis, and eight infants with eczema. They found significantly greater intestinal permeability among those with either gastroenteritis or eczema.

Researchers from Paris' Cochin-St Vincent de Paul Hospital (Kalach *et al.* 2001) studied 64 children with cow's milk allergy symptoms, and found that higher intestinal permeability levels were also associated with anemia.

Researchers from London's Middlesex Medical School tested intestinal permeability among eight patients with food-intolerance using EDTA testing. While fasting levels were normal, after they ate the sensitive foods, permeability levels changed some, but not that significantly.

Researchers from Paris' Saint-Vincent de Paul Hospital (Barau and Dupont 1990) tested intestinal permeability using the lactulose and mannitol test with 17 children with irritable bowel syndrome (IBS). Of the 17, nine tested positive to IgE food allergies. Among these, permeability levels increased when the children were given foods they were sensitive to, illustrating the link between IBS, food allergies and intestinal permeability among many IBS sufferers.

Russian researchers (Sazanova *et al.* 1992) studied 122 children, four months old to six years old with food intolerances. Symptoms included atopic dermatitis among 52 children, and chronic diarrhea among 70 children. They found antibodies to food antigens among all the children. They also found chronic gastroduodenitis (duodenum and stomach inflammation) among every child with atopic dermatitis and among 95% of those with chronic diarrhea. They observed that lactase deficiencies and microorganism growth in the duodenum increased the levels of intestinal permeability and subsequent allergy response.

Increased Intestinal Permeability Immune Mechanisms

Once permeability is increased in the intestinal tract, there is no telling what the immune system will begin responding to. At this point it is likely that the immune system is greatly burdened by the many strange and different molecular structures now gaining entry into internal tissues and the bloodstream. What is known is that once permeability is increased, a self-perpetuating cycle of increased permeability and immune response produces more intestinal dysfunction and more immune response (Heyman 2005).

Researchers from Ontario's McMaster University (Berin *et al.* 1999) studied the role of cytokines in intestinal permeability. They found that interleukin-4

(IL-4) increased intestinal permeability and increased horseradish peroxidase (HRP) transport through intestinal walls. They found that IL-4 was inhibited by the soy nutrient genistein, and anti-IL-4 antibodies also reduced the HRP transport. The researchers concluded that: *"We speculate that enhanced production of IL-4 in allergic conditions may be a predisposing factor to inflammation by allowing uptake of luminal antigens that gain access to the mucosal immune system."*

Research has indicated that CD23 encourages the transport of intestinal IgE and allergens across intestinal epithelium. This opens a gateway for antigen-bound IgE to move across (transcytose) the intestinal cells. This sets up the immune response of histamine and atopic environmental conditions (Yu 2009).

Researchers from the University of Cincinnati College of Medicine (Groschwitz *et al.* 2009) determined that mast cells are critical to the regulation of the intestinal barrier function. The type and condition of the mast cells seems to affect the epithelial migration through intestinal cells.

Researchers from the Cincinnati Children's Hospital Medical Center (Forbes *et al.* 2008) found that interleukin-9 appears to help stimulate, along with mast cells, increased intestinal permeability. The researchers found that this *"IL-9- and mast cell-mediated intestinal permeability"* activated conditions for food allergen sensitization.

Thus we can conclude that food sensitivities – including gluten sensitivity – are symptoms of increased intestinal permeability.

What Causes Increased Intestinal Permeability?

The causative forces of increased permeability are a bit complicated. Infections, toxins, pharmaceuticals, probiotic deficiencies, breast milk deficiencies, metabolic stress and others have been identified as potential causes of increased intestinal permeability.

Accordingly, French INSERM researchers (Desjeux and Heyman 1994) concluded that increased protein permeability in milk allergies follows what they called *abnormal immunological response.* This abnormal immune response, they observed, leads to mucosal inflammation and a dysfunction of intestinal cellular endocytic processes (endocytosis is the process the cells undertake when they engulf or absorb amino acids and polypeptides).

The researchers based this conclusion on the observation that the milk protein beta-lactoglobulin stimulated lymphocytes that released increased levels of cytokines tumor necrosis factor-alpha (TNF alpha) and gamma interferon. The cytokines stimulated an inflammatory response that in turn disturbed the intestinal cell wall barrier.

In other words, first an irritating toxin, abnormal macromolecule or other stressor disrupts the intestinal mucous membrane. This produces inflammation, which in turn opens gaps in the intestinal barrier.

On a biochemical level, electrogenic chloride secretion is involved in an ion transport chain that stimulates the inflammatory prostaglandin E2 (PGE2) response within the intestinal mucosa. This secretion is balanced by the chloride channel blocker diphenylamine-2-carboxylate in healthy persons. In unhealthy persons, inflammatory cytokines alter the balance among intestinal barrier cells, with the effect of increasing permeability.

Medical researchers from the University Hospital in Groningen, The Netherlands (van Elburg *et al.* 1992) point out that the intestinal immunity mechanisms, which include IgA immunoglobulin and cell-mediated immune factors – and the brush barrier in general – do not completely mature until after about two years of age. Until this time, the barrier is sensitive to toxins and feeding problems.

Researchers from the Medical University of South Carolina (Walle and Walle 1999) found that mutagens formed when frying meat are implicated in opening the transport process in intestinal permeability. These mutagens, such as phenylimidazo-pyridine, were studied for their possible transport across human Caco-2 intestinal cells. The absorption was characterized as *"extensive and linear."* Equilibrium exchange tests showed that the mutagens form substrates with intestinal transporters. This indicates that these fried meat byproducts directly increase intestinal permeability.

A biochemistry researcher from Germany's Otto-von-Guericke University (Schönfeld 2004) discovered that dietary phytanic acid increases intestinal permeability through a function of ionic exchange and disruption of mitochondrial energy production. Damage to mitochondria may also explain the production of the inflammatory cytokine IL-4 within intestinal cells.

Researchers from the Department of Pediatrics at Italy's University of Federico II (Raimondi *et al.* 2008) found that bilirubin modifies the intestinal barrier. They also found among infants that cow's milk protein intolerance had higher levels of bilirubin and higher stool excretion. Those infants that had higher levels of bilirubin in the first year also had a greater risk of contracting cow's milk allergy.

To this, the French INSERM researchers added that stomach and upper intestinal infections with microorganisms such as *Helicobacter pylori* also increase intestinal permeability. Their observations led them to conclude that this was caused by an increased burden upon the immune system, and the resulting increase in inflammatory cytokines.

Medical researchers from Finland's University of Helsinki (Kuitunen *et al.* 1994) studied permeability using beta-lactoglobulin from cow's milk with 20 infants through eight months old or until they began weaning from breast milk. In one week after they weaned from breast milk, bovine beta-lactoglobulin levels were found in the bloodstream among 38% of the infants.

After two weeks, 21% retained beta-lactoglobulin in the bloodstream. The researchers concluded that: *"The gut may often be transiently permeable to BLG when cow's-milk-based formula is started."*

INSERM researchers from the Hospital Saint-Lazare (Heyman *et al.* 1988) studied intestinal permeability with milk allergy among infants. They tested 33 children ages one month to 24 months, which included 18 healthy infants and 15 with milk allergies, using the protein marker horseradish peroxidase and jejunal biopsies. No absorption permeability was seen in the control children over two months of age, illustrating that *"gut closure probably occurred earlier in life."* However, milk allergy children had about eight times the permeability levels than the control children.

The connection may lie in the health condition of the mother. French doctors (de Boissieu *et al.* 1994) reported that in one case, a 1-month-old breast-fed boy who had regurgitation, diarrhea, feeding difficulties, and malaise – typical of food sensitivities. They conducted intestinal permeability tests on mother and baby. These illustrated that the mother's breast milk induced intestinal permeability in the baby. The child's symptoms continued without improvement after the mother eliminated dairy products from her own diet. Then the mother withdrew egg and pork from her diet. This resulted in an almost immediate disappearance of allergy symptoms in the child. The doctors tested the child again for intestinal permeability after provocation with mother's milk (the same test done previously). Intestinal permeability levels were normal. The doctors concluded that allergens can be transferred from mother to baby through breast milk.

After extensive research, medical scientists from the Department of Internal Medicine at France's University Hospital suggest that the risk factors for severe anaphylaxis include agents that produce increased intestinal permeability – which they indicated include alcohol, aspirin, beta-blockers and angiotensin-converting enzyme (ACE) inhibitors.

Researchers from Rush University's Division of Gastroenterology and Nutrition and the Rush-Presbyterian-St. Luke's Medical Center in Chicago (DeMeo *et al.* 2002) has proposed that the gastrointestinal tract maintains one of the body's biggest areas that offers exposure to the outside environment. This is because everything we eat ends up at the intestinal wall. The Rush University researchers illustrated in their research that disruptions to the gut barrier follow injury to these mechanisms.

They further explained that this injury takes place from a number of causes, including non-steroidal anti-inflammatory drugs, free radical oxidation, adenosine triphosphate depletion (metabolic stress) and damage to the epithelial cell cytoskeletons that regulate tight junctions. They also pointed out evidence that associates gut barrier damage to immune dysfunction and sepsis

– infection from microorganisms. This of course alludes to the defenses provided by our probiotic microorganisms, which keep populations of infective microorganisms minimized – as we'll discuss in detail later.

Medical researchers from the University of Southampton School of Medicine (Macdonald and Monteleone 2005) have suggested that this epidemic of intestinal permeability among industrialized nations has been creating genetic mutations that produce greater levels of permeability among successive generations. This of course, provides the link between greater levels of allergies among those with allergic parents.

Thus we can conclude that intestinal permeability is not simply a creative explanation for allergies made without substantiation. It is a scientifically proven fact.

Is IIPS always involved in gluten sensitivities?

But intestinal permeability may not be a big factor in non-celiac non-wheat allergy gluten sensitivities This was found in a study of 42 celiac disease patients tested together with 26 people who were non-celiac gluten sensitive along with 39 healthy control subjects.

The researchers qualified the gluten intolerant patients by conducted a food challenge. The gluten intolerant patients were also screened and confirmed that none had any positive antibodies to tTG or gliadin as did the celiac patients. The gluten intolerant patients were also screened for any intestinal mucosa issues – they all had healthy intestinal cells and no sign of inflammation. Those who had any of these issues were excluded from the study.

The researchers used the lactulose/mannitol ratio test to determine intestinal permeability. They also conducted biopsies of each patient before and after testing.

The researchers found the celiac disease patients had significantly greater intestinal permeability compared with the healthy control group. However, the gluten sensitive group did not have increased intestinal permeability compared with the healthy group.

This doesn't mean there weren't differences. The gluten intolerant group had different L/M ratio characteristics, indicating there was something different taking place with respect to their intestinal walls.

But remember that the gluten intolerant group had also been screened out to exclude anyone who had any signs of intestinal inflammation. This would certainly also exclude those with greater intestinal permeability as well. They excluded anyone with symptoms of inflammatory bowel disease.

As we've shown, gluten sensitivities are often related to inflammatory conditions such as IBS and others – and these have been related to increased intestinal permeability.

But this study illustrates that non-celiac, non-wheat allergy gluten sensitivities may not always involve increased intestinal permeability.

And this is important because while there is a definite association between IIPS and celiac disease and wheat allergies – we cannot necessarily say all gluten sensitivities involve IIPS.

But because celiac disease and wheat allergies are verifiable conditions with conclusive mechanisms, and gluten sensitivities are to this date unverified as to any particular mechanism – we can state clearly that IIPS is related to gluten sensitivities that have been verified as inflammatory immune-system related disorders.

The other gluten intolerance symptoms, as we've discussed, can be related to a number of other issues – as we will lay out in this chapter.

Candida Overgrowth

Overgrowths of yeasts like *Candida albicans* can also contribute to or be a primary cause for wheat intolerances and even wheat allergies in progressive cases. *Candida albicans* can grow in our guts and elsewhere conjunctively with *Staphylococcus aureus*. This often results in the accelerated growth of both pathogenic microorganisms.

Yeast overgrowths also often accompany the overgrowths of bacteria such as *E. coli* and *B. fragilis*.

This can result in a tremendous burden for the immune and probiotic systems as they try to defend against the incursion of the combined fungi and bacteria infections, along with the various waste streams they produce.

We see this lethal combination of microorganisms involved in many of the fatalities from other outbreaks. The deaths typically occur in immunosuppressed patients with concurrent bacteria infections.

This type of immunosuppression is also related to food sensitivity.

As the immune system becomes overloaded with a microorganism invasion, it will often respond with an acute inflammatory response, simply because the system is already on alert mode. This produces a number of inflammatory-type symptoms.

This shouldn't be confused with baker's yeasts. Baker's yeast (*Saccharomyces cerevisiae*) is typically healthy and even probiotic for most people. It is commonly used to prepare a variety of foods, including many breads. *S. cerevisiae* is also found within the colons of healthy people, and is thus considered as a probiotic microorganism.

Like any microorganism, however, there must exist a balance between the species and strains within the gut in order the maintain health. Persons without that balance, or who have become infected with overgrowths of other not-so-probiotic yeast colonies such as *Candida spp.*, may become sensitive to foods containing yeast. Yeast sensitivities may also yield or be a symptom of other intestinal problems.

Australian researchers from Ninewells Hospital and Medical School (McKenzie *et al.* 1990) studied IgG antibodies in 15 Crohn's disease patients, 15 patients with ulcerative colitis, and 15 healthy subjects. They exposed the subjects to 12 strains of yeast (*Saccharomyces cerevisiae*). They found the Crohn's patients had heightened IgG antibodies to 11 of the 12 *S cerevisiae* strains.

However, to state that baking yeasts cause gluten sensitivities would be unfair. However, for those who have Candida overgrowth and poor probiotic populations, baker's yeast can imbalance these populations even further, producing dysbiosis, which is related to increased intestinal permeability and a lack of enzymes available to break down the gluten proteins before they are presented to the intestinal walls.

Mucoid Plaque

Mucin and mucus are the substances that line our intestines – providing a layer of protection over intestinal walls. These are produced by the body to protect the intestinal walls from the acidic environment of the intestine and colon. Much of this mucin and mucus is secreted by Brunner's glands located in the duodenum. These glands are stimulated by changes in pH. They harmonically work to balance the pH of the intestinal tract, as an acidic environment will damage the intestinal wall.

Because the stomach produces various acids to break down food and kill microorganisms, the Brunner's glands typically provide just enough mucin and mucous to balance everything and provide enough protection.

However if the food we eat itself has too much acidic quality – such as overly-processed foods with high acid content – these glands will produce more mucus and mucin to counteract the acidity. This extra production provides the glue for the plaque throughout the intestinal and colon walls.

How do we know if we have mucoid plaque? The first sign is the size of our stool. If the stool is runny and not solid, or perhaps pencil-thin as a norm, then it is likely there is a build up of mucoid plaque preventing our stools from forming correctly. Another giveaway is chronic constipation or irregular bowel movements. Bloating also indicates a strong possibility of mucoid plaque build-up.

And this directly relates to gluten sensitivity because this build up of mucoid plaque will harm colon and intestinal cells, and in general, produce an inflammatory environment within the digestive tract.

Remember that a build up of mucin and mucoid plaque will accompany a build up of toxic byproducts such as lipopolysaccharides, which are basically endotoxins – the toxic waste stream of pathogenic bacteria.

A diseased mucoid plaque layer will also slow the passage and elimination of toxic byproducts from the small intestines through to the colon and excretion in bowel movements. This will leave the small intestine environment with increased toxicity. As intestinal walls become exposed to this level of toxicity, an inflammatory situation is set up. Furthermore, the mucosal membranes protecting the intestinal wall become weaker, allowing more exposure to the intestinal cells by macromolecules, in addition to a decrease in enzymes produced by probiotic bacteria.

In addition, because a thickened mucoid plaque layer will cause an increased absorption of these endotoxins, symptoms that are often attributed to gluten sensitivity become likely: including bloating, headaches, chronic fatigue and so on. This has been illustrated in several studies.

For example, medical researchers from Thailand (Maes *et al.* 2012) tested 128 chronic fatigue patients with fibromyalgia. The researchers found that nearly all of the patients had inflammatory IgA responses to lipopolysaccharides, and the degree of their IgA sensitivity was directly associated with the severity of their chronic fatigue and fibromyalgia.

This is because, as explained earlier, the buildup of waste products and pathogenic bacteria within this layer of plaque will release bacteria endotoxins into our bloodstream, which will produce inflammatory responses around the body and in general, overload the body's detoxification systems and immune system.

Dietary Causes of Food Sensitivities

Remember that gluten sensitivity is a food sensitivity. The relationships that exist between food sensitivities and diet also relate to gluten sensitivities.

Our diets directly affect our immune system strength and the health of our intestines. As we will read in the studies below, our diet, our childhood diet, and the diet of our mother during pregnancy and breastfeeding plays a significant role in our risk of food sensitivities. The mechanisms, as we have been discussing, relate to the immune system and the health of our intestines. An exhausted immune system will inevitably react differently than a strong immune system to a perceived foreigner.

Let's look at some of the research supporting these conclusions:

Researchers from the University of Western Australia and the Princess Margaret Hospital (Jennings and Prescott 2010) reviewed the clinical data regarding diet and environmental changes with respect to autoimmunity and food allergies. They concluded that dietary factors such as omega-3 fatty acids, oligosaccharides, probiotics, vitamin D, retinoic acid and various antioxidants in foods stimulate and assist immune function and the development of the immune system; and inherently decrease the risk of food allergies.

In a study of 460 children and mothers on Menorca – a Mediterranean island in Spain – medical researchers from Greece's Department of Social Medicine and the University of Crete (Chatzi *et al.* 2008) found that children of mothers eating primarily a Mediterranean diet (a predominantly plant-based diet) had significantly fewer food and other allergies. In fact, the higher the adherence to the Mediterranean diet during pregnancy, the fewer the allergies among the children.

The same researchers (Chatzi *et al.* 2007) surveyed the parents of 690 children from ages seven through 18 years old in the rural areas of Crete. The children also were tested with skin prick tests for 10 common allergens. They found that consuming a Mediterranean diet reduced the risk of allergic rhinitis by over 65%. The risk of skin allergies and respiratory conditions (such as wheezing) also reduced, but by smaller amounts. They also found that a greater consumption of nuts among the children cut wheezing rates in half, while consuming margarine more than doubled the prevalence of both wheezing and allergic rhinitis.

Remember the research showing that food sensitivities directly relate to asthma occurrence. Asthmatic parents increase the risk of food sensitivities among their children. Children who outgrow their milk allergy are more likely to contract asthma a few years later. Those with early allergies have a greater likelihood of later food sensitivities than those who don't.

An international group of researchers from around the world (Nagel *et al.* 2010) reported in the International Study on Allergies and Asthma in Childhood (ISAAC) that asthma occurrence is related to diet. The group conducted cross-sectional studies between 1995 and 2005 in 29 locations within 20 different countries. In all, 50,004 children ages eight through twelve years old were analyzed.

This study revealed that those with diets containing large fruit portions had lower incidence of asthma. This link occurred among both affluent and non-affluent countries. Fish consumption in affluent countries (where vegetable intake is less) and cooked green vegetables among non-affluent countries were also associated with a lower asthma rates. In general, the consumption of fruit, vegetables and fish was linked with reduced rates of asthma throughout life.

Consuming the Mediterranean diet (a diet with plenty of plant-based foods and healthy oils) has clear results: It is linked with lower allergy and asthma rates.

These associations also confirm the well-researched relationship between a diet rich in antioxidants and strengthened immunity in general.

Lack of Phytonutrients

The connection between phytonutrient deficiency and food sensitivities has been confirmed by a plethora of research. Here are a few examples.

In a study by researchers from Korea's Kyung Hee University (Oh *et al.* 2010), atopic dermatitis – many related to food sensitivities – among young children was studied together with antioxidant intake. One hundred eighty children at an average age of five years old were studied. Several antioxidant-related nutrients were found to lower the risk of allergic dermatitis.

Beta carotene reduced the risk of atopic dermatitis by 56%. Vitamin E reduced the risk of atopic dermatitis by 67%. Folic acid reduced the risk by 63%. Iron reduced the risk of atopic dermatitis by 61%. Retinol and alpha-tocopherol reduced the risk by 26% and 36%, respectively. Vitamin C did not produce any reduction of risk.

Researchers from the Medical University of Vienna (Diesner *et al.* 2010) concluded after a study conducted inside a nursing home, that food sensitivities are under-diagnosed and under-estimated among elderly persons. They also recognized that deficiencies in certain micronutrients such as zinc, iron, vitamin D and others among the aging or elderly appear to contribute to allergy development.

The researchers commented that a less active digestive system resulting from gastritis or anti-ulcer medication could also be a contributing factor. Undigested or partially digested proteins may become subject to an immunoglobulin response.

Refined Foods

Processing of a food typically consists of chopping or pulverizing the food, heating it to high temperatures, distilling or extracting its contents, or otherwise isolating some parts of the food by straining off, clarifying or refining.

We discussed earlier how many foods in Western diets are processed, and thus lacking in their essential fibers and nutrients, producing disproportionate levels of simple carbohydrates. The research has shown that these can produce an increased risk of cardiovascular disease, insulin sensitivity and lack of glucose control.

We can also relate processed forms of flour are also part of the cause of the problem of gluten sensitivity. This is because these foods deliver a disproportionate amount of gluten-related proteins as compared to those whole versions containing a full array of nutrients, fiber and arabinoxylans, the later of which feeds our probiotics – and produce the enzymes that break down gluten proteins. When these are included, probiotics are nourished and become active by producing the enzymes which break down the macromolecules that we can become sensitive to.

We might add that while enriching refined flour certainly does help, it does not remove the imbalance that refining creates in the way of other content. In addition, the forms of B vitamins – such as folic acid – are not the forms our body is accustomed to. – as opposed to nature's version and the version whole wheat supply – folate.

Food processing is typically considered by humans as a good thing, because humans like to focus on one or two characteristics or nutrients of a food as making up that food's intrinsic value. In the end it is a value proposition, because all the energy and work required to produce the final food product must equal or be greater than the increase in the processed food's value.

Typically this increase in value is due to the food being sweeter, smoother or simply easier to eat or mix with other foods. In the case of oils or flours, the food extract is used for baking purposes, for example. In the case of sugar, which is extracted from a number of whole plants, including cane and beets, it is added to nearly every refined processed food.

Ironically, what is left behind in this value proposition is the food's real value. The fiber and nutrients are typically stripped away during food processing. As we've discussed, plant fiber is a necessary element of our diet, because it renders sterols and lignans that aid digestion and reduce LDL cholesterol. Many nutrients are attached to food fiber. Once the fiber is stripped away, the food's nutrients can be easily damaged by the heat of processing.

What is being missed in the value proposition of food processing is that nature's whole foods have their greatest value when minimally processed. When a food is over-processed, many of the molecular bonds that hold the food's fibers and polysaccharides are lost. As these bonds are lost, the remaining components can lose their buffering agents and become radicalized or unstable in the body. When some of these become unstable, they can form free radicals, requiring our bodies to neutralize them. This produces instability elsewhere in the body, and places a burden upon our immune system.

In other words, *whole foods* provide the nutrients our bodies need, in the combinations already provided by nature. In some cases, we might need to physically peel a food to get to its edible part. In other cases, such as in the case of grains, we may need to remove the husk and heat or cook the whole grains to soften the fibers to enable chewing and digestion. In the case of wheats, milling or cracking the whole grain (including the bran and the epicarp hair) will render a healthier flour.

Because many of our processed foods have been in our diet for many decades, it is difficult to prove that a diet of processed food produces more food allergies. In an attempt to test this hypothesis, a more historically recent processed food must be tested.

French researchers (Fremont *et al.* 2010) attempted this by studying the effects of processed flax. This is because foods containing processed flax are somewhat of a new phenomenon.

So they studied the introduction of processed flax into the French diet. They found that, in a study of 1,317 patients with allergies, those who were allergic to flax could be identified by their sensitivity to *extruded, heated flax,* rather than raw flax seed.

This of course indicates that the increase in flax allergies is likely related to the increase in *processed flax* rather than the increased availability of flax in general, as first hypothesized. Certainly, over time, as flax allergies proceed, there will be more allergies to raw flax. But now, while flax exposure is fairly recent, allergies to processed flax indicates that processing increases the risk of food allergies.

We can also see how processing increases diseases when we compare the disease statistics of developing countries with developed countries.

For example, like many developing countries, India now has more heart disease because of increased consumption of refined flours and fried foods. These processed foods damage intestinal health and promote free radicals. They are nutrient-poor. They burden and starve our probiotics. Frying foods also produces a carcinogen called acrylamide (Ehling *et al.* 2005).

Refined Sweeteners

The Western processed diet is also laden with refined sugars. Today, nearly every pre-cooked recipe found in mass market grocery stores contains refined sugar. Many brands now try to white-wash the massive sugar content of their products by calling their sugar content "all natural." This is a deception, because nature in the form of fiber has been unnaturally stripped away from their refined sugars. This is hardly a "natural" proposition.

Research has linked refined sugars to diabetes, obesity, kidney diseases, Candida and many other conditions (Lustig *et al.* 2012). This is hardly news to those who have investigated natural health literature.

Nature attaches sugars to complex fibers, polysaccharides and nutrients in such a way that prevents them from easily attaching to proteins. Sugars that are cooked and stripped of these complexes are assimilated too quickly, and drive the pancreas to produce and even overproduce insulin. This has the effect of stressing the pancreas. Refined sugars also stress the liver that feeds the pancreas, and stresses the detoxification processes that must metabolize the insulin, glucose and glycogen byproducts. All of this slows down the body's immunity and detoxification processes.

Refined sugars also feed pathogenic microorganisms. While our probiotics feed on oligosaccharides such as FOS, GOS and others, pathogenic microorganisms tend to feed on refined sugars. This is the case for Clostridium and Candida microorganisms – whose colonies are enlarged and promoted by sugar.

Glycation End Products

Refined sugars also become immediate unnatural glycation candidates within the body as they combine with proteins and become glycated.

As our digestive system combines refined sugars with proteins, many of the glycated proteins are identified as foreign by IgA or IgE antibodies in immune-burdened physiologies. Why are they considered foreign? Because glycated proteins and their AGE end products damage blood vessels, tissues and brain cells. In this case, the immune system is launching an inflammatory attack in an effort to protect us from our own diet!

There is no surprise that glycation among foods and in the body is connected with systemic inflammation. It is also no accident that the increased consumption of overly-processed foods and manufacturing processes that pulverize and strip foods of their fiber; and blend denatured proteins and sugars using high-heat processes has increased as our rates of inflammatory diseases have increased over the past century.

In fact, this connection between inflammatory diseases and processed foods has been observed clinically by natural physicians over the years. They may not have understood the precise mechanics, however. Many of these reputable health experts have categorized the effect of processed foods as one of acidifying the bloodstream. The concept was that denatured and over-processed foods produced more acids in the body.

This thesis did not go over too well among scientific circles, because the acidification mechanism was not scientifically confirmed, and there was no concrete mechanism.

Well this can now change, as we are providing the science showing both the mechanism and the evidence that glycation end products do produce acidification in terms of peroxidation radicals that damage cells and tissues.

We should note that a healthy form of natural glycation also takes place in the body to produce certain nutrient combinations. Unlike the radical-forming glycation formed by food manufacturing and refined sugar intake, this type of glycation is driven by the body's natural enzyme processes, resulting in molecules and end products the body uses and recognizes. When glycation is driven by the body's own enzyme processes, it is termed *glycosylation,* however.

Researchers from France's University of Burgundy (Rapin and Wiernsperger 2010) have confirmed that protein or lipid glycation produced by modern food manufacturers is linked to food sensitivities.

Glycation is produced during the manufacturing of food products, specifically when sugars and protein-foods are heated to extremely high temperatures during cooking or filling. During glycation, sugars bind to protein molecules. This produces a glycated protein and glycation end products, both of which have been implicated in cardiovascular disease, diabetes, some cancers, peripheral neuropathy and Alzheimer's disease (Miranda and Outeiro 2010).

In Alzheimer's disease, one of the products of a glycation reaction is the amyloid protein. Glycation end products introduced to the cerebrospinal fluid have been directly implicated in the process of amyloid plaque build up among brain cells.

Glycation also takes place within the body. This occurs especially in diets containing high levels of refined sugars combined with considerable amounts of cooked or caramelized proteins.

The Western diet contains an incredible amount of processed protein compared to traditional diets. Americans eat far beyond the amount of protein required for health. Studies indicate that Americans eat an average of 80-150 grams of protein a day. This is significantly higher than the 25-50 grams of protein consumed in most healthy traditional diets around the world (Campbell and Campbell 2006; McDougall 1999).

This amount of protein in the American diet is also significantly higher than even U.S. RDA levels. The U.S. recommended daily allowance for protein is 0.8 grams per 2.2 lbs of body weight. This converts to 54 grams for a person weighing 150 pounds. Americans eat on average nearly double that amount.

To this we can add the sugar-laden Western diet. Today, nearly every precooked recipe found in the mass market grocery stores contains refined sugar. Even processed organic foods contain organic cane syrup – a form of sugar that may not be as refined as white sugar, but is definitely refined, and stripped of the natural plant fibers in cane or beets.

Today, many brands are trying to white-wash the massive sugar content of their products by calling their sugar content "all natural." This is a deception, because nature in the form of fiber has been unnaturally stripped away from their refined sugar. This is hardly a "natural" proposition. Nature attaches sugars to complex fibers and nutrients in such a way that prevents them from easily attaching to proteins. Sugars that are cooked and stripped of their fibers become immediate glycation candidates within the body.

As our digestive system combines these sugars with proteins, many of the glycated proteins are identified as foreign by IgA, or IgE antibodies in immune-burdened or inflammatory intestines. Why are they considered foreign? Because, as we've mentioned, glycated proteins and their AGE end products damage blood vessels, tissues, brain cells and also stimulate cancerous cells. So the immune system is simply trying to protect us from our own diet!

There is no surprise that glycation among foods – and the glycation that occurs within the body as a result of the heavy consumption of refined proteins and sugars – is connected with the increase of allergies among Western societies over the past few decades. This has occurred with the increased consumption of overly-processed foods and manufacturing processes that pulverize and strip foods of their fiber; and blend denatured proteins and sugars using heating processes.

Food Additives

This is a large topic, because so many processed foods are chock full of many different artificial additives. These include hundreds of artificial food colors, preservatives, stabilizers, flavorings and a variety of food processing aids. A number of these additives have been found to cause sensitivities in some people.

Illustrating the effects that food additives can have, Australian researchers (Dengate and Ruben 2002) studied 27 children with irritability, restlessness, inattention and sleep difficulties. The researchers saw many of these symptoms subside after putting the children on the Royal Prince Alfred Hospital Diet, which is absent of food additives, natural salicylates, amines and glutamates.

Using preservative challenges, the researchers were also able to determine that the preservatives significantly affected the children's behavior and physiology adversely.

Researchers from Britain's University of Southampton (Bateman *et al.* 2004) screened 1,873 three-year old children for hyperactivity and the consumption of artificial food colors and preservatives. They gave the children 20 mg daily of artificial colors and 45 mg daily of sodium benzoate, or a placebo mixture. The additive group showed significantly higher levels of hyperactivity than the group that did not consume the artificial colors and preservative.

While these studies are not proof that these food additives are allergens, we can say that with confidence that they can cause food intolerances, as hyperactivity is considered a reaction to eating these "foods."

Once an additive has caused intolerance symptoms such as those from the research above, there is always the possibility that the immune system may begin to become sensitive to some of the foods these additives are associated with. This likelihood increases should the immune system become continually exposed to the foods together with the additives over a considerable period of time.

Sulfites

Sulfites provide a classic case of harmful additives. Yes, the sulfite ion will aggressively preserve a food. Sulfites can also produce wheezing, tightness of the throat and other symptoms almost immediately after eating foods preserved with them. However, the effects of sulfites may not be as significant as often portrayed. It may well be that many sulfite-sensitivities seen among wine drinkers are actually the product of the alcohol rather than the sulfites.

Illustrating this, researchers from Australia's Centre for Asthma (Vally *et al.* 2007) tested eight wine-sensitive subjects with sulfite wine and non-sulfite wine. The researchers found that the wine sensitivities were unlikely caused by the sulfites in the wine.

Today, sulfites are used to preserve many wines, dehydrated potatoes and numerous dried fruits. Sulfites include potassium bisulfite, sulfur dioxide, potassium matabisulfite and others. Often labels do not disclose the use of sulfites, because the preservative may have been used early in the processing of the raw ingredients instead of added into the finished product. In addition, under current U.S. labeling laws, if an ingredient such as sulfite is less than 10 parts per million, there is no requirement for putting the ingredient on the panel.

Sulfite sensitivity may be the result of B12 deficiency. In a study presented to the American Academy of Allergy and Immunology, 18 sulfite-sensitive persons were given sublingual B12. The B12 effectively blocked adverse reactions to sulfites in 17 of the 18 (Werbach 1996).

Monosodium Glutamate

Monosodium glutamate also gets a lot of attention for producing sensitivity symptoms. This has also been echoed among a number of studies.

To better understand this, Harvard researchers (Geha *et al.* 2000) set out to study the effects of MSG sensitivities in a multi-center study. They found that of 130 human volunteers who thought they were sensitive to MSG, 38% physically responded to MSG with allergic symptoms. However, 13% also responded to a placebo (they thought contained MSG). Subsequent retesting continued to show inconsistent responses among some of those who thought they were MSG-sensitive.

This led the researchers to conclude that people who believe they are sensitive tend to react more strongly to MSG, but their responses were not always consistent. This of course may be the result of differing levels of tolerance and periods of sensitivity – again depending upon immunity.

This research still confirms that MSG can cause sensitivity responses. Possibly MSG may be overhyped somewhat, but like so many other food additives, there is no doubt that it is not a natural part of our food supply.

However, when MSG comes into contact with yeast colonies such as Candida, there maybe another issue altogether, because yeast utilize the glutamates as stimulants. This may well be the link between MSG and intestinal issues, as those yeast colonies expand. In fact, some of the symptom complaints with those sensitive to MSG sound a lot like endotoxin responses.

Wheat Allergen Exposures

As we will show in this section, a person can become sensitive to wheats or gluten by becoming exposed to airborne or topic wheat allergen exposure.

When wheat proteins are breathed into the lungs and sinuses – especially when the immune system is overloaded – the body may react by forming allergic-type immunoglobulins.

We should add to this that a similar reaction can occur in response to a topical (skin) exposure to certain food proteins.

In both of these cases, however, we should note that airborne or skin exposure to other types of food proteins can also cause allergies to that food. This is notable among exposure to lipid transfer proteins – which relate to pollen exposure. These can result in food allergies to apples, peaches, kiwifruit, melon, cherries and many other fruits and vegetables.

But there are many other airborne exposures that can also produce food allergies to other foods besides wheats.

For example, Spanish allergy researchers (Prieto *et al.* 2010) found that lupin inhalation from manufacturing facilities caused sensitization to lupin proteins, which carried over to food sensitivities to lupin-related foods and lupin flour-containing foods.

Polish researchers (Swiderska-Kiełbik *et al.* 2010) found those who have occupational contact working with birds in zoos, facilities that slaughter birds, or pet birds, are significantly more likely to develop allergies to eggs, feathers and other related allergens.

Researchers from France's Nancy Central Hospital Immunology Clinic (Moneret-Vautrin *et al.* 1996) estimated that while food allergy-related asthma is less common than food allergy-related atopic dermatitis, there is an 8.5% incidence of food allergies among asthma sufferers. This also connects airborne sensitivities with food sensitivities.

Furthermore, the researchers pointed out that occupational exposure to inhaled food proteins is increasing. They advised that egg protein or feather inhalation is particularly risky. Among adults, food allergies are common after bronchi become sensitized to either food allergen inhalation or cross-reactive pollen allergens.

They also reported latex as a cross-allergen. They documented that intestinal permeability caused by viral infections, aspirin, alcohol, and other toxins is a typical precursor to these cross-reactive sensitizations.

This conclusion confirms the premise that immunosuppression caused by the exposure to the unnatural increase in synthetic toxins can produce increased sensitivity to food allergens, especially those available from abnormal situations.

Furthermore, research from Italy's University of Ferrara (Boccafogli *et al.* 1994), Japan's Yokohama City University Hospital (Maeda *et al.* 2010) and many others that indicated airborne allergens such as pollen can crossover to food allergies once sensitized.

We can conclude that the abnormal inhalation of proteins, either as pollens or from milled, cooked or ground foods, can increase the likelihood of food sensitivities related to those proteins or pollens (also proteins) inhaled. The risk is significantly higher among immunosuppressed people.

Whether it is through airborne or topical exposure: Later, when those proteins are eaten, a immunological response may result as the antibodies stimulate an allergic response – even if that protein or food is able to be properly digested.

Such immunological responses may occur with IgAs or IgEs, but severe cases are typical IgE related. Let's look at two such types of exposures.

Baker's Asthma

Studies over the past few decades have uncovered a condition that is prevalent among those who work with wheat flour – often termed baker's asthma. This is similar to respiratory diseases related to dust in many other occupations such as mining. Because breathing in practically any large particulate – whether it is from food, rocks or even sand – can produce an immune response to those substances.

The notable difference is that baking flour is also a food.

When a baker or mill worker breathes in too much flour dust over time or their immune system is otherwise overloaded, the body can produce IgEs to the microparticles. This response is similar to other particulates.

In some of the cases of wheat flour, the person may become allergic to eating wheat proteins. For example, researchers from Italy's University of Verona (Olivieri *et al.* 2013) tested 81 bakers who had allergic symptoms to baking flour. They used skin prick testing along with IgE testing.

They found that 28 of the bakers had positive skin prick sensitivity to wheat proteins, and 51 had IgE antibodies reactive to wheat proteins.

Many of the bakers showed allergic symptoms such as dermatitis (hives, rashes and/or eczema) and asthmatic issues, produced by their sensitivities.

Many with these baker's asthma wheat sensitivities also have allergic responses when wheat foods are eaten. In other words, wheat allergy.

Hydrolyzed Wheat Proteins

While digestive enzymes and those produced by probiotics hydrolyze proteins through enzymatic processes, manufacturers can synthetically break down proteins by extrusion, heating and blending with a variety of processing aids. These can also include enzymes. These processes synthetically break apart the proteins. As water is integrated into the process, synthetic hydrolysis results, leaving hydrolyzed amino and peptide substrates.

This produces what have been termed hydrolyzed wheat proteins. These synthetically hydrolyzed proteins are often used in skin lotions, makeup and otherwise topical creams. In sensitive people or those whose immune systems are overloaded, those hydrolyzed wheat proteins may produce wheat sensitivities when they are applied on the skin over time.

While this is using the word *synthetic* loosely – as some of the enzymes used to hydrolyze wheat proteins may be derived from bacteria – the purpose is to distinguish it from what our body does. Our digestive enzymes hydrolyze proteins – whether produced by bacteria or not – differently. In our bodies, the broken-off amino acids and small peptide combinations are bound to intestinal escorts and brought into the bloodstream. They are absorbed, in other words and immediately utilized by the body, while unneeded hydrolysis byproducts are escorted out through the colon.

When proteins are hydrolyzed during manufacturing, the hydrolyzed aminos and peptides and hydrolysis byproducts can become radicalized after they have been broken off. Unless of course they are handled appropriately – which is what processors of infant hydrolyzed protein formulas do.

To explain this further: When molecules are broken up, the parts still typically need to be chemically combined. This is related to their need to share electrons with other atoms – their covalency. They still need to be bound to something. So they seek those chemicals or tissues that will provide a means to share electrons. In the case of some hydrolyzed proteins and hydrolysis byproducts, if they come into contact with our skin or airways, they might threaten our tissues and provoke an immunological response. This is because their electron-sharing may disrupt the molecules of our tissues.

French laboratory researchers (Bouchez-Mahiout *et al.* 2010) found by using immunoblot testing that hydrolyzed wheat proteins from skin conditioners can produce hypersensitivity, which eventually crossed over to allergies to wheat proteins in foods.

In other words, hydrolyzed wheat proteins in skin treatments are not necessarily recognized by the immune system. Once the body becomes sensitized to these hydrolyzed wheat proteins from skin absorption, this sensitivity can cross over to sensitivity to similar wheat proteins in foods.

Researchers from France's Center for Research in Grignon (Laurière *et al.* 2006) tested nine women who had skin contact sensitivity to cosmetics containing hydrolyzed wheat proteins (HWP). Six were found to react with either skin hives or anaphylaxis to different products (including foods) containing HWP. The whole group also had IgE sensitivity to wheat flour or gluten-type proteins. The tests showed that they had become sensitive not only to HWP, but also to unmodified grain proteins. As they tested further, they found that reactions often occurred among larger wheat protein peptide aggregates.

The researchers concluded that the use of HWP in skin products can produce hypersensitivity not only to HWP, but this sensitivity can crossover to sensitivities to seemingly unrelated wheat proteins in foods.

This allergic response to hydrolyzed proteins does not only happen with wheats. Spanish researchers (Cabanillas *et al.* 2010) found that enzymatic hydrolysis of lentils and chickpeas produced allergens for four out of five allergic patients in their research.

The commercial enzymes used for hydrolysis by many food manufacturers may also stimulate allergic responses. Danish researchers (Bindslev-Jensen *et al.* 2006) tested 19 commercially available enzymes typically used in the food industry on 400 adults with allergies. It was found that many of the enzymes produced histamine responses among the patients.

Lipid Transfer Proteins

We mentioned LTPs with respect to other foods above, but wheat and cereal grasses can also provide lipid transfer proteins within their pollen. This can translate to food sensitivities to wheats.

LTPs are portions of pollen and food molecules that a weakened immune system can become sensitized to. Once a sensitization reaction occurs, these LTPs are then recognized by the immune system as being antigens, or invaders – effectively stimulating an allergic reaction every time a similar LTP-containing food is eaten. Worse, becoming sensitized to one type of LTP can also cross over to becoming sensitized to other LTPs in foods.

In one study from Italy (Asero *et al.* 2009) 25,601 allergy clinic patients throughout Italy were tested. Almost 50% had allergic skin reactions and 8.5% had IgE-mediated allergic reactions to food. Of these, 64% were female. Most of their food sensitivities were related to lipid transfer proteins.

The Italian study showed that pollen-related food LTP sensitivities occurred in a whooping 55% of all allergy sufferers among Italians. LTP allergy rates are seemingly lower among Northern European countries and the U.S. This is no surprise, since Italy is a big agricultural producer. It is considered by some to be the breadbasket of Western Europe.

However, the research is increasingly illustrating that LTP exposures may very well be at the root of many food sensitivities, including wheat.

In addition, most pollen-related food sensitivities are related to lipid transfer protein sensitization. Furthermore, the research has indicated a link between diet, lifestyle and pollen exposure.

It should be noted that Italy is an industrialized nation, but most of its urban population lives in the South. Thus it is no surprise that 96% of Type I food allergies among the group in the Asero research lived in the urban areas of Southern Italy. So while pollen-crops are grown throughout Italy, the greater per-capita pollen-related food allergy rates occur among those from urban areas – where processed, convenient foods are more readily consumed.

In a study by German researchers from the Paul-Ehrlich-Institute (Hartz *et al.* 2010), those with allergies to peach, cherry or hazelnuts were significantly sensitized to non-specific lipid transfer protein. As the three groups were compared, it became evident that becoming sensitized to LTP together with the allergic protein of peaches (Pru p3), produced a stronger potential of becoming allergic to hazelnuts and cherries. This is apparently because LTPs exhibit stronger IgE-binding capacity, and greater crossover capability.

LTPs are proteins that are intrinsically and complexly combined with other elements of a particular food. How does one become allergic to an LTP? Part of the issue is a stressed or weakened immune system during an exposure to the LTP epitope. This exposure typically accompanied by LTP penetration through thinned, weakened mucosal membranes of the airways.

Yes, just as our intestines are lined with protective mucosal membranes, our airways are too. These mucosal membranes are lined with – you guessed it – numerous probiotic bacteria – along with immune cells and mucin. These all work together to protect the airways from these sorts of intrusions – such as LPT or flour dust. But when these membranes are thinned or the person's immune system is otherwise overloaded, an LPT may penetrate and produce an immunological response.

Let's consider lipid transfer protein one (LTP1). This protein can be derived from barley during refining, and it is the notable protein component in beer foam. The refined LTP1 in beer foam is not like the LTP1 found within the barley grain, however. In its modified state, LTP1 produces a higher foam capacity than natural LTP1 from barley grain would produce. So beer producers have developed a more appealing "head" of foam, possibly at the expense of making available a protein the body can become sensitive to.

But what else are beer drinkers getting? They are consuming a modified version of LTP1. Does the body consider this a foreigner? Likely, because it *is* foreign. It has been modified. This LTP1 will have a slightly different molecular and magnetic configuration. Thus the body won't consider it a part of the natural diet.

Does this mean that beer is causing LTP type allergies? While beer allergies are not commonplace, they are increasingly occurring.

Beer allergies and anaphylaxis were studied by Israeli doctors and published in the *Journal of the Israel Medical Association* (Nusem and Panasoff

2009). As they tested for related allergens, they found that the cause of the beer allergies was not the alcohol, as there was no sensitivity to other alcohol beverages – only beer. They eventually concluded that the LTP allergen related to the barley refinement discussed above was at the root of the allergy syndrome.

Furthermore, researchers from Japan's Okayama Prefectural University (Hiemori *et al.* 2008) wanted to investigate the cause of the sudden rise in beer allergies among Japanese beer consumers. Again, they found that the allergen LTP 18-kDa IgE-binding proteins likely originated from the barley used in the beer.

Early Life Causes

We have touched upon the importance of maintaining probiotic colonies, but we will investigate this issue in more detail in the next chapter. For now, here are a couple of relationships between food sensitivities and our children.

C-Sections

In a C-section, the baby is denied passage through the vagina, which is typically (in healthy women) occupied with a plethora of healthy probiotic species. Thus while the baby passes through the birthing canal it picks up these bacteria, and they begin to colonize throughout the baby's body.

When there is a deficiency in this area, this can result in an allergic progression through life, unless the baby is inoculated otherwise – such as through breastfeeding and lots of hugs.

Researchers from the Netherlands' National Institute for Public Health and the Environment (Roduit et al 2009) studied the allergic status of 2,917 children with respect to whether they were born with a cesarean section. They tested 1,454 of the children for IgE antibodies for inhalants and food allergens at age eight. They found conclusively that babies born with cesarean section had a significantly increased risk of asthma and food sensitivities.

Researchers from Finland's National Institute for Health and Welfare (Metsälä *et al.* 2010) studied all children born in Finland between 1996 and 2004 that were diagnosed with cow's milk allergies. In all, 16,237 allergic children were found. Children born of cesarean section had an 18% greater risk of contracting milk allergies.

Researchers from the Germany's National Research Centre for Environment and Health and the Institute of Epidemiology (Laubereau *et al.* 2004) studied 865 healthy infants whose parents had allergies. They tested the babies at one, four, eight and twelve months old. They found that babies (147) born with cesarean section had over double the risk of sensitivities to allergens than their peers without C-section birth.

Breastfeeding

Research is increasing illustrating that breastfeeding is critical to the future possibility of food sensitivities. Plenty of research on breastfeeding has found that babies breast-fed from healthy mothers have a lower incidence of disease, higher rates of growth, and stronger immune systems.

The reasons for these include not only that breast milk contains a variety of proteins, fatty acids, vitamins, nucleotides and colostrum (a special immune system-stimulator). Breast milk from a healthy mother also contains a variety of important probiotics.

Researchers from Japan's Shiga Medical Center for Children (Kusunoki *et al.* 2010) surveyed 13,215 parents of children aged from seven to 15 years old. The study compared allergic rates among three types of infant feeding histories: exclusive breastfeeding; mixed formula and breastfeeding; and exclusive formula feeding. The results showed conclusively that exclusive breastfeeding produced significantly fewer cases of bronchial asthma.

Researchers from University of Cincinnati's Department of Internal Medicine (Codispoti *et al.* 2010) studied 361 children, 116 who had allergic rhinitis. They found that prolonged breastfeeding among African American children decreased the allergy risk by 20%.

Researchers from Spain's University of Granada (Martínez-Augustin *et al.* 1997) studied intestinal permeability during the first month of life, along with antibody production to milk proteins. The study fed either cow's milk formula for low-birth weight or the same formula supplemented with nucleotides matching human breast milk. Blood and urine samples were obtained at one, seven and 30 days of age. They found that (low allergy risk) blood IgG antibodies to cow milk protein beta-lactoglobulin were higher among the babies that were fed the formula with the breast milk nucleotides.

Researchers from Sweden's Institute of Environmental Medicine (Kull *et al.* 2010) studied 3,825 children over a period of eight years to determine the role of breast feeding and food allergies. They determined that children who were exclusively breast-fed for four months or more experienced a significantly lower risk of asthma for the first eight years of their lives – as compared to those breast-fed for less than four months. The exclusively breast-fed group also were observed to have significantly better lung function.

Newborns and infants have under-developed intestinal epithelial barriers, and their immune system is still developing. For this reason, it is a sensitive time for the intestinal tract. Breast milk has been shown to stimulate greater levels of IgA within the intestinal tract – thereby reducing the risk of allergies (Brandtzaeg 2010).

However, this association between breast feeding and milk allergies is more complicated. University of Helsinki researchers (Saarinen *et al.* 2000) studied breast-fed and formula infants. From a sampling of 6,209 infants, 824 were found to be exclusively breast-fed. They found that the cumulative incidence of cow's milk allergies was higher in the cow's milk formula group than among the exclusively breast-fed group (2.4% versus 2.1%). This also illustrated that exclusive breastfeeding does not necessarily eliminate the potential for becoming allergic to milk. We would postulate that this rate of milk allergies was due to the mother's own IgE sensitivities to milk and passing these along, as we've discussed.

It also appears that some early exposure to cow's milk may reduce sensitivity. Israeli researchers (Katz *et al.* 2010) from the Assaf-Harofeh Medical Center studied 13,019 infants. The rate of IgE-mediated cow's milk allergy among the population was 0.5%. The average age that cow's milk feeding was introduced was significantly different between the allergic children and those not allergic. The healthy infants were started on milk an average of 62 days after birth. Those infants with cow's milk allergies were started on milk an average of 116 days after birth. Only 0.05% of those infants who were given cow milk formula within the first two weeks of life contracted milk allergies. This is compared to 1.75% of those children who took cow's milk formula between 105 and 194 days after birth contracting allergy to cow's milk.

No breast milk can result in other issues. Researchers from Italy's Siena University (Garzi *et al.* 2002) found that of the about-20% of infants given formula (not fed with breast-milk) suffered from gastroesophageal reflux (GERD), about a third also suffered from milk allergies.

Scientists from the Center for Infant Nutrition at the University of Milan (Arslanoglu *et al.* 2008) found that short-chain galactooligosaccharides (scGOS) and long-chain fructooligosaccharides (lcFOS) (both present in healthy breast milk) can reduce the incidence of atopic dermatitis (AD) and infections through six months of age. They fed 134 infants either a prebiotic-supplemented formula or a placebo-supplemented formula. Follow-ups continued until age two. Atopic dermatitis, asthma, and allergic urticaria rates were significantly higher among the infants given the placebo formula. Formula with oligosaccharide prebiotics lowers the risk of allergies. This of course relates to the fact that prebiotics increase probiotic populations within the intestines.

The bottom line: Exclusive breastfeeding for around the first four months reduces food allergy risk in general.

Early Hygiene

We are bacteria-carriers. Our bodies are full of bacteria. And our intestines are bacteria fermentation tubes.

Bacteria are colonizers. When we attack our colonies with antiseptics and antibiotics we rob our bodies of its major source of immunity and inflammation reduction. Not to speak of its source of digestive enzymes.

Researchers from Finland's University of Turku (Kalliomäki and Isolauri 2002) concluded after a review of multiple studies that the sterile birthing environments among Western hospitals have reduced exposure to early microbes.

This, they hypothesized, is a key reason that sensitivity and atopic diseases such as eczema, allergic rhinitis and asthma are on the rise among these Western nations. This has been called the *Hygiene Hypothesis of Allergy.*

The Finnish researchers supported their hypothesis with immunological data illustrating that the immune system responds to microbial antigens, both pathogenic and non-pathogenic ones, with the expression of cytokines that balance the T-helpers produced by the infants.

In other words, with an increase in exposure to available pathogens – to a degree – comes a strengthened immune system. This is to a degree because too many pathogens can overwhelm the immune system.

This is supported by a number of studies confirming that children born and raised on farms have a lower incidence of food allergies (Hamelmann *et al.* 2008).

For example, Finnish researchers (Metsälä *et al.* 2010) found that a lower family socioeconomic status lowered the risk of contracting milk allergies by 35%. Having given birth to five or more babies previous to the child (more siblings) reduced the risk of cow's milk allergies by 29%. Lower economic status is associated with more exposure to nature's microbes, soils and other elements. Lower socioeconomic status among the Fins is also associated with farmers, who tend to be poorer than their city-dwelling peers.

In a study mentioned earlier, University of Cincinnati researchers (Codispoti *et al.* 2010) found in a study of 361 children that multiple children in the home during infancy decreased the risk of allergic rhinitis by 60%.

Medical researchers from Switzerland's University of Basel (Waser *et al.* 2007) conducted a study of 14,893 children between the ages of five and 13 from five different European countries. The testing group included 2,823 children from farms and 4,606 children attending Steiner Schools (known for their farm-based living and instruction). They found that children on the farms – particularly those who drank farm milk – had significantly fewer allergies and asthma. The reason, as we'll discuss, stems from the increase in probiotics among raw farm milk.

Dr. Oner Ozdemir, M.D. at the SEMA Research and Training Hospital in Turkey, characterizes the issue with an understanding of immune and probiotic mechanisms:

"Development of the child's immune system tends to be directed toward a T-helper 2 (Th2) phenotype in infants. To prevent development of childhood allergic/atopic diseases, immature Th2-dominant neonatal responses must undergo environment-driven maturation via microbial contact in the early postnatal period. Lactic acid bacteria and bifidobacteria are found more commonly in the composition of the intestinal flora of nonallergic children. Epidemiological data also showed that atopic children have a different intestinal flora from healthy children. Probiotics are ingested with live health-promoting microbes that can modify intestinal microbial populations in a way that benefits the host; and enhanced presence of probiotic bacteria in the intestinal microbiota is found to correlate with protection against atopy."

The Role of Obesity

The rates of obesity have increased as gluten sensitivities have increased among industrialized countries. Meanwhile, those countries that have low obesity levels also have low levels of gluten and other food sensitivities. This is a correlation, yes. But it is nonetheless important, because with obesity comes a certain overload upon the digestive system and immune system as the body deals with the over-abundance of food and accompanying toxins.

Currently, about 72 million Americans – nearly one-third of the population – are obese according to National Health and Nutrition Examination research. And over half of Americans are overweight.

As part of this National Health and Nutrition Examination research, scientists from the University of North Carolina (Visness *et al.* 2009) directly correlated obesity with the prevalence of food allergies among children. They defined obesity as being over the 95th percentile of weight; and overweight as being over the 85th percentile of weight for children between the ages of two and nineteen years old.

The researchers found that obese children had greater levels of atopic sensitivities, allergen-specific IgE levels and allergy symptoms. They also found that obese children had a 31% greater risk of having allergies, and overweight children had a 25% greater risk of having allergies.

Incidentally, the researchers also found that allergies correlated with increased levels of C-reactive protein, which is known to reflect a status of inflammation within the body. As we have discussed, an overly inflammatory status leads to a lower tolerance of foods due to the heightened state of sensitivity within the immune system.

Anxiety, Stress and Depression

Mood and stress are critical to the intestinal barrier function. French researchers (Ducrotté 2009) have illustrated that food sensitization can occur from a dysfunction of afferent neurons, which can produce disturbances among the *"brain-gut axis."*

In other words, the interplay between stress and digestive responsiveness can stimulate immune response and increased intestinal permeability. Research has showed that chronic stress also plays a primary role in the occurrence and continuance of irritable bowel syndrome. This of course involves various neural and sensory relationships, as well as neurotransmitters and their receptors (Buret 2006).

Researchers from Norway's University of Bergen Medical School (Lillestøl *et al.* 2010) found that anxiety and depression are often associated in food intolerance. They studied 130 food sensitive patients with 75 healthy volunteers. They found that 57% of the food sensitive patients had at least one psychiatric disorder. Anxiety disorders were seen among 34% and depression disorders were seen among 16%. Meanwhile, 89% of the patients had irritable bowel syndrome. The researchers concluded that, *"anxiety and depression are common in patients with IBS-like complaints self-attributed to food hypersensitivity. Anxiety disorders predominate."*

The conclusion is that stress and anxiety induces intestinal hypersensitivity, and a higher risk of food sensitivities.

Vitamin D and Sun Exposure

Multiple studies have found that food allergies are significantly greater among regions further from the equator and those with less sunlight exposure. In both Europe and the U.S., living in Southern regions significantly lowers incidence of food sensitivities with far fewer hospital visits for food allergies.

This link was confirmed in a European study of 17,280 adults from different countries by researchers from Australia's Monash Medical School (Woods *et al.* 2001). Among developed countries, 12% reported either having food allergies or food intolerances. Food allergy rates were higher among those living in Northern Europe as compared with Southern European countries.

Researchers from the Children's Hospital Boston (Rudders *et al.* 2010) studied allergic emergency room visits throughout the United States. They found those living in Southern regions had significantly lower incidence of food allergies and far fewer hospital visits for food allergies. The Northeast region had 5.5 visits per thousand, while the South had 4.9 visits per thousand.

This difference was even greater when the analysis was restricted to food sensitivities. The risk of food sensitivities was 33% higher for those living in the Northeast than those living in the sun-drenched South:

> *"These observational data are consistent with the hypothesis that vitamin D may play an etiologic role in anaphylaxis, especially food-induced anaphylaxis."*

Fetal vitamin D exposure is also related to food allergies. Researchers from Massachusetts General Hospital (Vassallo *et al.* 2010) found in a study of 1,002 patients with food allergies, that children born in the fall or winter had a significantly higher incidence of food allergies. The findings indicate UV-B exposure and subsequent vitamin D production was linked to food allergies.

This protection provided by vitamin D produced from sun exposure may or may not be provided by vitamin D supplementation. The author has done substantial research in this area, concluding that the sulfated version of 25(OH)D3 produced from sunlight has different properties from supplemented D2 or D3. This includes fat cell sequestration. The sun also has other beneficial effects. Refer to the author's book, *Healthy Sun* for more information.

Autoimmunity

Research indicates that the risk of developing (or already having) food sensitivities increases significantly for those with autoimmune diseases. There are many conditions now being defined as an autoimmune disease, and it appears that new ones are being added. Why?

About 3% of the U.S. population suffers from systemic or tissue-specific autoimmune disorders (Jacobson *et al.* 1995), with women making up about 85% (Walsh and Rau, 2000). A significant amount of research data confirms the conclusion that environmental exposures contribute significantly to autoimmune disease in general (Cooper *et al.* 2002; Hess 1997).

For example, researchers from Sweden's University Hospital in Uppsala (Lidén *et al.* 2010) found that many rheumatoid arthritis (RA) patients have food allergies. They surveyed 347 RA patients, and found that 27% of the RA patients reported that they had food intolerances. These included sensitivities to cow's milk, meat and wheat gluten. Further testing using oral tolerance parameters found that 22% had cow's milk intolerance, and 33% had wheat gluten intolerance.

Swiss researchers from the University Hospital in Zurich (Bentz *et al.* 2010) studied 79 Crohn's disease patients with 20 healthy subjects. Food-activated IgG antibodies were found to be significantly increased among the Crohn's patients. The scientists tested 40 additional patients to confirm the result. In total, they found that 83% of the patients maintained significant levels of IgG antibodies against processed cheese and yeast. When a diet that eliminated these foods was instituted, daily stool frequency (a common issue among Crohn's sufferers) significantly decreased compared with the control (sham) diet. Abdominal pain was reduced and Crohn's patients on the elimination diet reported increased well-being.

Intestinal diseases come with a variety of names, including intestinal hypersensitivity, inflammatory bowel disease, irritable bowel syndrome, Crohn's disease, colitis and many others. In practically every one of these conditions, there is a disruption of the intestinal barrier along the walls of the intestines. Because the intestinal barrier function responds to neural impulses from the vagus nerve and other sympathetic nerves, there is an association with stress.

As these neural impulses are activated by corticotrophin-releasing hormone (a stress response hormone), mucosal mast cells release tryptase, TNF-alpha, nerve growth factor and interleukins that directly disrupt the intestinal barrier function (Keita and Söderholm 2010).

As we've discussed, a dysfunctional barrier function causes permeability issues, which burden the immune system within the intestinal area and the body as a whole, as the body must respond to the entry of foreigners.

As the immune system responds to macromolecule entry into the epithelial layer, there are particular responses. The responses are similar between ulcerative colitis disease and Crohn's disease. Both show an increase in chloride and water secretion, which lead to an increase of intestinal wall permeability, along with a faster turnover (death) of intestinal wall cells. The cytokine that appears to stimulate this process in Crohn's disease in particular is tumor necrosis factor alpha (TNF-a). In ulcerative colitis, the same processes are stimulated by the cytokine interleukin-13 (IL-13) (Salim and Söderholm 2010).

Illustrating this, researchers from the Norway's University of Bergen Medical School (Lillestøl *et al.* 2010) studied 71 allergic patients. Of the group, 66, or 93%, had irritable bowel syndrome. Forty-three, or 61%, had atopic symptoms – primarily rhinoconjunctivitis. In addition, 43 were sensitized to inhalant allergens. Of the 71 patients, 41% (29) had food allergies. The researchers described the IgE-positive mast cells as *"armed."*

As we investigate autoimmunity in more detail, we unfold a number of relationships between autoimmunity and environmental factors. We also discover a strong link between autoimmunity and the viability of the immune system itself. This relationship becomes apparent as most autoimmune diseases occur during the middle age years or elderly years. The relationship between our environment and autoimmune disorders is also highlighted by the rise in autoimmune disease as our environment becomes increasingly contaminated with chemical toxins.

The Immunosciences Lab in California (Vojdani 2008) released a study that tested the fluids of 420 patients with a variety of autoimmune-type disorders.

These were screened for 96 different antibodies to a variety of different infectious microorganisms and proteins. A significant number of the autoimmune-patients tested positive to one or multiple *autoantibodies*. This leads to a thesis that some autoimmunity is related to a derangement of the immune system from previous infections, and/or the immune system has been overloaded with too many toxins.

We have discussed how the thymus can weaken with age, stress and toxic overload. The thymus is where T-cells are programmed with the antigen-programming called T-cell receptors or TCRs. These direct the T-cells to identify particular types of infected cells or toxins. The thymus accomplishes this through the major histocompatibility complex or the MHC as explained in the chapter on the immune system.

However, this MHC programming can be corrupted by stress and toxins. Over the years of toxic load bombardment and malnourishment, the thymus can begin to collapse and become increasingly unproductive. As this happens, the immune system's T-cells are not programmed with the most up-to-date instructions. Should the thymus not be productive, T-cells will not be appropriately programmed with the updated MHC and TCR information. They will become less tolerant and less adaptable.

Researchers are now suspecting that this lack of updated programming causes T-cells to begin attacking the body's own intestinal cells: Especially if those intestinal cells have become altered as a result of exposure to new toxins or macromolecules.

This is only logical, since over time the body's cells must adapt to all the stressors that we throw at them in order for our body to keep living in a toxic world. How else could we survive so many lethal toxic threats? As intestinal cells begin to adapt and change, they become increasingly unrecognizable if the immune system is working with older programming.

Today, our intestinal cells must learn to adapt to so many chemicals in our foods: preservatives, food dyes and overly processed and isolated ingredients. Our immune systems must learn to adapt to these plus chemicals in our immediate environment: formaldehyde, PCBs, plasticizers and petrochemicals. Our immune systems must learn to adapt to the stresses of our modern culture: not getting enough sleep, rushing for time, and dealing with money. For some of us, our intestinal cells must also learn to adapt to deficient water. For some of us, our cells must also learn to adapt to a lack of good nutrition. Any changing environmental element will require the cells and the immune system to adapt.

Over time, all these adaptations are reflected in our cells' gene sequences. These will also be reflected on the cell membrane.

In the case of the intrusion of a toxic chemical, for example, the immune system stimulates a detoxification event to clear the toxin. This may dispatch macrophages to take apart the toxin. Should the toxin not be cleared, the free radicals produced by the toxin or the toxin itself may enter and damage cells within the body. Once cells are invaded, the invaded cell genes adapt to the invasion in order to accommodate it.

Viruses are more specifically tuned to forcing genetic changes. In either case, the immune system will often initiate an inflammatory response and detoxification event the toxin and/or the invaded cells. This produces swelling, sneezing, coughing, watery eyes and so on.

However, should the cell adapt without a significant loss in function, the cell's genes make adjustments, which are communicated through to the thymus' MHC programming of T-cells. Since the T-cells have been given updated genetic information, the body is adapted to the intrusion.

We might compare this to how we adapt to weather. When there is hot weather, we will wear different clothes and move more slowly. During cold weather, we put on many more clothes and shiver more to create heat. During the wintertime, we adapt to the cold weather with many changes to our house and habits in order to stay warm.

As the cell adapts, it produces a reflective molecular signal on the cell membrane reflecting its change. This ligand can signal the TCR of the thymus that it is genetically different but functional.

This signal is comparable to a ship raising a flag that it has undergone change for other boats to see from far away. This 'flag' can be read by T-cells that are searching for cells that have been invaded. Should T-cells without updated programming 'read' such a signal on the surface, they dispatch the appropriate immune response. A large group of 'flagged' cells will likely cause a full-scale inflammatory attack against the region.

In the case of a lack of nutrients or water for extended periods, the DNA and RNA within the cell may be forced to adapt to a condition where the cell operates with less fuel. We could compare this to the ship raising a flag that it is trying to accommodate running out of fuel.

The first nutrient deficiency to damage the cell is oxygen. Without oxygen, our cells will starve for energy and will not be able to function. This can take place within minutes. The second most dangerous nutrient deficiency is water. Should the cell not have enough water, it will begin to deteriorate. We'll discuss this shortly.

Our DNA may also undergo direct damage from ionizing electromagnetism. This has been illustrated in the research on nuclear bomb victims. Electromagnetic ionizing waveforms originating from radiation from x-rays, CT-scans and so on will subtly stress the cell's ability to communicate within itself and with other cells. The cell must then adapt to these new environmental waveforms by making genetic accommodations. The need for chronic adjustment can result in the mutation of DNA. This mutation may also turn the cell into a cancerous cell.

In the same way, we find our bodies can accommodate many environmental toxins: Despite these toxins' ability to damage our cells and burden our immune system. Why have our bodies seemingly adapted to the avalanche of plastics and the plasticizers that come with them over the past three decades? The plethora of plastics have certainly increased our immune system burden, disrupted our hormones and damaged our livers. Yet many of us have little in the way outward allergies, sensitivities or other obvious symptoms of plastic use. The problem is that we cannot readily recognize the genetic accommodation to plasticizer toxicity. These may include hormone imbalances, chronic fatigue, reduced immunity, allergic reactions to natural elements like pollen and grass, and of course autoimmune conditions.

Our cells are adjusting to new environments all the time. For example, if we were to move to a warmer location – with greater UV radiation and contact with the sun's infrared rays – our cells will begin to operate with slower metabolism, allowing the body's core temperature to remain balanced. Though this might stress the cells somewhat, this sort of adapting mechanism is not considered harmful, because the sun's rays (except perhaps mid-day UV) are considered healthy to the body. However, should our body move into a 'sick' building – where it is exposed to toxic chemicals – our cells might react more violently, with allergies and physical stress, should our (burdened) cells be forced to adapt to a toxic environment. The same cells may have adapted to a change of weather nicely, but an overburdened cell can easily react negatively to a toxic environment.

As we will discuss further, conventional Western medicine's solution to autoimmune disorders is to try to stop the symptoms by interrupting the symptoms of inflammation and immune response. While this may temporarily slow the inflammatory response, this solution also can weaken the entire immune system by blocking the body's healing mechanisms. This puts more burdens on the body because the body cannot efficiently detoxify and heal itself from the offending toxins or pathogens. This chemical 'solution' ends up increasing the burden upon the body's already-overloaded immune system.

This pharmaceutical strategy would be analogous to punishing our dog because he barked at a thief who was invading our home.

Toxin Exposure and Immunosuppression

In addition to exposure from glyphosate and related surfactants in herbicides, there are other toxins that have the effect of stressing the immune system and our probiotic microbes. Let's discuss some of the toxin exposures that have been associated with increased risk of food sensitivities.

Tobacco

Tobacco smoke contains carbon monoxide, nicotine, aldehydes, ketones and hundreds of other toxins. These can easily burden the immune system with toxin overload. This is especially when it pervades the oxygen environment of a child, or the bloodstream of the mother.

Illustrating this, researchers from the Respiratory Diseases Department of France's Hospital of Haut-Lévèque in Bordeaux (Raherison *et al.* 2008), studied 7,798 children from six cities in France. The research found that children from parents (especially mothers) who smoked, had a significantly greater likelihood of having asthma and allergies than children from families that did not smoke.

Mold

An undue amount of mold can also overwhelm the immune system. Mold is related to asthma and rhinitis, and as we showed earlier, research indicates that the risk of food sensitivities increases among those with asthma and rhinitis.

This was confirmed by researchers from the National University of Singapore (Tham *et al.* 2007), who found that home dampness and indoor mold is linked to an increase in allergies among children. They studied 4,759 children from 120 daycare centers. After eliminating other possible effects, home humidity was significantly associated with increased rates of allergic rhinoconjunctivitis. As discussed earlier, allergic rhinoconjunctivitis is the inflammation of the conjunctiva and sinuses as a result of histamine release following an allergic immune response. As mold burdens the immune system, the body responds with hypersensitivity.

Mercury

Exposure to mercury has been suspected as a possible culprit in reducing immunity and thus increasing the risk of hypersensitivity.

This was illustrated in multicenter research from the Department of Medicine from Lavoro Medical Center in Bari, Italy (Soleo *et al.* 2002). Here researchers studied the effects of low levels of inorganic mercury exposure on 117 workers. They compared these with 172 general population subjects. There was no difference in the white blood cell count between the two groups. However, the exposed worker group had increased levels of CD4+ and CD8+ cytokines. CD4+ levels were significantly high. A significantly lower level of interleukin (IL-8) occurred among the exposed workers.

This research concluded that even low levels of environmental exposure to mercury (and likely other heavy metals) suppresses the immune system. As we've discussed, the increase in these cytokines and the burdening of the immune system in general increases the potential for an inflammatory intestinal response and subsequent food sensitivity.

Toxins and Immunosuppression

Clinical research by Professor John G Ionescu, Ph.D. has concluded that environmental pollution is clearly associated with the development of new sensitivities. Dr. Ionescu's research indicated that environmental noxious agents, including many chemicals, contribute to the total immune burden, producing increased susceptibility for intolerances.

Environmental toxins are also sensitizing in themselves, producing new trigger allergens. Professor Ionescu draws this conclusion from studying more than 18,000 atopic eczema patients:

> *"Beside classic allergic-triggering factors (allergen potency, intermittent exposure to different allergen concentrations, presence of microbial bodies dyand sensitizing phenols), the adjuvant role of environmental pollutants gains increasing importance in allergy induction."*

According to Dr. Ionescu, toxic inputs such as formaldehyde, smog, industrial waste, wood preservatives, microbial toxins, alcohol, pesticides, processed foods, nicotine, solvents and amalgam-heavy metals have been observed to be mediating toxins for new sensitization of a variety of atopic allergies.

Research has concluded that allergen responses are accelerated by pharmaceutical use because they stimulate histamine and/or acetylcholine. These provoke smooth muscle neuromediators, which stimulate rapid nutrient absorption within the intestines (Liu *et al.* 1977).

This is also consistent with findings of other scientists – as discussed earlier – that pharmaceuticals can increase intestinal permeability.

Immunosuppression may be a long word, but it really is very simple: The immune system has been overburdened and compromised by the combination of unnatural, synthetic or deranged foods or toxins. The chart below itemizes a few of these toxins that promote immunosuppression:

Major Modern Toxins

Source	Toxin
Antacids	Heavy Metals
Antiperspirant	Aluminum
Carpets, rugs	Molds, dander, lice, PC-4, latex
Cigarette Smoke	Carbon monoxide, nicotine, aldehydes, ketones
Cosmetics	Aluminum, phosphates and chemicals

Dental Fillings	Mercury, alloys, various chemicals
Dish soap	Perfumes, dyes, phosphates
Electric Blankets	EMFs, PC-4, various toxins
Food	Food colors, preservatives, trans-fats, pesticides, arachidonic acids, acrylamide, phytanic acid, artificial flavors
Soaps and Shampoos	Fragrances, chemicals, phosphates
House	Radon, formaldehyde, pollen, dust, mold, dander
Householder cleaners	Chlorine, various phosphates
Indoor Light	Blinking fluorescent lights
Industrial Plant or Freeway	Lead, mercury, carbon monoxide
IUDs	Copper
Old pillows	Lice eggs, dander, molds
Paints	Lead, arsenic, cadmium, various toxins
Pesticides	Neurotoxins, poisons
Pets	240 infectious diseases & parasites (65 from dogs/39 from cats)
Pipes	Lead, copper, deposits
Plastics	Plasticizers (see also tap water)
Pools and spas	Chlorine, various carbonates
Appliances	Electromagnetic frequencies
Restaurants	Parasites, pesticides, trans-fats
Pans	Aluminum, copper, lead
Stoves, Fireplaces	Carbon monoxide, arsenic, soot
Tap Water	Chlorine, microorganisms, pesticides, nitrates, pharmaceuticals
Toothpaste	Propylene glycol, microparticles, synthetic sweeteners
Work environment	Various toxins
Microorganisms	Various species

We aren't suggesting that any of these toxins will cause gluten sensitivity or even food sensitivity. But each can be seen as a contributing factor. And from an accumulated basis, increase the burden on our immune system.

For each of these toxins, the liver and immune system must launch a variety of macrophages, T-cells and B-cells to break them apart and escort them out of the body. This means that each toxin represents an additional load the immune system must carry.

We might compare this to moving dirt. A small handful of dirt can be carried around easily, and dispersed without much effort. However, a truckload of dirt is another matter completely. What do we do with a truckload of dirt? If we dumped it on our lawn, we'd have a hill of dirt that would bury the front of our house, preventing us from getting in or out of the house.

This is a useful comparison because while our bodies can handle a small amount of toxins quite easily, modern society is increasingly dumping toxic 'dirt' into our atmosphere, water and foods, effectively inundating our bodies by the 'truckload.'

With this increased burden, the research shows that the body's defenses are lowered. The mucosal membrane is thinned. The immune system is on alert and sensitive. In this immunosuppressed state, the body is more likely to overreact to macromolecules, LTPs or other food proteins such as gliadins.

Chapter Six

Probiotics and Gluten Sensitivities

As the reader will discover among the research provided in this chapter, probiotics provide not only a contributing cause but a potential solution to many food sensitivities, including gluten sensitivities.

Thus an entire chapter will specifically focus on how probiotic deficiencies can cause or contribute to food sensitivities and how probiotics can be used to resolve intestinal damage and return the gut to a more normal environment.

We'll also show how a lack of probiotics can directly cause other conditions promote food sensitivities – including Crohn's disease, irritable bowel syndrome (IBS), colitis and others.

Indicating how our intestinal bacteria specifically relates to gluten sensitivity, we can discuss a study from Sweden's University of Umeå (Myléus *et al.* 2012) that investigated the potential cause for a startling uptick in celiac disease among Swedish children between 2004 and 2007.

The researchers tested 954 children, with 373 cases of celiac disease in children, comparing them to healthy matched controls.

The celiac children developed celiac disease on average before one year old. The researchers found that those who had three or more infections during the first year were 50% more likely to develop celiac disease. And those who had cases of gastroenteritis were 80% more likely to develop celiac disease.

We will identify the mechanism for this association later on.

Let's start with some general information relating to our diets and our microbiome.

The Diet of Our Microbiome

The human genome contains about 20,000 or so gene sequences. But our microbiome – the combined genome of our probiotics – dwarfs our genome by many degrees. If we were to consider our body's entire genetic map as an apple pie, the sliver of the slice our genome would make up wouldn't be much wider than a human hair. Our microbiome would make up the rest.

At evidence is the research of the Human Microbiome Project, sponsored by the National Institutes of Health. An initial study that drew samples from 242 healthy humans found 11,174 different species of commensal bacteria and yeasts among the guts, mouths, skin and vaginas (women) of the subjects. And certainly this was not the entire count of microorganisms living among us.

Yet each of these species found can have up to 13,000 gene sequences, so we can imagine the size of our microbiome when we multiply the two numbers together.

Then our bodies contain about 100 trillion of these organisms, ten times the number of cells in our body.

As researchers have investigated the variations between gut bacteria enterotypes among different ethnicities and populations, our individual and cultural dietary choices can be linked to the makeup of our gut bacteria. Research from Yale University (Moeller and Ochman 2013) confirmed this. The researchers also detailed what has been discovered among chimpanzees from different locations – as common differences in gut bacteria are related to their particular diets and environments.

This aspect was not only confirmed in this study, but among many others. Multiple studies have shown that the makeup of ones gut bacteria is significantly related to ones diet now and in the past. In one, University of Pennsylvania researchers (Wu, *et al.* 2011) drew fecal samples from 98 healthy people, and compared their diets and long-term diets (the diets their families had) to the makeup of their intestinal bacteria.

The researchers found that ones diet significantly correlated with the nature of their gut's intestinal bacteria. They also found an even stronger correlation between the gut bacteria and their long-term diet, based upon their ethnic cultural foods and so on. But when their diets were changed, the researchers found that the makeup of their intestinal bacteria actually changed dramatically. They stated:

> *"A controlled-feeding study of 10 subjects showed that microbiome composition changed detectably within 24 hours of initiating a high-fat/low-fiber or low-fat/high-fiber diet."*

The Microbiome Enterotypes

The researchers also saw a pattern of two particular clusters of bacteria types, which they referred to as enterotypes. The two primary enterotypes were based upon larger populations of the genera Bacteroides or Prevotella.

Research has also found a third enterotype, Ruminococcus – based upon more of these populations – but this enterotype has been relegated as rare and not so prevalent among humans.

As the University of Pennsylvania researchers compared long-term dietary habits with each enterotype, they found that long-term Western diet and greater meat and fat consumption is associated with to the Bacteroides enterotype, while the Prevotella enterotype is associated with greater long-term consumption of high-fiber, plant-based diets among the cultures of those being tested.

The researchers also measured intestinal clearance – the time it takes for food to pass through the digestive tract – between the high-fiber diets with high-fat diets. They found that the transit time among high-fat diet subjects went up to a high of seven days, while the high-fiber subjects' transit time ranged from two to four days.

And changes within their gut microorganism composition occurred even within that time – as early as 24 hours from the time their diets were changed.

This enterotyping of the microbiome was also studied by Cornell University scientists (Koren *et al.* 2013), who also found the two clusters – Bacteroides and Prevotella enterotypes – prevalent among their test subjects.

And they also found that the two enterotypes were associated to the dietary habits of the subjects in the form of their ancestry. They found those descending from Western countries had a predominantly Bacteroides enterotype, while those who were from non-Western countries were primarily Prevotella in enterotype.

This of course relates to the Yale study, as the Western diet is most closely associated with Western countries – hence the term *"Western diet."*

Microbiome Enterotypes and Disease

While certainly the overgrowth of some Prevotella bacteria can cause problems – such as among dental caries – Prevotella species are known to reduce acidosis within the intestines. This was first discovered among cows, and supplementation with Prevotella species has been shown to significantly reduce and even eliminate acidosis among cows (Chiquette *et al.* 2012).

In another recent study, researchers from the University of Pittsburgh (Ou *et al.* 2013) analyzed fresh feces samples from 24 healthy Africans – 12 African Americans and 12 Native Africans between the age of 50 and 65 years old.

The researchers found that the Native Africans had predominantly Prevotella gut microbiota enterotypes, while the African Americans had predominantly Bacteroides enterotypes. The African Americans also had significantly fewer total microorganisms.

The researchers also found that the Native Africans also had higher levels of the healthier short-chain fatty acids, while the African Americans had higher levels of secondary bile acids – meaning their intestines were highly acidic compared to the Native Africans.

These relationships have been made with colon cancer: Higher levels of secondary bile acids are linked with greater incidence of colon cancer while higher levels of short-chain fatty acids – such as butyrate produced by healthy gut microorganisms – have been linked with reduced incidence of colon cancer. The researchers concluded:

> *"Our results support the hypothesis that colon cancer risk is influenced by the balance between microbial production of health-promoting metabolites such as butyrate and potentially carcinogenic metabolites such as secondary bile acids."*

And the difference between the two groups of Africans? Naturally, the African Americans ate predominantly a Western diet, while the Native Africans ate more fiber-rich plant-based foods.

This correlation was confirmed in an earlier study by some of the same University of Pittsburgh researchers. In this study (Ou *et al.* 2012), 12 African Americans who were examined and determined to be at high-risk of colon cancer were studied and compared to 10 Caucasian Americans (who ate a high-fat diet), together with 13 Native Africans, who ate primarily a low-fat diet greater in fiber-rich plant-based foods.

The researchers found that the levels of components found high in colon cancer cases – notably secondary colonic bile acids, deoxycholic acid and lithocholic acid – were higher among both the Caucasian Americans and the African Americans, who both ate a higher-protein, higher-fat Western diet. These were significantly higher than those levels of the Native Africans, who ate a diet with more plant-based foods.

The researchers wrote:

> *"Our results suggest that the higher risk of colon cancer in Americans may be partly explained by their high-fat and high-protein, low complex carbohydrate diet, which produces colonic residues that promote microbes to produce potentially carcinogenic secondary bile acids and less antineoplastic short-chain fatty acids."*

Again, intestinal bacteria that produce these cancer-related short-chain fatty acids are related to higher levels of the Bacteroides enterotype.

And research has shown that a switch to a plant-based diet can immediately and effectively alter the ratio of Bacteroides within the intestines. Research from the Republic of Korea's Kyung Hee University (Kim *et al.* 2013) found that changing ones diet to a plant-based diet for one month dramatically changed levels of their gut microbiota, along with improvements in blood glucose levels and hypertension symptoms.

The researchers tested six adults who were obese with type 2 diabetes and/or high blood pressure. They tested their gut microbiota initially, and after a month of a plant-based diet, they retested the subjects.

They found that the plant-based diet significantly reduced levels of pathobiotics such as the Enterobacteriaceae (such as *E. coli*). They had increased levels of healthy species (type XIVa and IV) of *B. fragilis* and Clostridium (which compete with the pathogenic, beta-lactamase producing versions). They also found decreased production of the colon-cancer producing short-chain fatty acids. The month-long diet also improved fasting glucose levels, hemoglobin A1c levels, reduced triglyceride levels, reduced LDL-cholesterol levels and resulted in weight loss.

The researchers stated:

> *"This study underscores the benefits of dietary fiber for improving the risk factors of metabolic diseases and shows that increased fiber intake reduces gut inflammation by changing the gut microbiota."*

The Rise of Pathogenic Bacteria

One of the most hardy and prevalent Bacteroides bacteria among the guts of humans is *Bacteroides fragilis*. When it is out of control, *Bacteroides fragilis* can be a highly pathogenic gram-negative bacteria. It has been linked to a number of inflammatory conditions within the gut and elsewhere.

Among scientific research on pathogenic bacteria in the gut, *B. fragilis* has been isolated the most in inflammatory infections. It has been shown to make up from 40-75% of those samples pulled from intestinal inflammatory conditions. And *B. fragilis* has been shown to be one of the most antibiotic-resistant bacteria within the gut – meaning that it will likely survive when other bacteria are killed by a course of antibiotics. These include penicillin, moxifloxacin and others (Snydman *et al.* 2010).

B. fragilis also has the distinction of being so hardy that it doesn't always show up in stools – especially during intestinal infections. This is because *B. fragilis* tends to be stronger than other gut bacteria, and will protect itself within colony capsules to avoid die off from competing bacteria. When *B. fragilis* escapes the confines of the intestines, infection rates skyrocket.

For this reason, intestinal-related infections known to be primarily caused by *B. fragilis* include appendicitis, irritable bowel syndrome, intestinal abscesses, polyps and others. Research has found that *B. fragilis* infections have a 19% mortality rate (Wexler 2007).

We should include obesity in this list as well. University of Antwerp scientists (Bervoets *et al.* 2013) tested the fecal microbiota of 26 overweight or obese children along with 27 lean children. The data found that obese children had nearly triple the content of *B. fragilis* as the lean children (17.3% versus 6.1%). This of course is compounded by the fact that *B. fragilis* does not show up as much in fecal testing as do other bacteria. So this means that *B. fragilis* is worse of a problem in obese individuals.

One of the characteristics of many *B. fragilis* strains is that they produce a chemical called beta-lactamase, which makes them resistant to many antibiotics.

And research by Mariat (*et al.* 2009) and others have found that ones gut microbiota will change as we age – with an increase in *E. coli* and other pathogenic bacteria – and will be different among obese or lean individuals. Obesity has been specifically found to relate to higher levels of *E. coli* and other pathogenic bacteria such as Clostridia and *B. fragilis*.

In fact, Clostridium bacteria and others have been implicated directly in celiac disease.

Researchers from Sweden's Umeå (Ou *et al.* 2009) tested 45 children with celiac disease together with18 healthy matched control children. The researchers did small intestine biopsies and determined that while both the healthy children and the celiac children had many of the same species of bacteria, many of the celiac children had greater species of Clostridium and Actinomyces species. They also found Prevotella species, but the Clostridium and Actinomyces species are known to be pathogenic.

The researchers also found these three among children within what is referred to as the *Swedish celiac disease epidemic,* which occurred between 2004 and 2007 in Sweden:

> *"Bacteria of all three genera were isolated from children born during the Swedish celiac disease epidemic. New Clostridium and Prevotella species and Actinomyces graevenitzii were tentatively identified."*

Notice they have isolated new species here. These are ones not previously identified, which means they can be more rigorous and pathogenic than previous strains and species found from these genera.

Other studies have found a relationship between higher levels of Clostridium and *B. fragilis* with poor health.

For example, researchers from Sweden's Lund University (Karlsson *et al.* 2012) tested twenty overweight or obese children who were between four and five years old, and compared these children with twenty healthy children.

The researchers conduced a DNA analysis of the children's intestinal microbiota (using the quantitative polymerase chain reaction test). They also conducted liver enzyme tests as well.

The researchers found that the obese/overweight children had higher levels of Enterobacteriaceae – which include *E. coli* as well as Klebsiella, along with more pathogenic genus' such as Salmonella and Shigella.

Borderline but greater levels of Clostridia and *B. fragilis* species were found among obese children in another study of 26 overweight children and 27 lean children. The researchers found that overweight children had significantly higher ratios of Firmicutes (inclusive of Clostridia) than did lean children (Bervoets *et al.* 2013). This study also found higher levels of *B. fragilis* and lower levels of a Bacteroides species that balance *B. fragilis* bacteria, *B. vulgatus.*

Clostridia bacteria include *Clostridium difficile* – one of the most vigorous pathogenic bacteria, responsible for many types of infections. Growing populations are often partnered with growth of Staphylococcus – including *Staphylo-*

coccus aureus – Bacillus species, and Enterococcus species –including numerous other pathogenic organisms.

In another study – this one comparing the gut microbiota of 16 type 1 diabetes children with 16 healthy children, researchers from Spain (Murri *et al.* 2013) found that the gut microbiota from the children with diabetes had significantly greater levels of Clostridium, Bacteroides and Veillonella bacteria – all known to be pro-inflammatory. And they had fewer populations of Lactobacillus and Bifidobacterium, which are important in a healthy gut.

Meanwhile the counts of Prevotella-type bacteria were significantly lower among the diabetes children.

They also found greater colonies of Clostridium were associated with higher levels of blood glucose – meaning problematic glucose metabolism.

Remember that the Bacteroides enterotype is associated with greater inflammation and overgrowth of *E. coli* and *B. fragilis*, while the Prevotella enterotype maintains a more balanced gut microbiota. It isn't that the Prevotella enterotype doesn't also contain plenty of *E. coli* and *B. fragilis* bacteria. In fact, the healthy gut is typically 1-2% *B. fragilis*.

But because Prevotella guts are better balanced and have faster transit times, the *E. coli* and *B. fragilis* species begin to overwhelm the gut: especially species that produce ESBL.

ESBL means *extended-spectrum beta-lactamase.* ESBL-positive (ESBL+) *Escherichia coli* are multidrug-resistant bacteria that can cause severe infections. Severe illnesses from ESBL+ *E. coli* are typically worse than normal *E. coli* infections.

When these bacteria produce greater amounts of beta-lactamase, they become stronger. This is because just as beta-lactamase helps the bacteria become antibiotic-resistant, the beta-lactamase also allows these same bacteria to become less controlled by other bacteria within the gut.

You see, bacteria control each other's populations through the production of their own unique antibiotics. And these antibiotic chemicals will allow that particular species to colonize itself into greater colonies by keeping back bacteria that compete for the same territory.

Beta-lactamase is like a defense shield that allows that particular species to be impervious to the other bacterial antibiotics.

Our Microbiome Inner World

We might compare the human gut to the world, with the various nations all competing with each other for territory. Those stable countries that are able to protect their borders (or utilize the protection of larger nations) will be able to maintain their territories. But every so often a nation of people produce a stronger weapon that endangers the borders and territories of the weaker nations. Unless those other countries figure out how to counteract that weapon, they will be taken over.

Most of the time there is a kind of stalemate between countries, as they accept each other. But if one aggressor country was to figure out how to protect itself from the bombing or nuclear threat of the rest of the countries – say with a nuclear shield defense system – that aggressor could take over other territories by gradually conquering the other nations without the threat of being controlled by the weapons of the other countries.

This is the situation with beta-lactamase. It is like the nuclear shield defense system. When pathogenic, inflammation-producing bacteria such as *E. coli* and *B. fragilis* are able to produce beta-lactamase, they suddenly have the ability to grow stronger and take over many territories of the intestinal tract normally controlled by more friendly bacteria.

And should these pathogenic bacteria escape through the walls of the intestines – infecting the intestinal walls, the appendix or the walls of the anus, they can cause serious infections. And should they enter the vagina or penis and infect the urethra, they can cause serious urinary tract infections and bladder infections.

So not only is toilet hygiene important (cleaning up what comes out), but what is put into the mouth is critical. Why? Because our diets are critical to determining the kind of bacteria our guts contain. And the longer we maintain that diet, the more likely we are to keep the Bacteroides from overgrowing our intestinal tract.

Probiotic Diversity and Diet

New human clinical research from France has found that the more genetic diversity our gut bacteria have, the lower our tendency for inflammation, obesity and metabolic dysfunction.

The research comes from France's Institut National de la Recherche Agronomique (National Institute of Agronomic Research or INRA). In a study that culminated from a decade of progressive research linking probiotics to obesity, over 75 prominent European researchers (Le Chatelier et a. 2013) assembled to gather and analyze the data from 292 patients.

The researchers tested 123 obese Danish people, along with 169 non-obese Danes. They conducted medical examinations on each individual, measuring not only their weight and body fat, but their level of insulin resistance, cholesterol levels, cardiovascular condition and general inflammation.

The researchers also tested the makeup of each individual's gut bacteria. This was done through DNA analysis, which tests the genetic diversity – read the number of different strains – of the probiotic bacteria living within the gut.

The researchers found that 23% of the entire group of 292 had low levels of diversity – which the researchers referred to as "bacterial richness." This 23% had an average of 380,000 genes, while the average gene count of those with more diverse bacteria had a count of 640,000 genes on average.

More importantly, the researchers found those with lower probiotic diversity had significantly greater levels of obesity, higher cholesterol levels, more insulin resistance and a greater level of inflammatory conditions.

Those with lower levels of probiotic diversity also would struggle more with their weight. The researchers noted:

> *"The obese individuals among the lower bacterial richness group also gain more weight over time."*

In their investigation of the strains of probiotics that directly lead to greater probiotic diversity, the researchers found that species of Faecalibacterium, Bifidobacterium, and Lactobacillus were associated with greater gene microbiota diversity. They also found that pathogenic microorganism genus' such as Bacteroides and Ruminococcus are linked with lower levels of genetic diversity.

It should be added that the former group of probiotic bacteria have been linked in the research as being anti-inflammatory, while those in the second (pathogenic) group have been associated in the research as being pro-inflammatory microorganisms.

Another French study (Cotillard *et al.* 2013) – a partner study within MetaHIT, a European Union-commissioned organization – focused upon solving obesity and metabolic disease among Western countries – also linked lower probiotic gene diversity with greater levels of inflammation.

In this study, 49 obese or overweight patients were tested for gene diversity among their intestinal bacteria. The researchers found that 40% of the group had lower levels of probiotic gene diversity, and these individuals also had greater levels of *"low-grade inflammation"* and general *"dys-metabolism"* as compared with the rest of the group.

This study also found that a healthier diet with fewer processed carbohydrates (read junk food) led to higher scores of genetic diversity. However, the dietary intervention did not work as well for those with lower levels of genetic diversity at the beginning of the study:

> *"Dietary intervention improves low gene richness and clinical phenotypes, but seems to be less efficient for inflammation variables in individuals with lower gene richness."*

In other words, a diet that aids the growth of healthy probiotics (rich in prebiotics) helps reduce inflammation in the gut. And it is inflammation in the gut – along the walls of our intestines – that directly relate to food sensitivities – as unhydrolyzed proteins come into contact with intestinal cells.

It is somewhat like a revolving door problem: When our diets do not feed and nurture our probiotic populations, they are not as active in producing the enzymes needed to break down macromolecules like gliadins and WGA.

This lack of probiotics also reduces the protective lining of our mucosal membranes that line our intestines. As the uncleaved proteins come into close contact with the less-protected intestinal cells, they stimulate an immune response. This immune response produces an inflammatory response which then increases the sensitivity of those intestinal cells.

This combined and revolving situation produces the bloating, irritable bowels and other symptoms known among gluten sensitivities.

And because of the inflammatory situation, our intestinal cells are damaged and exposed further. The exposed intestinal cells will allow some of these proteins access to the blood and inner tissues. This is when the problem heightens and becomes more of a systemic (allergic) response to the food.

The evidence of these mechanisms is offered below.

Probiotics and Food Tolerance

We discussed this earlier: Our first major encounter with large populations of bacteria comes when our baby body descends the cervix and emerges from the vagina. During this birthing journey – assuming a healthy mother – we are exposed to numerous species of future resident probiotics. This first inoculation provides an advanced immune shield to keep populations of pathobiotics at bay. The inoculation process does not end here, however.

Because we get much of our bacteria as we pass through the vagina, cesarean section babies have significantly lower colonies of healthy bacteria. *Bifidobacterium infantis* is considered the healthiest probiotic colonizing infants. Some research has indicated that while 60% of vagina-birth babies have *B. infantis* colonies, only 9% of C-section babies are colonized with probiotics, and only 9% of those are colonized with *B. infantis.* This means that less than one percent of C-section babies are properly colonized with *B. infantis,* while 60% of vagina births are colonized with *B. infantis.* (The remaining 40% would indicate an unhealthy vagina.)

Our body establishes its resident strains during the first year to eighteen months. Following the inoculation from the vagina, these are accomplished from a combination of breastfeeding and putting everything in our mouth, from our parent's fingers to anything we find as we are crawling around the ground. These activities can provide a host of different bacteria – both pathobiotic and probiotic.

Mother's colostrum (early milk) can contain up to 40% probiotics. This will be abundant in bifidobacteria, assuming the mother is not taking antibiotics. Healthy strains of bifidobacteria typically colonize our body first and set up an environment for other groups of bacteria, such as the lactobacilli, to more easily become established.

Picking up a good mix of cooperative probiotic species is a crucial part of the establishment of our body's immune system. Some of the probiotic strains we ingest as infants may become permanent residents. They will continue to line the digestive tract to protect against infection while learning to collaborate with our immune system.

As our digestive tracts begin to become fully functional, interstitial and intercellular lymphocytes build up around our intestinal walls and mucosal membranes. However, these immune defenses only become functional when they are stimulated by the colonizing bacteria we gained from mother and the world around us. This probiotic stimulation renders the production of regulatory cytokines and immunoglobulins such as IgA.

These work together with our probiotics to seal up and defend our intestinal tissues from macromolecules and other potential allergens. IgA coats our intestinal cells and quietly removes allergens before they can invade our intestinal cells.

In other words, food tolerance is established early in life as the body begins to respond to probiotic bacteria. This is called *down regulation of systemic immunity.* Food tolerance marks the beginning of the maturity of the digestive tract. In other words, in order to become independent of mother, the baby body's immune system must recognize the good guys from the bad guys. Probiotics are the mediators for this discernment.

Imagine moving to a new location among the U.S. territories during the 1800s in the United States. The territories were full of different threats of various kinds. As we build our new log home and begin to settle in, we begin to try to distinguish between the creatures that will hurt us and those that won't. Say we are lucky enough to meet up with a frontiersman before we start building. The frontiersman has lived in 'these parts' for several decades. He begins telling us about what to 'watch out for' among the region. He also shows us how to prevent the bears from coming around and how to defend ourselves from the bears should they invade our new home. With his assistance, we can go about building our home and prepare for those threats.

Without his assistance, it would become difficult to determine what we should be defend ourselves from. As a result, we might just shoot some very harmless (and even helpful) creatures, while allowing some dangerous creatures (such as bears) too much proximity.

Oral tolerance is like being able to distinguish between the good creatures and the bad ones. Our probiotics "show" our bodies what molecules are nutritious and what molecules should be blocked and destroyed by the immune system. How and why does this take place? Our probiotic bacteria are living beings.

For millions of generations, these species have been living among our ancestors. Therefore, they have learned by experience what makes us healthy and what can make us sick. This information has been handed down through their generations through genetic evolution. In fact, it is more practical than that: What makes us sick likely also makes them sick.

Therefore, our probiotics can properly guide our immune system in terms of what is good for us and what is bad for us. Our immune system will then "mark" those "bad guys" for future responses when it comes into contact with them.

Of course, this does not exist in a vacuum, as our body's own DNA and immune system cells also will help our bodies recognize the good guys and bad guys. But without healthy probiotics, which our immune system has relied on for millions of years, there is no training.

Should our family's probiotics not be available for this training, we are in trouble. Caesarian sections, for example, will prevent our bodies from coming into contact with mother's probiotics from the birthing canal. Should we then be deprived of her breast milk, we will also miss out on these important probiotics that help train our immune system.

This scenario can result in a variety of situations. Our immune system may launch against the wrong things, including "good" proteins that give us nourishment. It may also launch against even the slightest difference in our air or what we might touch. This is called *sensitization*. The body's immune system becomes overly sensitized to things it should become tolerant to.

The other thing that can happen without the right probiotics is that that baby's brush barrier will not form properly, with the right mix of tight junctions and desmosomes. The intestines may then let into the body large molecules and toxins that the immune system knows it cannot handle. Once the immune system "sees" these invaders, it will launch an inflammatory attack in order to purge them, while alerting the body that it has been invaded (Pierce and Klinman 1977).

Illustrating this, researchers from Finland's University of Tampere Medical School (Majamaa and Isolauri 1997) found that the probiotic *Lactobacillus* GG (ATCC 53103) promotes IgA immunity, prevents increased intestinal permeability, and helps control antigen absorption. They gave Lactobacillus GG with whey formula or whey without probiotics to 27 children with atopic eczema and cow's milk allergy. They also gave Lactobacillus GG to mothers of 10 breast-fed infants with atopic eczema and cow's milk allergy.

The atopic dermatitis symptoms improved significantly during the one-month study period among infants and mothers treated with the probiotics. Probiotic-treated infants also showed decreased levels of alpha 1-antitrypsin while the non-probiotic group did not. The probiotic-treated groups also had lower levels of intestinal permeability. The researchers concluded:

> *"These results suggest that probiotic bacteria may promote endogenous barrier mechanisms in patients with atopic dermatitis and food allergy, and by alleviating intestinal inflammation, may act as a useful tool in the treatment of food allergy."*

This role played by probiotics to mediate and moderate potential allergens appears critical during the first few months of life, when the mucosal epithelial layer, the intestinal barrier and the immune system are all still in development. Probiotics increase plasma levels IL-10 and total IgA in children with allergic predisposition. Both of these immunoglobulins are central to intestinal immunity and preventing intestinal permeability and the hypersensitive allergic response.

University of Helsinki researchers (Salmi *et al.* 2010) studied 35 infants with atopic eczema, of which 16 had milk allergies. They gave the infants Lactobacillus rhamnosus GG or a placebo. After four weeks, they found that the intestinal organic acids of the milk allergy children began to look more like the non-allergic infants.

Researchers from Germany's Royal Veterinary and Agricultural University (Rosenfeldt *et al.* 2004) wanted to find out if probiotics could reverse intestinal inflammation and strengthen intestinal barrier function in 41 allergic children. Probiotics *Lactobacillus rhamnosus* 19070-2 and *Lactobacillus reuteri* DSM 12246 were given to the children for six weeks – who displayed symptoms of moderate and severe allergic atopic dermatitis. Intestinal permeability was quantified using the lactulose-mannitol test. Gastrointestinal symptoms were also analyzed. Before the probiotic treatment, the researchers found that lactulose-to-mannitol ratios were high, indicating increased intestinal permeability. After the probiotic treatment, the probiotic group's lactulose-to-mannitol ratios were significantly lower.

The probiotic group also experienced a significant decrease in gastrointestinal symptoms and eczema symptoms. The researchers concluded:

> *"The study suggests that probiotic supplementation may stabilize the intestinal barrier function".*

Remember the research from the University of Turku (Kalliomäki and Isolauri 2002) mentioned earlier. This clinical trial showed that probiotic supplementation reduced atopic eczema risk by 50% among children. They concluded by saying:

> *"Probiotics have also been shown to reverse increased intestinal permeability and to reduce antigen load in the gut by degrading and modifying macromolecules."*

As infants wean from breast milk, they can also pick up a host of probiotic colonies from drinking raw milk or by feeding on yogurt or kefir. These will introduce still new probiotics into the intestines. The probiotics will all help increase baby's oral tolerance and further develop the intestinal barrier.

The fact that the health of our intestinal walls is directly related to our probiotics has been shown in many other studies.

For example, researchers from the Vanderbilt University School of Medicine (Yan *et al.* 2006) found that epithelial damage to intestinal cells was mediated (reduced) by *Lactobacillus rhamnosus* GG. Other studies such as one from Korea's Chosun University Medical School (Bai *et al.* 2005) have shown that other probiotics such as *Lactobacillus paracasei, Lactobacillus reuterrii* and *Saccharomyces cerevisiae* reduce intestinal permeability.

Killing Probiotics

Remember earlier discussions related to the dramatic increase in food sensitivities including gluten sensitivities and even celiac disease over the past 3-4 decades.

And remember the research on children involved in the Swedish celiac disease epidemic. Those who had infections and gastroenteritis were significantly more likely to develop celiac disease.

This together with the understanding that probiotics are not only necessary for intestinal health but they mediate inflammation brings together the most probable causative element: The killing of our probiotics through antibiotic and antimicrobial strategies.

Just consider the dramatic over-utilization of prescriptive and over the counter antibiotics, antifungals, antivirals, antiseptic soaps and cleaning disinfectants. Just consider the use of antibiotics in our animal and dairy industries. All of this ends up in the same place: Our digestive tracts, where they slaughter our intestinal probiotics.

And in the case of the Swedish children, consider that any infant infection these days is prescribed with antibiotics.

The use of antibiotics has soared over the past few decades – suspiciously over the same period that food sensitivities have also soared. Today, over

3,000,000 pounds of pure antibiotics are taken by humans annually in the United States. This is complemented by the approximately 25,000,000 pounds of antibiotics given to animals each year.

Meanwhile, many of these antibiotics either are given in vain or are ineffectual. The Centers for Disease Control stated:

> *"Almost half of patients with upper respiratory tract infections in the U.S. still receive antibiotics from their doctor." This said, the CDC also warns that "90% of upper respiratory infections, including children's ear infections, are viral, and antibiotics don't treat viral infection. More than 40% of about 50 million prescriptions for antibiotics each year in physicians' offices were inappropriate."*

In addition to the die-off of our intestinal probiotics, the growing use of antibiotics has created a Pandora's box of *superbugs*. As bacteria are repeatedly hit with the same antibiotic, they learn to adapt. Just as any living organism does (yes, bacteria are alive), bacteria learn to counter and resist repeatedly utilized antibiotics.

As a result, many bacteria today are stronger and more resistant to antibiotics and probiotics. This means they can overpopulate our intestinal tracts, causing a variety of intestinal problems – including damage to our intestinal cells.

This is because bacteria tend to adjust to their surroundings. If they are attacked enough times with a certain challenge, they are likely to figure out how to avoid it and thrive despite it.

This has been the case for a number of other new antibiotic-resistant strains of bacteria. They have simply evolved to become stronger and more able to counteract these antibiotic measures.

This phenomenon has created *multi-drug resistant organisms*. Some of the more dangerous MDROs include species of *Enterococcus, Staphylococcus, Salmonella, Campylobacter, Escherichia coli*, and others. Superbugs such as MRSA are only the tip of the bacterial iceberg.

Another growing infectious bacterium is *Clostridium difficile*. Research has connected the Clostridium genera to celiac disease. These bacteria will infect the intestines of people of any age. Among children, this is one of the world's biggest killers – causing acute, watery diarrhea. It is also a growing infection – known and unknown – among adults.

Every year *C. difficile* infects tens of thousands of people in the U.S. according to the Mayo Clinic. Worse, *C. difficile* are increasingly becoming resistant to antibiotics and infections from clostridia are growing in incidence each year.

Medical researchers from the Norwegian University of Science and Technology (Mai *et al.* 2010) found that early antibiotic use increased the likelihood of allergies at age eight. Over 3,300 children were studied for antibiotic use and respiratory conditions at the ages of two months, one year, four years and eight years old.

Of all groups, 43% of the children received antibiotics. A third of the children had a respiratory infection, including pneumonia, bronchitis or otitis. The researchers found those who used antibiotics during their first year of life had increased rates of wheeze and eczema by age eight.

Other research as we have quoted, link higher rates of wheeze with greater incidence of food sensitivities.

Intestinal Dysbiosis

Dysbiosis is a state where the body has an imbalance between probiotic populations and pathogenic bacteria populations. In other words, the system is being overrun by the pathogenic bacteria and there are not enough probiotics in place to control their populations.

What many do not realize is that practically the same symptoms many will attribute to gluten intolerance are also symptoms of dysbiosis.

When the body is lacking probiotics, or is overgrown with pathobiotic populations, there is typically an intestinal infection of some type. The extent of the infection, of course, depends upon the type of pathogenic bacteria present, and their populations in proportion to probiotic populations.

Many disorders can be traced back to dysbiosis. Some are direct and obvious, and some are not so obvious, and often appear as other disorders. In general, most digestive disorders are either caused by or accompanied by a lack of balanced intestinal probiotic populations. There are several types of dysbiosis.

We can usually detect *putrefaction dysbiosis* from the incidence of slow bowel movement. Symptoms of putrefaction dysbiosis include depression, diarrhea, fatigue, memory loss, numbing of hands and feet, sleep disturbances, joint pain and muscle weakness.

Many of these disorders and others are often due directly to the overgrowth of pathobiotics and their endotoxins. The bacteria are burdening the blood stream with endotoxin waste products and neurotoxins; infecting cells, joints, nerves, brain tissues and other regions of the body.

Another overgrowth issue is *fermentation dysbiosis*. This is often evidenced by bloating, constipation, diarrhea, fatigue, and gas; and the faulty digestion of carbohydrates, grains, proteins and fiber. This is also a result of pathobiotic overgrowth, but in this type of dysbiosis, yeasts are prevalent among the overgrowth populations. As we know from baking bread, yeast will ferment quickly in warm, humid environments.

A body with low probiotic populations will create havoc for the immune system. *Deficiency dysbiosis* is related to an absence of probiotics, leading to damaged intestinal mucosa. This can lead to irritable bowel syndrome, food sensitivities, and intestinal permeability. The lack of probiotics allows the intestinal wall to come into contact with foreign molecules. This can open up the junctions between the intestinal cells. This can in turn lead to the entry of these toxins along with larger more complex food particles into the bloodstream – such as larger peptides and protein molecules – as we have discussed.

Because these molecules are not normally found in the blood stream, the immune system identifies them as foreigners. The body then launches an inflammatory immune response, leading to *sensitization dysbiosis.* Linked to probiotic deficiency, sensitization dysbiosis causes food and chemical sensitivities, acne, connective tissue disease and psoriasis. Intestinal permeability has also been suspected in a variety of lung and joint infections.

And it is this latter form of dysbiosis that is significantly linked to gluten sensitivities.

The obvious signs of dysbiosis include hormonal imbalances and mood swings, high cholesterol, vitamin B deficiencies, frequent gas and bloating, indigestion, irritable bowels, easy bruising of the skin, constipation, diarrhea, vaginal infections, reduced sex drive, prostate enlargement, food sensitivities, chemical sensitivities, bladder infections, allergies, rhinovirus and rotavirus infections, influenza, and various histamine-related inflammatory syndromes such as rashes, asthma and skin irritation.

Illustrating the connection between probiotics and allergic skin response, Denmark children ages one to thirteen years old who were diagnosed with atopic dermatitis were given freeze-dried *L. rhaminosus* 19070-2 and *L. reuteri* DSM 122460 probiotics for six weeks. The children were then examined for symptoms. Among the probiotic groups, 56% reported improved eczema symptoms, compared to 15% among the control groups (Rosenfeldt *et al.* 2003).

Furthermore, the infection of various parts of the body – either from pathogenic bacteria or their endotoxins – can cause various ailments typically associated with autoimmune or degenerative etiologies. Autoimmune type diseases of the liver, the urinary tract, the joints, gums and ears, heart and lungs can directly result from any of the above forms of dysbiosis.

An example of this is Grave's disease – considered a classic autoimmune disorder caused seemingly by the immune system attacking healthy cells of the thyroid gland. Tests have shown that some 80% of Grave's sufferers test positive for *Yersinia enterocolitica* antibodies.

Dysbiosis is often accompanied by an overgrowth of the bacteria, *Yersinia enterocolitica.* Yersina endotoxins can attach to thyroid cells, stimulating the over-production of thyroid hormone. This is precisely one of the symptoms of

Grave's disease, typically considered a classic autoimmune disorder, just as celiac disease is considered an autoimmune disorder.

Clinical Findings on Probiotics and Allergies

Probiotics mechanisms have been increasingly connected to inflammatory and allergic responses. Iinflammatory and allergic responses are typical among wheat allergies and some gluten intolerance cases.

They play a critical role in maintaining the epithelial barrier function of the intestinal tract. We've shown that allergies increase with intestinal permeability. Without an adequate intestinal barrier, larger food molecules, endotoxins and microorganisms can enter the bloodstream more easily. These increase the body's total toxin burden, making the immune system more sensitive.

Finnish researchers (Ouwehand *et al.* 2009) gave 47 children with birch pollen allergies *Lactobacillus acidophilus* NCFM and *Bifidobacterium lactis* Bl-04 or a placebo for four months, beginning before the birch pollen season. The probiotic group had significantly less sinus congestion, and lower numbers of nasal membrane eosinophils.

Researchers from Finland's University of Turku (Kirjavainen *et al.* 2003) gave 35 infants with milk allergies *Lactobacillus* GG or a placebo for 5.5 months. The researchers concluded that:

> *"Supplementation of infant formulas with viable but not heat-inactivated LGG is a potential approach for the management of atopic eczema and cow's milk allergy."*

The British medical publication *Lancet* published a study (Kalliomäki *et al.* 2001) where 132 children with a high risk of atopic eczema were given either a placebo or *Lactobacillus rhamnosus* GG during their first two years of life. While 31 of 68 of the children receiving the placebo contracted atopic eczema, only 14 of 64 children receiving the probiotic developed atopic eczema by the end of the study.

University of Helsinki researchers (Viljanen *et al.* 2005) treated 230 milk-allergic infants *Lactobacillus* GG, four probiotic strains, or a placebo for four weeks. Among IgE-sensitized allergic children, the LGG provoked a reduction in symptoms while the placebo group did not.

Researchers from Sweden's Umeå University (West *et al.* 2009) fed Lactobacillus F19 or a placebo to 179 infants with allergic eczema from four months to 13 months old. The placebo group had double the incidence of eczema at 13 months than the probiotic group. The probiotic group as a whole also tested with more balanced Th1/Th2 ratios – with greater Th1 levels than the placebo group.

Allergy Hospital researchers from Helsinki University (Kuitunen *et al.* 2009) gave a probiotic blend of two lactobacilli, bifidobacteria, propionibacteria and prebiotics, or a placebo to mothers of 1,223 infants with a high risk of allergies during the last month of pregnancy term. Then they gave their infants the dose from birth until six months of age. They evaluated the children at five years of age for allergies.

Of the 1,018 infants who completed the dosing, 891 were evaluated after five years. Allergies among the cesarean-birth children were nearly half in the probiotic group compared to the placebo group (24.3% versus 40.5%).

University of Milan researchers (Arslanoglu *et al.* 2008) found that a mixture of prebiotics galactooligosaccharides (GOS) and fructooligosaccharides (FOS) reduces allergy incidence. A mix of these or a placebo were given with formula for the first six months after birth to 134 infants. The incidence of dermatitis, wheezing, and allergic urticaria in the prebiotic group was half of what was found among the placebo group. The researchers concluded:

> *"The observed dual protection lasting beyond the intervention period suggests that an immune modulating effect through the intestinal flora modification may be the principal mechanism of action."*

Researchers from Finland's National Public Health Institute (Piirainen *et al.* 2008) found that *Lactobacillus rhamnosus* GG fed to pollen-allergic persons for 5-½ months resulted in lower levels of pollen-specific IgE, higher levels of IgG and higher levels of IgA in the saliva. This is consistent with lower sensitivity, greater immunity, and a greater tolerance for pollens and foods.

Researchers from the Medical School at Finland's University of Tampere (Majamaa and Isolauri 1997) gave *Lactobacillus* GG (ATCC 53103) or placebo to 27 infants allergic to milk. The probiotic group showed significant improvement of allergic symptoms after one month of treatment. This and levels of fecal tumor necrosis factor-alpha gave cause for the researchers to conclude:

> *"These results suggest that probiotic bacteria may promote endogenous barrier mechanisms in patients with atopic dermatitis and food allergy, and by alleviating intestinal inflammation, may act as a useful tool in the treatment of food allergy."*

Probiotics balance levels of pro and anti-inflammatory cytokines. They reduce antigens by digesting or otherwise modifying proteins and other food molecules. Probiotics can reverse increased intestinal permeability among children with food allergies. They enhance IgA responses, which are often dysfunctional in food allergy children. Probiotics also normalize the gut microenvironment (Laitinen and Isolauri 2006).

Probiotics improve the intestinal barrier function. They reduce the production of proinflammatory cytokines (Miraglia del Giudice and De Luca 2004).

Research from Sweden's Linköping University (Böttcher *et al.* 2008) gave *Lactobacillus reuteri* or a placebo to 99 pregnant women from gestational week 36 until infant delivery. The babies were followed for two years after birth, and analyzed for eczema, allergen sensitization and immunity markers. Probiotic supplementation lowered TGF-beta2 levels in mother's milk and babies' feces, and slightly increased IL-10 levels in mothers' colostrum. Lower levels of TGF-beta2 are associated with lower sensitization and lower risk of IgE-associated eczema.

German researchers (Grönlund *et al.* 2007) tested 61 infants and mother pairs for allergic status and bifidobacteria levels from 30-35 weeks of gestation and from one-month old. Every mother's breast milk contained some type of bifidobacteria, with *Bifidobacterium longum* found most frequently. However, only the infants of allergic, atopic mothers had colonization with *B. adolescentis.* Allergic mothers also had significantly less bifidobacteria in their breast-milk than non-allergic mothers.

Japanese scientists (Xiao *et al.* 2006) gave 44 patients with Japanese cedar pollen allergies *Bifidobacterium longum* BB536 for 13 weeks. The probiotic group had significantly decreased symptoms of rhinorrhea (runny nose) and nasal blockage versus the placebo group. The probiotic group also had decreased activity among plasma T-helper type 2 (Th2) cells and reduced symptoms of Japanese cedar pollen allergies. The researchers concluded that the results:

> *"suggest the efficacy of BB536 in relieving JCPsis symptoms, probably through the modulation of Th2-skewed immune response."*

Researchers from the Wellington School of Medicine and Health Sciences at New Zealand's University of Otago (Wickens *et al.* 2008) studied the association between probiotics and eczema in 474 children. Pregnant women took either a placebo, *Lactobacillus rhamnosus* HN001, or *Bifidobacterium animalis* subsp *lactis* strain HN019 starting from 35 weeks gestation, and their babies received the same treatment from birth to two years old. The probiotic infants given *L. rhamnosus* had significantly lower incidence of eczema compared with infants taking the placebo. There was no significant difference between the *B. animalis* group and the placebo group, however.

Researchers from Japan's Kansai Medical University Kouri Hospital (Hattori *et al.* 2003) gave 15 children with atopic dermatitis either *Bifidobacterium breve* M-16V or a placebo. After one month, the probiotic group had a significant improvement of allergic symptoms.

Japanese scientists (Ishida *et al.* 2003) gave a drink with *Lactobacillus acidophilus* strain L-92 or a placebo to 49 patients with perennial allergic rhinitis for eight weeks. The probiotic group showed significant improvement in runny nose and watery eyes symptoms, along with decreased nasal mucosa swelling and redness compared to the placebo group. These results were also duplicated in a follow-up study (2005) of 23 allergy sufferers by some of the same researchers.

Researchers from Tokyo's Juntendo University School of Medicine (Fujii *et al.* 2006) gave 19 preterm infants placebo or *Bifidobacterium breve* supplementation for three weeks after birth. Anti-inflammatory serum TGF-beta1 levels in the probiotic group were elevated on day 14 and remained elevated through day 28. Messenger RNA expression was enhanced for the probiotic group on day 28 compared with the placebo group. The researchers concluded:

> *"These results demonstrated that the administration of B. breve to preterm infants can up-regulate TGF-beta1 signaling and may possibly be beneficial in attenuating inflammatory and allergic reactions in these infants."*

Scientists from Britain's Institute of Food Research (Ivory *et al.* 2008) gave *Lactobacillus casei* Shirota (LcS) to 10 patients with seasonal allergic rhinitis. The researchers compared immune status with daily ingestion of a milk drink with or without live *Lactobacillus casei* over a period of five months. Blood samples were tested for plasma IgE and grass pollen-specific IgG by an enzyme immunoassay. Patients treated with the *Lactobacillus casei* milk showed significantly reduced levels of antigen-induced IL-5, IL-6 and IFN-gamma production compared with the placebo group. Levels of specific IgG also increased and IgE decreased in the probiotic group. The researchers concluded:

> *"These data show that probiotic supplementation modulates immune responses in allergic rhinitis and may have the potential to alleviate the severity of symptoms."*

Researchers from the Skin and Allergy Hospital at the University of Helsinki (Kukkonen *et al.* 2007) studied the role of probiotics and allergies with 1,223 pregnant women carrying children with a high-risk of allergies. A placebo or lactobacilli and bifidobacteria combination with GOS was given to the pregnant women for two to four weeks before delivery, and their babies continued the treatment after birth. At two years of age, the infants in the probiotic group had 25% fewer cases of eczema and 34% few cases of atopic eczema.

The same researchers from the Skin and Allergy Hospital and Helsinki University Central Hospital (Kukkonen *et al.* 2009) studied the immune effects of feeding probiotics to pregnant mothers. In all, 925 pregnant mothers were given a placebo or a combination of *Lactobacillus rhamnosus* GG and LC705, *Bifidobacterium breve* Bb99, and *Propionibacterium freudenreichii* ssp. *shermanii* for four weeks prior to delivery. Their infants were given the same formula together with prebiotics, or a placebo for six months after birth. During the infants' six-month treatment period, antibiotics were prescribed less often among the probiotic group by 23%. In addition, respiratory infections occurred less frequently among the probiotic group through the two-year follow-up period (even after treatment had stopped) compared to the placebo group (an average of 3.7 infections versus 4.2 infections).

Finnish scientists (Kirjavainen *et al.* 2002) gave 21 infants with early onset atopic eczema a placebo or *Bifidobacterium lactis* Bb-12. Serum IgE concentration correlated directly to *Escherichia coli* and bacteroide counts, indicating the association between these bacteria with atopic sensitization. The probiotic group had a decrease in the numbers of *Escherichia coli* and bacteroides after treatment.

Sonicated *Streptococcus thermophilus* cream was applied to the forearms of 11 patients with atopic dermatitis for two weeks. This led to a significant increase of skin ceramide levels, and a significant improvement of their clinical signs and symptoms – including erythema, scaling and pruritus (Di Marzio *et al.* 2003).

Japanese researchers (Odamaki *et al.* 2007) gave yogurt with *Bifidobacterium longum* BB536 or plain yogurt to 40 patients with Japanese cedar pollinosis for 14 weeks. *Bacteroides fragilis* significantly changed with pollen dispersion. The ratio of *B. fragilis* to bifidobacteria also increased significantly during pollen season among the placebo group but not in the *B. longum* group. Peripheral blood mononuclear cells from the patients indicated that *B. fragilis* microorganisms induced significantly more Th2 cell cytokines such as interleukin-6, and fewer Th1 cell cytokines such as IL-12 and interferon. The researchers concluded:

> *"These results suggest a relationship between fluctuation in intestinal microbiota and pollinosis allergy. Furthermore, intake of BB536 yogurt appears to exert positive influences on the formation of anti-allergic microbiota."*

Scientists from the Department of Oral Microbiology at Japan's Asahi University School of Dentistry (Ogawa *et al.* 2006) studied skin allergic symptoms and blood chemistry of healthy human volunteers during the cedar pollen season in Japan. After supplementation with *Lactobacillus casei*, pro-inflammatory activity of cedar pollen-specific IgE, chemokines, eosinophils and interferon-gamma levels all decreased among the probiotic group.

Researchers from the School of Medicine and Health Sciences in Wellington, New Zealand (Sistek *et al.* 2006) gave *Lactobacillus rhamnosus* and *Bifidobacteria lactis* or placebo to 59 children with established atopic dermatitis. They found that food-sensitized atopic children responded significantly better to probiotics than did other atopic dermatitis children.

French scientists (Passeron *et al.* 2006) found that atopic dermatitis children improved significantly after three months of *Lactobacillus rhamnosus* treatment, based on SCORAD (symptom) levels of 39.1 before and 20.7 afterward.

Scientists from Finland's National Public Health Institute (Piirainen *et al.* 2008) gave a placebo or *Lactobacillus rhamnosus* GG to 38 patients with atopic eczema for 5.5 months – starting 2.5 months before birch pollen season. Saliva and serum samples taken before and after indicated that allergen-specific IgA levels increased significantly among the probiotic group versus the placebo group (using the enzyme-linked immunosorbent assay (ELISA)). Allergen-specific IgE levels correlated positively with stimulated IgA and IgG in saliva, while they correlated negatively in the placebo group. The researchers concluded:

> *"L. rhamnosus GG displayed "immunostimulating effects on oral mucosa seen as increased allergen specific IgA levels in saliva."*

Children with cow's milk allergy and IgE-associated dermatitis were given a placebo or *Lactobacillus rhamnosus* GG and a combination of four other probiotic bacteria (Pohjavuori *et al.* 2004). The IFN-gamma by PBMCs at the beginning of supplementation was significantly lower among cow's milk allergy infants. However, cow's milk allergy infants receiving *L. rhamnosus* GG had significantly increased levels of IFN-gamma, showing increased tolerance.

The British medical publication *Lancet* published a study (Kalliomäki *et al.* 2003) where 107 children with a high risk of atopic eczema were given either a placebo or *Lactobacillus rhamnosus* GG during their first two years of life. Fourteen of 53 children receiving the probiotic developed atopic eczema, while 25 of 54 of the children receiving the placebo contracted atopic eczema by the end of the study.

In a study from the University of Western Australia School of Pediatrics (Taylor *et al.* 2006), 178 children born of mothers with allergies were given either *Lactobacillus acidophilus* or a placebo for the first six months of life. Those given the probiotics showed reduced levels of IL-5 and TGF-beta in response to polyclonal stimulation (typical for allergic responses), and significantly lower IL-10 responses to vaccines as compared with the placebo group. These results illustrated that the probiotics had increased allergen resistance among the probiotic group of children.

Researchers from the Department of Otolaryngology and Sensory Organ Surgery at Osaka University School of Medicine in Japan (Tamura *et al.* 2007) studied allergic response in chronic rhinitis patients. For eight weeks, patients were given either a placebo or *Lactobacillus casei* strain Shirota. Those with moderate-to-severe nasal symptom scores at the beginning of the study who were given probiotics experienced significantly reduced nasal symptoms.

Probiotics and Intestinal Permeability

We have discussed the mechanisms related to increased intestinal permeability and gluten sensitivities. We will summarize those mechanisms here and relate the issue more closely with probiotics.

Our probiotics line the walls of our intestines and move around our mucosal membrane. Here they police the intestinal cells and excrete acids that help manage the pH of the mucosal membrane. Should probiotic colonies be damaged by toxins, infection, antibiotics or poor dietary choices, their symbiotic relationship with our intestines can come to an end or become severely limited. This effectively thins the mucosal membrane and leaves the intestinal cells more exposed to food particles and toxins.

Should our probiotic colonies become scarce and our mucosal membrane thins, larger peptides, toxins and even invading microorganisms are allowed to have contact with the intestinal cells. This irritates the intestinal cells, producing an inflammatory immune response. This inflammatory immune response in turn damages the ability of the intestinal brush barrier to keep larger food proteins or toxins from invading our tissues and bloodstream.

Again, the intestinal brush barrier as a whole includes the mucosal layer of enzymes, probiotics and ionic fluid. This forms a protective surface medium over the intestinal epithelium. It also provides an active nutrient transport mechanism. It contains glycoproteins and other ionic transporters, which attach to nutrient molecules, carrying them across intestinal membranes. However, this mucosal membrane is supported and stabilized by the grooves between the intestinal microvilli.

This support is provided by four mechanisms existing between the intestinal microvilli: tight junctions, adherens junctions, desmosomes and probiotics. The tight functions form a bilayer interface between cells, controlling permeability. Zonulin appears to be one of the mediators for regulating the tight junctions.

Desmosomes are points of interface between the tight junctions. The adherens junctions keep the cell membranes adhesive enough to stabilize the junctions. These junction mechanisms together regulate permeability at the intestinal wall.

In healthy intestines, the microvilli gaps are policed by billions of probiotic colonies. These perform a variety of maintenance tasks. They help process and break down incoming food molecules. They excrete acids to manage the environment. They secrete various nutrients. They control pathogenic bacteria that can threaten the region. They also communicate closely with the immune system to help signal invasions.

This symbiotic relationship gives the brush barrier its triple-filter mechanism that essentially screens for molecule size, ionic nature and nutrition quality. Before a molecule can come into contact with the intestines, tissues or bloodstream, it must pass through these filter mechanisms.

Should the probiotics become damaged, the entire mucosal brush barrier begins to break down. You might say that our probiotics provide the "glue" that keeps everything working smoothly.

The health of our probiotics and the health of the brush barrier can be threatened by a number of factors. Alcohol is one of the most irritating substances to our probiotics and the mucosal brush barrier in general (Bongaerts and Severijnen 2005).

In addition, many pharmaceutical drugs, notably NSAIDs, have been identified as damaging to probiotics and the mucosal brush barrier integrity. Foods with high arachidonic fatty acid capability; low-fiber, high-glucose foods; and high nitrite-forming foods have been suspected for their ability to inhibit growth of our probiotics. They also can compromise the mucosal chemistry. Toxic substances such as plasticizers, pesticides, herbicides, chlorinated water and food dyes are also suspected. Substances that increase PGE-2 response also negatively affect permeability (Martin-Venegas *et al.* 2006).

In addition, the overuse of antibiotics can cause a die-off of our resident probiotic colonies. When intestinal probiotic colonies are reduced, pathogenic bacteria and yeasts can outgrow the remaining probiotic colonies. Pathogenic bacteria growth invades the brush barrier, introducing an influx of endotoxins (the waste matter of these microorganisms) into the bloodstream together with some of the microorganisms themselves.

Many distinguished scientists around the world have now attributed the breakdown of the mucosal brush barrier and the influx of macromolecules as the major cause for the increasing occurrence of food sensitivities in Western society. Healthy intestinal barriers prevent allergic response because they limit the entry of large food molecules into the body's tissues and bloodstream.

A food that has been a source of nutrition for many years can suddenly be identified by the immune system as a threat if its proteins get into the body's tissues before being properly broken down to size. This unfortunate circumstance results not only in the possibility of allergic response to some foods: Nutritional deficiencies can also result. Research is finally confirming these mechanisms (Laitinen and Isolauri 2005; Fasano and Shea-Donohue 2005).

Inflammatory responses resulting from increased intestinal permeability have now been linked to sinusitis, allergies, psoriasis, asthma, arthritis and other inflammatory conditions. Food sensitivities are simply one condition among others.

The research has also revealed a link between intestinal permeability and liver damage (Bode and Bode 2003). Alcohol consumption has also been associated with intestinal permeability (Ferrier *et al.* 2006).

Let's look at the research linking intestinal permeability to probiotics:

In a study by scientists from China's Qilu Hospital and Shandong University (Zeng *et al.* 2008), 30 irritable bowel syndrome patients with intestinal wall permeability were given either a placebo or a fermented milk beverage with *Streptococcus thermophilus, Lactobacillus bulgaricus, Lactobacillus acidophilus* and *Bifidobacterium longum.* After four weeks, intestinal permeability reduced significantly among the probiotic group.

Researchers from Greece's Alexandra Regional General Hospital (Stratiki *et al.* 2007) gave 41 preterm infants of 27-36 weeks gestation a formula supplemented with *Bifidobacterium lactis* or a placebo. After seven days, bifidobacteria counts were significantly higher, head growth was greater. After 30 days, the lactulose/mannitol ratio (marker for intestinal permeability) was significantly lower in the probiotic group as compared to the placebo group. The researchers concluded that:

> *"bifidobacteria supplemented infant formula decreases intestinal permeability of preterm infants and leads to increased head growth."*

Granada medical researchers (Lara-Villoslada *et al.* 2007) gave *Lactobacillus coryniformis* CECT5711 and *Lactobacillus gasseri* CECT5714 or a placebo to 30 healthy children after having received conventional yogurt containing *Lactobacillus bulgaricus* and *Streptococcus thermophilus* for three weeks. The supplemented yogurt significantly inhibited *Salmonella cholerasuis* adhesion to intestinal mucins compared to before probiotic supplementation. The probiotic supplementation also increased IgA concentration in feces and saliva.

German scientists (Rosenfeldt *et al.* 2004) gave *Lactobacillus rhamnosus* 19070-2 and *L. reuteri* DSM 12246 or a placebo to 41 children. After six weeks of treatment, the frequency of GI symptoms were significantly lower (10% versus 39%) among the probiotic group as compared to the placebo group. In addition, the lactulose-to-mannitol ratio was lower in the probiotic group, indicating to the researchers:

> *"probiotic supplementation may stabilize the intestinal barrier function and decrease gastrointestinal symptoms in children with atopic dermatitis."*

Researchers from the People's Hospital and the Jiao Tong University in Shangha (Qin *et al.* 2008) gave *Lactobacillus plantarum* or placebo to 76 patients with acute pancreatitis. Intestinal permeability was determined using the lactulose/rhamnose ratio. Organ failure, septic complications and death were also monitored. After seven days of treatment, microbial infections averaged 38.9% in the probiotic group and 73.7% in the placebo group. Furthermore, only 30.6% of the probiotic group colonized potentially pathogenic organisms, as compared to 50% of patients in the control group. The probiotic group also had significantly better clinical outcomes compared to the control group. The researchers concluded that: *"Lactobacillus plantarum can attenuate disease severity, improve the intestinal permeability and clinical outcomes."*

Researchers from the Department of Medical Microbiology at the Radboud University Nijmegen Medical Centre in The Netherlands (Bongaerts and Severijnen 2005) studied the intestinal permeability connection in food allergies with great focus. They came to the conclusion that:

> *"Adequate probiotics can (i) prevent the increased characteristic intestinal permeability of children with atopic eczema and food allergy, (ii) can thus prevent the uptake of allergens, and (iii) finally can prevent the expression of the atopic constitution. The use of adequate probiotic lactobacilli, i.e., homolactic and/or facultatively heterolactic l-lactic acid-producing lactobacilli, reduces the intestinal amounts of the bacterial, toxic metabolites, d-lactic acid and ethanol by fermentative production of merely the non-toxic l-lactic acid from glucose. Thus, it is thought that beneficial probiotic micro-organisms promote gut barrier function and both undo and prevent unfavorable intestinal micro-ecological alterations in allergic individuals."*

Probiotics, IBS and Crohn's

As we discussed earlier, the risk of food sensitivities increases substantially with irritable bowel syndrome (IBS), Crohn's disease, and other intestinal conditions. And gluten sensitivities are often linked with IBS symptoms.

Crohn's and IBS are often considered autoimmune diseases. However, the concept that the body's immune system is attacking itself for no reason is illogical. There are reasons the immune system might target cells from within the body. These can range from the cells being damaged by environmental toxins, endotoxins, oxidative (free) radicals, viruses, to the immune system itself being damaged. How do probiotics intermix within these possibilities?

The research illustrates that probiotics directly attack foreign invaders like bacteria, viruses and fungi before they can damage the cells of the intestinal walls. Probiotics can also bind to oxidative radicals formed by many types of toxins. Probiotics will also line the intestinal cells, creating a barrier for toxins to enter the blood. They secrete lactic acid and other biochemicals that prevent endotoxin microorganisms from flourishing. Probiotics will also signal the immune system with the identities of pathogens, and then assist in their eradication.

Deficiencies of probiotics in the intestines usually result in overgrowths of pathogenic microorganisms like *Clostridia* spp., *E. coli, H. pylori* and *Candida* spp. These damage the cells of the intestinal wall and produce endotoxins that poison intestinal cells. These can damage the brush barrier of the intestines and result in intestinal permeability and an increased risk of food sensitivities.

Here is some research supporting these conclusions:

Researchers from the Medical University of Warsaw (Gawrońska *et al.* 2007) investigated 104 children who had functional dyspepsia, irritable bowel syndrome, or functional abdominal pain. They gave the children either placebo or *Lactobacillus rhamnosus* GG. for four weeks. The probiotic group had overall treatment success (25% versus 9.6%) compared to the placebo group. The IBS probiotic group had even more treatment success compared to the placebo IBS group (33% versus 5%). The probiotic group also had significantly reduced pain frequency.

French researchers (Drouault-Holowacz *et al.* 2008) gave probiotics or a placebo to 100 patients with irritable bowel syndrome. Between the first and fourth weeks of treatment, the probiotic group had significantly less abdominal pain (42% versus 24%) than the placebo group.

Researchers from Poland's Curie Regional Hospital (Niedzielin *et al.* 2001) gave *Lactobacillus plantarum* 299V or placebo to 40 IBS patients. IBS symptoms significantly improved for 95% of the probiotic patients versus just 15% of the placebo group.

Forty IBS patients took *Lactobacillus acidophilus* SDC 2012, 2013 or a placebo for four weeks in research at the Samsung Medical Center and Korea's Sungkyunkwan University School of Medicine (Sinn *et al.* 2008). The probiotic group had a 23% reduction in pain and discomfort while the placebo group showed no improvement.

Scientists from Italy's University of Parma (Fanigliulo *et al.* 2006) gave *Bifidobacterium longum* W11 or rifaximin (an IBS medication) to 70 IBS patients for two months. The probiotic patients reported a fewer symptoms and greater improvement than the rifaxmin patients. The researchers commented:

> *"The abnormalities observed in the colonic flora of IBS suggest, in fact, that a probiotic approach will ultimately be justified."*

Researchers from the University of Helsinki (Kajander *et al.* 2008) treated 86 patients with IBS with either a placebo or a combination of *Lactobacillus rhamnosus* GG, *L. rhamnosus* Lc705, *Propionibacterium freudenreichii* subsp. *Shermanii* JS and *Bifidobacterium animalis* subsp. *lactis.* After five months, the probiotic group had a significant reduction of IBS symptoms, especially with respect to distension and abdominal pain. The researchers concluded:

> *"This multispecies probiotic seems to be an effective and safe option to alleviate symptoms of irritable bowel syndrome, and to stabilize the intestinal microbiota."*

Scientists from the Canadian Research and Development Centre for Probiotics and The Lawson Health Research Institute in Ontario (Lorea Baroja *et al.* 2007) studied 20 IBS patients, 15 Crohn's patients, five ulcerative colitis patients, and 20 healthy volunteers. All subjects were given a yogurt supplemented with *Lactobacillus rhamnosus* GR-1 and *L. reuteri* RC-14 for 30 days. IBS inflammatory markers were tested in the bloodstream. CD4(+) CD25(+) T-cells increased significantly among the probiotic IBS group. Tumor necrosis factor (TNF)-alpha(+)/interleukin (IL)-12(+) monocytes decreased for all the groups except the IBS probiotic group. Myeloid DC decreased among most probiotic groups, but was also stimulated in IBS patients. Serum IL-12, IL-2(+) and CD69(+) T-cells also decreased in probiotic IBS patients. The researchers also concluded:

> *"Probiotic yogurt intake was associated with significant anti-inflammatory effects..."*

Researchers from the General Hospital of Celle (Plein and Hotz 1993) gave *Saccharomyces boulardii* or placebo to 20 Crohn's disease patients with diarrhea flare-ups. After ten weeks, the probiotic group had a significant reduction in bowel movement frequency compared with the control group. The control group's bowel movement frequency rose in the tenth week and then subsided to initial frequency levels – consistent with flare-ups.

In another study from Finland (Kajander *et al.* 2005), a placebo or combination of *Lactobacillus rhamnosus* GG, *L. rhamnosus* LC705, *Bifidobacterium breve* Bb99 and *Propionibacterium freudenreichii* subsp. *shermanii* JS was given to of 103 patients with IBS. The total symptom score (abdominal pain + distension + flatulence + borborygmi) was 7.7 points lower among the probiotic group. This represented a 42% reduction in the symptoms of the probiotic group compared with a 6% reduction of symptoms among the placebo group.

In a study from Yonsei University College of Medicine in Korea (Kim *et al.* 2006), 40 irritable bowel syndrome patients were given either a placebo or a combination of *Bacillus subtilis* and *Streptococcus faecium* for four weeks. The severity and frequency of abdominal pain decreased significantly in the probiotic group.

Researchers from Sweden's Lund University Hospital (Nobaek *et al.* 2000) gave 60 patients with irritable bowel syndrome either a placebo or daily rosehip drink with *Lactobacillus plantarum* for four weeks. Enterococci levels increased among the placebo group but were unchanged in the test group. Flatulence was significantly reduced among the probiotic group compared with the placebo group. At a 12-month follow-up, the probiotic group maintained significantly better overall GI symptoms and function than the placebo group.

New York scientists (Hun 2009) gave 44 IBS patients either a placebo or *Bacillus coagulans* GBI-30 for eight weeks. The probiotic group experienced significant improvements in abdominal pain and bloating symptoms versus the placebo group.

Scientists at Ireland's University College in Cork (O'Mahony *et al.* 2005) studied 77 irritable bowel syndrome patients with abnormal IL-10/IL-12 ratios – indicating a proinflammatory, Th1 status. The patients were given a placebo, *Lactobacillus salivarius* UCC4331 or *Bifidobacterium infantis* 35624 for eight weeks. IBS symptoms were logged daily and assessed weekly. Tests included quality of life, stool microbiology, and blood samples to test peripheral blood mononuclear cell release of inflammatory cytokines interleukin (IL)-10 and IL-12. Patients who took *B. infantis* 35624 had a significantly greater reduction in abdominal pain and discomfort, bloating and distention, and bowel movement difficulty, compared to the other groups. IL-10/IL-12 ratios – indicative of Th1 proinflammatory metabolism – were also normalized in the probiotic *B. infantis* group.

Researchers from the Umberto Hospital in Venice in Italy (Saggioro 2004) studied probiotics on seventy adults with irritable bowel syndrome. They were given 1) a placebo; 2) a combination of *Lactobacillus plantarum* and *Bifidobacterium breve*; or 3) a combination of *Lactobacillus plantarum* and *Lactobacillus acidophilus* for four weeks. After 28 days of treatment, pain scores measuring different abdominal regions decreased among the probiotic groups by 45% and 49% respectively, versus 29% for the placebo group. The IBS symptom severity scores decreased among the probiotic groups after 28 days by 56% and 55.6% respectively, versus 14% among the placebo group.

Sixty-eight patients with irritable bowel syndrome were treated at the TMC Hospital in Shizuoka, Japan (Tsuchiya *et al.* 2004) with either placebo or a combination of *Lactobacillus acidophilus*, *Lactobacillus helveticus* and *Bifidobacteria* for twelve weeks. The probiotic treatment was either "effective" or "very effective" in more than 80% of the IBS patients. In addition, less than 5% of the probiotic group reported the treatment as "not effective," while more than 40% of the placebo patients reported their placebo treatment as "not effective." The probiotic group also reported significant improvement of bowel habits.

Researchers from Britain's University of Manchester School of Medicine (Whorwell *et al.* 2007) gave a placebo or *Bifidobacterium infantis* 35624 to 362 primary care women with irritable bowel syndrome in a large-scale, multicenter study. After four weeks of treatment, *B. infantis* was significantly more effective than the placebo in reducing bloating, bowel dysfunction, incomplete evacuation, straining, and the passing of gas.

Scientists from Denmark's Hvidovre Hospital and the University Hospital of Copenhagen (Wildt *et al.* 2006) gave 29 colitis-IBS patients either *Lactobacillus acidophilus* LA-5 and *Bifidobacterium animalis* subsp. *lactis* BB-12, or a placebo for twelve weeks. The probiotic treatment group had a decrease in bowel frequency from 32 per week to 23 per week. Furthermore, the probiotic group had an average reduction in the frequency of liquid stools from six days per week to one day per week.

Scientists at Poland's Jagiellonian University Medical College (Zwolińska-Wcisło *et al.* 2006) tested 293 ulcer patients, 60 patients with ulcerative colitis, 12 patients with irritable bowel syndrome and 72 patients with other gastrointestinal issues. Compared to placebo, *Lactobacillus acidophilus* supplementation resulted in a lessening of symptoms, a reduction of fungal colonization, and increased levels of immune system cytokines TNF-alpha and IL-1 beta.

Medical researchers from Finland's University of Helsinki (Kajander *et al.* 2007) sought to understand the mechanism of probiotics' proven ability to reduce IBS symptoms. They gave either a placebo or a combination of *Lactobacillus rhamnosus* GG, *Lactobacillus rhamnosus* Lc705, *Propionibacterium freudenreichii* subsp. *shermanii* JS and *Bifidobacterium breve* Bb99 to 55 irritable bowel syndrome patients. After six months of treatment, composition of feces and intestinal microorganism content illustrated a significant drop in glucuronidase levels in the probiotic group compared to the placebo group. The researchers concluded that there was a complexity of different factors, and so far unknown mechanisms explaining:

> *"the alleviation of irritable bowel syndrome symptoms by the multispecies probiotic."*

Probiotics and Other Digestive Problems

Other digestive symptoms such as bloating, indigestion, and cramping are often reported with gluten sensitivity.

Occasional indigestion, bloating and cramping is also found in developing cases of dysbiosis followed by antibiotic use, poor diet, or an overgrowth of specific pathogenic microorganisms.

Enzyme deficiency can be caused by probiotic deficiencies. Probiotics produce a number of enzymes, including protease and lypase – necessary for the break down of proteins and fats. We have discussed how probiotics produce the enzymes that break down gliadins and glutenins.

Poor digestion is often the result of a lack of these and other enzymes. Gastrointestinal difficulties in general are often caused by dysbiosis. This can include an overgrowth of yeasts, pathogenic bacteria or both. Here are a few of the many studies showing that digestion can improve with probiotic use:

French researchers (Guyonnet *et al.* 2009) fed *Bifidobacterium lactis* DN-173010 with yogurt strains for two weeks to 371 adults reporting digestive discomfort. After two weeks, 82.5% of the probiotic group reported improved digestive symptoms compared to 2.9% of the control group.

Another group of French scientists (Diop *et al.* 2008) gave 64 volunteers with high levels of stress and incidental gastrointestinal symptoms either a placebo or *Lactobacillus acidophilus* Rosell-52 and *Bifidobacterium longum* for three weeks. At the end of the three weeks, the stress-related gastrointestinal symptoms of abdominal pain, nausea and vomiting decreased by 49% among the probiotic group.

Probiotics, Polyps, Diverticulosis and Diverticulitis

Polyps, diverticulosis and diverticulitis are abnormalities within the intestines or colon. They have been associated with Crohn's, IBS and ulcerative colitis, as well as increased food sensitivities. They also have been seen forming seemingly without other disease pathologies.

Diverticulosis is the bulging of sections of the intestines. When a bulging area weakens and bursts, that is called diverticulitis. A polyp, on the other hand, is a growth on the inside of the intestinal wall. These may be either benign or cancerous. All of these conditions are associated with intestinal probiotics, because healthy probiotic colonies are essential to the health of the intestinal wall. We can see the evidence from the research:

Scientists from Sweden and Ireland (Rafter *et al.* 2007) gave placebo or *Lactobacillus rhamnosus* GG and *Bifidobacterium lactis* Bb12 to 43 polyp patients (who also had surgery for their removal) for 12 weeks. The probiotics significantly reduced colorectal proliferation and improved epithelial barrier function (reducing intestinal permeability) among the polyp patients. Testing also showed decreased exposure to intestinal genotoxins among the probiotic polyp patient group.

Researchers from The Netherlands' University Hospital Maastricht (Goossens *et al.* 2006) gave *Lactobacillus plantarum* 299v or a placebo to 29 polyp patients twice a day for two weeks. Fecal sample examinations and biopsies were collected during colonoscopy. *L. plantarum* 299v significantly increased probiotic bacteria levels from fecal tests and from rectal biopsies. Ascending colon populations were not significantly greater, however.

Researchers from the Digestive Endoscopy Unit at Italy's Lorenzo Bonomo Hospital (Tursi *et al.* 2008) treated 75 patients with symptomatic diverticulosis. Mesalazine and/or *Lactobacillus casei* DG were given for 10 days each month. Of the 71 patients that completed the study, 66 (88%) were symptom-free after 24 months. The researchers concluded that mesalazine and/or *Lactobacillus casei* were effective in maintaining diverticulosis remission for an extended period, assuming continued treatment.

Probiotics and Ulcers

Ulcers often relate directly to food sensitivities because ulcer symptoms can worsen after eating certain foods. Also, some food sensitivities are a direct result of an ulcerated condition in the stomach or duodenum – allowing undigested food molecules access to upper intestinal cells. Some food intolerances are the direct result of an ulcer, as gastric cells become inflamed.

Until only recently, medical scientists and physicians were certain that ulcers were caused by too much acid in the stomach and the eating of spicy foods. This assumption has been debunked over the past two decades, as researchers have confirmed that at least 80% of all ulcers are associated with *Helicobacter pylori* infections.

While acidic foods and gastrin produced by the stomach wall are also implicated by symptoms of heartburn and acid reflux, we know that a healthy stomach has a functional barrier that should prevent these normal food and gastric substances from harming the cells of the stomach wall. This barrier is called the mucosal membrane. This stomach's mucosal membrane contains a number of mucopolysaccharides and phospholipids that, together with secretions from intestinal and oral probiotics, protect the stomach cells from acids, toxins and bacteria invasions.

Helicobacter pylori damage the mucosal membrane that protects the stomach's gastric cells, and directly irritate the tissues. This damage produces the symptoms of heartburn.

As doctors and researchers work to eradicate *H. pylori,* which infects billions of people worldwide, they are finding that *H. pylori* is becoming increasingly resistant to many of the antibiotics used in prescriptive treatment. Research from Poland's Center of Gastrology (Ziemniak 2006) investigated antibiotic use on *Helicobacter pylori* infections: 641 *H. pylori* patients were given various antibiotics typically applied to *H. pylori*. The results indicated that *H. pylori* had developed a 22% resistance to clarithromycin and 47% resistance to metronidazole. Worse, a 66% secondary resistance to clarithromycin and metronidazole was found, indicating *H. pylori*'s increasing resistance to antibiotics.

H. pylori bacteria do not always cause ulcers. In fact, only a small percentage of *H. pylori* infections actually become ulcerative. Meanwhile, there is some evidence that *H. pylori* – like *E. coli* and *Candida albicans* – may be a normal resident in a healthy intestinal tract, assuming they are properly balanced and managed by strong legions of probiotics.

There is strong evidence that confirms the ability probiotics have in controlling and managing *H. pylori* overgrowths. We will also see that probiotics have the ability to arrest ulcerative colitis and even mouth ulcers:

Researchers from the Academic Hospital at Vrije University in The Netherlands (Cats *et al.* 2003) gave either a placebo or *Lactobacillus casei* Shirota to 14 *H. pylori*-infected patients for three weeks. Six additional *H. pylori*-infected subjects were used as controls. The researchers determined that *L. casei* significantly inhibits *H. pylori* growth. This effect was more pronounced for *L. casei* grown in milk solution than in the DeMan-Rogosa-Sharpe medium (a probiotic broth developed by researchers in 1960).

Mexican hospital researchers (Sahagún-Flores *et al.* 2007) gave 64 *Helicobacter pylori*-infected patients antibiotic treatment with or without *Lactobacillus casei* Shirota. *Lactobacillus casei* Shirota plus antibiotic treatment was 94% effective and antibiotic treatment alone was 76% effective.

Researchers from the Department of Internal Medicine and Gastroenterology at Italy's University of Bologna (Gionchetti *et al.* 2000) gave 40 ulcerative colitis patients either a placebo or a combination of four strains of lactobacilli, three strains of bifidobacteria, and one strain of *Streptococcus salivarius* subsp. *thermophilus* for nine months. The patients were tested monthly. Three patients (15%) in the probiotic group suffered relapses within the nine months, versus 20 (100%) in the placebo group.

Italian scientists from the University of Bologna (Venturi *et al.* 1999) also gave 20 patients with ulcerative colitis a combination of three bifidobacteria strains, four lactobacilli strains and *Streptococcus salivarius* subsp. *thermophilus* for 12 months. Fecal samples were obtained at the beginning, after 10 days, 20 days, 40 days, 60 days, 75 days, 90 days, 12 months and 15 days after the (12 months) end of the treatment period. Fifteen of the 20 treated patients achieved and maintained remission from ulcerative colitis during the study period.

British researchers from the University of Dundee and Ninewells Hospital Medical School (Furrie *et al.* 2005) gave 18 patients with active ulcerative colitis either *B. longum* or a placebo for one month. Clinical examination and rectal biopsies indicated that sigmoidoscopy scores were reduced in the probiotic group. In addition, mRNA levels for human beta defensins 2, 3, and 4 (higher in active ulcerative colitis) were significantly reduced among the probiotic group. Inflammatory cytokines tumor necrosis factor alpha and interleukin-1alpha were also significantly lower in the probiotic group. Biopsies showed reduced inflammation and the regeneration of epithelial tissue within the intestines among the probiotic group.

Scientists from Italy's Raffaele University Hospital (Guslandi *et al.* 2003) gave *Saccharomyces boulardii* or placebo to 25 patients with ulcerative colitis unsuitable for steroid therapy, for four weeks. Of the 24 patients completing the study, 17 attained clinical remission – confirmed endoscopically.

Researchers from Switzerland's University Hospital in Lausanne (Felley *et al.* 2001) gave fifty-three patients with ulcerative *H. pylori* infection milk with *L. johnsonii* or placebo for three weeks. Those given the probiotic drink had a significant *H. pylori* density decrease, reduced inflammation and less gastritis activity from *H. pylori.*

Lactobacillus reuteri ATCC 55730 or a placebo was given to 40 *H. pylori*-infected patients for four weeks by researchers from Italy's Università degli Studi di Bari (Francavilla *et al.* 2008). *L. reuteri* effectively suppressed *H. pylori* infection, decreased gastrointestinal pain, and reduced other dyspeptic symptoms.

Scientists from the Department of Internal Medicine at the Catholic University of Rome (Canducci *et al.* 2000) tested 120 patients with ulcerative *H. pylori* infections. Sixty patients received a combination of antibiotics rabeprazole, clarithromycin and amoxicillin. The other sixty patients received the same therapy together with a freeze-dried, inactivated culture of *Lactobacillus acidophilus*. The probiotic group had an 88% eradication of *H. pylori* while the antibiotic-only group had a 72% eradication of *H. pylori*.

Scientists from the University of Chile (Gotteland *et al.* 2005) gave 182 children with *H. pylori* infections placebo, antibiotics or probiotics. *H. pylori* were completely eradicated in 12% of those who took *Saccharomyces boulardii*, and in 6.5% of those given *L. acidophilus*. The placebo group had no *H. pylori* eradication.

Researchers from Japan's Kyorin University School of Medicine (Imase *et al.* 2007) gave *Lactobacillus reuteri* strain SD2112 in tablets or a placebo to 33 *H. pylori*-infected patients. After four and eight weeks, *L. reuteri* was significantly decreased *H. pylori* among the probiotic group.

In a study of 347 patients with active *H. pylori* infections (ulcerous), half the group was given antibiotics and the other half was given antibiotics with yogurt (*Lactobacillus acidophilus* HY2177, *Lactobacillus casei* HY2743, *Bifidobacterium longum* HY8001, and *Streptococcus thermophilus* B-1). The yogurt plus antibiotics group had significantly more eradication of the *H. pylori* bacteria, and significantly fewer side effects than the antibiotics group (Kim *et al.* 2008).

Lactobacillus brevis (CD2) or placebo was given to 22 *H. pylori*-positive dyspeptic patients for three weeks before a colonoscopy by Italian medical researchers (Linsalata *et al.* 2004). A reduction in the UBT delta values and subsequent bacterial load ensued. *L. brevis* CD2 stimulated a decrease in gastric ornithine decarboxylase activity and polyamine. The researchers concluded:

> *"Our data support the hypothesis that L. brevis CD2 treatment decreases H. pylori colonization, thus reducing polyamine biosynthesis."*

Thirty *H. pylori*-infected patients were given either probiotics *Lactobacillus acidophilus* and *Bifidobacterium bifidum* or placebo for one and two weeks following antibiotic treatment by British researchers (Madden *et al.* 2005). Those taking the probiotics had a recovery of normal intestinal microflora, damaged during antibiotic treatment. The researchers also observed that those taking the probiotics throughout the two weeks showed more normal and stable microflora than did those groups taking the probiotics for only one out of the two weeks.

Researchers at the Nippon Medical School in Tokyo (Fujimori *et al.* 2009) gave 120 outpatients with ulcerative colitis either a placebo; *Bifidobacterium longum;* psyllium (a prebiotic); or a combination of *B. longum* and psyllium (synbiotic) for four weeks. C-reactive protein (pro-inflammatory) decreased significantly only with the synbiotic group, from 0.59 to 0.14 mg/dL. In addition, the synbiotic therapy resulted in significantly better scores on symptom and quality-of-life assessments.

Scientists from the Department of Medicine at Lausanne, Switzerland's University Hospital (Michetti *et al.* 1999) tested 20 human adults with ulcerative *H. pylori* infection with *L. acidophilus johnsonii*. The probiotic was taken with the antibiotic omeprazole in half the group and alone (with placebo) in the other group. The patients were tested at the start, after two weeks of treatment, and four weeks after treatment. Both groups showed significantly reduced *H. pylori* levels during and just following treatment. However, the probiotic-only group tested better than the antibiotic group during the fourth week after the treatment completion.

Medical scientists from the Kaohsiung Municipal United Hospital in Taiwan (Wang *et al.* 2004) studied 59 volunteer patients infected with *H. pylori*. They were given either probiotics (*Lactobacillus* and *Bifidobacterium* strains) or placebo after meals for six weeks. After the six-week period, the probiotic treatment *"effectively suppressed H. pylori,"* according to the researchers.

In the Polish study mentioned earlier (Ziemniak 2006), 641 *H. pylori* patients were given either antibiotics alone or probiotics with antibiotics. The two antibiotic-only treatment groups had 71% and 86% eradication of *H. pylori,* while the antibiotic-probiotic treatment group had 94% eradication.

Researchers from the Cerrahpasa Medical Faculty at Istanbul University (Tasli *et al.* 2006) gave 25 patients with Behçet's syndrome (chronic mouth ulcers) six *Lactobacillus brevis* CD2 lozenges per day at intervals of 2-3 hours. After one and two weeks, the number of ulcers significantly decreased.

Probiotics and Inflammation

As we've discussed earlier, when the immune system is prone to inflammatory response, it will respond with more hypersensitivity to macromolecules and other food elements that gain entry to the intestinal wall.

This is specifically associated with gluten sensitivities.

In such a condition, the immune system is overreacting. Research has confirmed that these conditions are characterized by an increase in T-cell helper-2 cells (Th2); outside of their normal balance with Th1 cells. This sets up the hair-trigger immune system.

Research shows that probiotics produce a balance among the immune system. Let's see some of the evidence:

Researchers from the Department of Clinical Sciences at Spain's University of Las Palmas de Gran Canaria (Ortiz-Andrellucchi *et al.* 2008) studied the ability of *Lactobacillus casei* DN114001 to modulate immunity factors among lactating mothers and their babies. *L. casei* or a placebo was given to expecting mothers for six weeks. T helper-1 and T helper-2 (Th1/ Th2) levels were tested from breast-fed colostrum, early milk (10 days) and mature milk (45 days).

Allergic episodes among the newborns were also observed throughout their first six months of life. Among the probiotic group, T-cell and B-cell levels were increased, and natural killer cells were significantly increased. Furthermore, Th1/Th2 ratios were more balanced (anti-inflammatory) among the probiotic group.. Levels of the proinflammatory cytokine TNF-alpha was decreased in maternal milk. Significantly fewer gastrointestinal issues occurred among the breast-fed children of the probiotic mother group as well.

Japanese scientists (Hirose *et al.* 2006) gave *Lactobacillus plantarum* strain L-137 or placebo to 60 healthy men and women, average age 56, for twelve weeks. Increased Con A-induced proliferation (acquired immunity), increases in IL-4 production by CD4+ T-cells, and a more balanced Th1:Th2 ratio was seen in the probiotic group. Quality of life scores were also higher among the probiotic group.

The Gluten-Probiotic Conclusion

In the last chapter we illustrated a number of studies proving that probiotics specifically break down gliadin and glutenin proteins – and even AWG. This naturally prevents the exposure of the intestinal cells to those uncleaved proteins. We have illustrated how even celiac disease patients can tolerate breads and other gluten foods that have been fermented with probiotics.

In this chapter we showed conclusively that probiotics can reverse a host of conditions that have been associated with gluten sensitivities – from bloating to indigestion to IBS to Crohn's to intestinal permeability to inflammation.

This should indicate two clear findings:

1) Dysbiosis – the lack of adequate probiotics and/or overgrowth of pathogenic microorganisms – lies at the root of many digestive ailments that have been attributed to gluten sensitivities.
2) Dysbiosis is one of the clearest contributing causes for gluten sensitivities.

"Contributing causes" is used because the digestive tract does not exist within a vacuum. There are other factors typically involved – some of which may actually contribute to dysbiosis and others that are the result of dysbiosis. This is added to factors unrelated to probiotics as we laid out in the previous chapter.

Let's add another study to the mix to drive the point home:

Researchers from Argentina's University of Buenos Aires (Smecuol *et al.* 2013) studied 22 adult celiac disease patients. They were randomly divided into two groups. Before every meal, one group was given two capsules of *Bifidobacterium infantis* (Natren life start superstrain) consisting of 2 billion CFUs per capsule. The other group received placebo capsules. The trial lasted three weeks.

Those celiac patients who received the probiotics had significantly fewer symptoms of indigestion, constipation and acid reflux. There was no difference in symptoms among the placebo group. The celiac patients given the probiotics also had significantly lower IgA tissue transglutaminase antibodies and lower IgA deamidated gliadin protein epitopes (DGP) antibodies. This of course means their sensitivity levels to gliadins had decreased – even though they were eating gluten.

We can thus conclude from this evidence, combined with the other research establishing the relationship between gluten sensitivities and our gut microbiome; that a healthy, balanced immune system with strong probiotic populations should produce a *normal* response to any food macromolecule.

As we've discussed, probiotic responses are multivariate. Probiotics will:

- ✓ Establish an anti-inflammatory environment within the intestinal tract
- ✓ Secrete enzymes to break down or break apart macromolecule proteins such as gliadins
- ✓ Help maintain healthy mucosal membrane to protect the intestines from any macromolecule exposure

- ✓ Calm and neutralize inflammatory responses
- ✓ Help signal the repair of damaged or inflamed intestinal walls

In a healthy digestive tract, should probiotics not handle the invader, the immune system will initiate a mucosal IgA response that causes immune cells to surround and expunge the invader *before it gains access to the cells and tissues of the intestinal wall.*

During the whole time, assuming a healthy diet and lifestyle, the intestinal wall in a healthy gut will maintain sufficient mucopolysaccharides for the proper mucous membrane layer. With probiotics, this will maintain a "moat" to prevent foreign bodies or large macromolecules from gaining access to the intestinal wall and blood stream.

Should a foreigner gain access for any reason in a healthy, balanced immune system, the response will be immediate and *balanced.* Among intestinal cells, probiotics mediate inflammatory responses by secreting substances that help heal intestinal cells and better protect them.

And in those cases where foreigners slip through the mucosal lining and interface with intestinal cells, the healthy immune system will produce IgA and IgE antibodies to the foreigner, and will attach and help direct the break down of the invader where ever it dwells. The liver then sends out scavengers to collect and send the unneeded parts out of the body. All this can occur without symptoms of a inflammatory response in a healthy body.

Once this interplay has been recorded and arranged for any future interfacing, a healthy immune system, through the IgG system, will begin to develop a tolerance to the protein. It will also design a strategy to better prevent the invader from getting in next time. It will program mast cells, IgAs and probiotics to help prevent a future incursion.

These responses will both be localized and broadcast throughout a healthy immune system. And they occur every minute of the day in a healthy body. Unbeknownst to us, our bodies have thousands of antibodies formed against so many foreigners, and those foreigners are being removed every minute of the day.

The burdened immune system – weakened and overwhelmed with intruders of different types – must sound the inflammatory alarm and turn on all the sirens, even if the intruder is a simple protein macromolecule.

Chapter Seven

Natural Solutions for Gluten Sensitivities

Dealing with any food sensitivity – whether a tolerance or allergy – is no easy job. As any food-sensitivity sufferer will tell you, elimination diets are particularly difficult. They are wrought with danger. One slip up, be it accepting bite of some food from a friend (who doesn't know the allergen is in the food) or eating some restaurant food with unknown ingredients can lead to disaster, even death for a severely allergic person.

We might compare this to walking on razor blades.

Food intolerance is typically not so severe. Here some breaks in elimination might bear some renewed symptoms. Or they might not.

Illustrating how difficult elimination diets are, researchers from The Netherlands' University of Groningen Medical Center (Vlieg-Boerstra *et al.* 2006) assessed whether and to what degree children could actually eliminate a popular allergen food. Among 38 children who were practicing a strict allergen avoidance diet, allergenic foods were inadvertently in the diets of 34% of the children for sure, and likely in the diets of another 37%. Only 29% of the children were able to strictly avoid their respective allergens.

In another study, researchers from University of Southampton's School of Medicine (Monks *et al.* 2010) surveyed 18 teenagers with severe food allergies. They found that most of the teenagers ate foods labeled *"may contain"* their allergen, because they thought that it is unlikely the food actually contained the allergen. Furthermore, many only carried adrenaline in definite risk situations, and some did not even know how to deal with a reaction.

So we must ask: Is it more difficult to deal with a food sensitivity and do nothing to correct it than to undertake the necessary steps to reverse the sensitivity?

This of course bears another question: How likely is reversing the sensitivity? To this, many medical professionals simply dismiss any method as impossible.

This is despite the scientific evidence pointing to real solutions. This is despite thousands of years of traditional medicine's use of natural herbs to reverse food sensitivities. This is despite the many hypersensitive people who have been helped by some of these solutions.

This is also despite the fact that the majority of food-sensitive children outgrow their food sensitivities, and many adults outgrow their sensitivities after some time. How can so many people outgrow them if reversing a food sensitivity is impossible? Is it simply chance? Is outgrowing a food sensitivity simply a random freak of nature?

This does not mean these solutions offered here are guaranteed to work for everyone. Each of us has an individual physiology. As such, it could be that a particular strategy will work for one person but not another. And the research supports this.

However, this doesn't mean that because one solution does not work, another won't. Here we offer a variety of methods that can be combined or systematically done one after another, incrementally.

The overall strategy incorporated within this chapter seek to reduce sensitivities by first:

- ✓ Switching to a diet of predominantly organic foods
- ✓ Reducing toxin intake to lower our immune burden
- ✓ Healing and reducing intestinal permeability
- ✓ Reducing inflammation and the inflammatory response to certain foods.
- ✓ Strengthening the immune system using foods, herbs and other strategies.
- ✓ Rebuilding the mucosal lining of the intestinal cells.
- ✓ Increasing enzymatic activity to properly break down proteins and other macro molecules within our foods.
- ✓ Improving colon health to allow waste products to be effectively and efficiently removed.
- ✓ Increasing probiotic colonization to help police and protect our intestinal walls and produce proteolytic enzymes.

These strategies will create a stronger foundation from which the body will be able to:

- ✓ Digest all foods better
- ✓ Break down gliadin and glutenin proteins
- ✓ Become tolerant to wheat- and gluten-based foods
- ✓ Become tolerant to other healthy foods possibly sensitive to
- ✓ Become generally stronger and more resistant to inflammation

The above strategies are best taken on during an elimination period – where gluten foods are eliminated from the diet for a limited period of time – from 60 days to one year depending upon the state of ones diet, immunity, symptoms and so on.

Once the above objectives are met, this chapter will outline a process called oral tolerance – where wheat or gluten-containing foods are slowly reintroduced back into the diet. Or in some cases, introduced for the first time.

Remember that for a person with severe allergic responses or someone with any other medical condition should seek the consultation of a personal healthcare practitioner.

Reversing Increased Intestinal Permeability

As we've discussed extensively in this text, the scientific evidence points to the fact that increased intestinal permeability is not just a correlation with gluten sensitivity: Rather, IIP is a causative element involved in a majority of gluten sensitivities.

As we've shown, food sensitivities including gluten sensitivity involve or are worsened by the weakening and breakdown of the intestinal mucosal membrane and intestinal barrier. Once the barrier has broken down, toxins and food macromolecules can come into contact with intestinal tissues and the bloodstream. As this takes place, the immune system launches an attack and identifies and remembers (*'fingerprints'*) the foreigners using immunoglobulins.

Assuming a weakened or overloaded immune system, the food macromolecule can stimulate a systemic immune system response.

Once *fingerprinted,* IgE or IgA immunoglobulins are programmed to look for those food proteins on an ongoing basis. Every exposure will cause a lock on, stimulating the systemic immune response. This mechanism has been described over and over in the research, and has been verified through peer-reviewed clinical studies as we've shown in this text.

Now the question is how to rebuild the mucosal membrane and the intestinal barrier to prevent the exposure.

Two chapter ago we have discussed a variety of toxins that can weaken the immune system. Most of these toxins are also implicated in the weakening of the mucosal membrane and intestinal barrier. Is this a coincidence?

The fact is, the intestinal barrier is *part* of the body's immune system. It is the body's most important first and/or second line of defense against invading microorganisms and toxins. This barrier also prevents larger, undigested food molecules from penetrating the body's tissues and invoking a hypersensitive response.

Removing exposure to toxins to the extent possible is the first step. As we discussed the research, alcohol, NSAIDS, nitrites, plasticizers, pesticides, herbicides, chlorinated water and food additives are a good place to start. See the toxin table a couple of chapters ago for more toxins.

We have also showed that probiotics help prevent and even reverse intestinal permeability. These include:

> *Streptococcus thermophilus, Lactobacillus bulgaricus, Lactobacillus acidophilus, Bifidobacterium longum, Bifidobacterium lactis, Lactobacillus coryniformis, Lactobacillus gasseri, Lactobacillus rhamnosus,*

Lactobacillus reuteri, Lactobacillus plantarum, Bifidobacterium infantis

In addition, throughout this chapter we will lay out numerous other strategies, most of which will also help reduce intestinal permeability.

These will include dietary strategies, supplements, herbs, colon rebuilding and lifestyle and environmental strategies. While some of these may not directly heal the barrier, most will contribute to their repair and/or the removal of the of the elements that weaken the mucosal membrane and brush barrier.

We must remember that the cells within the intestines have some of the fastest turnover rates of all the body's cells. Most of these cells will divide and be replaced by new cells within a week. While this doesn't necessarily mean we can heal the intestinal brush barrier within that short a period of time, it does mean that gradually, over several generations of intestinal cells, the brush barrier can gradually be rebuilt.

We'll start with specific foods and supplements that can reverse intestinal permeability, starting from the early diet.

Early Diet Strategies

As we've laid out in this book, significant research has illustrated that gluten sensitivities – and any other food sensitivity – can be the result of missteps in a child's early diet.

In the last chapter we discussed the science that illustrates the importance of breast feeding for the infant. The bottom line is that breast milk gives the child a host of immune cells, cytokines and immunoglobulins that fine tune the baby's immune system. Additionally, breast milk gives the child a host of probiotics that help colonize the intestinal tract and boost the immune system. Breast milk also delivers special nutrients to nourish both baby and its intestinal probiotics with prebiotic nutrition.

The combination of these elements feed and nurture the baby, helping the mucosal membrane and the intestinal barrier mature. At the end of the day, the child's immune system is handicapped without breast feeding. While there are some fine replacements for breast milk, nothing is quite as good as the real thing – from a healthy mother.

We might suggest that if the mother is unable to feed, there are breast milk banks that supply donated breast milk to mothers who cannot breast feed. Currently there are eleven banks in the U.S. and Canada. They require a prescription from a pediatrician, but this should not be difficult because most pediatricians advocate breast milk. These breast milk banks accept and store donated breast milk from lactating mothers under the rules and guidelines of the *Human Milk*

Banking Association of North America. Breast milk providers are medically screened and the breast milk is also tested for diseases, alcohol and quality.

In addition, there are several natural lactation inducement strategies to consider. Unfortunately, these are outside the scope of this text.

Introducing Cow's Milk and Solid Foods

Research has illustrated that children who become sensitive to cow's milk early may later become sensitive to gluten.

Cow's milk or solid foods should not be introduced too early. This is because an infant's intestinal wall barrier has not matured enough, leaving the intestinal cells exposed to larger peptides and proteins that can stimulate a food sensitivity – including a gluten sensitivity.

At the same time, some early exposure has benefits, especially when it comes to cow's milk. Early exposure can mean the immune system becomes more tolerant, but that is only if the intestinal barrier has matured to a point where the mucosal membrane, IgAs and desmosomes are all in place to prevent allergen exposure to the tissues and bloodstream.

For these reasons, many physicians suggest that mothers should wait four months before introducing cow's milk to their babies. Is this advice backed up with clinical evidence, however? Let's look at some of the research:

Researchers from Israel's Allergy and Immunology Institute and the Assaf-Harofeh Medical Center (Katz *et al.* 2010) surveyed the feeding history of 13,019 infants. Those children with apparent milk allergies were challenged and tested with skin prick testing. They found that .5% or 66 of the 13,019 children had active milk allergies. They also found those children with milk allergies were introduced to milk at an average age of 116 days, while the infants without milk allergies were introduced to milk at an average age of 62 days.

Furthermore, the risk of becoming allergic to milk among infants who were introduced to milk in the first 14 days was .005%, while the risk of developing milk allergies when given milk between 105 days and 194 days was 1.75%. The researchers concluded that the early introduction of milk along with breastfeeding can prevent milk allergies.

We should add that these results did not include the effects of natural raw milk from grass-fed cows or even goats. These sources of milk might have significantly different results due to the fact that these milks contain natural probiotics and a host of immune factors that more closely match mother's breast milk. Extrapolating from the research we'll lay out later, raw cow's milk will likely do more to support the intestinal barrier than pasteurized cow's milk.

Early Cow's Milk Alternatives

This brings us to an often temporary, yet common problem for parents: Their infant or young child becomes sensitive to milk or other formula ingredient. Or perhaps their child has increased risk because the mother has food allergies or asthma.

Scientists around the world have focused a great amount of research upon this problem. This has resulted in several options, depending upon the sensitivity. Here we will lay out the research, and let the parent and their health professional apply the specific situation. Remember that parents should also consult their health practitioner prior to implementing any of these feeding strategies.

For children with milk sensitivities, there are several choices. Here are some of the choices we'll discuss in this section:

- Soy formulas
- Rice milk formulas
- Almond milk formulas
- Goat milk
- Donkey milk
- Sheep milk
- Hydrolyzed formulas (milk, soy, rice, casein)
- Partially-hydrolyzed formulas
- Amino acid formulas
- Omega-3 additives (with any formula)

Not all, but the majority of children with milk sensitivity will tolerate soy formula. Finish researchers (Klemola *et al.* 2002) found from testing 170 milk-allergic children that all but about 10% tolerated the soy formula. The other 10% tested sensitive to the soy formula.

Soy formulas are typically rich in protein. Still, some believe that they simply do not provide the nutrition for subtle brain development. The newest solution has been hydrolyzed formulations. Here the proteins are hydrolyzed in a way that approximates what is done in a healthy intestinal tract. Because larger macromolecules can seep through immature intestinal barriers and stimulate sensitivity, hydrolyzed proteins can provide a possible temporary feeding solution for an allergic child.

Hydrolyzed milk formulas are now recommended for babies with high allergy risk, especially if breastfeeding is impossible. Partially hydrolyzed formulas will also break down larger allergen-proteins like beta-LG into smaller peptides. When they are broken down enough, they become indistinguishable to the immune system because they are in amino acid or smaller peptide form. These partially hydrolyzed formulas appear to significantly reduce allergenicity to casein protein as well (Nentwich *et al.* 2001).

Hydrolyzed milk formulations may also reduce allergy risk in general, especially among those who are genetically susceptible. Researchers from the Marien-Hospital in Wesel, Germany (von Berg *et al.* 2003) studied 2,252 infants between 1995 and 1998 who had a genetic atopic risk for milk allergies. For one year, the infants were fed either cow's milk, a partially hydrolyzed whey formula, an extensively hydrolyzed whey formula, or an extensively hydrolyzed casein formula. Both the hydrolyzed casein formula and the partially hydrolyzed whey formula caused less allergies among the children compared to the cow's milk formula.

Finnish researchers (Seppo *et al.* 2005) gave 168 milk-allergic infants with an average age of eight months either hydrolyzed whey formula or soy formula. Both groups tolerated the two formulas quite well. They also found that both supported normal growth and nutritional status through two years old.

Spanish hospital researchers (Ibero *et al.* 2010) fed hydrolyzed casein milk formula to 67 milk-allergy children aged between one month and one year old. The formula was tolerated by 98.5% of the children.

Italian researchers (Fiocchi *et al.* 2003) found that children who were both allergic to cow's milk and soy tolerate and thrived from a hydrolyzed rice formula.

Another group of Italian researchers (D'Auria *et al.* 2003) studied 16 milk-allergic infants. They also found that rice hydrolysate formula renders normal growth and nutrition, along with *"adequate metabolic balance"* using standardized growth indices (Z scores) and biochemical nutrient testing.

Pediatrics researchers from The Netherlands' Wilhelmina Children's Hospital (Terheggen-Lagro *et al.* 2002) gave thirty milk-allergic children extensively hydrolyzed casein-based formula. They found that this was well tolerated by the children.

Italian researchers (Giampietro *et al.* 2001) found, in a two-center study of 32 milk-allergic children, that the majority successfully tolerated two extensively hydrolyzed whey-based formulas.

Researchers from Brazil's San Paolo Hospital (Agostoni *et al.* 2007) tested four different types of feeding with 125 infants with allergies. After being fed breast milk for four months or more, the infants were weaned to either soy formula, a casein hydrolysate formula, a rice hydrolysate formula, or were exclusively breastfed for the remainder of the year. Both the hydrolysates (casein- and rice-based) were accompanied by better weight compared to the soy formula – which fared the worst out of the feeding strategies.

In a research review (Alexander and Cabana 2010), infants fed with partially hydrolyzed whey protein formula had a 44% reduced likelihood of developing allergic symptoms, as compared with children who fed with milk formula.

Hydrolyzed formulas have proved to reduce allergy risk better than partially-hydrolyzed formulas, however. In a study from Denmark (Halken *et al.* 2000), 595 children were either breast fed or given formula from June 1994 to July 1995. Of the 595, 478 children finished the study.

Of these, 232 ended up being breast-fed; 79 were fed an hydrolyzed casein formula; 82 were fed an extensively hydrolyzed whey formula; and 85 were fed a partially hydrolyzed whey formula. Cow's milk allergy rates were highest among those fed partially hydrolyzed formula. Extensively hydrolyzed formula was more effective in preventing milk allergies.

Researchers from the University of Milan Medical School (Terracciano *et al.* 2010) tested 72 children with an average age of 14 months, and followed up over a 26 month period. They gave the children either hydrolyzed rice formula, extensively hydrolyzed milk formula or a soy formula. Surprisingly, they found that children not exposed to milk protein residue become tolerant to milk earlier than children fed hydrolyzed milk. The researchers felt that this was due to the substantial change in the protein among hydrolyzed milks.

Cow's milk hydrolysates can also produce allergens, however, French researchers (Ammar *et al.* 1999) discovered.

Researchers from Italy's University of Palermo (Carroccio *et al.* 2000) divided up a group of infants who were sensitive to cow's milk and/or hydrolyzed proteins into two groups. The 21 hydrolyzed protein-intolerant infants were fed donkey milk. The 70 cow's milk-intolerant infants were given casein-hydrolyzed milk.

The children were followed up after four years to see if either method produced more or less food sensitivities. All of the donkey milk infants suffered from multiple food sensitivities, whereas 28% (20) of the hydrolyzed-casein milk drinkers had food sensitivities. Four out of seven of the patients receiving donkey milk were also intolerant to sheep milk. Three of the 21 donkey milk drinkers became intolerant to the donkey milk. The good news is that 52% of the donkey milk drinkers became tolerant to milk over the four year period. Even better, 78% of the hydrolyzed-casein group became milk-tolerant over the four years.

Almond milk may also be a good alternative. Researchers from Italy's University of Messina (Salpietro *et al.* 2005) tested almond milk feeding on a group of 52 infants aged five to nine months who had milk allergies. They compared this to soy milk formula. They found that while supplementation with soy-based formula and hydrolyzed milk protein formulas both caused sensitivities in 23% and 15% respectively, none of the children developed sensitivities to almond milk. The researchers also found the almond milk to be safe and nutritious.

A newer option is amino acid formula. An amino formula contains an array of individual amino acids rather than hydrolyzed proteins. Amino acids are the fundamental building blocks for protein production. Mount Sinai School of Medicine researchers (Sicherer *et al.* 2001) tested 31 children with milk allergies with a pediatric amino acid-based formula and compared this with tolerance to hydrolyzed milk formula. Of the 31 children, 13 did not tolerate the hydrolyzed formula, while almost all of the children tolerated the amino acid formula. The amino formula also maintained normal growth rates among the children.

In addition, German researchers (Niggemann *et al.* 2001) found that among 73 milk-allergic infants, an amino acid-based formula fared better than extensively hydrolyzed cow's milk formula in terms of growth and health of the infants after six months.

A newer development is an amino acid-based formula combined with docosahexaenoic acid (DHA) and arachidonic acid – at levels that closely resemble those of breast milk. In a study of 165 allergic infants, Duke University Medical Center researchers (Burks *et al.* 2008) found that this amino acid/EFA formula was hypoallergenic, and provided a safe alternative to breast milk.

Swedish researchers (Furuhjelm *et al.* 2009) also found that consuming DHA during pregnancy decreases the risk of childhood allergy.

The American Academy of Pediatrics (AAP), the European Society of Pediatric Gastroenterology and Nutrition (ESPGAN) and the European Society of Pediatric allergy and Clinical Immunology (ESPACI) all concur that any of these alternative formulas should be tested using the double-blind placebo-controlled challenge tests on allergic children or children with a high risk of milk or other food allergies.

We should also note that once the infant's intestinal barrier matures, specific oral tolerance programs – as outlined later – may be instituted to establish tolerance, again supervised by a health professional.

Solid Food Introduction Strategies

Introducing solid foods is an important milestone. This text will not profess the best method. Rather, we'll lay out some of the research and let the mother and pediatrician decide. While some suggest that the order of foods introduced is important, others, including some researchers, have shown that the order is not important.

What is known is that most children are exposed to their sensitive foods at home or through breast feeding, and early solid food exposure can often lead to a sensitivity. This means that early solid foods are probably better being low-sensitivity, easily-digested plant-based foods such as squashes, fruits and other simple foods – rather than the more common allergen foods. This is supported by research. Also, introducing common allergenic solid foods into children's diets is best done a bit later, gradually and in small increments (Vlieg-Boerstra *et al.* 2008).

Illustrating this, Dutch researchers (Kiefte-de Jong *et al.* 2010) found that by two years of age, about 12% of children are constipated. Furthermore, those children with constipation were more likely to have been introduced to gluten prior to six months of age.

Feeding solid foods prior to three months old appears to increase allergies, but so does feeding any solid foods after seven months old. Researchers have confirmed, for example, that feeding grains before three months or after seven months increases the child's risk of celiac disease and/or wheat allergies (Guandalini 2007). From this we can assess from the research that a safe strategy is to gradually increase solid foods during the fifth or sixth month, accompanied by breast milk feeding through the first year.

General Diet Strategies

Much of the literature on gluten sensitivities is geared strictly towards the elimination of sensitive foods. In other words: *avoid those foods at any cost,* and *get used to it,* because it's a life sentence.

This text offers the research and evidence concluding that the body can be trained to tolerate those healthy foods providing needed nourishment such as proteins, vitamins, fiber and so on – including healthy foods containing gluten.

Note the emphasis on healthy. This is critical, as the evidence shows that our overly-processed food diet is part of the reason for our sensitivities in the first place. As we have discussed, eating refined flour will retain much of the gluten protein content without the fiber and other elements that feed and stimulate our intestinal probiotics to produce the enzymes needed to break down those gluten proteins.

This also means converting to an organic diet. This will immediately lower our consumption of pesticides and herbicides such as glyphosate – directly linked to decreased probiotic bacteria populations.

Outside of the switch to organic foods – which should be undertaken immediately – remember that significant dietary changes done too quickly or otherwise incorrectly can have negative health consequences and even dangerous effects on a person with food sensitivities.

A person may very well be sensitive to some of the foods discussed here. Therefore, it is suggested that while making changes to the diet, eliminating sensitive foods until the process is complete is advisable.

Note also with respect to the information here, that organic foods contain more beneficial nutrients than conventionally grown foods.

Plant-Based Foods

Increasing intake of plant-based foods is critical to rebuilding the strength of our intestinal tract because these foods contain numerous polyphenols and antioxidants that serve to help buffer radicals and help repair damage among intestinal cells.

Furthermore, the research clearly shows that people eating more plant-based foods have significantly lower incidence of allergies of any type. This is because plant-based foods discourage inflammatory responses. Plant-based foods are wholesome and nutritious. They also feed our probiotics with complex polysaccharides called prebiotics. They are also a source of fiber – critical for intestinal health.

Research on plant-based diets has revealed that plant-based foods produce longer life, reduce cancer (especially colon cancer) and heart disease, and have fewer food sensitivities and intestinal problems. And plant-based protein offers an easily digestible source of protein.

Certainly this is not to say everyone can immediately accept a completely plant-based diet. This is to say that a diet that contains more plant-based foods than is currently the norm among Western industrialized countries will reduce inflammation and assist the healing of the intestinal tract.

Whole Foods and Antioxidants

More specifically, certain plant-based foods are significantly antioxidant, immunity-strengthening and helpful for healing include *polyphenols* and *sterols* from vegetables; *lycopene* and other phytochemicals from tomatoes; *quercetin* and *sulfur/allicin* from garlic, onions and peppers; *pectin* and *rutin* from apples and other fruits; *phytocyanidins* and antioxidant *flavonoids* such as *apigenin* and *luteolin* from various greenfoods; and *anthocyanins* from various fruits and even oats.

Some sea-based botanicals like kelp also contain antioxidants as well. Consider a special polysaccharide compound from kelp called *fucoidan.* Fucoidan has been shown in animal studies to significantly reduce inflammation (Cardoso *et al.* 2009; Kuznetsova *et al.* 2004).

Procyanidins are found in apples, currants, cinnamon, bilberry and many other foods. The extract of *vitis vinifera* seed (grapeseed) is one of the highest sources of bound antioxidant proanthrocyanidins and leucocyanidines called *procyanidolic oligomers,* or "PCOs." Pycnogenol also contains significant levels of PCOs.

Research has demonstrated that PCOs have protective and strengthening effects on tissues by increasing enzyme conjugation (Seo *et al.* 2001). PCOs also increase vascular wall strength (Robert *et al.* 2000).

Oxygenated carotenoids such as *lutein* and *astaxanthin* also have been shown to exhibit strong antioxidant activity. Astaxanthin is derived from the microalga *Haematococcus pluvialis,* and lutein is available from a number of foods, including spirulina.

Nearly every plant-food has some measure of some of these botanical constituents. They alkalize the blood and increase the detoxification capabilities of the liver. They help clear the blood of toxins. Foods that are particularly detoxifying and immunity-building include fresh pineapples, beets, cucumbers, apricots, apples, almonds, zucchini, artichokes, avocados, bananas, beans, leafy greens, berries, casaba, celery, coconuts, cranberries, watercress, dandelion greens, grapes, raw honey, corn, kale, citrus fruits, watermelon, lettuce, mangoes, mushrooms, oats, broccoli, okra, onions, papayas, parsley, peas, radishes, raisins, spinach, tomatoes, walnuts, and many others.

For example, the flavonoids *kaempferol* and *flavone* have been shown to block mast cell proliferation by over 80% (Alexandrakis *et al.* 2003). Sources of kaempferol include Brussels sprouts, broccoli, grapefruit and apples.

Diets with significant fiber levels also help clear the blood and tissues of toxins to support the immune system. Fiber in the diet should range from about 35 to 45 grams per day according to the recommendations of many diet experts. Six to ten servings of raw fruits and vegetables per day should accomplish this – which is even part of the USDA's recommendations. This means raw, fibrous foods can be at every meal.

Good fibrous plant sources also contain healthy *lignans* and *phytoestrogens* that help balance hormone levels, and help the body make its own natural corticoids. Foods that contain these include peas, garbanzo beans, soybeans, kidney beans and lentils.

Garlic, cayenne and onions can be added to any cooked dishes to add inflammation-inhibiting *quercetin* and other antioxidants. Cooked beans or grains can be spiced with turmeric, ginger, basil, rosemary and other anti-inflammatory spices such as cayenne.

Over the past few years, research has discovered that red, purple and blue fruits have tremendous antioxidant and anti-inflammatory benefits. Continued studies have concluded that oxidative species – free radicals – are at the root of much of the damage that burdens the immune system and triggers allergic inflammatory responses. Oxidative species come from poor diets and chemical toxins – exacerbated by stress.

The greatest and most efficient way to neutralize these oxidative radicals comes from fresh botanical foods. The method scientists and food technologists have used to measure the ability a particular food has to neutralize free radicals is the *Oxygen Radical Absorbance Capacity Test* (ORAC). This technical laboratory study is performed by a number of scientific bodies, including the USDA and specialized labs such as Brunswick Laboratories in Massachusetts.

Research from the USDA's Jean Mayer Human Nutrition Research Center on Aging at Tufts University has suggested that a diet high in ORAC value may protect blood vessels and tissues from damage that can result in inflammation (Sofic *et al.* 2001; Cao *et al.* 1998). These tissues, of course, include the intestines.

This research and others have implicated that damage from free radicals also contributes to many disease mechanisms, which burden the immune system and result in hypersensitivity. Although antioxidants cannot be considered treatments for any disease, many studies have suggested that increased antioxidant intake supports immune function and detoxification, allowing the body to better respond with greater tolerance. Many researchers have agreed that consuming 3,000 to 5,000 ORAC units per day can have protective benefits.

ORAC Values of Selected (Raw) Fruits (USDA, 2007-2008)

Cranberry	9,382		Pomegranate	2,860
Plum	7,581		Orange	1,819
Blueberry	6,552		Tangerine	1,620
Blackberry	5,347		Grape (red)	1,260
Raspberry	4,882		Mango	1,002
Apple (Granny)	3,898		Kiwi	882
Strawberry	3,577		Banana	879
Cherry (sweet)	3,365		Tomato (plum)	389
Gooseberry	3,277		Pineapple	385
Pear	2,941		Watermelon	142

There is tremendous attention these days on two unique fruits from the Amazon rain forest and China called *acai* and *goji berry* (or wolfberry) respectively. A ORAC test documented by Schauss *et al.* (2006) gives acai a score of 102,700 and a test documented by Gross *et al.* (2006) gives goji berries a total ORAC of 30,300. However, subsequent tests done by Brunswick Laboratories, Inc. gives these two berries 53,600 (acai) and 22,000 (goji) total-ORAC values.

In addition, we must remember that these are the dried berries being tested in the later case, and a concentrate of acai being tested in the former case. The numbers in the chart above are for fresh fruits. Dried fruits will naturally have higher ORAC values, because the water is evaporated – giving more density and more antioxidants per 100 grams. For example, in the USDA database, dried apples have a 6,681 total-ORAC value, while fresh apples range from 2,210 to 3,898 in total-ORAC value. This equates to a two-to-three times increase from fresh to dried. In another example, fresh red grapes have a 1,260 total-ORAC value, while raisins have a 3,037 total-ORAC value. This comes close to an increase of three times the ORAC value following dehydration.

One of the newest additions to the new high-ORAC superfruits is the maqui superberry. This is small purplish fruit grown in Chile. It is about the size of an elderberry (another good antioxidant fruit).

Part of the equation, naturally, is cost. Dried fruit and concentrates are often more expensive than fresh fruit. High-ORAC dried fruits or concentrates from açaí, goji or maqui will also be substantially more expensive than most fruits grown domestically (especially for Americans and Europeans). Our conclusion is that local or in-country grown fresh fruits with high total-ORAC values produce the best value. Local fresh fruit offers great free radical scavenging ability, support for local farmers, and pollen proteins we are most likely more tolerant to.

By comparison, spinach – an incredibly wholesome vegetable with a tremendous amount of nutrition – has a fraction of the ORAC content of some of these fruits, at 1,515 total ORAC. It should be noted, however, that some (dehydrated) spices have incredibly high ORAC values. For example, USDA's database lists ground turmeric's total ORAC value at 159,277 and oregano's at 200,129. However, while we might only consume a few hundred milligrams of a spice per day, we can eat many grams – if not pounds – of fruit per day.

Quercetin

A number of studies have shown that quercetin inhibits the release of the inflammatory mediator histamine (Kimata *et al.* 2000). Foods rich in quercetin include onions, garlic, apples, capers, grapes, leafy greens, tomatoes and broccoli. In addition, many of the herbs listed earlier contain quercetin as an active constituent.

In other words, quercetin stimulates and yet balances immune response and helps stabilize the intestinal mucosal membrane. In one study, quercetin was given to Wistar rats after they were sensitized to peanuts. After a week, the rats were given either the quercetin or a placebo for four weeks. After the treatment period, the rats' histamine levels and allergen-specific IgE levels fell. More importantly, the quercetin completely inhibited anaphylaxis among the treated rats, while the untreated rats experienced no change (Shishehbor *et al.* 2010).

Over the past few years an increasing amount of evidence is pointing to the conclusion that foods with quercetin slow inflammatory response and autoimmune derangement. Researchers from Italy's Catholic University (Crescente *et al.* 2009) found that quercetin inhibited arachidonic acid-induced platelet aggregation. Arachidonic acid-induced platelet aggregation is seen in allergic inflammatory mechanisms.

Researchers from the University of Crete (Alexandrakis *et al.* 2003) found that quercetin can inhibit mast cell proliferation by up to 80%.

Organic foods contain higher levels of quercetin. A study from the University of California-Davis' Department of Food Science and Technology (Mitchell *et al.* 2007) tested flavonoid levels between organic and conventional tomatoes over a ten-year period. Their research concluded that quercetin levels were 79% higher for tomatoes grown organically under the same conditions as conventionally-grown tomatoes.

Methylmethionine

One of the more productive whole foods that promote healthy mucosal membranes is cabbage. Cabbage contains a unique constituent, s-methylmethionine, also referred to as vitamin U. Through a pathway utilizing one of the body's natural enzymes, called Bhmt2, s-methylmethionine is converted to methionine and then to glutathione in a series of steps.

In this form, glutathione has been shown to stimulate the repair of the mucosal membrane within the stomach and intestines. This rebuilding of the mucosal membrane is critical to replenishing the intestinal barrier that is depleted in many food sensitive people. Glutathione has also been shown to increase liver health.

Raw cabbage or cabbage juice has been used as a healing agent for ulcers and intestinal issues for thousands of years among traditional medicines, including those of Egyptian, Ayurvedic and Greek systems. The Western world became aware of raw cabbage juice in the 1950s, when Garnett Cheney, M.D. conducted several studies showing that methylmethionine-rich cabbage juice concentrate was able to reduce the pain and bleeding associated with ulcers.

In one of Dr. Cheney's studies, 37 ulcer patients were treated with either cabbage juice concentrate or placebo. Of the 26-patient cabbage juice group, 24 patients were considered "successes," achieving an astounding 92% success rate.

In another study, medical researchers from Iraq's University Department of Surgery (Salim 1993) conducted a double-blind study of 172 patients who suffered from gastric bleeding caused by nonsteroidal anti-inflammatory drugs (NSAIDs). They gave the patients either cysteine, methylmethionine sulfonium chloride (MMSC) or a placebo. Those receiving either the cysteine or the MMSC stopped bleeding. Their conditions became *"stable"* as compared with many in the control group, who continued to bleed.

Research has showed that this effect is due to the fact that s-methylmethionine stimulates the healing of cell membranes among the leaves and stems of plants that have been damaged. This is a similar story as most antioxidants. Plants produce antioxidants to help to protect them from damage from the sun, insects and diseases. It just so happens that what protects plants also helps heal humans.

Astragalus, mustard, asparagus, onions, green tea, corn, soy, Brussels sprouts and broccoli also contain limited quantities of s-methylmethionine.

Pasteurized Milk

One food that may present an issue for the digestion of gluten foods is pasteurized milk. Pasteurized milk will typically contain a higher amount of casein because it has not been properly broken down (hydrolyzed) by those probiotics that naturally live within the breast milk of cows.

When milk is drank raw or within yogurt or kefir, much of the casein will be hydrolyzed and thus not present a problem. Otherwise, it may indeed present an issue for the digestion of gluten-containing foods.

At least one of the reasons for this was found in a study from Switzerland's University Vaudois and the University of Lausanne (Juillerat-Jeanneret *et al.* 2011). The research found that casein inhibited the enzyme actions of prolyl-amino-peptidases, prolyl-amino-dipeptidases, and prolyl-endopeptidases laboratory testing. Remember that these enzymes – particularly prolyl-endopeptidase – are enzymes that digest gliadins and glutenins.

Casein is also the protein often responsible for milk allergies, and can produce congestion and increased inflammation in those whose digestive tracts cannot adequately break casein down.

And a number of probiotics produce the enzymes that break down casein, as we've discussed. In pasteurized milk, these casein-cleaving probiotics are absent.

For these reasons, eating gluten-containing grains with pasteurized milk is not advised. Yogurt, kefir or certified raw milk are better choices.

Mineral Strategies

Magnesium deficiency has been found to be at the root of a number of intestinal conditions. Allergies appear to be one of them. This is because magnesium is a critical element used by intestinal cells, and magnesium is used within the mucosal membranes.

A body deficient in magnesium will likely be immunosuppressed. Animal studies have illustrated that magnesium deficiency leads to increased IgE counts, and increased levels of inflammation-specific cytokines. Magnesium deficiency is also associated with increased degranulation among mast cells, which stimulates the allergic response.

Clinical studies have confirmed that ingesting magnesium salts also appear to improve allergic skin reactions (Błach *et al.* 2007).

Other research has reported that dietary sulfur can significantly relieve allergy symptoms. In a multi-center open label study by researchers from Washington state (Barrager *et al.* 2002), 55 patients with allergic rhinitis were given 2,600 mg of methylsulfonylmethane (MSM) – a significant source of sulfur derived from plants – for 30 days. Weekly reviews of the patients reported significant improvements in allergic respiratory symptoms, along with increased energy. Other research has suggested that sulfur blocks the reception of histamine among histamine receptors.

Good sources of sulfur include avocado, asparagus, barley, beans, broccoli, cabbage, carob, carrots, Brussels sprouts, chives, coconuts, corn, garlic, leafy green vegetables, leeks, lentils, onions, parsley, peas, radishes, red peppers, soybeans, shallots, Swiss chard and watercress.

The other macro- and trace-minerals should not be ignored, however. For example, research has shown that zinc modulates T-cell activities (Hönscheid *et al.* 2009).

Numerous holistic doctors now prescribe full-spectrum mineral combinations for food sensitivities. Many have attested to the ability of these minerals to balance the inflammatory response and stimulate healthy mucosal membranes.

Good sources of the full spectrum of trace and macro minerals include mineral water, whole rock salt, spirulina and vegetables.

Fat Strategies

The types of fats we eat relate directly to gluten and other food sensitivities because some fats are pro-inflammatory while others are anti-inflammatory. This doesn't mean that the pro-inflammatory fats are necessarily bad. Rather, we must have a *balance* of fats between the pro- and anti-inflammatory ones, with the balance teetering on the anti-inflammatory side.

The fat balance of our diet is also important because our cell membranes are made of different lipids and lipid-derivatives like phospholipids and glycolipids. An imbalanced fat diet therefore can lead to weak cell membranes, which leads to cells less protected and more prone to damage by oxidative radicals – and increased intestinal permeability.

Illustrating this, Danish researchers (Willemsen *et al.* 2008) tested the intestinal permeability/barrier integrity of incubated human intestinal epithelial cells with different dietary fats. The different fats included individual omega-6 oils linolenic acid (LA), gamma linolenic acid (GLA), DGLA, arachidonic acid (AA); a blend of omega-3 oils alpha-linolenic acid (ALA), eicosapentaenoic acid (EPA), docosahexaenoic acid (DHA); and a blend of fats similar to the composition of human breast milk fat.

The DGLA, AA, EPA, DHA and GLA oils reduced interleukin-4 mediated intestinal permeability. LA and ALA did not. The blend with omega-3 oils, *"effectively supported barrier function,"* according to the researchers. They also concluded that DGLA, AA, EPA and DHA – all long chain polyunsaturated fats – were *"particularly effective in supporting barrier integrity by improving resistance and reducing IL-4 mediated permeability."*

Arachidonic acids in moderation are important for nutrition, and we all need them, especially in early feeding as infants. They are important factors in the inflammatory process – but in the right quantity. For this reason, our bodies convert linoleic acid to arachidonic as needed.

As we showed with the research earlier, a typical Western diet can oversupply arachidonic acid. Because arachidonic acid stimulates the production of pro-inflammatory prostaglandins and leukotrienes in the enzyme conversion process, too much leads to a tendency for our bodies to over-respond during an inflammatory event. Worse, a system overloaded with arachidonic acid makes halting the inflammatory process more difficult.

Interestingly, carnivorous animals cannot or do not readily convert linoleic acid (found in many common plants) to arachidonic acid, but herbivore animals do convert linoleic acid to arachidonic acid, as do humans. This conversion – on top of an animal-protein heavy diet – produces high arachidonic acid levels. On the other hand, a diet that is balanced between plant-based monounsaturates, polyunsaturates and some saturates will balance arachidonic acids with the other fatty acids.

Here is a quick review of the major fatty acids and the foods they come from:

Major Omega-3 Fatty Acids (EFAs)

Acronym	Fatty Acid Name	Major Dietary Sources
ALA	Alpha-linolenic acid	Walnuts, soybeans, flax, canola, pumpkin seeds, chia seeds
SDA	Stearidonic acid	hemp, spirulina, blackcurrant
DHA	Docosahexaenoic acid	Body converts from ALA; also obtained from certain algae, krill and fish oils
EPA	Eicosapentaenoic acid	Converts in the body from DHA
GLA	Gamma-linolenic acid	Borage, primrose oil, spirulina

Major Omega-6 Fatty Acids (EFAs)

Acronym	Fatty Acid Name	Major Dietary Sources
LA	Linoleic acid	Many plants, safflower, sunflower, sesame, soy, almond especially
AA	Arachidonic acid	Meats, salmon
PA	Palmitoleic acid	Macadamia, palm kernel, coconut

Major Omega-9 Fatty Acids

Acronym	Fatty Acid Name	Major Dietary Sources

EA	Eucic acid	Canola, mustard seed, wallflower
OA	Oleic acid	Sunflower, olive, safflower
PA	Palmitoleic acid	Macadamia, palm kernel, coconut

Major Saturated Fatty Acids

Acronym	Fatty Acid Name	Major Dietary Sources
Lauric	Lauric acid	Coconut, dairy, nuts
Myristic	Myristic acid	Coconut, butter
Palmitic	Palmitic acid	Macadamia, palm kernel, coconut, butter, beef, eggs
Stearic	Stearic acid	Macadamia, palm kernel, coconut, eggs

Essential fatty acids

EFA's are fats necessary for adequate health. Eaten in the right proportion, they can also lower inflammation and speed healing. EFA's are long-chain polyunsaturated fatty acids – longer than the linolenic, linoleic and oleic acids. The major EFAs are omega-3s – primarily alpha linolenic acid (ALA), gamma-linoleic acid (GLA), docosahexaenoic acid (DHA) and eicosapentaenoic acid (EPA). EPA and DHA are found in algae, mackerel, salmon, herring, sardines, sablefish (black cod); and omega-6s – primarily linoleic acid, (LA), palmitoleic acid (PA) and arachidonic acid (AA). The term *essential* was originally given with the assumption that these types of fats could not be assembled or produced by the body – they must be taken directly from our food supply.

This assumption, however, is not fully correct. While it is true that we need *some* of these from our diet, our bodies readily convert linoleic acid to arachidonic acid, and ALA to DHA and EPA. Therefore, these fats can be considered essential in some sense, but we do not necessarily have to consume each one of them.

Monounsaturated Fats

Monounsaturated oils are high in omega-9 fatty acids like oleic acid. A monounsaturated fatty acid has one double carbon-hydrogen bonding chain. Oils from seeds, nuts and other plant-based sources have the largest quantities of monounsaturates. Oils that have large proportions of monounsaturates such as olive oil are known to lower inflammation when replacing high saturated fat in diets. Monounsaturates also aid in skin cell health and reduce atopic skin responses.

Monounsaturated fatty acids like oleic acid have been shown in studies to lower heart attack risk, aid blood vessel health, and offer anti-carcinogenic potential. The best sources of omega-9s are olives, sesame seeds, avocados, almonds, peanuts, pecans, pistachio nuts, cashews, hazelnuts, macadamia nuts, several other nuts and their respective oils.

Polyunsaturated Fats

Polyunsaturated fats have at least two double carbon-hydrogen bonds. They come from a variety of plant and marine sources. Omega-3s ALA, DHA and EPA simply have longer chains with more double carbon-hydrogen bonds. ALA, DHA and EPA are known to lower inflammation and increase artery-wall health. These *long-chain* omega-3 polyunsaturates are also considered critical for intestinal health.

The omega-6 fatty acids are the most available form of fat in the plant kingdom. Linoleic acid is the primary omega-6 fatty acid and it is found in most grains and seeds.

Saturated Fats

Saturated fats have multiple fatty acids without double bonds (the hydrogens "saturate" the carbons). They are found among animal fats, and tropical oils such as coconut and palm. Milk products such as butter and whole milk contain saturated fats, along with a special type of healthy linoleic fatty acid called CLA or *conjugated linoleic acid.*

The saturated fats from coconuts and palm differ from animal saturates in that they have shorter chains. This actually gives them – unlike animal saturates – an antimicrobial quality.

Trans Fats

Trans fats are oils that either have been overheated or have undergone hydrogenation. Hydrogenation is produced by heating while bubbling hydrogen ions through the oil. This adds hydrogen and repositions some of the bonds. The "trans" refers to the positioning of part of the molecule in reverse – as opposed to "cis" positioning. The cis positioning is the bonding orientation the body's cell membranes work best with. Trans fats have been known to be a cause for increased radical species in the system; damaging artery walls; contributing to inflammation, heart disease, high LDL levels, liver damage, diabetes, and other metabolic dysfunction (Mozaffarian *et al.* 2009). Trans fat overconsumption slows the conversion of LA to GLA.

It should be noted that CLA is also a trans-fat, but this is a trans fat the body works well with – it is considered a healthy fat.

Arachidonic Acid

The science and research on arachidonic acid was discussed on pages 111-112 and elsewhere. AA is an essential fatty acid, and research has shown that it is essential for infants while they are building their intestinal barriers. However, as we discussed, AA is pro-inflammatory, and too much of it as we age increases the burden on our immune systems, and tends to push our bodies towards hypersensitivity.

As we discussed, AA content is highest among animal meats, fish, fried foods and heavily-processed foods. Plant-based foods contain little or no AA.

The Anti-inflammatory Omega-3s

Research has illustrated that DHA obtained from fish oils and DHA from algae have significant therapeutic and anti-inflammatory effects. The research is so well-known that we hardly need to quote it here.

ALA is the primary omega-3 fatty acid the body can most easily assimilate. Once assimilated, the healthy body will convert ALA to omega-3s, primarily DHA, at a rate of about 7-15%, depending upon the health of the liver. One study of six women performed at England's University of Southampton (Burdge *et al.* 2002) showed a conversion rate of 36% from ALA to DHA and other omega-3s. A follow-up study of men at Southampton showed ALA conversion to the omega-3s occurred at an average of 16%.

DHA readily converts to EPA by the body. EPA degrades quickly if unused in the body. It is easily converted from DHA as needed. Our bodies store DHA and not EPA.

It appears that the anti-inflammatory effects of DHA in particular relates to a modulation of a gene factor called NF-kappaB. The NF-kappaB is involved in signaling among cytokine receptors. With more DHA consumption, the transcription of the NF-kappaB gene sequence is reduced. This seems to reduce inflammatory signaling (Singer *et al.* 2008).

Because much of the early research on the link between fatty acids and inflammatory disease was performed using fish oil, it was assumed that both EPA and DHA fatty acids reduced inflammation. Research from the University of Texas' Department of Medicine/Division of Clinical Immunology and Rheumatology (Rahman *et al.* 2008) has clarified it is DHA that is primarily implicated in reducing inflammation. DHA was shown to inhibit RANKL-induced pro-inflammatory cytokines, and a number of inflammation steps, while EPA did not.

The process of converting ALA to DHA and other omega-3s requires an enzyme produced in the liver called delta-6 desaturase. Some people – especially those who have a poor diet, are immune-suppressed, or burdened with toxicity such as cigarette smoke – may not produce this enzyme very well. As a result, they may not convert as much ALA to DHA and EPA.

For those with low levels of DHA – or for those with problems converting ALA and DHA – DHA microalgae can be supplemented. These algae produce significant amounts of DHA. They are the foundation for the DHA molecule all the way up the food chain, including fish. This is how fish get their DHA, in other words. Three algae species – *Crypthecodinium cohnii, Nitzschia laevis* and

Schizochytrium spp. – are now in commercial production and available in oil and capsule form.

Microalgae-derived DHA is preferable to fish or fish oils. Fish and fish oils typically contain saturated fats and may also – depending upon their origin – contain toxins such as mercury and PCBs (though to their credit, many producers also carefully distill their fish oil). However, we should note that salmon contain a considerable amount of arachidonic acid as well (Chilton 2006). And finally, algae-derived DHA does not strain fish populations.

One study (Arterburn *et al.* 2007) measured pro-inflammatory arachidonic acid levels within the body before and after supplementation with algal DHA. It was found that arachidonic acid levels decreased by 20% following just one dose of 100 milligrams of algal DHA.

In a study by researchers from The Netherlands' Wageningen University Toxicology Research Center (van Beelen *et al.* 2007), all three species of commercially produced algal oil showed equivalency with fish oil in their inhibition of cancer cell growth. Another study (Lloyd-Still *et al.* 2007) of twenty cystic fibrosis patients concluded that 50 milligrams of algal DHA was readily absorbed, maintained DHA bioavailability immediately, and increased circulating DHA levels by four to five times.

In a randomized open-label study (Arterburn *et al.* 2008), researchers gave 32 healthy men and women either algal DHA oil or cooked salmon for two weeks. After the two weeks, plasma levels of circulating DHA were bioequivalent.

We should include that ALA, the plant-based omega-3 oil, also produces anti-inflammatory activity. In studies at Wake Forest University (Chilton *et al.* 2008), for example, flaxseed oil produced anti-inflammatory effects, along with borage oil and echium oil (both also containing GLA).

Gamma Linoleic Acid

As mentioned earlier, a wealth of studies have confirmed that GLA reduces or inhibits the inflammatory response. Leukotrienes produced by arachidonic acid stimulate inflammation, while leukotrienes produced by GLA block the conversion of polyunsaturated fatty acids to arachidonic acid. This means that GLA reduces the inflammatory response.

A healthy body will convert linoleic acid into GLA readily, utilizing the same delta-6 desaturase enzyme used for ALA to DHA conversion.

From GLA, the body produces *dihomo-gamma linoleic acid,* which cycles through the body as an eicosinoid. GLA aids in skin health, and down-regulates the inflammatory and hypersensitivity allergic response.

In addition to conversion from LA, GLA can be also obtained from the oils of borage seeds, evening primrose seed, hemp seed, and from spirulina. Excellent food sources of LA include chia seeds, seed, hempseed, grapeseed, pumpkin seeds, sunflower seeds, safflower seeds, soybeans, olives, pine nuts, pistachio nuts, peanuts, almonds, cashews, chestnuts, and their respective oils.

The conversion of LA to GLA (and ALA to DHA) is reduced by trans-fat consumption, smoking, pollution, stress, infections, and various chemicals that affect the liver.

The Healthy Fat Balance

In a meta-study by researchers from the University of Crete's School of Medicine (Margioris 2009), numerous studies showed that long-chain polyunsaturated omega-3s tend to be anti-inflammatory while omega-6 oils tend to be pro-inflammatory.

This, however, simplifies the equation too much. Most of the research on fats has also shown that most omega-6s are healthy oils. Balance is the key. Let's look at the research:

In a study by researchers from the University of Guelph in Ontario (Tulk and Robinson 2009), eight middle-aged men with metabolic disorder were tested for the inflammatory effects resulting from changing their fat content proportion between omega-3 and omega-6. The men were divided into two groups, one eating a high saturated fat diet with a proportion of 20:1 between omega-6 and omega-3, and the other eating a diet of 2:1 (high omega-3 diet). Both groups were tested before and after the diet change. Testing after the diet change showed that the high omega-3 diet did not change the inflammatory marker tests.

The proportion between omega-6s and omega-3s is thus recommended to be about one or two to one (1-2:1). The current Western American diet has been estimated to be about twenty to thirty to one (20-30:1) for the proportion between omega-6 and omega-3. This imbalance (of too much omega-6 and too little omega-3) has been associated with a number of inflammatory diseases, including arthritis, heart disease, ulcerative colitis, Crohn's disease, and others. When fat consumption is out of balance, the body's metabolism will trend towards inflammation. This is because omega-6 oils convert more easily to arachidonic acid than do omega-3s. AA seems to push the body toward the processes of inflammation (Simopoulos 1999).

We also know that reducing dietary saturated fats and increasing omega-6 polyunsaturated fats reduces inflammation, cardiovascular disease, high cholesterol and diabetes (Ros and Mataix 2008).

The relationships were cleared up in a study performed at Sydney's Heart Research Institute (Nicholls *et al.* 2008). Here fourteen adults consumed meals either rich in saturated fats or omega-6 polyunsaturated fats. They were tested following each meal for various inflammation and cholesterol markers. The results showed that the high saturated fat meal increased inflammatory activities and decreased the liver's production of HDL cholesterol; whereas HDL levels and the liver's anti-inflammatory capacity were increased after the omega-6 meals.

What this tells us is that the omega-3/omega-6 story is complicated by the saturated fat content of the diet and subsequent liver function. High saturated fat diets increase (bad) LDL content and reduce the anti-inflammatory and antioxidant capacities of the liver. Diets lower in saturated fat and higher in omega-6 and omega-3 fats encourage antioxidant and anti-inflammatory activity.

We also know that diets high in monounsaturated fats – such as the Mediterranean Diet – are also associated with significant anti-inflammatory effects. Mediterranean diets contain higher levels of monounsaturated fats like oleic acids (omega-9) as well as higher proportions of fruits and vegetables, and lower proportions of saturated fats (Basu *et al.* 2006).

High saturated fat diets are also associated with increased obesity, and a number of studies have shown that obesity is directly related to inflammatory diseases – including allergies as we've discussed. High saturated fat diets and diets high in trans fatty acids have also been clearly shown to accompany higher levels of inflammation and inflammatory factors such as IL-6 and CRP (Basu *et al.* 2006).

Noting the research showing the relationships between the different fatty acids and inflammation, and the condition of the liver (which can be burdened by too much saturated fat), scientists have logically arrived at a model for dietary fat consumption for a person who is either dealing with or wants to prevent inflammation-oriented diseases such as food sensitivities:

Omega-3	25%-30% of dietary fats
Omega-6+Omega-9	40%-50% of dietary fats
Saturated	5%-10% of dietary fats
GLA	10%-20% of dietary fats
Trans-Fats	0% of dietary fats

Herbal Medicine for Gluten Sensitivities

There are numerous herbs that have been utilized in traditional medicine for modifying hypersensitivity and increasing the immune system's tolerance. Herbs that accomplish this are called *adaptogens*. Here we will discuss many adaptogens that have been shown among research and/or clinical use among traditional medicines, to alter hypersensitivity to foods and other allergens. Best to consult with your personal health practitioner before implementing herbal medicines.

Here we will also lay out a wealth of clinical research that illustrates these effects along with other beneficial properties. This is generally because nature's herbs will typically contain tens if not hundreds of medicinal constituents, each one stimulating our metabolism and immune system in unique and even synergistic ways.

Herbal medicine works differently than pharmaceuticals designed to shut off a particular symptom. The proper use of herbal medicine can lead to changes in the way the immune system responds in general.

An ideal way to utilize herbal medicine by a person who has a food sensitivity is to dose with an appropriate herbal formulation during an elimination diet. After some time, oral tolerance therapy may be conducted, overseen by a health professional for those with severe reactions.

Here we will summarize some of the herbs that traditional doctors from different disciplines have utilized to curb allergic responses to foods, or in some way modify the immune system's responsiveness. In some cases, the herb will be utilized to strengthen the immune system. In other cases, the herb will be used to damper the nervous system or otherwise reduce hypersensitivity.

This presentation of the science and traditional use of medical herbs is not simply the personal opinion of the author. Rather, this discussion utilizes the medical science and research of numerous researchers, scientists and physicians trained in herbal medicines.

Here the traditional clinical use of herbal medicine has been derived from a number of *Materia Medica* texts from various traditions or otherwise documented clinical uses of these herbs upon large populations over thousands of years. Unless otherwise noted in the text, this information utilized the following reference materials (see Reference section for complete citation):

> Agarwal *et al.* 1999; Bensky *et al.* 1986; Chopra *et al.* 1956; Ellingwood 1983; Fecka 2009; Foster and Hobbs 2002; Frawley and Lad 1988; Gray-Davidson 2002; Griffith 2000; Gundermann and Müller 2007; Halpern and Miller 2002; Henih and Ladna 1980; Hobbs 2003; Hoffman 1990; Konrad *et al.* 2000; Lad 1984; LaValle 2001; Lininger *et al.* 1999; Mabey 1988; Mehra 1969; Melzig 2004; Miceli *et al.* 2009; Mindell and Hopkins 1998; Murray and Pizzorno 1998; Nadkarni and Nadkarni 1908/1975; Newall *et al.* 1996; Newmark and Schulick 1997; O'Connor and Bensky 1981; Potterton 1983; Schulick 1996; Schauenberg and Paris 1977; Schutz *et al.* 2006; Shi *et al.* 2008; Shishodia *et al.* 2008; Sung *et al.* 1999; Thieme 1996; Tierra 1992; Tierra 1990; Tiwari 1995; Tisserand 1979; Tonkal and Morsy 2008; Vila *et al.* 2002; Weiner 1969; Weiss 1988; Mi-

celi *et al.* 2009; Wang and Huan 1998; Williard 1992; Williard and Jones 1990; Wood 1997.

The Food Allergy Herbal Formula (FAHF)

Mount Sinai School of Medicine researchers have been testing a traditional formula made of Chinese medicine herbs for about ten years now. The blend, dubbed the *Food Allergy Herbal Formula* (or FAHF), has undergone a variety of studies on mice, even though the formula and its derivatives have been used on humans for thousands of years in Chinese medicine. A human phase I study using FAHF-2, focused on its safety. A phase II (drug) trial is now underway. The FAHF formula contains the following herbs:

- Ling-Zhi (Chi) (*Ganoderma lucidum*)
- Fu-Zi (Zhi) (*Radix lateralis aconiti*)
- Wu-Mei (*Fructus pruni mume*)
- Chuan-Jiao (*Pericarpium zanthoxyli bungeani*)
- Xi-Xin (*Herba cum radice asari*)
- Huang-Lian (Chuan) (*Rhizoma coptidis*)
- Huang-Bai (*Cortex phellodendri*)
- Gan-Jiang (*Rhizoma zingiberis officinalis*
- Gui-Zhi (*Ramulus cinnamomi cassiae*)
- Ren-Shen (Hong) (*Radix ginseng*)
- Dang-Gui (Shen) (*Corpus radix*)

FAHF-2 is the same formula, *minus* Fu-Zi and Xi-Xin.

As we discuss this formulation research, remember that traditional Chinese physicians have prescribed the complete FAHF formula or similar formulations using many of the same herbs for thousands of years – *and still do.*

The first Mount Sinai study (Li *et al.* 2001) sensitized mice to fresh whole peanuts by introducing the cholera toxin, followed by a boosting. They then fed the mice the FAHF-1 herbal formula for seven weeks. After the seven weeks, the FAHF-1 completely halted peanut-induced anaphylactic reactions in the mice. It also significantly reduced histamine release and lymphocyte proliferation, and reduced peanut-specific IgEs within two weeks of treatment. These tolerance levels remained for four weeks after the treatment was stopped. Cytokines IL-4, IL-5, and IL-13 synthesis were also decreased among the FAFH-1 mice.

The second published Mount Sinai study on FAFH (Srivastava *et al.* 2005) came four years later and also tested mice with induced peanut allergies. This used the revised FAHF-2 herbal formula, which removed two herbs, Fuzi and Xixin, as noted earlier. They found that the FAHF-2 also successfully blocked peanut allergy anaphylaxis, as well as rendered long term peanut tolerance.

Among the FAHF-2 mice, there were no anaphylactic reactions, and histamine/body core temperatures decreased. They also observed a down-regulation of Th-2 response.

Another Mount Sinai study, this one two years later (Qu *et al.* 2007), found that, once again, peanut-specific IgE levels fell while IgG2a levels increased after dosing with FAHF-2. Reduced IL-4 and IL-5, and a modulation of the all-important inflammatory T helper Type I cell (Th1) and Th2 within the intestines, illustrated how this herbal combination modulated the immune system and increased tolerance.

Yet another FAHF-2 study by Mount Sinai Medical School researchers followed three years later (Kattan *et al.* 2008). Once again, the FAHF-2 formula proved successful in mice by reducing peanut anaphylaxis. This time, they also tested the individual herbs to see if they could isolate a single herb or constituent responsible for the activity.

This proved unsuccessful. Although most of the herbs had some positive effects upon histamine, cytokines and allergic symptoms, the formula worked in combination. In the end, the researchers admitted that the formula, *"may work synergistically to produce the curative therapeutic effects produced by the whole formula."* In other words, the herbs alone did not have the same synergistic effect the combination formula had.

Now let's think about this for a second. Here is a team of medical researchers from one of the world's most respected medical schools, failing to understand precisely what part of a formula – that has undergone ten years of laboratory and animal research – is the active element. What does this tell us about nature, and the wisdom of those Traditional Chinese medicine physicians who devised such a formula?

Furthermore, remember that these research teams did not fall off the turnip truck. They were experienced researchers with M.D. degrees and Ph.D.s. Some were professors of medicine at one of the world's most prestigious medical schools. Why did these physicians have to resort to an ancient Chinese herbal remedy? Perhaps these Traditional Chinese medicine physicians and healers had an understanding about the body and the application of herbal medicine that modern medicine has yet to comprehend.

The next Mount Sinai study focused on the *mechanisms* of the formulation (Srivastava *et al.* 2009). This time, mice with induced peanut allergies received FAHF-2 each day for seven weeks, while receiving periodic oral challenges with peanuts over a period of 36 weeks. They also gave some mice T-cell- or IFN-gamma- reducing antibodies during that period. Once again, they found that the FAHF-2 treatment protected mice from anaphylaxis, this time for more than 36 weeks after the treatment was stopped.

Furthermore, their testing revealed up to a 50% reduction of peanut-specific IgE levels, and up to a 60% increase in IgG levels, which continued long after the treatment period. In other words, the FAHF-2 formula modified their immune systems. The conclusion of the researchers:

> *"Food Allergy Herbal Formula-2 provides long-term protection from anaphylaxis by inducing a beneficial shift in allergen-specific immune responses mediated largely by elevated CD8(+) T-cell IFN-gamma production."*

Finally, nearly ten years after beginning research on the formula, human clinical studies have begun. Researchers from New York's Mount Sinai School of Medicine (Wang *et al.* 2010) tested 19 food allergy patients with FAHF-2. The herbal formula significantly decreased interleukin (IL-5) levels among the active treatment group after seven days of treatment. In culture, the herbal product also increased interferon gamma and IL-10 levels. The researchers determined that FAHF-2 was safe for humans – something that Chinese medicine has known for centuries.

One must wonder why these studies, for a combination of herbs that have been consumed by humans for thousands of years and are regularly taken as supplements, took ten years of mice research to achieve clinical testing? Could Chinese traditional healers be poisoning their patients?

Meanwhile, millions of people suffer from anaphylaxis and die each year of food allergies. Why has the research moved so slow?

One reason is that research such as this requires funding. Funding human studies in Western science research is not cheap. For this reason, researchers must typically follow a rigorous process of animal studies before human studies will be funded. These protocols are even more strict if the human studies aim to be approved by the FDA for distribution as drugs. It is one thing to study an herbal supplement on humans – as many are. But it is quite another protocol to be seeking clearance as a drug. As the researchers aimed to achieve drug clearance by the FDA for the FAHF formulation, FDA-approved phase one and phase two studies became necessary.

Note that a pharmaceutical developed by a billion-dollar drug company won't take ten years to get out of animal research. This is because there is significant investment and income at stake for a pharmaceutical company. Plus a pharmaceutical can be patented. Herbs cannot be patented. So there is a value proposition.

Certainly the efforts of the researchers who have promoted the research should be commended. They see the wisdom of applying for drug approval to allow the herbal formula to reach the mainstream of physicians and patients. At the same time, we must question the logic of the application of these protocols to products that already have thousands of years of application in traditional medicine. Furthermore, the herbal formulation and slight variations are already commercially available. Physicians could prescribe them today. While clinical testing is appropriate, there is little reason the research could not have gone to human testing immediately. Since the formulation is made up of herbs with a history of safety, the need for extended animal and drug testing is curious.

All of the herbs in the FAHF formulation, and combinations thereof, are also available for purchase without a prescription. However, because herbs are considered supplements and not medicines, suppliers cannot advertise that the formula treats any particular disease in many Western countries, including the United States. Supplement laws in the United States and most Commonwealth countries strictly regulate how herbs and herbal formulas can be labeled and advertised.

In the U.S., for example, this herbal formulation would be limited to descriptions that it provides support for the immune system. This follows "structure/function" statements required by dietary supplement act of 1994.

Furthermore, as we investigate (and demystify) the herbs in FAHF, we find that many of these have been quite commonly used elsewhere in Eastern and Western herbal medicine. Many are even commonly used as culinary herbs. Using the traditional texts mentioned and some of the research, let's review some of the FAHF herbs and their properties, beginning with the two eliminated from the formula by the Sinai researchers:

Xi-Xin

Xi-Xin's botanical name is *Herba asari,* and also called Chinese wild ginger (not to be confused with common ginger, which is also in the FAHF formula). The entire plant is used, but its roots have significant usefulness. It is pungent and warming, and widely used in Chinese and Ayurveda medicine to provide heat and help clear the body of phlegm and congestion. It is said to slow the histamine response while stimulating the immune system's detoxification routines. TCM doctors often prescribe it alone with aconitum to help relieve congestion. It is also sometimes combined with peppermint herb to help clear headaches and nasal congestion.

Fu-Zi

Fuzi's botanical name is *Aconitum carmichaelii,* and it is also referred to as *Radix Aconiti Carmichaeli Praeparata* among Chinese medicine. It is also commonly called aconitum, or monkshood by herbalists. It is a well-known herb among Chinese medicine and Ayurveda. There are many related species. The rationale for excluding this herb from the formula is likely because unprocessed aconitum can be lethally poisonous.

However, Ayurvedic and Chinese herbal formulations utilize aconitum only after it has been thoroughly steamed with ginger. This precise process of extraction makes aconitum a safe herbal medicine as prescribed by traditional doctors.

This toxin-extracted aconitum has been used for thousands of years for clearing obstructions and blockages among the organs and channels. It is used for chills, colds and congestion.

A number of traditional texts have documented its anti-inflammatory and anti-arthritic effects.

In its raw form, aconitum is used among herbalists strictly for external purposes. As a liniment, aconitum is considered useful for rheumatism and neuralgia.

It is also used in homeopathy in infinitesimal (significantly diluted) doses.

The type of aconitum utilized in the original FAHF formula is most certainly the processed version. It was also extremely diluted to reduce any potential of toxicity. Nonetheless, we should issue the appropriate warning about aconitum: *This is a lethal poison and should only be given by an health professional who is expert in its safe usage*.

Ling-Zhi

This is none other than *Ganoderma lucidum,* also known as reishi – a popular medicinal mushroom. It is known for significantly modulating the immune system.

Reishi contains many constituents, including steroids, triterpenes, lipids, alkaloids, glucosides, coumarin glycoside, choline, betaine, tetracosanoic acid, stearic acid, palmitic acid, nonadecanoic acid, behenic acid, tetracosane, hentriacontane, ergosterol, sitosterol, ganoderenic acids, ganolucidic acids, lucidenic acids, lucidone and many more.

Ling-Zhi strengthens the immune system and modulates the body's tolerance and responses to allergens. Reishi has been shown to increase production of IL-1, IL-2 and natural killer cell activity. A number of studies have shown that reishi significantly modulates IgE responses. It has been shown to lower IgE levels specific to allergens, and reduce histamine levels. It has also been shown to improve lung function and has been used traditionally for bronchitis and asthma.

Research from Japan's University of Toyama (Andoh *et al.* 2010) found that reishi relieves skin itching and rash in several tests with mice.

Wu-Mei

Prunus mume (Seib et Zucc) is referred to as *Fructus pruni mume* in Chinese medicine. It is also called *omae* in Korea, *ume* or *umeboshi plum* in Japan, which translates, quite simply, to 'dark plum,' 'black plum,' or 'mume.' It is, quite simply, the fruit of a special variety of plums.

This plum is treasured for its immune-stimulating properties. The Chinese *Materia Medica* describes it as able to alleviate coughing and lung deficiencies. It has a strongly astringent property, and thus helps to cleanse the digestive tract and halt diarrhea. Research documented in the *Medica* has indicated that it stimulates bile production, is anti-microbial, and has been able to relieve fever, nausea, abdominal pain and vomiting.

Chuan-Jiao

This is the fruit from *Zanthoxylum simulans* which is also sometimes referred to as *Fructus Zanthoxyli Bungeani* or *Pericarpium zanthoxyli bungeani* in Traditional Chinese medicine. More precisely, this herb is also referred to as Sichuan pepper. The tree is also called prickly ash, and is grown around the world. The small peppers that come from the prickly ash tree can be dried and ground or used fresh.

Chuan-jiao is also referred to as fagara, sansho, Nepal pepper, Szechwan pepper, or even dried prickly ash. Some of these may simply be relatives of the Sichuan pepper.

Because it is very spicy and hot, it is often used in Sichuan dishes – known for their spiciness. Chuan-jiao contains limonene, geraniol and cumic alcohol, among with a number of other medicinal constituents.

In Traditional Chinese medicine, cuan-jiao is known to remove abdominal pain, vomiting, nausea and parasites – especially roundworm. It is also used as a skin wash for eczema, and has a mild diuretic effect.

Huang-Lian

This is from the species *Coptis chinnensis.* It is often referred to as *Rhizoma coptidis* in Chinese medicine. Its common names include gold thread or golden thread. In Ayurveda, other species of *Coptis* spp. are also considered gold thread.

Materia Medica of Traditional Chinese medicine document that gold thread removes heat associated with histamine responses that affect the eyes, throat and skin. It is also helpful for digestion. Applied topically, it has been used to calm skin rash, and has been used to treat boils and abscesses.

In Ayurveda, gold thread is considered a bitter and tonic herb that reduces fever (antipyretic). It is also reputed to belong in the same category as goldenseal.

Huang-Bai

This is from the plant with the botanical name *Phellodendron amurense* or *Phellodendron chinense.* It is also called *Cortex phellodendri* in Traditional Chinese medicine. One of huang-bai's most common Western names is the Amur cork tree. Others have simply called this tree the cork tree.

In a study by researchers from Taiwan's National Changhua University (Tsai *et al.* 2004), huang-bai in combination with another herb qian- niuzi (Pharbitis) was found to significantly effect the ion transport mechanisms within the cells of the intestinal wall. Other clinical documentation has confirmed that it can reduce blood pressure, slow contraction reflexes within the intestines, and modulate the central nervous system. Ointments of huang-bai have been used traditionally for treating eczema as well.

Gan-Jiang

This is *zingiberis officinalis,* also called *Rhizoma zingiberis officinalis* in Traditional Chinese Medicine. It is quite simply common ginger root.

Ginger is extensively used in both Chinese and Ayurvedic medicine. It is also commonly used in Western herbalism and a number of other traditional medicines around the world.

Ginger is one of the most versatile food-spice-herbs known to humanity. In Ayurveda – the oldest medical practice still in use – ginger is the most recommended botanical medicine. As such, ginger is referred to as *vishwabhesaj* – meaning "universal medicine" – by Ayurvedic physicians.

An accumulation of studies and chemical analyses has determined that ginger has at least 477 active constituents. As in all botanicals, each constituent will stimulate a slightly different mechanism – often moderating the mechanisms of other constituents. Many of ginger's active constituents have anti-inflammatory and/or pain-reducing effects. These include a number of gingerols and shogaols.

Clinical evaluation has documented that ginger blocks inflammation by inhibiting lipoxygenase and prostaglandins in a balanced manner. This allows for a gradual reduction of inflammation and pain without the negative GI side effects that accompany NSAIDs. Ginger also stimulates circulation, inhibits various infections, and strengthens the liver.

Properties of ginger supported by traditional clinical use describe it as analgesic, anthelmintic, anticathartic, antiemetic, antifungal, antihepatotoxic, antipyretic, antitussive, antiulcer, cardiotonic, gastrointestinal motility, hypotensive, thermoregulatory, analgesic, tonic, expectorant, carminative, antiemetic, stimulant, anti-inflammatory, antimicrobial and more.

Ginger has therefore been used as a traditional treatment for bronchitis, rheumatism, asthma, colic, nervous disorders, colds, coughs, migraines, pneumonia, indigestion, respiratory ailments, fevers, nausea, colds, flu, ulcers, hepatitis, liver disease, colitis, tuberculosis and many digestive ailments to name a few.

Gui-Zhi

This is *Cinnamomum cassia*, also referred to as *Ramulus cinnamomi cassiae* in Traditional Chinese Medicine. It is commonly called cinnamon – a delicious culinary spice present in most kitchens.

Cinnamon is used in just about every traditional medicine. The bark is often used, although the twigs are also utilized. According to Western herbalism, Ayurvedic Medicine and Traditional Chinese Medicine, it is useful for colds, sinusitis, bronchitis, dyspepsia, muscle tension, toothaches, the heart, kidneys, and digestion. It is also thought to strengthen circulation in general. It is considered stimulant, expectorant, diuretic, analgesic and alterative. In other words, it is immune-system modulating. It also apparently dilates blood vessels and warms the body according to these traditional disciplines.

Dang-Gui

This is *Angelica sinensis,* also referred to as *Corpus radix angelicae sinensis* in Traditional Chinese Medicine. In Western herbology it is sometimes referred to simply as angelica. It is also called dong quai.

This herb is considered antispasmodic, which means it reduces hypersensitivity. The root is usually used, and it is a very popular herb for balancing the female reproductive system and irregular menstruation. It is considered a tonic in general, and has been used in traditional medicine for colds, fevers, inflammation, arthritis, rheumatic issues and anemia.

Ren-Shen (Hong)

Panex ginseng is a traditional remedy for allergies with thousands of years of use. Panax ginseng will come in white forms and red forms. The color depends upon the aging or drying technique used.

The ginseng in the FAHF formula is termed *Radix* ginseng or *Ren Shen* because it is *Panex ginseng.* Depending upon how the ginseng is cured, there are several types of *Ren Shen.*

When ginseng is cultivated and steamed it is called 'red root' or *Hong Shen.* Ginseng root will turn red when it is oxidized or processed with steaming. Some feel that red root is better than white, but this really depends upon the age of the root and how it was processed. Soaking ginseng in rock candy produces a white ginseng that is called *Bai Shen.* This soaking seems odd, but it also has been known to increase some of its constituent levels such as superoxide and nitric oxide. When the root is simply dried, it is called 'dry root' or *Sheng Shaii Shen.* Korean red ginseng is soaked in a special herbal broth and then dried.

There are a number of species within the *Panax* genus, most of which also contain most of the same adaptogens, referred to as gensenosides. Most notable in the *Panex* genus is American ginseng, *Panax quinquefolius.*

Eleutherococcus senticosus, often called Siberian ginseng, is actually not ginseng. While it also contains adaptogens (eleutherosides), these are not the gensenoside adaptogens within *Panex* that have been observed for their adaptogenic properties.

Researchers from Italy's Ambientale Medical Institute (Caruso *et al.* 2008) tested an herbal extract formula consisting of *Capparis spinosa, Olea europaea, Panax ginseng* and *Ribes nigrum* (Pantescal) on allergic patients. They found that allergic biomarkers, including basophil degranulation CD63 and sulphidoleukotriene (SLT) levels were significantly lower after 10 days. They theorized that these biomarkers explain the herbal formulation's *"protective effects."*

Researchers from Japan's Ehime University Graduate School of Medicine (Sumiyoshi *et al.* 2010) tested *Panax ginseng* on mice sensitized to eggs. After the oral feedings, they found that the ginseng significantly reduced allergen-specific IgG Th2 levels. It also increased IL-12 production, and increased the ratio of Th1 to Th2 among spleen cells. In addition, it enhanced intestinal CD8, IFN-gamma, and IgA-positive counts. The researchers concluded:

> *"Red Ginseng roots may be a natural preventative of food allergies."*

Ku-Shen

The small shrub *Sophora flavescens* is known to substantially modulate the immune system. It has also been shown to slow tumor progression (Li *et al.* 2010).

Among other constituents, it contains prenylated flavonoids, quinolizidine alkaloids (such as matrine), dehydromatrine, flavascensine and a number of other alkaloids (Liu *et al.* 2010; Jung *et al.* 2010). Research has shown it to inhibit several cytokines involved in the inflammatory sequence, notably IL-6 and TNF-alpha. It also blocks the release of the pain precursor, substance P (Liu *et al.* 2007; Xiao et al 1999).

This co-opted Chinese herb has also been extensively used in Traditional Hawaiian herbal medicine for asthma. In further research, this Polynesian medicine, it has been shown to reduce allergy responses among the lung passages (Massey *et al.* 1994).

Gan-Cao

Glycyrrhiza uralensis is also called Chinese licorice. It is not the common licorice (*Glycyrrhiza glabra*) known in Western and Ayurvedic herbalism, however. It is known in Chinese medicine as giving moisture and balancing heat to the lungs. It has thus been extensively used to stop coughs and wheezing. It also is known to clear fevers. Either taken internally or topically, it is known to ease carbuncles and skin lesions. It is also soothing to the throat and eases muscle spasms. This makes the root antispasmodic.

One of Chinese licorice's active constituents is isoliquiritigenin. This has been shown to be a H2 histamine antagonist (Stahl 2008). Chinese licorice has been shown to prevent the IgE binding that signals the release of histamine. This essentially disrupts the histamine inflammatory process while modulating immune system responses (Kim *et al.* 2006).

Chinese licorice also contains glactomannan, triterpene saponins, glycerol, glycyrrhisoflavone, glycybenzofuran, cyclolicocoumarone, glycybenzofuran, cyclolicocoumarone, licocoumarone, glisoflavone, cycloglycyrrhisoflavone, licoflavone, apigenin, isokaempferide, glycycoumarin, isoglycycoumarin, glycyrrhizin and glycyrrhetinic acid (Li *et al.* 2010; Huang *et al.* 2010).

This combination of constituents gives Chinese licorice aldosterone-like effects. This means that the root stimulates the production of the steroidal corticoids. Animal research has confirmed that Chinese licorice is anti-allergic, and decreases anaphylactic response. It also balances electrolytes and inflammatory edema (Lee *et al.* 2010; Gao *et al.* 2009).

Ayurvedic Food Sensitivity Formulations

Ayurvedic doctors have been prescribing herbal medicine to their food-sensitive patients for thousands of years. There is a wealth of information provided in the Sanskrit and Materia Medica texts that have been passed down through the centuries.

Texts that include tenets on Ayurveda include the Arshnashaka, Kricch-Hridroganashak, Mehnashaka, Kasa-swasahara, Pandunashaka, Kamla-Kushta-Vataraktanashaka, Rasayana, Sangrahi, Balya, Agnideepana, Tridoshshamaka, Dahnashaka, Jwarhara, Krimihara and Prameha. This information had a tradition of acceptance and clinical application among literally hundreds of millions of patients over the centuries.

Ayurvedic doctors were highly esteemed and respected among Asia and the world for thousands of years. In fact, the medicines of Arabia, China, Europe, Greece and Rome borrowed many of their basic principles and uses of herbal medicines from Ayurveda. And of course, these medical traditions also practiced those principles on millions of patients over the centuries. We can conclude that Ayurveda has had a rich history of clinical use, success and safety.

Because of this history of safety, little thought was given to double-blind studies until recent years. This history of thousands of years of success and safety of Ayurvedic herbs did not indicate the need for clinical research until Ayurveda was challenged by modern medicine. The age of pharmaceuticals has challenged Ayurvedic formulations, just as they have challenged Chinese formulations. And just as Chinese formulations are proving successful in double-blind, placebo-controlled research, Ayurvedic medicine has also proved successful and safe in clinical research.

However, Ayurvedic medicine research has been trailing Chinese medicine over the past few years. Traditional Chinese medicine has enjoyed research funding over the past decade or so from the Chinese government, and more recently from a few Western medical schools. As a result, while Ayurvedic formulations have such a rich tradition of success, we must rely primarily upon the tradition texts for clinical documentation, with only a smattering of clinical research for additional substantiation.

For example, Indian researchers (Amit *et al.* 2003) tested an anti-food allergy botanical formula on rats. The combination proved to block histamine activity in this study.

This Ayurvedic formula contains the following seven herbs:

- Amalaki (*Phyllanthus emblica*)
- Haritaki (*Terminalia chebula*)
- Bihitaki (*Terminalia bellerica*)
- Sirisha (*Albizia lebbeck*)
- Black pepper (*Piper nigrum*)
- Ginger (*Zingiber officinale*)
- Long pepper (*Piper longum*)

Each of these have been used traditionally for inflammation and immune dysfunction. Let's discuss a few of these and other Ayurvedic herbs useful for food sensitivities. Note, however, that ginger was reviewed previously as Gan-Jiang.

Ayurvedic Triphala

Triphala is a combination of three Ayurvedic herbs: *Terminalia chebula, Terminalia bellirica* and *Emblica officinalis*. These three are also termed haritaki, bihitaki and amalaki, respectively. They are also called *"three fruits"* which is the direct translation of triphala. This combination has been utilized for thousands of years to rejuvenate the intestines, regulate digestion and create efficiency within the digestive tract.

The 'three fruits' also are said to produce a balance among the three doshas of *vata, pitta* and *kapha*. Each herb, in fact, relates to a particular *dosha:* haritaki relates to *vata*, amalaki relates to *pitta* and bibhitaki relates to *kapha*. The three taken together comprise the most-prescribed herbal formulations given by Ayurvedic doctors for digestive issues.

This use has been justified by preliminary research. For example, in a study by pharmacology researchers from India's Gujarat University (Nariya *et al.* 2003), triphala was tested on rats that had suffered intestinal damage and intestinal permeability from methotrexate.

After being given the triphala, the researchers found that the triphala:

> *"significantly restored the depleted protein level in brush border membrane of intestine, phospholipid and glutathione content and decreased the myeloperoxidase and xanthine oxidase level in intestinal mucosa of methotrexate-treated rats."*

The triphala also produced a *"significant decrease in permeation clearance."* This of course means that the triphala significantly reduced intestinal permeability.

The traditional texts and the clinical use of triphala today in Ayurveda has confirmed these types of intestinal effects in humans.

We might want to elaborate a little further on Haritaki in particular. *Terminalia chebula* has been used by Ayurvedic practitioners specifically for conditions related to asthma, coughs, hoarseness, abdominal issues, skin eruptions, itchiness, and inflammation. It is also called He-Zi in traditional Chinese medicine.

Research has found that haritaki contains a large number of polyphenols, including ellagic acids, which have significant antioxidant and anti-inflammatory properties (Pfundstein *et al.* 2010).

Black Pepper

While *Piper nigrum* is considered Ayurvedic, it is probably one of the most common spices used in Western foods. In fact, the world probably owes its use of black pepper in foods to Ayurveda.

Black pepper is used in a variety of Ayurvedic formulations because of its anti-inflammatory action. Ayurvedic doctors describe black pepper as a stimulant, expectorant, carminative (expulsing gas), anti-inflammatory and analgesic. It has been used traditionally for rheumatism, bronchitis, coughs, asthma, sinusitis, gastritis and other histamine-related conditions. It is also thought to stimulate a healthy mucosal membrane among the stomach and intestines.

Black pepper used as a spice to increase taste is certainly not unhealthy, but it takes a significantly greater and consistent dose to produce its anti-inflammatory effects.

A traditional Ayurvedic prescription for gastroesophageal reflux or GERD, for example, is to take black pepper in a warm glass of water first thing in the morning. This initial dose of black pepper, according to Ayurveda, stimulates mucosal secretion, and thickens the mucosal membranes of the stomach and intestines.

Long Pepper

The related Ayurvedic herb, *Piper longum* has similar properties and constituents as black pepper. It is used to inhibit the inflammation and histamine activity that results in lung and sinus congestion. Like *P. nigrum, P. longum* is also known to strengthen digestion by stimulating the secretion of the mucosal membrane within the stomach and intestines. It is also said to stimulate enzyme activity and bile production.

Sirisha

Albizia lebbeck has been used in Ayurveda for allergies for thousands of years. It comes from the Siris tree, and contains a variety of glycosides, flavonoids, tannins and saponins. It has also been used in Ayurveda to treat inflammation, lung issues and skin issues.

Guduchi

Guduchi's botanical name is *Tinospora Cordifolia*. This climbing shrub, at home in tropical regions of India and China, has been utilized for thousands of years to modulate the immune system and increase tolerance. In other words, it is an adaptogen. Among Western herbalists this herb is referred to as heartleaf moonseed.

The guduchi plant contains a number of alkaloids, aliphatic compounds, diterpenoid lactones, glycosides, sesquiterpenes, phenolics, steroids, and various polysaccharides. Ayurvedic physicians report that the medicinal properties of guduchi are anti-allergic, antispasmodic, anti-arthritic, anti-inflammatory, antioxidant, anti-stress and hepato-protective (protects the liver).

Guduchi contains two researched constituents called tinosporide and cordioside. These have been shown to significantly modulate the immune system, including NK cells, B-cells, T-cells. It was shown to increase the production of cytokines IL-1Beta, IL-6, IL-12, IL-18 INF-alpha and TNF-alpha (Kapil and Sharma 1997; Nair *et al.* 2004).

Guduchi has been used extensively for asthma, chronic coughs, allergic respiratory conditions and allergic rhinitis. Researchers from India's Indira Gandhi Medical College (Badar *et al.* 2005) gave *T. cordifolia* extract or placebo to 75 allergic rhinitis patients for eight weeks. Of the guduchi extract-treated group, 83% reported complete relief from sneezing associated with allergies. The guduchi treatment also produced complete relief of nasal discharges in 69% of the group, and relief of nasal obstruction in 61%. There was no relief in most of the placebo group. The researchers also found that pro-inflammatory eosinophil and neutrophil counts decreased, and inflammatory goblet cells were absent in nasal smears among the guduchi-treated group.

Additionally, numerous animal and laboratory studies over recent years have confirmed the immune-modulating, liver-protective, antioxidant and anti-inflammatory effects of guduchi (Upadhyay *et al.* 2010).

Boswellia/Frankincense

Boswellia species include *Boswellia serratta, Boswellia thurifera,* and *Boswellia spp.* (other species). Boswellia contains a variety of active constituents, including a number of boswellic acids, diterpenes, ocimene, caryophyllene, incensole acetate, limonene and lupeolic acids.

The genus of *Boswellia* includes a group of trees known for their fragrant sap resin that grow in Africa and Asia. Frankincense was famously used in ancient Egypt, India, Arabia and Mesopotamia thousands of years ago as an elixir that relaxed and healed the body's aches and pains. The gum from the resin was applied as an ointment for rheumatic ailments, urinary tract disorders, and on the chest for bronchitis and general breathing problems. It is classified in Ayurveda as bitter and pungent.

Over the centuries, boswellia has been used as an internal treatment for a wide variety of ailments, including bronchitis, asthma, arthritis, rheumatism, anemia, allergies and a variety of infections. Its properties are described as stimulant, diaphoretic, anti-rheumatic, tonic, analgesic, antiseptic, diuretic, demulcent, astringent, expectorant, and antispasmodic.

In two studies, boswellic acids extracted from boswellia were found to have significant anti-inflammatory action. The trials revealed that boswellia inhibited the inflammation-stimulating LOX enzyme (5-lipoxygenase) and thus reduced the production of inflammatory leukotrienes (Singh *et al.* 2008; Ammon 2006).

Another study (Takada *et al.* 2006) showed that boswellic acids inhibited cytokines and suppressed cell invasion through NF-kappaB inhibition.

In an animal study by researchers from the University of Maryland's School of Medicine (Fan *et al.* 2005), boswellia extract exhibited significant anti-inflammatory effects. The report also concluded that, *"these effects may be mediated via the suppression of pro-inflammatory cytokines."*

In an *in vitro* study also from the University of Maryland's School of Medicine (Chevrier *et al.* 2005), boswellia extract proved to modulate the balance between Th1 and Th2 cytokines. This illustrated boswellia's ability to strengthen the immune system and increase tolerance.

Turmeric

Turmeric, or *Curcuma longa,* has been extensively used as a medicinal herb for many centuries, and this predicated its use as a curry food spice – as Ayurveda has long incorporated healing herbs with meals. Turmeric is a root (or rhizome) and a relative of ginger in the *Zingiberaceae* family.

Just as we might expect from a medicinal botanical, turmeric has a large number of active constituents. The most well known of those are the curcuminoids, which include curcumin (diferuloylmethane, demethoxycurcumin, and bisdemethoxycurcumin). Others include volatile oils such as tumerone, atlantone, and zingiberene; as well as polysaccharides and a number of resins.

As stated in a review from the Cytokine Research Laboratory at the University of Texas (Anand 2008), multiple studies have linked turmeric with *"suppression of inflammation; angiogenesis; tumor genesis; diabetes; diseases of the cardiovascular, pulmonary, and neurological systems, of skin, and of liver; loss of bone and muscle; depression; chronic fatigue; and neuropathic pain."*

Indeed, turmeric has been used for centuries for arthritis, inflammation, gallbladder problems, diabetes, wound-healing, liver issues, hepatitis, menstrual pain, anemia, and gout. It is described as alterative, antibacterial, carminative and stimulating. It also is known for its wound-healing, blood-purifying and circulatory powers. Studies have illustrated that curcumin has about 50% of the effectiveness of cortisone, without its damaging side effects (Jurenka 2009).

A number of studies have proved over the past decade that turmeric and/or its key constituents such as curcumin halt or inhibit both inflammatory COX and LOX enzymes. Curcumin has specifically been shown to inhibit IgE signaling processes, and slow mast cell activation (Aggarwal and Sung 2009; Thampithak *et al.* 2009; Sompamit *et al.* 2009; Kulka 2009).

In a study by researchers at the UK's University of Reading (Bundy 2004), 500 human volunteers with irritable bowel syndrome took either one or two tablets of a standardized turmeric extract for eight weeks. After the eight-week period, the prevalence of IBS dropped by 53% for the one-tablet group and reduced by 60% for the two-tablet group. Pain severity scores also dropped significantly.

In another study on 45 patients with peptic ulcers (Prucksunand 2001), ulcers were completely resolved and absent in 76% of the group taking turmeric powder in capsules.

Other studies have also shown similar positive gastrointestinal effects of turmeric. We can conclude from the evidence that turmeric strengthens the mucosal membranes within the digestive tract.

Coriander/Cilantro/Parsley

Coriandrum sativum is documented in Ayurvedic medicine as an anti-allergy herb. This is also cilantro, which is also sometimes called Chinese parsley. It is related to Italian parsley, with many of the same constituents. Coriander is taken as fresh or juiced fresh, and it has been used by Ayurvedic practitioners primarily for allergic skin rashes and hay fever.

Fresh Italian parsley can readily be found in supermarkets and farmers' markets. While often used as a garnish (for looks and/or to clean the breath), a therapeutic quantity of parsley is about a *bunch*. A bunch of parsley is about two ounces or about ten stalks together with their branches and leaves. A bunch can be added to a salad or put into a soup. Parsley can be delicious with tomatoes, vinegar and olive oil. And of course, it can also freshen the breath.

Fennel Seed

Fennel (*Foeniculum vulgare*) contains anetholes, caffeoyl quinic acids, carotenoids, vitamin C, iron, B vitamins, and rutins. Ayurvedic and traditional herbalists from many cultures have used fennel to relieve digestive discomfort, gas, abdominal cramping, bloating and irritable bowels; and to treat food sensitivities. Fennel stimulates bile production. Bile digests fats and other nutrients. Inadequate fat breakdown can result in macromolecules, including larger protein combinations.

The constituent anethole is known to suppress the inflammatory TNF alpha, slowing excessive immune response. The combination of anethole and antioxidant nutrients such as rutin and carotenoids are known to strengthen immune response while increasing tolerance.

Fennel is not appropriate for pregnant moms, because it has been known to promote uterine contractions. As with any herbal supplement, fennel should be used under the supervision of a health professional. Anyone with a birch allergy should also be aware that they may be sensitive to fennel. (The same goes for cumin, caraway, carrot and others).

Cumin

Cuminum cyminum has a long history of use among European and Asian herbalists. It is described as antispasmodic and carminative, so it tends to soothe inflammatory responses. Like fennel, cumin has been used traditionally to ease indigestion, abdominal cramping and gas.

Cumin contains mucilage, gums and resins, which appear to give it its ability to stimulate and strengthen the mucosal membrane of the digestive tract. This may well be its central benefit for food sensitivities. Those sensitive to celery should avoid cumin.

Bishop's weed or Khella

Bishop's weed (*Trachyspermum ammiis*) is also called khella or khellin among Middle-Eastern herbalists. It is also referred to as Ajwain weed or *Ammi visnaga* among Ayurvedic practitioners and traditional herbalists. Some also refer to it as *Carum copticum,* Spanish toothpick, toothpick weed, *Daucus vis-*

naga and honeyplant. The plant is related to celery and parsley, and blooms with clusters of fragile white flowers. From the flower heads come a fruit and seeds known for their medicinal properties.

Bishop's weed has a long tradition of use among Ayurvedic medicine and Egyptian medicine, especially for coughs, bronchitis and hypersensitivity. It's use was mentioned in the *Ebers Papyrus*, written more than 3,000 years ago.

Often the fruit and seeds are crushed to produce a brown oil, which is called omam. The oil can also be infused into creams and tinctures. Omam water is also produced from Bishop's weed. To make omam water, the seeds are simply soaked in water.

Bishop's weed has been shown to inhibit histamine release (Weiss 1988). It also opens the bronchi and is considered spasmolytic (stops spasms), anticholinergic (blocks acetylcholine), and vagolytic (inhibits vagus nerve responses).

It most important constituents include thymol, isothymol, pinene, cymene, cromoglycate, terpinene and limonene. The fruits contain coumarins and furocoumarins. Khellin and visnagin are considered the more active compounds in bishop's weed.

Bishop's weed is also antimicrobial. Its antispasmodic traits may be due to its ability to dilate the bronchial passages and blood vessels without stimulation. These actions make it useful for allergies and inflammation response.

Khella's traditional uses thus include coughing, asthma, bronchitis, heart pain and muscle spasms. It has also been used for wound healing, headaches and urinary conditions. While side effects are few, Bishop's weed has been said to increase the skin's sensitivity to the sun.

There is little research on bishop's weed proving its usefulness. However, sodium cromoglycate – thought to be one of its more active anti-allergic constituents – has been extensively studied and proven effective for allergies and asthma.

Disodium cromoglycate was developed by Dr. Roger Altounyan, an asthma sufferer. It is used in many cases as a drug for asthma and allergy patients as an alternative to steroids. Dr. Altounyan derived the drug by isolating sodium cromoglycate from khella. Disodium cromoglycate has undergone extensive clinical drug studies, and is considered one of the more effective anti-allergic pharmaceutical drugs – and probably the most prescribed drug for allergies behind prednisone. Disodium cromoglycate stabilizes mast cells and smooth muscle fibers. This is effected through modulation of calcium and other ions involved in cell membrane permeability. This effect also alters the degranulation process, thus inhibiting histamine (González Alvarez and Arruzazabala 1981).

Job's Tears

Job's tears' genus-species name is *Coix lachryma-jobi* (L. var. ma-yuen Stapf). Job's tears are an ancient grain known to grow primarily in Asia. This grass is native to the tropical regions of Southern Asia, but has been increasingly cultivated as an ornamental grass around the world.

Researchers from National Taiwan University (Chen *et al.* 2010) tested the anti-allergic activity of Job's tears in the laboratory. They found that an extract of Job's tears suppressed mast cell degranulation and inhibited histamine release. It also suppressed the release of inflammatory mediators IL-4, IL-6 and TNF-A. The researchers concluded that Job's tears inhibited the body's physiological allergic response.

Pine Bark

The bioflavonoid-rich extract from French maritime pine bark (*Pinus pinaster*) called pycnogenol® has been the subject of numerous studies showing anti-allergy, antioxidant and anti-inflammatory effects.

In a German study (Belcaro *et al.* 2008), pycnogenol lowered C-reactive protein levels – known to increase during inflammation and allergies – after 156 patients were given 100 milligrams of pycnogenol or placebo for three months. The average CRP decrease was from 3.9 to 1.1 after treatment. This is 300%+ reduction in this inflammation marker.

Researchers from Loma Linda University's School of Medicine (Lau *et al.* 2004) gave 60 asthmatic children from 6-18 years old pycnogenol or placebo for three months. The pycnogenol group experienced a significant reduction of asthma symptoms, and an increase in pulmonary function. Pycnogenol also allowed the patients to reduce or discontinue the use of inhalers significantly more than the placebo group.

In a study of allergic rhinitis to birch pollen, 38 allergic patients were given pycnogenol several weeks before the start of the 2009 birch allergy season. The pycnogenol reduced allergic eye symptoms by 35% and sinus symptoms by 20%, compared to the placebo group. Better results were found among those who took pycnogenol 7-8 weeks before the birch pollen season began (Wilson *et al.* 2010).

Researchers from Ireland's Trinity College (Sharma *et al.* 2003) found that pycnogenol inhibited the release of histamine from mast cells. This effect appeared to come from the significant bioflavonoid content of the pycnogenol.

Dandelion

Dandelion species include *Taraxum officinale, Taraxum mongolicum,* and *Taraxum spp.* Dandelion contains hundreds of active constituents, which include beta-carboline alkaloids, beta-sitosterol, boron, caffeic acid, calcium, coumaric acid, coumarin, four steroids, furulic acid, gallic acid, hesperetin, hesperidin, indole alkaloids, inulin, iron, lupenol, lutein, luteolin, magnesium, mannans, monoterpenoids, myristic acid, palmitic acid, potassium, quercetins, rufescidride, sesquiterpenes, silicon, steroid complexes, stigmasterol, syringic acid, syringin, tannins, taraxacin, taraxacoside, taraxafolide, taraxafolin-B, taraxasterol, taraxasteryl acetate, taraxerol, taraxinic acid beta-glucopyranosyl, benzenoids, triterpenoids, violaxanthin, vitamin A (7,000 IU/oz), Bs, C, D, K and zinc among others (Williams *et al.* 1996; Hu and Kitts 2003; Hu and Kitts 2004; Seo *et al.* 2005; Trojanova *et al.* 2004; Leu *et al.* 2005; Kisiel and Michalska 2005; Leu *et al.* 2003; Michalska and Kisiel 2003; Kisiel and Barszcz 2000).

Taraxum is derived from the Greek words *taraxos* meaning 'disorder' and *akos* meaning 'remedy.' Dandelion is a common weed with a characteristic beautiful yellow flower that assumes a globe of seeds to spread its humble yet incredible medicinal virtues. Its hollow stem is full of milky juice, with a long, hardy root; and leaves that taste good in a spring salad. Dandelion is one of the most well known traditional herbs for all sorts of ailments that involve toxicity within the blood, liver, kidneys, lymphatic system and urinary tract. Dandelion has been listed in a variety of herbal formularies around the world for many centuries.

Dandelion's use was expounded by many cultures from the Greeks to the Northern American Indians – who used it for stomach ailments and infections. It is also used for the treatment of viral and bacterial infections as well as cancer. The latex or milky sap that comes from the stem has a mixture of polysaccharides, proteins, lipids, rubber, and metabolites such as polyphenoloxidase. The latex has been used to heal skin wounds and protect those wounds from infection – also the sap's function when the plant is injured.

Dandelion is known to protect and help rebuild the liver. The famous herbalist Culpeper documented that it *"has an opening and cleansing quality and, therefore, very effectual for removing obstructions of the liver, gall bladder and spleen and diseases arising from them, such as jaundice."* It is known to stimulate the elimination of toxins and clear obstructions from the blood and liver. This is thought to be the reason why dandelion helps clear stones and scarring from kidneys, gallbladder and bladder. It has also been used to treat stomach problems, and is thought to reduce blood pressure.

In ancient Chinese medicine, it has been recommended for issues related to the imbalance between liver enzymes and pancreatic enzymes. It has been used in traditional treatments for hypoglycemia, hypertension, urinary tract infection, skin eruptions, breast cancer, appetite loss, flatulence, dyspepsia, constipation, gallstones, circulation problems, skin issues, spleen and liver complaints, hepatitis and anorexia.

Dandelion is also thought to increase the flow of bile, necessary for the digestion of fats and other food constituents.

A study by researchers at Canada's University of British Columbia (Hu and Kitts 2004) found that dandelion extract suppressed the inflammatory mediator prostaglandin E2 (PGE2) without causing cell death. Further tests indicated that COX-2 was inhibited by the luteolin and luteolin-glucosides in dandelion.

In another study by Hu and Kitts (2005), nitric oxide was inhibited. Reactive oxygen species – free radicals – were also significantly reduced by dandelion – attributed to the plant's phenolic acid content. This in turn prevented lipid oxidation – one of the mechanisms in heightened LDL (bad cholesterol) levels and artery inflammation.

In a 2007 study from researchers at the College of Pharmacy at the Sookmyung Women's University in Korea (Jeon *et al.* 2008), dandelion was found to reduce inflammation, leukocytes, vascular permeability, abdominal cramping, pain and COX levels among exudates.

Dandelion was also found to stimulate fourteen different strains of bifidobacteria – important components of the intestinal immune system as we've discussed at length (Trojanova *et al.* 2004).

Another study found that dandelion extract significantly prevented cell death in Hep G2 (liver) cells, while stimulating TNF and IL-1 levels – illustrating its ability to arrest or slow liver disease and stimulate healing (Koo *et al.* 2004).

Other studies have illustrated that dandelion inhibits both interleukin IL-6 and TNF-alpha – both inflammatory cytokines (Seo *et al.* 2005).

Dandelion was shown to stimulate the liver's production of glutathione (GST) – an important antioxidant (Petlevski *et al.* 2003).

Dandelion increased the liver's production of superoxide dismutase and catalase, increasing the liver's ability to purify the blood of toxins and allergens (Cho *et al.* 2001).

Pro-inflammatory leukotriene production was decreased with an extract of dandelion (Kashiwada *et al.* 2001).

Dandelion illustrated the ability to inhibit inflammatory IL-1 cytokines (Kim *et al.* 2000) and Takasaki *et al.* (1999).

In a study of 24 patients with chronic intestinal colitis, pains in the large intestine vanished in 96% of the patients by the 15th day after being given a blend of herbs including dandelion (Chakurski *et al.* 1981).

Goldenrod

Goldenrod includes several varieties, including *Solidago virgaurea, Solidago altissima* and *Solidago canadensis*. Goldenrod's constituents include quinine, dictyopterol, cadinene, caffeic acid, caffeoylquinic acids, ent-germacra, kaempferols, limonene and methyl caffeoyl, neochlorogenic acid, quercetin, quercetrin, quinate, rutin, saponins, sesquiterpenes, solicanolide, and several tannins among others. (Bradette-Hébert *et al.* 2008; Choi 2004; Vila *et al.* 2002; Sung *et al.* 1999; Bader *et al.* 1996; Bongartz and Hesse 1995)

Belonging to the daisy family, goldenrod is a perennial bushy plant indigenous to North America and many other places in the world. Its Latin name is derived from *solido* which means to 'make whole or strengthen.' The leaves and flowers are used for medicinal purposes.

Goldenrod has been used for many centuries for inflammatory conditions. It was used by early Americans and North American Indians for rheumatism, colds, headaches, sore throats, and neuralgia (pain). American Indians also used a mouthwash of goldenrod for toothaches. The flowers were chewed for sore throats.

Traditional herbalists have documented goldenrod's anti-inflammatory effects and wound-healing abilities. It has also been used traditionally for rheumatism, flatulence, arthritis, gout, prostatitis and eczema. Goldenrod has also been observed increasing glomerulus filtration and decreasing albumin levels. Thus it has been used for issues of nephritis, unuria and oliguria.

Goldenrod's medicinal properties are considered anti-inflammatory, antimicrobial, diaphoretic, antidiarrhoeic, carminative, stimulant, diuretic (increases urine output), analgesic, antiseptic, antispasmodic (reduces spasms), antioxidant, antifungal and antiedematous (reduces swelling). The flowers are typically used for medicinal purposes.

A German review of multiple clinical studies indicated that significant anti-inflammatory and pain-relieving effects were accomplished when dosages of goldenrod were comparable to NSAID use – with few of the adverse effects of NSAIDs (Klein-Galczinsky 1999).

In several randomized, placebo-controlled and double-blind clinical studies, goldenrod significantly reduced pain and inflammation in rheumatic diseases (Gundermann and Müller 2007).

Goldenrod was also found to boost immune response and promote cytotoxicity to tumor cells (Wu *et al.* 2008, Plohmann *et al.* 1997).

Goldenrod proved spasmolytic (reduced spasms), antihypertensive and diuretic in other investigations (von Kruedener *et al.* 1995).

Goldenrod proved to be a potent free radical scavenger in a study from Canada's McGill University (McCune and Johns, 2002).

A 60% ethanol extract of goldenrod showed anti-inflammatory activity similar to diclofenac (a well-known NSAID).

Goldenrod also stimulates glutathione activity (Apáti *et al.* 2006). The essential oil from goldenrod produced antimicrobial activity against a number of bacteria and yeasts (Morel *et al.* 2006).

Plant Corticoids

Corticosteroids systemically reduce allergic symptoms and response by blocking histamine release. For this reason, prednisone and similar cortisone drugs are the most-prescribed drugs for allergies. Prednisone and methylprednisone mimic the actions of cortisol produced by the adrenal gland. Cortisol's and cortisone's main mechanism is to slow or shunt the inflammatory response and suppress the immune system. Thus it is used for a wide range of inflammatory conditions.

However, because prednisone acts like a hormone, it significantly alters moods. This may begin with mild frustration or annoyance over trivial things. With consistent use, this can turn into rage, depression, mania, personality changes and psychotic behavior. Other side effects include weight gain, high blood pressure, sodium retention, headaches, ulcers, cataracts, irregular menstruation, elevated blood sugar, growth retarding, osteoporosis, wound healing impairment, moon face (puffiness of the face), glaucoma, bruising, buffalo hump (rounded upper back), and thinning of the skin.

In addition, over time, prednisone dosing can reduce the body's own production of cortisol. Furthermore, increased doses are usually required to maintain the same suppression of symptoms. This can result in an inflammatory and immunosuppressed situation should the prednisone dosing be reduced or withdrawn (Todd *et al.* 2002).

The body produces cortisol and other corticoids using a complex adrenal process that begins with the body's production of cholesterol (not the same as the dietary cholesterol obtained from animal diets). The body uses plant-based phytosterols to produce the steroidal compounds that stimulate cortisone production through the adrenal glands. In other words, the best raw materials for cortisone production come from a healthy plant-based diet of phytosterols. Let's discuss some of the many plants that provide these natural raw materials.

For many years, the pharmaceutical industry utilized wild yam (*Dioscorea floribunda* and *D. floribunda*) to produce the raw corticoid ingredient diosgenin. Diosgenin was utilized to produce progesterone and other steroid drugs. In the human body, the diosgenin in wild yam is a steroid, and is converted into progesterone and DHEA.

As wild yam production could not keep pace with pharmaceutical steroid demand, stigmasterols and sitosetrols from soy and solasodine from *Solanum dulcamara* became the preferred source of corticoid precursors for the pharmaceutical industry.

Many foods, especially those containing seeds, are good sources of phytosterols.

Mallow

As long as we are discussing allergic skin responses, we should mention *Malva sylvestris,* also called mallow. This herb has been used in decoctions in European herbalism for allergic skin responses and eczema. For this reason, Swiss doctors during the World Wars were known to apply compresses onto skin rashes with good success.

Evening Primrose

Another herb known by traditional herbalists to be beneficial for allergic skin responses is evening primrose, or *Oenothera spp.* The seeds are rich in gamma-linolenic acid (GLA) – a fatty acid known to slow inflammatory responses of prostaglandins, especially those relating to skin hypersensitivity. The oil from evening primrose can be applied directly onto the skin and taken internally. Evening primrose oil has thus been used successfully in cases of allergic eczema, for example.

Wild Pansy

This herb, botanical name *Viola tricolor,* has been used traditionally in Western herbal medicine for eczema. Its wonderful colorful flowers are difficult to miss in grasslands across North America and Europe. Wild pansy is known to be high in saponins, as many other anti-allergic herbs are.

Saponins are the glycosides such as triterpenes – active compounds in many of the medicinal plants we've discussed in this chapter. Ginseng is a rich source of saponins, for example.

Wild pansy's saponins are drawn out via simple tea infusion. This can be applied externally onto skin rashes, as well as taken internally.

Red Seaweed

Red seaweed has been used for thousands of years to treat inflammation-oriented conditions, including bronchitis and hypersensitivity. Researchers from the National Taiwan Ocean University (Kazłowska *et al.* 2010) studied the ability of the red seaweed *Porphyra dentata*, to halt allergic responses. The researchers found that a *Porphyra dentata* phenolic extract suppressed nitric oxide production among macrophages using a NF-kappa-Beta gene transcription process. This modulated the hypersensitivity immune response on a systemic level. The phenolic compounds within the red algae have been identified as catechol, rutin and hesperidin.

Other Anti-inflammatory Herbs

A number of other herbs also contain anti-inflammatory properties. These work in different ways, and while they may or may not specifically modulate food sensitivities, they can help strengthen the immune system, and thus reduce the inflammatory process the provokes hypersensitivity. Thus they can contribute to the modulation of the immune system, allowing us to begin tolerating foods that were not previously tolerated. Here is a quick overview of some of the most well-known (and most available) of these anti-inflammatory herbs:

Basil (*Osimum basilicum*) contains ursolic acid and oleanolic acid, both shown in laboratory studies to inhibit inflammatory COX-2 enzymes.

Rosemary (*Rosmarinus officinalis*) contains ursolic acid, oleanolic acid and apigenin – a few of the many constituents in this important botanical – shown to inhibit inflammatory enzymes in laboratory studies.

Oregano (*Origanum vulgare*) contains at least thirty-one anti-inflammatory constituents, twenty-eight antioxidants, and four significant COX-2 inhibitors (apigenin, kaempherol, ursolic acid and oleanolic acid).

Garlic (*Allium sativum*) probably deserves a larger section, but that information could easily encompass a book in itself (as was well documented by Paul Bergner: *The Healing Power of Garlic,* 1996). Garlic is an ancient medicinal plant with a wealth of characteristics and constituents that stimulate the immune system, protect the liver, purify the bloodstream, reduce oxidative species, reduce LDL cholesterol, reduce inflammation, and stimulate detoxification systems throughout the body. This is supported by a substantial amount of rigorous scientific research.

Garlic is also one of the most powerful antibiotic-antimicrobial plants known. A fresh garlic bulb has at least five different constituents known to inhibit bacteria, fungi and viruses. This antibiotic capability, however, is destroyed by heat and oxygen. Therefore, eating freshly peeled bulbs are the most assured way to retain these antibiotic potencies.

Cooked, aged or dehydrated garlic powder also has a variety of powerful antioxidants, but little of its antibiotic abilities. Garlic is also a tremendous sulfur donor as well. The combination of garlic's antibiotic, antioxidant, anti-inflammatory and immune-building characteristics make it a *must* food for any inflammatory condition.

The Herbal Conclusion

Certainly this is an extensive list of herbs and herbal formulations that have been shown in research and clinical use among traditional medicines to have adaptogenic and/or tonic properties.

Choosing the right herb and/or formula for a particular sensitivity can thus be a little tricky. For this reason, a seasoned expert in herbal formulations can offer specific suggestions relating to ones constitution and precise level of sensitivities.

That said, one of the strategies that many traditional physicians have utilized is to select those herbs that target the symptoms of the patient. While this might be compared to "treating the symptoms," as some pharmaceutical strategies are accused of, herbal medicines work on a much deeper level as we've discussed. While an herb's primary constituents might be productive with particular symptoms, the rest of the herb's constituents will likely also modulate the immune system's tolerance. This is its adaptogenic ability. These are the effects we have also seen among the research on herbal medicines. This *"from the outside in"* strategy produces a deeper correction of the systemic immunity issues often at the root of the problem.

We also see in many of these herbs, their ability to stimulate a healthy mucosal membrane and strengthen the intestinal barrier. These illustrate a strategy of treating from both directions: *outside-in* and *inside-out.*

Therefore, in the case of a food allergy where the primary reaction is respiratory – coughing, lung congestion, and so on – the traditional herbalist might select those anti-allergic herbs listed above that are known for their respiratory responses.

Likewise, a person with food allergy-related skin reactions might be given those herbs known to help atopic skin responses.

Concurrently, the herbalist might select those herbs discussed above that modulate and strengthen the intestinal barrier and intestinal mucosal membranes to reduce the exposure of the allergen on the intestinal tissues and bloodstream.

Enzyme Strategies

As we've shown in this text, enzymes are critical components for breaking down macromolecule proteins that can cause food sensitivities. While we are increasing our probiotic colonies, strengthening the immune system and reviving our digestive system, mucosal membranes and intestinal brush barriers; we can also take some of the heat off our immune system by supplementing with naturally-produced proteolytic enzymes to help break down some of the proteins and peptides that our bodies have become sensitized to.

Proteolytic enzymes are produced by plants, probiotics, and our own gastric, liver and bile systems. For those with compromised digestive systems, these enzymes may not be as available as they should. In these cases, the supplementation of natural enzymes can be extremely effective.

For example, chemical engineering researchers from Stanford University (Ehren *et al.* 2009) evaluated the breakdown of gluten-related proteins using two enzymes produced by probiotic microorganisms: Aspergillopepsin (ASP) produced from *Aspergillus niger* and dipeptidyl peptidase IV (DPP-IV) produced from the probiotic *Aspergillus oryzae* were tested.

The two enzymes were tested on gluten-type peptides in a simulation of conditions that would resemble the digestion of whole gluten and whole-wheat bread. They found that ASP and DPP-IV collectively and effectively cleaved (broke down) the gluten-type proteins in the study.

Another study – this also from Stanford University (Gass *et al.* 2007) – tested two proteases for the ability to digest and break down whole wheat gluten. The researchers utilized glutamine-specific endoprotease (EP-B2) which was produced from barley and a prolyl endopeptidase (SC PEP) which was produced from the bacteria *Sphingomonas capsulate*. They tested the enzymes on gluten in the laboratory and also tested them on sensitive rats.

Another study from Amsterdam's VU University Medical Center (Tack *et al.* 2013) tested 14 celiac patients who ate toast with 7 grams of gluten content each day with a prolyl endoprotease supplement made from *Aspergillus niger*. The supplement was well-tolerated and the patients were able to consume the toast.

The researchers found that the combination of enzymes "extensively" broke down the gluten proteins, and allowed the digestion of the glutens. They stated:

> *"By combining 2 enzymes with gastric activity and complementary substrate specificity, it should be possible to increase the safe threshold of ingested gluten, thereby ameliorating the burden of a highly restricted diet for patients with celiac sprue."*

While these enzymes can be produced by probiotics as we've proven earlier, they may also be supplemented in the form of enzymes. There are multiple enzyme suppliers who provide formulations specifically intended to help bread down glutenin and gliadin proteins.

Utilizing commercial enzymes from a reputable enzyme manufacturer is a smart choice for someone who is gluten sensitive. But a more sustainable approach is to colonize the probiotics that produce these enzymes.

That brings us right into our next strategy.

Prebiotic and Probiotic Strategies

Probiotic Foods

We've discussed in depth that probiotics and their enzymes can prevent and even help resolve food sensitivities. Here is another angle on that research: Eating fermented versions of foods that we are sensitive to.

The rationale is that probiotics will change the structure of foods as they ferment the food. In many cases they produce enzymes that digest and break down macromolecular versions of the sugars and proteins that we might be sensitive to. They will present to the digestive tract a different, often more digestible form of the nutrient along with numerous enzymes that aid in further digestion and assimilation.

Fermented foods also deliver to the digestive tract colonies of probiotics that can colonize and continue to help break down those food macromolecules that often cause sensitivities. While fermented foods may only present temporary residents, they will typically endure for a couple of weeks, and during that time provide numerous benefits. During that two weeks, we can eat another meal of the fermented food to help replenish those colonies.

Illustrating this, researchers from the Department of Food Science and Human Nutrition at the University of Illinois (Frias *et al.* 2008) studied the sensitivity response (or, as the researchers termed it, *"immunoreactivity"*) of soybeans in the cracked bean form and in the flour state before and after fermentation with probiotics. They fermented some of the cracked beans and flour with *Aspergillus oryzae, Rhizopus oryzae, Lactobacillus plantarum,* and *Bacillus subtilis.* These are fermenting bacteria are commonly used to make various probiotic cultured foods such as tempeh and sauerkraut.

The researchers used ELISA tests and the Western blot test to quantify IgE immunoglobulin response with human plasma. They found that all of the fermentation processes dramatically decreased the immunoreactivity of the soybeans and flours. Soy flour fermented with *L. plantarum* exhibited the highest reduction, with a 96-99% lower immunoreactivity levels. *R. oryzae* and *A. oryzae* reduced immunoreactivity by 66% and 68% respectively. *B. subtilis* produced from 81% to 86% reduction in immunoreactivity to the soy.

In addition, a positive side effect of the fermentation was the improvement of the protein quality of the soy products. After fermentation with *R. oryzae,* for example, levels of the amino acids alanine and threonine were increased, making the soy products more nutritious!

The bottom line is that this research illustrates what healthy colonies of probiotics can do within the intestinal tract. Probiotics process foods. During their processing, they reduce the immune system's sensitivity to the foods. This is a subtle process related to the probiotics' activity. Now why would probiotics increase the tolerance for otherwise-sensitive foods? Think about it. Let's say that you are living in a house that is too cold. Would you let the cold continue until you freeze to death? No. You would work hard to get the house warm enough so you could continue to survive and maybe even live in comfort. It is a survival issue. In the same way, symbiotic bacteria that are living within our intestines want to remain alive and comfortable, and make their stay as hospitable as possible. In order to do that, they help process nutrients in such a way that works best for our bodies. This keeps us healthy, which also keeps them healthy.

Here is a sampling of some of the world's favorite probiotic foods:

Traditional Yogurt

Traditional yogurt is produced using *L. bulgaricus* and *S. thermophilus.* Commercial preparations sometimes include L. acidophilus, but the use of *L. acidophilus* in yogurt will rarely result in the final product containing *L. acidophilus.* This is because *L. bulgaricus* is a hardy organism, and it will easily overtake *L. acidophilus* within a culture. Note also that in commercial yogurt preparations that are pasteurized after culturing, there are few or no living probiotics remaining after pasteurization. Some manufacturers culture the milk after pasteurization. This will result in a healthy probiotic culture.

Traditional Kefir

Kefir is a traditional drink originally developed in the Caucasus region of what is now considered Southern Russia, Georgia, Armenia and Azerbaijan. Kefir uses fermented milk mixed with kefir grains that resemble little chunks of cauliflower. Kefir typically contains *L. bulgaricus* and *S. thermophilus.* Cow's milk is most used, but sheep's milk, goat's milk or deer milk can also be used.

Traditional Buttermilk

Buttermilk is a soured beverage that was originally curdled from cream. Traditional buttermilk utilized the acids that probiotic bacteria produce for curdling. Today, forced curdling is done using commercially available acidic products such as lemon juice or vinegar. This however, does not result in the probiotic cultures of traditional buttermilk, unless of course, raw probiotic milk is utilized as a base.

This also goes for butter and cottage cheese. Both were probiotic foods until modern dairies decided that there was no value in the probiotics that naturally occur from grass-fed cows.

Traditional Kimchi

Kimchi is a fermented cabbage with a wonderful history from Korea. Kimchi was considered a ceremonial food served to emperors and ambassadors. It was also highly regarded as a healing and tonic food. There are a variety of different recipes of kimchi, depending upon the region and occasion. *Lactobacillus kimchii* is the typical probiotic colonizer, but others have also been used.

Traditional Miso

Miso is an ancient fermented food from Japan. A well-made miso will contain over 160 strains of aerobic probiotic bacteria. This is because the ingredients are perfect prebiotics for these probiotics. Miso is produced by fermenting beans and grains. Soybeans are often used, but other types of beans are also used. *Aspergillus oryzae* or koji is typically used as a fermenting base. When other beans other than soy are used, they will produce different varieties of miso. Shiromiso is white miso, kuromiso is black miso, and akamiso is red miso. They are each made with different beans. There are also various other miso recipes, many of which are highly guarded by their makers.

Traditional Shoyu

Shoyu is a traditional form of soy sauce made by blending a mixture of cooked soybeans and wheat, again with koji, or *Aspergillus oryzae*. The combination is fermented for an extended time. The aging process for shoyu is dependent upon the storage temperature and cooking methods used, and is also regarded as a secret by many producers.

Traditional Tempeh

Tempeh is an aged and fermented soybean food. It is extremely healthy and contains a combination of probiotics and naturally metabolized soy. Tempeh is made by first soaking dehulled soybeans for 10-12 hours. The beans are then cooked for 20 minutes and strained. The dry, cooked beans are then mixed with a tempeh starter containing *Rhyzopus oryzae, Rhizopus oligosporus* or both. The flattened and aged cake will be full with white mycelium (fungal roots) when it is ready. This tasty food can then be eaten raw, baked, or toasted.

Traditional Kombucha Tea

Traditional kombucha tea is an ancient beverage from the orient. Its use dates back many centuries; and was used by China and Taiwanese emperors, as well as Russian, and Eastern Europe peoples, where its reputation grew.

Recent research has revealed that kombucha was originally derived from kefir grains developed for fermentation. The kefir was exported to China, where the grains were added to tea with sugar rather than milk. The result was a combination of probiotic bacteria and yeasts that can include (depending upon the evolution of the mother culture) *Acetobacter xylinum, Acetobacter xylinoides, Glucobacter bluconicum, Acetobacter aceti, Saccharomycodes Ludwigii, Schizosaccharomyces pombe,* and *Picha fermentans* – and possibly some other species.

The fermenting of these organisms renders a beverage that is full of nutrients and enzymes as well as healthy probiotics. While the probiotic count may not be as high as yogurt or kefir, the range of probiotics will be wider.

Traditional Lassi

Lassi is a traditional beverage once enjoyed by kings and governors in ancient India. Lassi is still very popular in India. It is quite simple to make, as it is made with yogurt, fruit and spices. Quite simply, it is a blend of diluted yogurt with fruit pulp – often mango is used in the traditional lassi. A little salt, turmeric and sweetener give it a sweet-n-salty taste. Other spices are also sometimes used. Sugar is often added in today's versions, but honey and/or fruit would be preferable, health-wise.

Traditional Sauerkraut

Sauerkraut is a traditional German fermented food. It is made quite simply, by blending shredded cabbage and pickling salt with *Lactobacillus plantarum* and *L. brevis* fermentation cultures.

More information on probiotic foods, supplements and the science of probiotics may be found in the author's two books on probiotics: *Probiotics–Protection Against Infection* (2009), and *Oral Probiotics* (2010).

Raw vs. Pasteurized Milk

Remember the study by researchers at Switzerland's University of Basel (Waser *et al.* 2007). The researchers studied of 14,893 children between the ages of five and 13 from five different European countries, including 2,823 children from farms and 4,606 children attending a Steiner School (known for its farm-based living and instruction). The researchers found that drinking farm milk was associated with decreased incidence of allergies and asthma. In other words, the raw milk was found to be the largest single determinant of this reduced allergy and asthma incidence among farm children. Why?

Raw milk from the cow contains a host of bacteria. In a healthy, mostly grass-fed cow, these bacteria are primarily probiotics. This is because a grass diet provides prebiotics that promote the cow's own probiotic colonies. Should the cow be fed primarily dried grass and dried grains, probiotic counts will be reduced, and replaced by pathogenic bacteria. As a result, most non-grass fed herds must be given lots of antibiotics to help keep their bacteria counts low. Probiotics, on the other hand, naturally keep bacteria counts down.

As a result, the non-grass fed cow's milk will have higher pathogenic bacteria counts than grass-fed cows. This means that the milk itself will also have high counts. When the non-grass-fed cow's milk is pasteurized, the heat kills most of these bacteria. The result is a milk containing dead pathogenic bacteria parts. These are primarily proteins and peptides, which get mixed with the milk and are eventually consumed with the milk.

In other words, pasteurization may kill the living pathogenic bacteria, but it does not get rid of the bacteria proteins. This might be compared to cooking an insect: If an insect landed in our soup we could surely cook it until it died. But the soup would still contain the insect parts.

Now the immune system of most people, and especially infants with their hypersensitive immune system, is trained to attack and discard pathogenic bacteria. And how does the body identify pathogenic bacteria? From their proteins.

In the case of pasteurized commercial milk, the immune system can still identify heat-killed microorganism body parts and proteins and launch an immune response against these proteins. This was shown in research from the University of Minnesota two decades ago (Takahashi *et al.* 1992).

It is not surprising that weak immune systems readily reject pasteurized cow's milk. In comparison, raw milk has far fewer microorganism content in general, most of which are probiotic in content. This was confirmed by tests done by a local California organic milk farm, who tested their raw milk against standardized tests from conventional milk farms.

In addition, pasteurization breaks apart or denatures many of the proteins and sugar molecules. This was illustrated by researchers from Japan's Nagasaki International University (Nodake *et al.* 2010), who found that when beta-lactoglobulin was conjugated with dextran-glycylglycine, its allergenicity decreased. This occurred by shielding epitope reception on cell membranes. A dextran is a very long chain of glucose molecules – a polysaccharide. In this case, the polysaccharide is joined with the amino acid, glycine.

This is not surprising. Natural whole cow's milk contains special polysaccharides called oligosaccharides. They are largely indigestible polysaccharides that feed our intestinal bacteria. Because of this trait, these indigestible sugars are called prebiotics.

Whole milk contains a number of these oligosaccharides, including oligogalactose, oligolactose, galacto-oligosaccharides (GOS) and transgalactooligosaccharides (TOS). These polysaccharides provide a number of benefits. Not only are they some of the more preferred food for probiotics: they also reduce the ability of pathogenic bacteria like *E. coli* to adhere to intestinal cells.

These oligosaccharides also provide bonds that reduce the incidence of beta-lactoglobulin, through the combination of being food for probiotics and the availability of the buffering effect of long-chain polysaccharides on radical molecules.

This reduction of beta-lactoglobulin has been directly observed in humans and animals after supplementation with probiotics (Taylor *et al.* 2006; Adel-Patient *et al.* 2005; Prioult *et al.* 2003).

Galacto-oligosaccharides are produced by conversion from enzymes in healthy cows and mothers.

The Benefits of Raw Whole Milk

While some children are sensitized to milk, milk should not be ignored as a healthy food for infants in most cases. Cow's milk contains many of the nutrients found in mother's milk. These include a host of vitamins, proteins, nucleotides, minerals, probiotics, immunoglobulins and healthy fatty acids. Raw milk also helps support the intestinal barrier.

Researchers from the University of Malawi College of Medicine (Brewster *et al.* 1997) – in Southeastern Africa – tested intestinal permeability and disease progression among 533 kwashiorkori-ridden children. Kwashiorkori is a protein- assimilation disease often seen among children in poor countries, and is typically accompanied by increased intestinal permeability.

The researchers compared a local mix of maize-soya-egg to the standard milk diet given in kwashiorkor treatment. Intestinal permeability significantly improved among the milk diet group. Fatalities among the milk group were 14% versus 21% among the maize group. The maize group also experienced more infections and gained less weight compared to the milk group.

Raw whole milk is a substantial food for children, and pregnant or lactating mothers, assuming that:

- The milk comes from cows that have been primarily grass-fed. When cows eat grass, they nourish their natural probiotic colonies. They also have stronger immune systems with which to battle pathogenic microorganisms. This means that the milk that comes out will have more probiotics and fewer pathogens. When cows are grass-fed they also receive more sunlight, which increases the health of their own immune systems. Just as in the case of a healthy mother, when cows' immune systems are stronger, they will produce more nourishing milk, which is healthier for the milk consumer.
- The cows receive no synthetic or genetically modified growth hormones. Growth hormones injected into cows have been shown to produce higher levels of IGF-1 in the milk and human body after drinking milk from growth hormones-injected cows. The American Public Health Association stated in a 2009 Policy Release regarding the use of growth hormones in dairy cows, after a review of the evidence, that, *"elevated IGF-1 levels in human*

blood are associated with higher rates of colon, breast, and prostate cancers." Indeed, researchers from the University of Cincinnati's College of Medicine (Biro *et al.* 2010) studied 1,239 girls from 6-8 years old. They found that girls in this age group are reaching puberty at double the rate they did just ten years ago.

- The cows receive little or no antibiotics. These antibiotics will travel through the milk into the body. Here they can weaken the immune system and set up a greater susceptibility of antibiotic-resistant microorganisms.
- The milk (from grass-fed cows) is not pasteurized. Pasteurization kills all the beneficial microorganisms cows provide that promote healthy probiotics in the gut.

At least within the United States, the consumer should check to be sure that the dairy is registered with the state and undergoes continuous microorganism control. This means the state tests the milk periodically. Also the dairy should test every batch of milk and should be able to supply their customers with test results. These should show coliform counts less than 10 bacteria per mL of milk (also the same as pasteurized milk).

For those readers whose states ban the sale of raw milk; organic milk, yogurt and kefir are probably the best alternatives. Organic milk from a smaller dairy will typically come from predominantly grass-fed cows. They will also not receive hormones or antibiotics (organic cows can receive antibiotics if they are sick, but must then be separated from the milking herd for a significant period of time).

Note that lactose-intolerant persons should do fine with fresh raw milk from an organic dairy. This is not a guarantee, but the owner of one of the largest raw milk dairies in California has informed the author that many of his raw milk customers are lactose-intolerant.

How does this work? The probiotics in the cow have large colonies of lactobacilli. These species love to break down lactose and they produce lactase. They also consume a number of the polysaccharides in raw milk.

If pasteurized milk is the only option, it can be mixed with yogurt or kefir to increase its probiotic benefit and digestion. This will supply the microorganisms that can help break down the lactose and proteins in the milk to better prepare it for digestion.

Note that as for this and any other information, the reader should consult their health provider before making any significant changes to their diet. Any experimentation with raw milk or any other severely sensitized food should be done in the supervision of a health expert prepared to deal with severe allergic responses.

Why the big disclaimer again? This is because while this information is based upon science, food sensitivities can still be tricky and unique. It always pays to be cautious, moderate and careful.

All of this said, finding raw milk that is inspected and certified (recommended) may be difficult for many of us. Yogurt and kefir are good alternatives. These milk-derived foods will supply milk's many benefits while delivering much-needed prebiotics and probiotics.

The Prebiotic Diet

One of the most important factors in establishing a healthy environment for our probiotic colonies is making sure they have the right mix of nutrients available. The nutrients our probiotic families favor are called prebiotics.

More specifically, some foods are particularly beneficial for *bifidobacteria, lactobacilli* and other probiotic populations. These are the oligosaccharides, fructooligosaccharides, galactooligosaccharides, and transgalactooligosaccharides – also referred to as inulin, FOS, GOS and TOS.

Even two or three grams of one of these prebiotics will dramatically increase probiotic populations assuming healthy colonies. Inulin, FOS, GOS and TOS are also antagonistic to toxic microorganism genera such as *Salmonella, Listeria, Campylobacter, Shigella* and *Vibrio.* These and other pathogenic bacteria tend to thrive from refined sugars as opposed to the complex saccharides of inulin, FOS, GOS and TOS.

Oligosaccharides are short stacks of simple yet mostly indigestible sugars (from the Greek *oligos*, meaning "few"). If the sugar molecule is fructose, the stacked molecule is called a fructooligosaccharide. If the sugar molecule is galactose, the stacked molecule is called a galactooligosaccharide. These molecules are very useful for human cells and probiotics because they can be processed directly for energy as well as be combined with fatty acids to create cell wall structures and cellular communication molecules. These nutrients also provide energy and nourishment to our probiotic colonies.

The oligosaccharides inulin and oligofructose are probably the most recognized prebiotics. Inulin is a naturally occurring carbohydrate used by plants for storage. It has been estimated that more than 36,000 plant species contain inulin in varying degrees (Carpita *et al.* 1989). The roots often contain the greatest amounts of inulin.

Commercial sources of inulin include Jerusalem artichoke, agave cactus and chicory. Chicory, the root of the Belgian endive, is known to contain some of the highest levels of both inulin at 15-20%, and oligofructose at 5-10%. Inulin from agave has been described as highly branched. This gives it a higher solubility and digestibility than inulin derived from Jerusalem artichoke or chicory.

Notable prebiotic FOS-containing foods include beets, leeks, bananas, tree fruits, soybeans, burdock root, asparagus, maple sugar, whole rye and whole wheat among many others. Bananas contain one of the highest levels of FOS. Bananas are thus a favorite food for both humans and probiotics.

GOS and TOS are natural byproducts of milk. They are produced as lactose is enzymatically converted or hydrolyzed within the digestive tract. This process can also be done commercially. Before much of the recent research on prebiotics was performed, nutritionists simply thought of GOS and TOS as indigestible byproducts of milk.

A lesser known yet important prebiotic is the polysaccharide arabinoxylan-oligosaccharide. This is a component of wheat bran. We will discuss this further in our chapter on grains.

It is the longer-chain polysaccharides that provide the most benefit to our probiotics. These are contained in whole, plant fiber foods.

On the other hand, foods that have been stripped of these important plant fibers, creating refined simpler sugars, feed the more aggressive disease-causing bacteria and yeasts such as Staphylococcus and Candida.

Another element in plant foods providing prebiotic nutrition for probiotics is the polyphenol group. Polyphenols are groups of biochemicals produced in plants such as lignans, tannins, resveratrol, and flavonoids. There is some uncertainty as to which of these are most helpful to probiotic populations.

Some prebiotics have interesting side effects. For example, there seems to be a relationship between oligofructose inulin and calcium absorption. Inulin has been shown to improve calcium absorption by 20%, and yogurt supplemented with TOS has increased calcium absorption by 16% (van den Heuvel *et al.* 2000)

Galactooligosaccharides have another side effect that is important to note. Dr. Kari Shoaf and fellow researchers at the University of Nebraska (Shoaf *et al.* 2006) found in laboratory tests that galactooligosaccharides reduce the ability of *E. coli* to attach to human cells within tissue cultures. This effect was isolated from GOS' ability to nourish probiotics. This means that GOS provides more than nutrition to our probiotic colonies. This once considered useless indigestible nutrient also helps keep *E. coli* and other pathogenic bacteria from attaching to our cells. A nice package deal indeed.

FOS and GOS have been known to cause digestive disturbance in rare cases. Such a digestive disturbance is likely caused by dysbiosis, however.

Conclusively, a preponderance of scientific literature indicates that probiotics thrive from a diet of plant-based natural foods with plenty of phytonutrients, while overly processed, sugary and meat diets tend to promote pathogenic bacteria and their disease-causing endotoxins.

Probiotic Supplementation

The supplementation of probiotics can accomplish three mutually-advantageous objectives:

1) Help rebuild the intestinal wall mucosal membranes. Because the mucosal membranes protect the intestinal cells, healthy membranes will provide a stronger barrier between any macromolecules and contact with the intestinal cells, which can provoke inflammation as we've discussed.
2) Provide a basis for an environment that promotes the colonization of our resident species of probiotics, many of which will – if they are fed and activated – produce the enzymes such as prolyl endopeptidase that break down gluten proteins.
3) Directly provide the species that produce these enzymes. This can be done both short-term and long-term. While supplemented strains will not necessarily stay in the gut past two weeks or so after supplementation ends, continued periodic supplementation can provide the enzymes necessary for gluten digestion.

We've illustrated several studies that have proven these points. In one we have yet to discuss, Spanish researchers (Alvarez-Sieiro *et al.* 2014) tested two strains of *Lactobacillus casei* and found each produced prolyl endopeptidase in different parts of the colon.

In general, a supplementation plan should include those species that will encourage gut health and aid in food sensitivities.

After reviewing hundreds of clinical studies, some quoted in this book and many more discussed in the author's *Probiotics–Protection Against Infection*, here is a summary of those probiotics shown useful for one type of food sensitivity or another (refer to the author's probiotics text mentioned above for reference specifics):

Lactobacillus acidophilus

Lactobacillus acidophilus is by far the most familiar probiotic to most of us, and is also by far the most-studied probiotic species to date. They are one of the main residents of the human gut, although supplemented strains may still be transient. In addition to helping digest lactose, probably the most important benefit of *L. acidophilus* is their ability to inhibit the growth of pathogenic intestinal microorganisms such as *Candida albicans, Escherichia coli, Helicobacter pylori, Salmonella, Shigella* and *Staphylococcus* species.

The research has found that L. acidophilus help digest milk, reduce stress-induced GI problems; inhibit *E. coli*, reduce various intestinal infections, reduce intestinal permeability, control *H. pylori*, reduce inflammation, reduce dyspepsia, help relieve IBS and colitis, inhibit and control Clostridium spp., inhibit Bacteroides spp., and inhibit Candida spp. overgrowths.

Lactobacillus helveticus

L. helveticus was made popular by cheese-makers from Switzerland. The Latin word *Helvetia* refers to Switzerland. *L. helveticus* is used to make Swiss cheese and other cheese varietals, as it produces lactic acid but not other probiotic metabolites that can often make cheese taste bitter or sour.

Lactobacillus salivarius

L. salivarius are residents of most humans. They are found in the mouth, small intestines, colon, and vagina. They are hardy bacteria that can live in both oxygen and oxygen-free environments. *L. salivarius* is one of the few bacteria species that can also thrive in salty environments. *L. salivarius* produce prolific amounts of lactic acid, which makes them hardy defenders of the teeth and gums. They also produce a number of antibiotics, and are speedy colonizers.

Lactobacillus casei

L. casei are transient bacteria within the human body, but are residents of cow intestines. Thus they are readily found in naturally raw milk and colostrum. *L. casei* have been reported to reduce allergy symptoms and increase immune response. This is accomplished by their regulating the immune system's CHS, CD8 and T-cell responsiveness – an effect seen among immunosuppressed patients. *L. casei* are also competitive bacteria that will overtake other probiotics in a combined supplement. So it is best to supplement *L. casei* individually.

Lactobacillus rhamnosus

Much of the research on this species has been done on a particular strain, *L. rhamnosus* GG. *L. rhamnosus* GG have been shown in numerous studies to significantly stimulate the immune system and inhibit allergic inflammatory response as noted earlier. This is not to say, however, that non-GG strains will not perform similarly. In fact, studies with *L. rhamnosus* GR-1, *L. rhamnosus* 573/L, and *L. rhamnosus* LC705 strains have also showed positive results. The GG strain is trademarked by the Valio Ltd. Company in Finland and patented in 1985 by two scientists, Dr. Sherwood Gorbach and Dr. Barry Goldin, who also led most of the exhaustive research on this strain.

Lactobacillus reuteri

L. reuteri is a species found residing permanently in humans. As a result, most supplemented strains attach fairly well, though temporarily, and stimulate colony growth for resident *L. reuteri* strains. *L. reuteri* will colonize in the stomach, duodenum and ileum regions. *L. reuteri* will also significantly modulate the immune response of the gastrointestinal mucosal membranes. This means that *L. reuteri* are useful for many of the same digestive ailments that *L. acidophilus* are also effective for. *L. reuteri* also have several other effects, including the restoration of our oral cavity bacteria. They also produce a significant amount of antibiotics.

Lactobacillus plantarum

L. plantarum has been part of the human diet for thousands of years. They are used in numerous fermented foods, including sauerkraut, gherkins, olive brines, sourdough bread, Nigerian ogi and fufu, kocha from Ethiopia, sour mifen noodles from China, Korean kimchi and other traditional foods. *L. plantarum* are also found in dairy and cow dung.

This species has been shown to stimulate the production of enzymes that break down gluten proteins.

L. plantarum is a hardy strain. The bacteria have been shown to survive all the way through the intestinal tract. Temperature for optimal growth is 86-95 degrees F. *L. plantarum* are not permanent residents, however. When supplemented, they vigorously attack pathogenic bacteria, and create an environment hospitable for incubated resident strains to expand before departing. *L. plantarum* also produce lysine, and a number of antibiotics including lactolin. They also strengthen the mucosal membrane and reduce intestinal permeability.

Lactobacillus bulgaricus

We owe the *bulgaricus* name to Ilya Mechnikov, who named it after the Bulgarians – who used the bacteria to make the fermented milks that produced the original kefirs apparently related to their extreme longevity. In the 1960s and 1970s Russian researchers, notably Dr. Ivan Bogdanov and others, began focused research on *L. bulgaricus*. Early studies indicated antitumor effects. As the research progressed into Russian clinical research and commercialization, it became obvious that even heat-killed *L. bulgaricus* cell fragments have immune system stimulating benefits.

L. bulgaricus bacteria are transients that assist in *bifidobacteria* colony growth. They significantly stimulate the immune system and have antitumor effects. They also produce antibiotic and antiviral substances such as bulgarican and others. *L. bulgaricus* bacteria have also been reported to have anti-herpes properties. *L. bulgaricus* require more heat to colonize than many probiotics – at 104-109 degrees F.

The research has shown that L. bulgaricus will help increase absorption of dairy (lactose).

Bifidobacterium bifidum

These are normal residents in the human intestines, and by far the largest residents in terms of colonies. Their greatest populations occur in the colon, but also inhabit the lower small intestines. Breast milk typically contains large populations of *B. bifidum* along with other bifidobacteria. *B. bifidum* are highly competitive with yeasts such as *Candida albicans*. As a result, their populations may be decimated by large yeast overgrowths. This will also result in a number of endotoxins, including ammonia, being leached out of the colon into the bloodstream. As a result, *B. bifidum* populations are extremely important to the health of the liver, as has been illustrated in the research. They produce an array of antibiotics such as bifidin and various antimicrobial biochemicals such as formic acid. *B. bifidus* populations can also be severely damaged by the use of pharmaceutical antibiotics.

Bifidobacterium infantis

B. infantis are also normal residents of the human intestines – primarily among children. As implicated in the name, infants colonize a significant number of *B. infantis* in their early years. They will also colonize in the vagina, leading to the newborn's first exposure to protective probiotic bacteria. For this reason, it is important that pregnant mothers consider probiotic supplementation with *B. infantis*. *B. infantis* are largely anaerobic, and thrive within the darkest regions, where they can produce profuse quantities of acetic acid, lactic acid and formic acid to acidify the intestinal tract.

We discussed the research in the previous chapter illustrating that this particular species will allow celiac patients to digest gluten-containing foods with less inflammation and other symptoms. It also reduced IgA antibody levels among the celiac patients that took the probiotic supplement – as we discussed.

Bifidobacterium longum

B. longum are also normal inhabitants of the human digestive tract. They predominate the colon but also live in the small intestines. They are one of our top four bifidobacteria inhabitants. Like *B. infantis,* they produce acetic, lactic and formic acid. Like other bifidobacteria, they resist the growth of pathogenic bacteria, and thus reduce the production of harmful nitrites and ammonia. *B. longum* also produce B vitamins. Healthy breast milk contains significant *B. longum.*

Bifidobacterium animalis/B. lactis

B. animalis was previously thought to be distinct from *B. lactis,* but today they are considered the same species with *B. lactis* being a subspecies of *B. animalis*. *B. lactis* has also been described as *Streptococcus lactis*. They are transient bacteria typically present in raw milk. They are also used as starters for traditional cheeses, cottage cheeses and buttermilks. They are also found among certain plants.

Bifidobacterium breve

B. breve are also normal inhabitants of the human digestive tract – living mostly within the colon. They produce prolific acids, and also B vitamins. Like the other bifidobacteria, they also reduce ammonia-producing bacteria in the colon, aiding the health of the liver. Latin *brevis* means short.

Streptococcus thermophilus

Streptococcus thermophilus are common participants in yogurt making. They are also used in cheese making, and are even sometimes found in pasteurized milk. They will colonize at higher temperatures, from 104-113 degrees F. This is significant because this bacterium readily produces lactase, which breaks down lactose.

Like many other supplemented probiotics, *S. thermophilus* are temporary microorganisms in the human body. Their colonies will typically inhabit the system for a week or two before exiting (unless consistently consumed). During that time, however, they will help set up a healthy environment to support resident colony growth. Like other probiotics, *S. thermophilus* also produce a number of different antibiotic substances, including acids that deter the growth of pathogenic bacteria.

Saccharomyces boulardii

S. boulardii are yeasts (fungi). This is a yeast often used in bread making and is a central component of most sourdough starters.

S. boulardii render a variety of preventative and therapeutic benefits to the body. Yet should this or another yeast colony grow too large, they can quickly become a burden to the body due to their dietary needs (primarily refined sugars) and waste products. *S. boulardii* are known to enhance IgA – which, as we've discussed, will typically reduce IgE atopic sensitivities.

S. boulardii also help control diarrhea, and have been shown to be helpful in Crohn's disease and irritable bowel issues. *S. boulardii* have also been shown to be useful in combating cholera bacteria (*Vibrio cholerae*).

Probiotic Supplement Considerations

The main consideration in probiotic supplementation is consuming live organisms. These are typically labeled as "CFU" which stands for *colony forming units*. In other words, live probiotics will produce new colonies once inside the intestines. Dead ones will not. So the key is keeping the probiotics alive while in the capsule and supplement bottle, until we are ready to consume them. Here are a few considerations about probiotic supplements:

Capsules

Vegetable capsules contain less moisture than gelatin or enteric-coated capsules. Even a little moisture in the capsule can increase the possibility of waking up the probiotics while in the bottle. Once woken up, they will starve and die. Enteric coating can minimally protect the probiotics within the stomach, assuming they have survived in the bottle. Some manufactures use oils to help protect the probiotics in the stomach. In all cases, encapsulated freeze-dried probiotics should be refrigerated (no matter what the label says) at all times during shipping, at the store, and at home. Dark containers also better protect the probiotics from light exposure, which can kill them.

Powders

Powders of freeze-dried probiotics are subject to deterioration due to increased exposure to oxygen and light. Powders should be refrigerated in dark containers and sealed tightly to be kept viable. They should also be consumed with liquids or food, preferably dairy or fermented dairy. If used as to insert into the vagina, a douche mixture with water and a little yogurt is preferable.

Caplets/Tablets

Some tablet/caplets have special coatings that provide viability through to the intestines without refrigeration. If not, those tablets would likely be in the same category as encapsulated products, in terms of requiring refrigeration.

Shells or Beads

These can provide longer shelf viability without refrigeration and better survive the stomach. However, because of the size of the shell, these typically come with less CFU quantity, increasing the cost of a therapeutic dose. Another drawback may be that the intestines must dissolve this thick shell. An easy test is to examine the stool to be sure that the beads or shells aren't coming out the other end whole.

Lozenges

These are new and exciting ways to supplement with probiotics. A correctly formulated chewable or lozenge can inoculate the mouth, nose and throat with beneficial bacteria to compete with and fight off pathogenic bacteria as they enter or reside in our nose, throat, mouth and even lungs. However, the probiotics in a lozenge will not likely survive the stomach acids and penetrate the intestines.

Still, lozenges are an excellent way to protect against new infections and prevent sore throats when we are traveling or working in enclosed spaces. The bacteria in a lozenge or chewable ease out as we are sucking or chewing, leaving probiotics dispersed throughout our gums and throat, rendering increased immunity. This type of supplement should still be kept sealed, airtight and cool. Refer to the author's book *Oral Probiotics* (2010) for detailed information regarding species and strategies for oral probiotic lozenges.

Liquid Supplements

There are several probiotic supplements in small liquid form. One brand has a long tradition and a hardy, well-researched strain. A liquid probiotic should be in a light-sealed, refrigerated container. It should also contain some dairy or other probiotic-friendly culture, giving the probiotics some food while they are waiting for delivery.

Probiotic Hydrotherapy

This method of supplementation is probably the best way to implant live colonies of probiotics into the lower colon. Colon hydrotherapy (or colonic) is one of the healthiest things we can do for preventative and therapeutic health. Colon hydrotherapy is performed by a certified colon hydrotherapist who uses specialized (and sanitary) equipment to flush out the colon. This colon flushing usually takes about 30 minutes. Once the process is complete, the hydrotherapist can "insert" a blend of probiotics into the tube and "pump" the probiotics directly into our colon. Colon hydrotherapy is a wonderful treatment recommended for most anyone, especially those with disorders related to autoimmunity, allergies and food sensitivities.

Colonic treatments are relatively inexpensive, especially for their benefit. Two to three colonics a year is often recommended for ultimate colon health. Those with sensitive or irritable bowels should consult with their health professional before submitting to a colonic, however.

Probiotic Dosage

A good dosage for intestinal probiotics for prevention and maintenance can be ten to fifteen billion CFU (*colony forming units*) per day. Total intake during an illness or therapeutic period, however, will often double or triple that dosage. Much of the research shown in this text utilized 20 billion to 40 billion CFU per day, about a third of that dose for children and a quarter of that dose for infants. (*B. infantis* is often the supplement of choice for babies.)

Supplemental oral probiotic dosages can be far less (100 million to two billion), especially when the formula contains the hardy *L. reuteri*.

People who must take antibiotics for life-threatening reasons can alternate doses of probiotics between their antibiotic dosing. The probiotic dose can be at least two hours before or after the antibiotic dose. (Always consult with the prescribing doctor first.)

Remember that these dosages depend upon delivery to the intestines. Therefore, a product that passes into the stomach with little protection would likely not deliver well to the intestines. Such a supplement would likely require higher dosage to achieve the desired effects.

Antibacterial Strategies

This may see odd to end this section with, but it is critical. The fundamental lesson in gluten sensitivity from the accumulation of evidence is that it is the overuse of antibiotics, antiseptics and other antimicrobials that has given rise to the imbalances existing among our probiotic populations and the subsequent inability to break down gliadin and glutenin proteins.

To this we can add that this very same problem – the overuse of antibacterials – is the foundation for many other intestinal disorders among our population, most of which have risen substantially as antibiotics have become abused.

The word *abused* is used because there may well be appropriate uses for antibiotics – when there is a potentially lethal infection that cannot be stopped using either probiotic or nature's antibacterials – many of which have been shown to outperform antibiotics.

So this book is not advising against appropriate use of antibiotics in such situations. It is, however, recommending against the use of antibiotics when not necessary.

And even then, supplementing with probiotics in between doses has been found to not only be more effective, but able to help retain some of those resident species that can be lost with antibiotic use.

Furthermore, as we discussed the evidence showing how healthy oral bacteria will break down (hydrolyze) gliadin proteins, it is now evident that using antiseptic mouthwashes and toothpaste would not be recommended.

Rather, healthy oral hygiene and the use of oral probiotics in cases of bacterial imbalances are prudent. This is discussed in detail in the author's books, *Oral Probiotics.*

Colon Health Strategies

Remember our discussions of mucoid plaque build up within the colon. Not only will mucoid plaque build up create an inflammatory environment within the small intestines: It will also produce some of the same symptoms, such a chronic fatigue, headaches and bloating attributed to gluten sensitivity.

We have also discussed the need for dietary fiber, and the well-accepted recommendation that an adult should consume between 25 and 40 grams of fiber per day, with about 75% of that in the form of insoluble fiber.

Whole wheat is perfect for this, because wheat provides a good source of insoluble fiber. Fiber content from whole wheat bread is about 80% insoluble and 20% soluble. Pumpernickel bread is about 55% insoluble. In other words, whole wheat is one of the more readily available forms of insoluble fiber.

Eating whole wheat versions of these wheats is important. Whole wheat spaghetti, for example, will contain 2.7 grams of fiber in a serving, while white spaghetti only contains about 0.9 grams per serving. For whole wheat bread versus white bread, we are talking over double, 1.5 grams versus 0.6 grams in a slice.

Certainly while a gluten-sensitive person is rebuilding their intestinal health during the gluten-elimination phase, other fibrous foods are preferred.

Other foods high in insoluble include green leafy vegetables, flax seeds, psyllium husks, apples and sunflower seeds. Various other whole grains such as oats and rice are also good fiber sources. Refer to earlier fiber discussion.

In other words, enough fiber in our diet is necessary to both avoid and help remedy a buildup of mucoid plaque within the colon.

Our stools should take place twice or at least once per day – every day. The stool should look solid and husky: Missile-shaped is best and about (depending upon age and size) an inch to two inches in diameter. The longer the stool, the better shape the colon is probably in. Shorter "plops" indicate mucoid plaque build up with small colon lumen.

The exception is that sometimes a meal with lots of leafy greens can result in a cow patty-type bowel movement. Nothing wrong with this.

The easiest solution for mucoid plaque build-up is a combination of fiber, plant-based foods, a balanced fat diet, probiotic foods and a periodic hydrotherapy colonic. A colonic is a flushing out of the lower colon utilizing a hydrotherapy colonic machine.

A colonic machine will push water in and out of the colon, washing away the plaque and debris along the colon walls. For difficult cases, this may take 2-3 visits to accomplish. We will typically experience tremendous results after just one treatment though.

This treatment has proven very successful among natural therapists.

And a number of well-known physicians utilized colonic hydrotherapy in the early to mid twentieth century experienced success treating various illnesses with colon cleansing. Dr. John Kellogg, Dr. William Koch, Dr. Eugene Blass, Dr. J.H. Tilden and Dr. Bernard Jensen and Sir Arbuthnot Lane – King of England's surgeon – all had notable success in treating patients with colon cleansing.

In 1929, Dr. J.F. Burgess, a professor at McGill University and dermatologist at the Montreal General Hospital reported in the Canadian Journal of Medicine that his research led him to believe that "alimentary toxins" (build-up of colonic bacteria and plaque) were one of the most important factors in eczema (Burgess 1930).

William Lintz, M.D. successfully treated 472 patients who suffered from allergies with colon cleansing.

Dr. J.H. Tilden successfully treated hundreds of patients with pneumonia during the early 1900s by cleansing their bowels followed by a good diet.

Allan Eustis, M.D., a Tulane University of Medicine professor in 1912, is said to have cured 121 cases of bronchial asthma with colon cleansing.

D. Rochester, M.D. of the University of Buffalo's School of Medicine, made a statement in 1906 saying that after 23 years of observation, he believed that intestinal toxemia is the underlying cause of asthma.

Harvey Kellogg, M.D. once said:

> *"Of the 22,000 operations that I have personally performed, I have never found a single normal colon, and of the 100,000 that were performed under my jurisdiction, not over 6% were normal."*

Lifestyle and Environment Strategies

Hydration

One might think that hydration is completely unrelated to gluten sensitivities. This is absolutely false.

The intestinal mucosal membrane is primarily water. In a dehydrated state, this mucosal membrane thins. It is for this reason that research on water drinking has found that many ulcerated conditions can be cured simply by drinking adequate water (Batmanghelidj 1997).

The immune system is also irrevocably aligned with the body's water availability. The immune system utilizes water to produce lymph fluid. Lymph fluid circulates immune cells throughout the body so that they can target specific intruders. The lymph is also used to escort toxins out of the body.

Water in general is needed to speed the removal of toxins, from every organ and tissue system.

Water also increases the availability of oxygen to cells. Water balances the level of free radicals. Water flushes and replenishes the digestive tract. Thus, water is necessary for the proper digestion of food. The gastric cells and intestinal wall cells require water for proper functioning.

Water is also intimately involved in the release of histamine. Research has revealed that increased levels of histamine are released during periods of dehydration, in order to help provide water balance within the bloodstream, tissues, kidneys and other organs.

A rule of thumb accepted by many experts, and consistent with government studies, would be to drink one-half ounce of water per pound of body weight per day.

Drinking just any water is not advised. Chlorinated, fluoridated municipal water is not advised without a filter.

Care must be taken to drink water that is naturally mineralized. Research has confirmed that distilled water and soft water are not advisable. Please refer to the author's book, *Pure Water* for the specific research on this, as well as information on which types of water and filtration methods are the healthiest.

Exercise

Gluten sensitivities are directly related to the health of the immune system and exercise is directly related to immunity. Is there evidence for this?

Nutrition researchers from The Netherlands' Wageningen University (Chin *et al.* 2000) found that as elderly people became more frail, their immune systems weakened and they became more sensitive to certain foods. The researchers studied 112 elderly subjects with an average age of 79 years old.

The research compared the effects of vitamin supplementation and exercise with food sensitivities. They found that vitamin supplementation slowed the level of food sensitivity among the elderly men and women.

We are not surprised about the vitamin supplementation. While even antioxidant vitamins such as C and E have been shown to strengthen the body's immune system, isolated vitamins do not have the cofactors and buffers needed for a balanced effect. This is also why studies on isolated vitamins such as E have been inconclusive.

Nature produces several forms of vitamin E, which includes alpha-, beta-, gamma- and delta-tocopherols. When these are isolated they do not have the same effects as when they are naturally presented in foods. Also, we might add that elderly persons often do not absorb isolated nutrients very well. Food-based nutrition is the best strategy, although sometimes isolated nutrients become necessary in order to avoid a deficiency.

As far as exercise goes, this is one of the most assured ways of strengthening the immune system and thus increasing tolerance. When we exercise, we contract muscles. Muscle contraction is what circulates (or pumps) lymph around the body through the lymph vessels. This is because the lymphatic system does not have a heart like the circulatory system has. The lymphatic system relies on muscle contraction for circulation.

Lymph circulation is critical because while immune cells are also circulated through the blood, much of our immune cells, cytokines and immunoglobulins are circulated through the lymph. Lymph also carries out of the body those broken-down toxins and cell parts after the immune system has done its job. And research has revealed that parts of the lymphatic system also houses and incubates probiotics in ducts such as the vermiform appendix (Randal, *et al.* 2007).

And of course exercise also circulates oxygen, nutrients and immune cells throughout the body using the bloodstream. The bloodstream also carries out of the body those detoxification byproducts as well. Exercise also stimulates the thymus gland, and speeds up healing of the intestinal cell walls. In all, exercise is one of the best and cheapest therapies available to boost immunity and tolerance.

One of the healthiest forms of exercise is called high-intensity training (HIIT). This is when high-intensity bursts of exercise are alternated with resting or slower activity. Sports that include short bursts of sprinting such as soccer, basketball and tennis are good examples of HIIT.

Environmental Strategies

As we mentioned earlier, a number of studies over the past decade have found that children living in rural areas were less likely to have allergies, including food sensitivities. For years, doctors and researchers have been supposing that this effect was coming from the increased exposures to the various allergens. In other words, the theory has been that the immune system becomes more tolerant when it is exposed to increased levels of potential toxins.

Remember the research from Switzerland's University of Basel on children from farms, found that farm living and farm milk lowered allergies. While we can attribute some of this effect to the natural probiotics in raw farm milk, rural living and the increased plant-food diets of the Steiner children also indicate lifestyles that decrease allergy rates among children.

Remember also the other studies quoted earlier that showed that food sensitivities were higher in industrialized countries and among those living in urban areas.

The hypothesis that the more exposure to toxins, the more tolerant the immune system becomes has come under scrutiny. This would mean those living in cities should be more tolerant to smog and other pollutants, and thus should have even lower levels of asthma than those living in rural regions where smog exposure is reduced.

A number of studies have shown the opposite. For example, a study done by the Arizona Health Care Cost Containment System (Smith *et al.* 2010) found that urban residents had a 55% greater likelihood of asthma than rural residents. The study followed 3,013 persons.

The real issue here is that the immune system of a human has evolved over millions of years along with nature. The healthy immune system is genetically set up to ultimately recognize nature's toxins and deal with them appropriately through IgA responses and liver detoxification systems.

Occasionally, the natural immune system launches a hyper-inflammatory response to an invasion of viruses and/or bacteria. These are dealt with appropriately; and the immune system memorizes the invader. This memory serves to protect the body from a reinvasion, typically without the need for hyper-inflammation.

However, our increasingly synthetic environments are corrupting and overloading the immune system, producing hypersensitivity. They are overloading the liver and immune system with a variety of chemical toxins that the immune system and its probiotic helpers have never encountered at these levels.

This barrage is producing immune system fallout. Normal processes of mucosal membranes and intestinal wall barriers are being destroyed. This in turn damages the body's ability to properly break down nutrients, leaving the intestinal wall exposed to macromolecules new to the immune system.

The destruction of the mucosal membranes of the mouth and digestive tract also weakens the body's IgA response. Out of desperation, the immune system responds with hypersensitivity, sometimes even to elements that were consumed for decades.

Urban industrialized areas expose people to environments with an increased amount of these synthetic toxins. This is one of the reasons that undeveloped countries and urban areas have less gluten sensitivity – even though some of these populations eat as much or more gluten foods than Western countries.

Pharmaceuticals and Alcohol

Alcohol and many pharmaceuticals can damage our intestinal cells and even destroy many of our resident probiotic species and strains.

This is not limited to antibiotics and fungicide medications either. There are numerous medications that slow or otherwise damage probiotics and/or damage the health of our mucous membranes and/or intestinal walls.

Illustrating this and the role probiotics play, researchers from Italy's Catholic University (Montalto *et al.* 2004) studied the health of the tight junctions between intestinal cells and aspirin. They found that aspirin increased intestinal permeability by damaging the tight junctions between intestinal cells – indicated by zonulin levels.

They also found that Lactobacillus acidophilus significantly protected the tight junctions against damage from aspirin.

After exhaustive research on the relationships between lifestyle and leaky gut, medical scientists from the Department of Internal Medicine at France's University Hospital (Moneret-Vautrin and Morisset 2005) found that increased intestinal permeability is associated with the use of alcohol, aspirin, beta-blockers and angiotensin-converting enzyme (ACE) inhibitors.

Oral Immunotherapy

A natural solution that has proved successful for resolving many food allergies – as well as food intolerances – is called *specific oral tolerance induction,* or SOTI. In SOTI, very small amounts of the offending food are periodically fed to the allergic subject, with gradual increases over time.

The body becomes tolerant to a previously-considered foreigner or allergen through a number of responses. One of the ways is through the production of mesenchymal stromal cells. These are produced in the bone marrow, and modulate the cytokine communications of T-cells. Researchers from Italy's University of Pavia (Ciccocioppo *et al.* 2014) found that mesenchymal stromal cells significantly modified gliadin-specific T-cells from celiac disease patients.

The application of oral immunotherapy for gluten sensitivities and gluten intolerances is clear, though much of the research below is discusses other food allergies. The reason this is applicable is that gluten sensitivities – if they are allergic – utilize the immunoglobulin response, which can be trained to produce a tolerance to that offending allergen. And because many cases of non-allergic gluten sensitivities can lead to allergenicity, the application is similar – in order to increase tolerance.

With respect to zero tolerance, research has shown that small amounts of gluten are not harmful even to active celiac disease patients. A 90-day study of 49 celiac patients from the University of Maryland School of Medicine (Catassi *et al.* 2007) found that all patients were able to tolerate up to 50 milligrams per day but less than 50 milligrams (taken via capsule) was advised. None of the groups – who took either 10 milligrams or 50 milligrams of gluten per day – had increased T-cell counts. However, there was some difference in villi height – indicating a little response – in the 50 milligram per day group. Only one person who took the 10 milligrams per day had a clinical response.

As we will see from the research following, oral immunotherapy is a frequent treatment among European doctors for food sensitivity sufferers – and with great success. As of 2003, over a third of allergies were treated with immunotherapy in Europe (Canonica *et al.* 2003). Today that rate is significantly higher.

Sublingual immunotherapy is another method of SOTI. Here clinically-tested tablets that contain extracts of the allergic substance are given with exact dilution rates. The tablet is taken under the tongue until it dissolves.

Nasal immunotherapy has also been used with success, although it has been observed being primarily beneficial for rhinitis symptoms.

These methods are all considered safer than *subcutaneous injection*, because subcutaneous injection can sometimes produce acute responses, especially among children.

Doctors in the U.S. do not utilize immunotherapy anywhere near the degree that doctors do in Europe. Besides not being well-accepted by most physicians, the FDA does not recognize immunotherapy, and Medicare does not provide insurance for immunotherapy treatment. Many other insurers follow Medicare's lead in not insuring immunotherapy.

This is quite simply a disservice to the millions of food sensitivity sufferers in North America. Possibly this discussion might help change that.

Specific immunotherapy has been established for pollen-food sensitivities in many studies. Swiss researchers (Bucher *et al.* 2004) used specific immunotherapy for 27 birch pollen-allergic subjects that either had allergies to apple or hazelnut. Fifteen of the 27 volunteers were given immunotherapy and the others were controls. They were given increasing doses of one gram to 128 grams of either fresh apples or ground hazelnuts over a year's time. After the year, 87% of the immunotherapy group (13) increased tolerance of apple or hazelnuts with no adverse symptoms. The average amount of increase in the allergen food was about 20 grams – ranging from 12 grams to 32 grams.

Researchers from the Allergology Department of Rome's Catholic University (Patriarca *et al.* 2003) gave 59 food-allergy patients oral tolerance treatment (SOTI) with standard protocols. A randomized control group followed a strict elimination diet. Of the SOTI-treated patients, 83% completed the oral tolerance protocol and became tolerant to the foods they were sensitive to. During the protocol, 51% experienced some mild responses.

Researchers from Italy's University of Trieste (Longo *et al.* 2008) tested SOTI treatment with 60 children with severe milk allergies. The children were five years old or more. They were split into two groups of 30 children each. One group started SOTI immediately, starting with very small amounts of milk. The second group stayed on a milk-free diet for a year. After the year was finished, In other words, 90% of the SOTI group became tolerant of milk: 36% of the SOTI group were completely milk-tolerant and another 54% could drink limited amounts of milk. In the elimination diet group, every person in the group was still sensitive to cow's milk after the one year.

Researchers from France's University Hospital of Nancy (Morisset *et al.* 2007) tested SOTI with 60 milk allergy children, aged between 13 months and 6.5 years old; and 90 egg allergy children, ages 12 months to eight years old. They were randomized, and given either allergen elimination diets or gradual SOTI desensitization by feeding small amounts of the allergen. After six months, skin prick testing and IgE testing revealed that sensitivities continued in only 11% of the milk SOTI group, and 30% of the egg SOTI group, This means the success rates were 89% and 70%, respectively.

Allergy researchers from the University of Rome (Meglio *et al.* 2004) gradually desensitized (SOTI) 21 milk allergy children within six months by feeding increasing amounts of milk daily, with a goal of 200 ml per day of eventual tolerance. Within the six months, 71% of the children (15 of 21) accomplished the 200ml daily intake. Of the rest, three (14%) were able to tolerate 40-80 ml per day, and only three of the 21 children (14%) failed the SOTI treatment completely. This rendered a total success rate of 86%.

Researches from Italy's University of Trieste (Longo *et al.* 2008) found that even children with extreme allergic responses to milk could significantly benefit from oral immunotherapy protocol. They divided 60 severely-allergic (to milk) children five years old or higher into two groups. The first group of 30 was given immediate oral immunotherapy of gradually increasing amounts of milk for one year. The other group remained on a milk elimination diet throughout the year. After the year, 11 become completely tolerant to milk while 16 of the children became partially tolerant. That means that out of the 30 *severely allergic* children, 90% (27 out of 30) became tolerant to milk to one degree or another.

Researchers from Humboldt University in Berlin (Rolinck-Werninghaus *et al.* 2005) found that children given graduated doses of allergens achieved maximum dose tolerance after 37, 41 and 52 weeks using SOTI. They also found those subjects put on a second elimination diet from the allergen had moderate systemic allergic responses when given the allergen again. This showed that while tolerance can be achieved with gradual dosing; the previously-sensitive food should be eaten periodically in order to maintain tolerance. The researchers concluded that: *"Regular allergen intake seems necessary to maintain the established tolerance."*

Allergy unit researchers from Italy's University of Messina (Caminiti *et al.* 2009) tested IgE-milk allergy children with the SOTI oral tolerance protocol. They gave 13 children either a randomized double-blind desensitization with milk or soy formula as placebo, or an open version of the protocol. The SOTI children were given one drop of whole milk diluted 1:25 the first week.

The dose was doubled every week until they had achieved a 200 mL dose on week 18. Of the 13 children, 10 received the milk protocol in total. Seven of the ten achieved the 200 mL of milk tolerance. Only two children failed the protocol because of severe reactions, while one patient accomplished partial milk tolerance (64 mL) during the study. The soy children were still allergic to milk at the end of the study.

Researchers from Rome's Catholic University (Patriarca *et al.* 2007) conducted SOTI oral immunotherapy desensitization with 42 children who were as old as 16 years and had been diagnosed with a variety of food allergies. Ten patients – the control group – were treated with an elimination diet. The immunotherapy consisted of gradually increasing the dose of the allergen. Of the allergic children who started, 86% completed the protocol and became tolerant. Allergen-specific IgE levels decreased significantly, and allergen-specific IgG significantly increased among the entire immunotherapy group.

Spanish researchers (Fernández-Rivas eta l. 2009) found that after six months of sublingual SOTI therapy that peach allergy patients were able to tolerate from three to nine times the amount of peach they could tolerate before the trial.

Immunotherapy research has finally reached the Americas, with similar success:

Duke University Medical Center researchers (Hofmann *et al.* 2009) tested SOTI oral tolerance immunotherapy among 28 patients with peanut allergies. They guided and observed as patients gradually increased doses daily, and recorded symptoms after each dose increase. Twenty of the 28 allergy patients (71%) completed the study – becoming tolerant. In the beginning, 79% experienced mild upper respiratory tract symptoms, and 68% experienced abdominal symptoms.

The initial escalation day resulted in the mild wheezing of 18% of the subjects. Mild symptoms on successive days fell to 46%, and only 3.5% had significant reactions during home dosing. Only 1.2% had upper respiratory tract symptoms and 1.1% had skin symptoms. *"Allergic reactions with home doses were rare,"* commented the researchers.

Cambridge University medical researchers (Clark *et al.* 2009) studied SOTI oral immunotherapy in four children allergic to peanuts. Peanut flour doses were increased from five mg to 800 mg of peanut protein using twice-weekly increases in doses. After six weeks, peanut dose maximum thresholds went from 1/40th to 1/4th of one peanut (5-50 mg) to at least 10 peanuts (approximately 2,380 mg) during challenges after the oral immunotherapy was completed. This translated to 48-times, 49-times, 55-times and 478-times the amount of peanuts tolerated by the four children than before the treatment.

Johns Hopkins University School of Medicine researchers (Skripak *et al.* 2008) tested 20 children (between the ages of six and 17 years old) who were allergic to milk with SOTI oral tolerance immunotherapy or placebo. They dosed using three phases: a build-up day with an initial dose of 0.4 mg of milk protein; gradually increased daily doses to 50 mg; which then continued daily but with eight weekly increases to a maximum of 500 mg per day. This dose was then continued daily for three to four months. Of the 12 patients who completed the SOTI treatment (12 of the milk dosing group completed along with seven in the placebo group):

The SOTI group went from a baseline of 40 mg of milk tolerance in the beginning of the treatment to a whopping 5,140 mg average (the range was 2,540 mg to 8,140 mg), while the placebo group remained at an average of 40 mg sensitivity. Their conclusion: *"Milk OIT appears to be efficacious in the treatment of cow's milk allergy."*

In earlier North American studies, researchers from Johns Hopkins University School of Medicine (Fleischer *et al.* 2004) evaluated 68 peanut allergy patients during a food elimination program followed by a gradual SOTI oral tolerance program.

Out of the 68, 47 became tolerant to peanuts. After becoming tolerant, 23 of the 47 stayed in the study and continued consuming concentrated peanut foods at least once per month, and another 15 stayed in and ate peanuts infrequently. After some time, only three of 15 among the infrequent peanut consumers suffered peanut allergy rebounds. Of the 23 patients who remained in the study and ate peanuts at least monthly, none had a rebound of allergy.

University of Colorado Health Sciences Center researchers (Leung *et al.* 2004) gave 84 peanut allergy sufferers placebo or different doses of peanut subcutaneously once every four weeks for sixteen weeks. After the protocol, the tolerance levels among the peanut 'vaccine' group went from a low of 178 mg to 2,627 mg for the highest peanut 'vaccine' dose, compared to 710 in the placebo group. This translates to an increase in tolerance from about ½ a peanut (178 mg) to nearly nine peanuts (2,805 mg).

New strategies in immunotherapy have been gaining increasing attention in research over the past few years. These include *homologous protein immunotherapy*, which utilizes a homologous (or similar) protein to produce tolerance of a particular food. For example, soybeans have been used to increase tolerance to peanuts. Other targeted anti-IgE therapy strategies include *altered peptide immunotherapy* (Scurlock and Jones 2010).

Oral food challenge testing does sometimes result in a severe reaction and even the need to use epinephrine to quell the response. Researchers from New York's Mount Sinai School of Medicine (Järvinen *et al.* 2009) reviewed food challenges in New York between 1999 and 2007. They found that 34% involved reactions, 4% of which required epinephrine. This is a good reason for those with severe allergies to conduct SOTI under physician supervision.

Just because there are reactions does not mean SOTI treatment is not efficacious. Remember that the treatment alleviates *future* severe reactions. It can save many from future anaphylaxis and even death.

Researchers from the Mount Sinai School of Medicine (Nowak-Wegrzyn and Fiocchi 2010) reviewed the research on SOTI and concluded that tolerance is achieved in approximately 50-75% of children treated (although we can see that the European research reached levels closer to 85%-90%). They concluded that:

> *"Side effects are common both during the initial dose escalation and during home dosing. Most reactions are mild (oral pruritus, abdomi-*

nal discomfort, and rashes) and decrease in frequency with the longer duration of OIT. Severe reactions treated with epinephrine have been reported during home dosing. Factors associated with increased risk of reactions to previously tolerated doses during home dosing include exercise, viral infection, dosing on empty stomach, menses, and asthma exacerbation."

Even if a course of immunotherapy is not completely successful initially, immunotherapy also offers other benefits. According to much of the research, immunotherapy seems to substantially strengthen the immune system in general (Kamdar and Bryce 2010).

We should note that most of the research on oral tolerance immunotherapy was conducted without changes to strengthen the immune system as we are suggesting. As we introduced throughout this chapter, there are a number of strategies that can strengthen the immune system's tolerance, including dietary changes and specific herbs. This strategy will decrease the burden on our immune system as well as increase our immune system strength.

This translates to renewed tolerance – also referred to as *adaptogenic.*

Applying SOTI to Gluten Sensitivities

Applying SOTI means introducing a very small amount of the offending food into the diet.

Depending upon the severity of the allergy or intolerance, the amount of food introduced should be very minute – such as one small cooked wheat berry or small amount of cooked whole wheat bread or flour.

It is important that the wheat is cooked – as this will deactivate any active WGA lectins and any phytates in the wheat.

It is important that the gluten food be a whole wheat product, not a refined flour product. It is also recommended that if it is a bread or muffin, that the bread is made from healthy ingredients, and not loaded with refined sugars and aluminum.

It is also advisable to utilize a food or supplement program to supply those probiotics that produce the enzymes to break down gliadin proteins. Such a probiotic food or supplement can be consumed with or prior to the consumption of the gluten food for best results.

The amount of probiotics will largely depend upon the species and format, but at least a few billion CFUs is typically recommended. See previous discussion on probiotic supplementation and don't be shy in terms of contacting your health professional for advice.

When to Implement SOTI

The sections described in this chapter before this SOTI section should be applied to prepare the physiology for a maximum tolerant response to SOTI. This should obviously include the elimination of gluten-containing foods for that period.

To make this protocol described in this chapter easy to refer back to, let's call it the *Adams Gluten Protocol.*

Once the immune system is stronger, the intestinal tract is better equipped, healthy probiotic colonies are established, our mucosal membranes are healthier and the body's inflammation response is balanced; our body's ability to break down the macromolecules in our foods and tolerate sensitive food macromolecules will grow.

This occurs because not only can the digestive tract handle and break down our foods better when it is in better shape, but the immune system can *modulate* its response when it is less burdened by other challenges. When the immune system is balanced and stabilized, it is less likely to respond with hypersensitivity.

We might compare this to physical fitness. When we go to a gym and lift weights for awhile, our body will naturally become stronger and better able to lift heavier weights. This increased strength will also allow the body to avoid injury as well. This is because the human physiology is highly adaptable – but only when it is healthy.

This doesn't mean that everything will change within a few weeks. But if the environment is changing, as our intestinal cells turnover, the new cells will quickly learn to accommodate that new environment – making them stronger and better protected from being damaged by unhydrolyzed proteins.

Depending upon the person, this process can take from 60 days to a year to accomplish – *during which it is best to eliminate the offending foods from the diet to the degree possible.*

In this case, it means employing a gluten-free diet for a period of time while implementing the other strategies.

For anyone with a severe wheat allergy or celiac disease, the introduction of these strategies should accompany the supervision of a health professional experienced in these conditions.

The Healthy Gluten Diet

For a gluten-sensitive person, this section should follow a gluten elimination phase, during which time ones immune system is strengthened and the intestinal health is established, and an oral immunotherapy routine is undertaken to the point where the person can eat a reasonable amount of gluten food at a sitting – such as a slice of bread.

In other words, this section discusses strategies related not only to reincorporating healthy gluten foods back into the diet. It also spells out a long-term approach to eating these foods.

Why is this important? Firstly, we do not want to repeat those mistakes that produced our gluten sensitivity in the first place. And we don't want to eat those foods that can cause or exacerbate those symptoms that are rightly or wrongly being attributed to gluten.

This means, first, converting our diet to organic foods. Yes, there can be some exceptions. But for the most part, the foods we eat should all be grown organically, which means they will not contain glyphosates or any other herbicide or pesticide residue that might interfere with our probiotic populations.

Know Your Wheat Food

As mentioned in the second chapter, part of the misunderstanding about gluten intolerance comes from the fact that much of the grain we are consuming in the Western diet is refined and lacks the essential nutrients, fibers and phytochemistry our bodies need to remain healthy.

To this we can add the issue of how conventional (non-organic) commercial wheat is grown. Today's conventional farmer begins by turning over the rich layers of soil to expose its nutrients and denitrifying bacteria to the sun. Chemical fertilizers are then spread over the soil.

Many conventional wheat berry seeds are treated with fungicides for bunt, smut and other potential diseases. Then chemical pesticides are sprayed on and around the crop as it sprouts and grows.

While we differentiated between the development of Clearfield wheat and genetic modification earlier, soaking to-be-planted-for-food seeds in chemicals and then spraying chemicals on and around the wheat fields is not a healthy recipe – producing the potential of bioaccumulation of those chemicals by the plant itself, possibly moving to the wheat berry.

For this reason, organic wheat products are suggested. Organic growers will utilize seeds that have not been treated chemically. They will also utilize natural fertilizers. They will also better rotate and care for their soils, rendering a healthier food with more nutrients (yes, proven – but not enough room here to elaborate). Most importantly, organic growers will also not spray chemical herbicides or pesticides onto and around their crops.

This doesn't mean that all conventionally-grown grain is toxic or poisoned with chemicals. The wheat berry does not bioaccumulate chemical toxins that well due to the protective nature of the bran and its antioxidants. Plus many sprayings are done well before the crop begins to mature, and often well outside the planting area. But at the very least, organic is better for the planet and the health of the farm workers.

Much of today's grain foods are made with white flour. To make white flour, the bran and germ are separated from the endosperm using large steel rollers. This creates flour that is rich in gluten yet lacking many of the nutrients and healthy components discussed in this chapter.

Depending upon the mill, the germ and bran are typically sold for animal feed. Sometimes it is just spread out onto a dormant field.

This is a waste, because the bran and at least part of the germ can be blended back into the flour to make whole-wheat flour or close to it in the form of brown flour.

Or the wheat can be ground whole to produce a single whole wheat component flour. Sometimes this is referred to as *stone ground* but this labeling can also be deceptive.

Ancient peoples used two large stones to grind flour. This is where the term originates. Human ingenuity resulted in the gristmill, a stone-grinding apparatus developed to grind larger quantities at once. In both of these techniques, there was no separation of the bran and germ from the endosperm. Flour was ground-up wheat berries, and that's what our ancestors baked and thrived from for thousands of years.

Today, after the commercial white flour has been ground, it is sent off to a bakery. Today's industrialized bakeries are set up with automated baking and mixing equipment. The flour is dumped into large vats where it is typically mixed with water, often blended with a variety of dough softeners and additives, followed by either dried yeast or baking powder and often sugar, refined salt and other chemicals as preservatives and flavor enhancers.

The result: white bread, donuts, coffee cakes and so on.

These provide the cornerstone of much of the calories of the Western diet. And these sugary refined foods fuel our taste buds along with our significant obesity rates. In the U.S., for example, over 60% of the population is overweight and more than a third is obese. So much for the romantic wheat berry.

Most of us know when we strip the bran and the germ off the berry, we end up with a product that has little or no fiber. Do we realize that the bran and germ also contain much of wheat's many valuable nutrients? We discussed some of the incredible nutrient qualities of whole wheat earlier. Do we realize this nutrient content is primarily within the bran and the germ?

As discussed earlier, whole grains also have micronutrients and phytochemicals critical to our health. Grains contain a host of phytosterols, lignans, fatty acids, arabinoxylans, and alkylresorcinols in addition to thiamin, riboflavin, niacin, vitamin E, potassium, iron, magnesium, zinc, selenium, copper, chromium, manganese, molybdenum, selenium and iodine, among others.

Meanwhile, our white breads and coffee cakes are so depleted of these nutrients that federal law now requires they are enriched with some synthetic B vitamins and iron to give them some semblance of food.

And yes, eating these types of gluten-containing overly-processed foods can certainly produce inflammatory conditions. This has been shown in the research. These overly-processed foods have been robbed of the balance of nutrients delivered by whole grain. They are foods gone awry. They are fake grain foods – junk foods in disguise.

But let's not throw out the baby with the bath water.

As we'll describe below, there is a better way to consume wheat foods, and this produces health – not robs the body of metabolic health.

Raw or Cooked?

While raw whole foods are often more wholesome to the body, some foods must be cooked to make them digestible. This is the case for gluten-containing foods, as well as beans, rice and many others.

In most of these cases, phytates and other elements such as wheat germ agglutinins – which can impede the absorption of nutrients – are neutralized and minimized.

In some cases, baking or cooking a food that causes an allergic reaction can reduce its allergenicity. This is not true for all allergens, but certain allergens are broken down or hydrolyzed into molecules the body is not sensitive to. This may be more likely for food intolerances, but is dependent upon the specific sensitivity.

For example, German researchers (Worm *et al.* 2009) found that heat-treating and processing of hazelnuts reduces their allergenicity among hazelnut allergic people.

It can also depend upon the person and their tolerance as well. Researchers at Switzerland's University Hospital (Ballmer-Weber *et al.* 2002) gave patients with celery allergies raw celery, cooked celery (at 110 degrees for 15 minutes) and celery spice. Six out of 11 patients tested were sensitive to the minimally cooked celery. Five of five patients were sensitive to celery spice. The researchers also tried extended cooking of celery to see if that would change its sensitivity. In most cases, it didn't.

In the case of gluten-containing foods, this is absolutely applicable. As we discussed in the second chapter, both phytates and WGA are neutralized by cooking and storage, and whatever minimal amounts remaining are neutralized by our probiotics. Cooking also softens fibers and hydrolyzes some other proteins and macromolecules present in these foods.

Still, because our enzyme and probiotic metabolisms are each unique, and these will determine our level of sensitivity, cooking times for different foods might have to be adjusted. As we become more tolerant to foods previously sensitive to, we can test whether we are more tolerant to their cooked or raw versions. This can be tested using the protocols and safety nets discussed earlier. Once a level of tolerance is determined, the food can be slowly and gradually added back to the diet in the form the body is more tolerant to.

But in the case of gluten-containing grains, these foods are always better cooked because phytates and wheat germ agglutinin (WGA) are both broken down and neutralized by heat as mentioned.

What is more important to consider is how much cooking and processing we need to do. How much cooking is necessary? Yes, cooking some foods often increases their digestibility. This is particularly important with grain-based foods and beans. Cooking these foods will help break down their fibers and complex carbohydrates into more digestible forms.

Also, many vegetables are better cooked, or even better, steamed. Steaming vegetables with a covered pot will preserve more nutrients, while softening some of fibers that hold nutrients. Foods such as beets, asparagus, broccoli, rhubarb, squash and many others are delicious and nutritious after being steamed or lightly boiled in clean water.

Other plant foods are best eaten raw. These include lettuce, cucumbers, avocado and many others. Because the nutrients in these foods are not so tightly bound within the cell walls of the plants, they can be destroyed by the heat and/or easily separated from the food during cooking.

A healthy diet strikes a balance between raw and cooked foods. A perfect way to accomplish this at dinner time is with a salad that includes seeds; cooked grains and/or beans; and a nice sauce.

Breakfast and lunch can include lightly toasted sourdough whole/cracked wheat bread, fresh fruit; nuts; and fermented dairy with slightly cooked grains such as oats and barley.

Snacks can go raw or otherwise. Raw, boiled or lightly roasted nuts and seeds also make especially healthy and slow-digesting snacks with essential fatty acid content.

Dinners can include cooked grains and sourdough breads, and steamed or raw vegetables.

Choosing Gluten-based Foods

When it choosing wheat-based foods, the only ones to eat raw would be wheat grass. Anything that uses wheat berries, which includes wheat flour, should be well **baked** or otherwise **cooked.**

Again, this is because baking and cooking neutralizes phytates and WGA, along with some of the macromolecule count. Cooking reinforces and supports protein hydrolysis.

In other words, it is **not** recommended to eat wheat germ, wheat berries or wheat flour **raw.**

This is actually quite easy, because practically every food with wheat has been cooked. Flour is somewhat raw (typically heated), but flour is also typically cooked into breads, muffins, pancakes and so on. Even wheat germ is typically toasted. If the wheat germ is not toasted, then it should be toasted prior to eating it. Or put into a product to be baked.

Toasting bread or otherwise making sure that the bread is **thoroughly cooked** is a good idea as well. This extra bake or toasting will help to deactivate any remaining lectins (such as AWGs) and will help to hydrolyze some of the gluten proteins or prepare them for hydrolyzation within the intestinal tract. See toasting section below.

Using **organic wheat** and other organic ingredients is also recommended as mentioned above. By using organic wheat we will avoid glyphosate and any other chemical residues that may have been bioaccumulated within the grain, not to mention supporting the planet's health and the health of farm workers.

Using organic wheat will also mean the seeds to plant the grain are better seeds, and often organic wheat growers will use **heritage seeds** that have bypassed any chemical hybridization.

A grain-based product should also be **primarily whole wheat.** At least 50% if not 100%. Bakery breads labeled WHOLE WHEAT are usually made with 50% whole wheat flour and 50% white (ENRICHED) flour.

But if the product just says MADE WITH WHOLE WHEAT then the label should be checked more closely. If the label has ENRICHED FLOUR before the WHOLE WHEAT FLOUR, then a product with 100% whole wheat or the ENRICHED after the WHOLE WHEAT FLOUR on the label is preferable.

Sprouted grain breads and **sourdough breads** are significantly better than typical white bread or even commercial (50/50) whole wheat bread. This is both from a glycemic perspective and the proportional content of glutens compared to bran and germ.

Some bakery products use flour with the wheat germ or bran added back, and some add the germ and/or bran back in the kitchen. This is still good – and should be considered as practically whole wheat depending upon the amount of bran and germ added back. The is because the wheat germ and the bran are rendering the necessary product fiber – bran more than the wheat germ.

Thus it is best to choose only whole wheat cereals, pancakes and muffins.

However, we can also add bran and toasted/cooked germ to these to compensate for less whole wheat. Flax seeds and other fibrous ingredients can also help compensate for the lack of fiber. But in order to feed those probiotics that secrete enzymes that break down gliadins and glutenins, it is best to eat whole wheat with the bran.

Also, **refined sugars** should be avoided with wheat foods to the extent possible. This is because the sugars will fuel pathogenic probiotics, which will crowd out those probiotics that produce the enzymes that break down the gliadin – and protect our intestinal walls.

And depending upon the food, refined sugar added to grains can also result in glycation end products, which can harm the intestinal walls.

Refined sugar in general should be avoided. But given the amount of refined sugars in our food supply, it is best to just minimize them as much as possible, and make sure that there is plenty of (prebiotic) plant fiber included in meals that include refined sugar.

Other ingredients to avoid, especially for children:

- Ammonium chloride
- Ammonium sulfate
- Artificial food colors
- Azodicarbonamide
- Calcium disodium EDTA
- Calcium propionate (or Calcium propanoate)
- Calcium sorbate
- High fructose corn syrup (or corn syrup)
- Hydrogenated soybean oil (partially or not)
- Modified food starch
- Monocalcium phosphate
- Potassium sorbate
- Propylene glycol
- Sodium acid pyrophosphate
- Sodium aluminum phosphate
- Sodium benzoate
- Sodium bisulfite
- Sorbic acid
- Sorbitan thisterate
- Titanium dioxide

Which breads are best?

If there is a choice between sourdough bread and whole wheat bread, pick the sourdough bread. And if there is a choice between regular whole wheat bread and sprouted wheat bread, go with the sprouted wheat bread.

A study from Canada's University of Guelph (Mofidi *et al.* 2012) studied 23 overweight and obese men in two studies of various types of breads, including whole-grain bread with sourdough and sprouted grain bread made with sourdough yeast starter. The researchers took blood panels of the test subjects and found those eating the sprouted-grain breads had significantly lower blood glucose levels than those eating the whole-grain breads.

They also found the insulin sensitivity was greater after eating sprouted grain breads and multi-whole grain breads compared to sourdough white breads.

In another study, University of Guelph researchers (Najjar *et al.* 2009) tested ten overweight adult volunteers. They gave them 50 grams of four breads on four occasions, following by blood testing. They gave the volunteers white bread, whole wheat bread, sourdough bread or whole wheat barley bread each meal, and three hours later each subject ate a standard second meal. Blood tests were taken for three hours after the eating the bread and then two more hours after the second meal.

The researchers found that glucose and glucagon-like peptide-1 (GLP-1) levels were lower in the subjects after eating the sourdough bread. The area under the curve for glucose was also lower throughout the study testing for the sourdough bread eaters compared to all the other breads.

They also found that ultra-fine grind whole wheat breads did not reduce glucose levels compared to white bread.

Probably one of the best strategies for eating practically any gluten-based food that we can apply from the myriad of research documented in this book is eating **yogurt** or **kefir** alongside a meal that contains gluten.

This is actually an ancient Ayurvedic principle. For thousands of years, Vedic peoples have included yogurt with every meal. The use of yogurt with the meal contributes two important factors to our gut and the digestion of the meal:

- ✓ Probiotic colonies excrete numerous enzymes that digest glutens and other food proteins.
- ✓ Prebiotics such as GOS feed the probiotics in our gut.

With regard to prebiotics, GOS from the dairy will combine with the arabinoxylans from the whole wheat to provide a mix of food for those critical probiotics within our guts.

Making Bread for Gluten Sensitivity

Research has illustrated that **probiotic sourdough breads,** in fact, can be eaten by most celiac patients. In a study from Italy's University of Bari (Di Cagno *et al.* 2004) 17 celiac patients were tested with baker's yeast or a sourdough bread made with a lactobacilli sourdough starter formula. The researchers found that all 17 of the celiac patients tolerated the bread with no allergic reaction. A number of other studies as we pointed out earlier has confirmed this.

Here is the formula for the bread used by Di Cagno and associates:

The sourdough mix contained four species:

- *Lactobacillus alimentarius*
- *L. brevis*
- *L. sanfranciscensis*
- *L. hilgardii*
- 5% bakers yeast

The following flours were blended:

- 3 parts wheat flour
- 1 part oat flour
- 1 part millet flour
- 4 parts buckwheat flour

The dough was incubated at 37 degrees Celsius with the yeast mixture. Maltose was added as a sweetener.

Here is a wonderful recipe for 100% sprouted wheat bread contributed by Kenneth Buzbee:

> *"I use two 16oz bags of Einkorn wheat berries. I sprout the first bag for two days. Pop the sprouted berries in the food processor for 30 seconds. Add it to the sourdough starter and start sprouting the second bag. Two days later I process that with a teaspoon of Himalayan salt. Separate out the starter from the first batch for the next loaf and mix the two together. Put it in a covered cast iron Dutch oven while the oven preheats. Bake at 500 degrees for 15 minutes then 350 degrees for 40 minutes. Remove it from the oven and let it cool in the oven.*
> *It takes days to make but it's all time waiting. There's no work involved. The grain and the starter do all the heavy lifting. I just sit back and let them do what they want to do naturally."*

It should be noted that dough can be fermented (risen) for much longer than typical recipes call for. This can be extended to a day or even 2-3 days, especially when probiotics are added to the dough. This of course should be tested first, depending upon the recipe and flour content.

Adding probiotics to the dough mix with the yeast can easily be done in the home with any bread recipe. Simply add a commercial probiotic supplement or a good probiotic yogurt or kefir. Here is a list of species shown in research to produce gluten-hydrolyzing enzymes:

- ✓ *Bifidobacterium infantis*
- ✓ *B. lactis*
- ✓ *Lactobacillus brevis*
- ✓ *L. alimentarius*
- ✓ *L. sanfranciscensis*
- ✓ *L. hilgardii*
- ✓ *L. casei*
- ✓ *L. plantarum*

This said, other research has shown that numerous lactobacilli strains will produce gliadin-digesting enzymes. So a yogurt or kefir with good cultures of these can provide, at the very least, assistance to those enzyme-producing probiotics within our gut and/or sourdough starter.

Baking Powder

As mentioned above, when it comes to baking breads, rolls or any other gluten-based foods, it's best to use at least 50% if not more whole wheat flour and then use yeast or better, a sourdough mix rather than baking powder – which can contain aluminum or similar metals.

This isn't to say that baking powder is necessarily bad. It really depends upon the ingredients. Most baking powders contain sodium bicarbonate also called baking soda. Then they will contain some sort of acid salt. This is where the problem occurs.

Some brands will blend the bicarbonate with sodium aluminum sulfate – at up to and even more than a quarter (25%) of the total ingredients. This means a tablespoon of baking powder will contain a quarter tablespoon of an aluminum salt. Aluminum has been linked with nerve and brain cell issues. At minimum, aluminum will distort our body's mineral balance. Ironically, it may also produce some of the symptoms attributed to gluten sensitivity, such as bloating and fatigue.

In addition to the aluminum salt, commercial baking powders – especially double-acting versions – may contain calcium acid phosphate – monocalcium phosphate. This does not present the toxicity of sodium aluminum sulfate.

Aluminum-free baking sodas are readily available today. These will utilize monocalcium phosphate in total instead of any aluminum sulfate.

A natural baking powder can be easily made by blending baking soda with cream of tartar and cornstarch. In fact, baking soda alone – together with some yogurt for its acid content – will fulfill many baking needs that don't require a huge rising action.

While cooking alone will break down and neutralize phytates, WGA and gliadin macromolecules, yeast and sourdough are better because the yeast produce enzymes that break these down during the rising of the dough.

Baker's yeast is also a digestive aid. And a good baker's yeast is also a source of B vitamins and other nutrients.

Cooking Pasta and Other Wheat Foods

There are several considerations when cooking gluten-containing foods such as pasta, couscous, bulgur and others. Cooking these foods in boiling water has several positive functions:

- ✓ It reduces phytate content: Following milling, heating during packaging, boiling a pasta should remove any remaining phytates. (Most pastas are heated during durum flour production and dried at fairly high temperatures during the process of making the pasta, eliminating most.) Whatever might be left will be decimated by healthy probiotic bacteria.
- ✓ It reduces trypsin-inhibitor content: Same as phytates
- ✓ It softens and even hydrolyzes some proteins: While water alone doesn't have proteases that will completely break down proteins, some hydrolysis in the presence of whole salt can take place with heat for some proteins, preparing for their further break down in the gut. In many cases, proteins encapsulate starches. For these mixed molecules, hydrolysis can break apart the protein-encapsulated molecules, allowing each to be better broken down during digestion.
- ✓ It makes starches more digestible: Boiling pasta will also soften many polysaccharide chains and convert them into smaller chains.

This last point might also backfire if the pasta is cooked too much. If the pasta is allowed to cook and soften too much, too many of the polysaccharides can turn into simpler starches, which can digest faster. This can produce a situation that is similar to eating white flour – increased glycemic response.

The best way to avoid this is to first utilize whole wheat pasta whenever available. Whole wheat pasta will contain more fiber and a balance of polysaccharides, some of which will be more resistant to breaking down into simple chains. These will slow the total assimilation of starches in the gut.

Whole wheat pasta also contains more phytonutrients. As we discussed earlier with regard to glycemic response, foods containing more nutrients will naturally be assimilated slower than foods that contain less nutrients. This is why, for example, raw honey and maple syrup will not cause the same glycemic response as white sugar or high-fructose corn syrup.

The other strategy with pasta and other boiled wheat foods is to find that mid-point between *al dente* and soft. In the author's opinion, *al dente* leaves proteins and starches that are not adequately softened during cooking. It is better to take the pasta just beyond *al dente* – just to the point where the pasta is softened throughout and not much further.

This can be determined simply with a fork. Instead of bothering with throwing the pasta up against the wall – a ridiculous proposal anyway: Simply pick up a little pasta in a cooking spoon and put a fork into one of the thicker pieces. If the fork cuts through the pasta with little resistance, it is ready. If the fork meets any resistance as it is pushed through, it isn't quite ready.

This can also be done with couscous as well, but will be more easily accomplished by pressing a few couscous grains between the finger and thumb. If the couscous mashes flat easily, it is ready. If it is still grainy, it is not ready.

Cooking bulgur and cracked or even complete wheat berries should be the same. It should be squishable-flat between the fingers.

Cooking bulgur or cracked wheat berries is probably easier and safer than whole wheat berries anyway. The water better penetrates the germ and helps hydrolyze or neutralize any remaining lectins.

Toast, eh?

Another consideration, at least at home, is to toast bread before eating it. We discussed this briefly earlier, but let's dig in a little more. Toasting bread, muffins or rolls will further neutralize any remaining lectins, phytates or trypsin-inhibitors not otherwise removed during dough fermentation or baking. This will help prepare the proteins for degradation in the gut.

While the author knows of no specific research testing toast and comparing it to non-toasted bread with respect to gluten sensitivity, there was an interesting study quoted in the enzyme section from Amsterdam's VU University Medical Center (Tack *et al.* 2013). The study tested 14 celiac patients who ate toast with 7 grams of gluten content each day. Half the patients took a prolyl endoprotease enzyme supplement while the other half took a placebo.

The interesting thing about this study is that both groups – even the celiac group taking the placebo – had few allergic symptoms during the two weeks eating the gluten-wheat toast. There were a few symptoms reported, but these were closely reported by two groups. By the researchers own observations, these were not significant.

The researchers said:

> *"During the efficacy phase, neither the placebo nor the AN-PEP [enzyme] group developed significant antibody titers. The IgA-EM concentrations remained negative in both groups."*

In their discussion, they also stated:

> *" the placebo arm did not show any deterioration after 2 weeks of gluten consumption."*

This result was certainly surprising to the researchers, who were convinced the celiac placebo group would react – at least immunologically – to eating seven grams of gluten per day. The author proposes that the extra cooking of the toast helped denature some of the gliadin proteins, rendering them less allergic.

A study confirming this possibility investigated the heating temperatures of pasta (De Zorzi *et al.* 2006) and tested them for digestion. The drying of the pasta at increased temperatures (up to 110 Celsius or 280 degrees F) denatured many of the gluten proteins. This denaturing of the proteins using heat allowed pepsin and pancreatin enzymes to completely break down the gluten proteins:

> *"… resulting in the disappearance of the main prolamin components."*

Because pepsin and pancreatin are produced by the gut in practically everyone, the research is encouraging. However, it doesn't necessarily mean toasting will remove all of the allergenicity of the gluten proteins for a celiac sufferer. Some allergenicity may certainly remain in smaller peptide forms, which, if not broken down further in the gut could produce a reaction. The above study confirmed this reality, as some IgE allergenicity still remained.

But toasting should render these proteins easier to break down in general, especially for a gluten intolerant person or a person who is supplementing with probiotics or otherwise going through the process of becoming more tolerant to gluten foods.

This would especially be the case with a sourdough bread where the sourdough yeasts and bacteria has already broken down the gluten to a large extent.

This doesn't mean we should burn our toast, however. Burning produces acrylamides, which are not that good for us. Acrylamides are known to contribute to cancer risk, especially the amounts produced during open flame roasting and frying.

In other words, potato chips or French fries are the worst according to research (Ahn *et al.* 2010). Other research (Jackson *et al.* 2005) has found that lightly-toasted (8 to 217 micrograms per kilogram) or even medium-toasted bread (10 to 214 micrograms per kilogram) has nearly a third of the acrylamide content than a dark toasted slice of bread (43 to 610 micrograms per kilogram).

This latter study indicates that French fries can have nearly ten times the acrylamide content (up to 2130 micrograms per kilogram).

Certainly acrylamides are not exclusive to gluten-containing foods, as the French fry example illustrates. The point is to keep our baking, frying and toasting of any food to minimized temperatures to avoid burning or darkening.

And the best way to seriously drop our acrylamide consumption is to curtail fried foods.

Ranking Some Wheat Foods

Below is a humble attempt to rank popular healthy wheat foods. The criteria for this ranking include ingredients, prebiotic content, glycemic index/load and others; ranked from best to the less acceptable. This is a rough gauge, not an absolute. And it is certainly not a complete list of wheat foods.

In fact, few of the grain foods on this list are particularly unhealthy. This is listing more healthy versus less healthy. White bread in itself is not unhealthy, assuming the bread doesn't have a bunch of other crap in it like high-fructose corn syrup and so on. Even white bread will contain protein, vitamins and minerals – even if much of the nutrient content was separated out with the bran and germ with some replaced with synthetic versions. But for the many reasons we've explained in this text, plain white bread is not as healthy as a sourdough whole wheat bread for example.

The exception here is the very bottom of the list, including cakes, cookies and donuts. Most of these are made with white cake flour – which has been finely ground and often supplemented with emulsifiers and dough conditions – along with sugar and aluminum baking soda, which makes them unhealthy choices. Cake flour will have less gluten, but also significantly less protein as a result. Cake flour also lacks bran and germ.

Donuts are also often made with cake flour. But they are also fried – making them likely one of the unhealthiest wheat foods.

This said, both cookies and cake can be made using whole wheat and even healthy sweeteners such as honey or maple syrup. These weren't listed because they are atypical (just as buckwheat pancakes are) but they can often be found at a healthy restaurant or health food store.

Donuts – even if they were made with whole wheat flour and a healthy sweetener – would still probably be at the bottom of the list because they are fried.

Note also that organic versions of these foods are recommended when available; understanding that sometimes organic isn't available – for example when traveling. The first "organic" on the list was added to illustrate this recommendation with the ultimate best form of wheat food. Also note unsweetened versions are assumed, and brands are avoided unless the product name is ubiquitous:

Wheat food ranking:

1) **Organic** cracked whole wheat sourdough bread made with probiotics
2) Wholemeal sourdough rye bread
3) Whole wheat sourdough bread
4) Whole wheat sourdough pizza
5) Whole wheat sourdough rolls
6) White sourdough bread, pizza, rolls
7) Pearled barley cooked
8) Whole kernel wheat cooked
9) Whole kernel rye cooked
10) Whole kernel durum wheat cooked

11) Whole durum wheat pasta
12) White durum wheat pasta
13) Barley kernel bread
14) Rye kernel (pumpernickel) bread
15) Wholegrain pumpernickel bread
16) Wholemeal rye bread
17) Bulgur cooked
18) Course wheat kernel bread
19) Sprouted whole wheat bread
20) Cracked whole wheat bread
21) Whole wheat pasta (spaghetti, linguine, capellini, macaroni, etc.)
22) Seven grain whole grain bread
23) Mixed grain bread
24) Traditional whole grain bread
25) Stone ground whole wheat bread
26) Whole wheat chapatti
27) Whole wheat flatbread
28) Whole wheat pita bread
29) Whole wheat roti
30) Whole wheat cous cous
31) Whole wheat porridge
32) Wholemeal Kurdish bread
33) High-fiber rye crisps
34) Stoned wheat crackers
35) Whole wheat pita chips
36) White cous cous
37) Whole wheat crisps
38) High-Bran Weetabix®
39) All-bran cereal
40) Mixed grain porridge
41) Whole meal barley cereal
42) Rye crisps
43) Muesli
44) Triscuit® wheat crackers
45) Wheetabix®
46) Shredded wheat®
47) Pasta (spaghetti, linguine, capellini, macaroni, etc.)
48) Whole wheat bagels
49) Whole wheat baguettes
50) Puffed wheat cereal
51) Roasted semolina
52) White bread
53) White bread stuffing
54) White bread bagels
55) White bread baguettes
56) White flour pancakes, muffins, rolls
57) White or cake flour cookies
58) White cake flour cakes
59) Angel food cake
60) White donuts

This list is not perfect, but it gives an idea of some of the healthier and unhealthier options for gluten-containing foods. As to the precise ranking of one food over the other there is certainly room to go either way, but this should help give a general idea.

The reason why bagels and baguettes rank near the bottom (below white bread) is because of their glycemic index and load numbers – substantially higher glycemic loads.

The whole wheat sourdoughs were ranked on top due to – as we've proven in this text – the ability of sourdough starters to substantially break down gliadin proteins. Even white sourdough is ranked better than most whole wheat breads for this reason.

Wheat Grass

Wheat grass is the young grass of the wheat species, *Triticum aestivum*. This food contains a plethora of vitamins, minerals, amino acids, phytonutrients, metabolic enzymes – including superoxide dismutase and cytochrome oxidase.

Early research by Dr. Charles Schnabel, Dr. George Kohler and Dr. A.I. Virtanen in the 1925-1950 era found that cereal grasses like wheatgrass achieved their highest nutrient content at around 18 days – right before the first jointing.

Wheat grass can increase blood hemoglobin levels. Wheat grass tablets decreased blood transfusion needs by 25% among 20 children requiring frequent blood transfusions in a clinical study.

Barley grass maintains similar properties. Research has found that barley grass is a potent free radical scavenger; significantly reduces total cholesterol and LDL-cholesterol; and inhibits LDL oxidation. Barley grass juice powder can have 14 vitamins, 18 amino acids, 15 enzymes, 10 antioxidants, 18 minerals and 75 trace elements.

Another wheat grass is Kamut grass. The khorasan wheat has higher protein levels than most wheat varieties, and contains higher zinc, selenium and magnesium content. Selenium is known for stimulating glutathione activity as we've discussed.

Wheat grasses will contain up to 70% chlorophyll. Chlorophyll has been shown by laboratory and clinical studies to be antiseptic and bacteriostatic. In other words, chlorophyll kills or repels pathogenic bacteria, making it useful for various internal infections.

Chlorophyll has also been shown to increase hemoglobin levels in cases of anemia, especially in combination with supplemental iron. For this reason, because the grasses contain iron, they make great blood content builders. For this very reason, many athletes have found that eating cereal grasses gives them a competitive edge when it comes to endurance and speed.

Wheat grass, barley grass and Kamut grass have been used with success for various healing and detoxification purposes. Nutritionists and alternative health professionals have recommended cereal grasses to alkalize the body – increasing the blood's ability to detoxify while boosting the productivity of the immune system. The combination of chlorophyll and antioxidant nutrients makes it the perfect way to protect the body against the stresses of our toxic world.

Wheat grasses have been shown to reduce inflammation and have beneficial effects upon the cardiovascular system as well. As the inflammation cascade is central to many disorders, cereal grasses are a great way to help deter or reduce the incidences of autoimmunity, allergies, and heavy metal toxicity.

As mentioned earlier, wheat grass may contain some of peptides similar to gliadins and glutenins eventually found in the wheat berries – but the grass does not contain gliadin and glutenin proteins.

So why is wheat grass recommended for someone who is sensitive to gluten? Because by consuming generous amounts of young wheat grass in the form of raw wheat grass or powdered, dehydrated wheat grass, a gluten-sensitive body will learn the nutritional benefits of the wheat plant. This learning process – if done when the immune system is strong and the intestinal tract is healthy – can help the body to become tolerant to gluten proteins.

Chewing Gluten Foods

A couple of chapters back we discussed some of the bacteria that reside in our mouth will break down gliadin and glutenin proteins. Thus it is critical to masticate any meals containing gluten well. This means eating calmly and slowly, and chewing each bite well before swallowing it.

Heck, digesting our food well in general requires good mastication.

If our bodies didn't have such a narrow, long windy digestive tract, mastication wouldn't be so important. Most of us have seen how snakes can swallow a mouse whole. This is because their digestive tracts are radically different from ours – they are wide and short, with powerful enzymes.

A masticated food mass mixed with chyme – food and saliva mixed with enzymes and oral bacteria – is called a bolus. As the bolus reaches our stomach, it should be more fluid than solid. This allows it better exposure to the stomach's gastrin and pepsinogen – to begin breaking it down and preparing it for the rest of its digestive journey. It also helps whatever unhydrolyzed gliadin and glutenin proteins remain to be exposed to those gluten-hydrolyzing enzymes produced by healthy probiotic colonies in our small intestines.

The right bolus is accomplished by chewing intently until the food can slide down the esophagus without the necessity of fluids. The bolus should have the consistency of a smoothie.

The salivary glands aid this process by infusing amylase into the food. Amylase is a potent enzyme that breaks down complex carbohydrates and fibers into more simple carbohydrates.

This also means that if we are washing our food down with liquids, we are not masticating them enough.

We might say the mouth is the first stomach.

While we are chewing, we can calmly breathe. Breathing while eating calms the body and slows the rush to swallow. It also gives the body a good dose of oxygen – a necessary element to aid digestion. And by oxidizing the bloodstream, which in turn supplies energy via the gastric arteries to the fundus glands, the pyloric glands and the cardiac glands lying within the stomach are nourished.

These glands produce the various digestive juices such as pyloric acid, gastric acid, pepsin converted from pepsinogen, and other enzymes. Balancing these are various hormones secreted by the mucosal cells of the stomach. Hormones such as *gastrin, somatostatin, enteroglucagon* and *inhibitory peptide* (or GIP) all work to balance the acidic content of the stomach.

Without a balanced secretion of these hormones the stomach is faced with the prospect of peptic ulcers and GERD – commonly known as *acid reflux.* A good supply of oxygen also helps relax the vagus nerve, which is involved in the stimulation and release of the various stomach enzymes and hormones from the stomach's glands, the liver and the gall bladder.

Smaller Meals and Lower Stress

The digestive tract was designed for small, frequent meals. If we can imagine foraging around the forest, eating fruits, nuts, leaves and berries as we find them, and then having a periodic group or family meal, this would probably best describe how our digestive tracts work. Most of our diet research has supported this fact as well. People who eat 4-6 smaller meals a day tend to keep the weight off more easily. This is primarily because the carbohydrate and fat parts of our meals are more thoroughly assimilated and more efficiently used, as opposed to converted to fatty acid molecules and stored into adipose cells for later use.

On the other hand, should we breathlessly stuff our food down, not only will we lack the oxygen to feed these glands and cells, but our mental intensity resonates through the limbic system through the vagus nerve. This biochemical cascade stops the flow of digestive enzymes. This physiological response is rooted in the survival situation. If a tiger started running towards us while we were eating, our bodies would respond by halting all digestive activities and redirecting that blood flow and nervous energy towards our muscles, eyes and other regions in order to escape the tiger. This might cause a bit of ingestion but it might save our body.

Preventing our body from responding to our anxieties means we have to put our anxieties away while we're eating. This means relaxing and breathing while we're eating. We might also consider meditative thinking or engaging in relaxing and pleasing discussions with other members at the table. Laughing is also good for digestion.

We are not simply speaking of our own body's production of enzymes here. We are also speaking of those probiotic species that produce the enzymes that break down many of the proteins and complex carbohydrates we eat.

These bacteria also do not respond well to stress. In fact, research has found that probiotic bacteria are most engaged when we are sleeping. This indicates that when we are under stress, our probiotics slow down. When we are relaxed, their activity increases.

Thus it makes sense to not only masticate our foods thoroughly: We must also eat calmly, and relax after eating in order to allow our probiotics to adequately energize and produce the enzymes needed to break down the gliadins and glutenins in our meals.

The Natural Rotary Diet

Once gluten foods are added back to the diet using SOTI, rotating foods is a great way to prevent future sensitivities.

The *"Rotary Diversified Diet"* was first proposed by Dr. Herbter Rinkel in 1934. The diet was intended to prevent food sensitivities and work with foods that a person had become sensitive to.

Dr. Rinkel's diet used a system of rotational cycles where different foods and food groups were alternated in a very disciplined manner. The principle used is that if a particular food or food group is too frequently eaten, the body may become intolerant to it. While the research absolutely proving this is sparse, Dr. Rinkel and many other physicians of his day, past and present, have observed this among their patients.

This however, does utilize some of the elements used in SOTI therapy.

The rotary system recognizes that similar foods that either cross-react, or have similar protein types (such as wheat and barley), could also cause similar sensitivities. Thus food groups are also separated by rotations in the diet.

The conventional rotary diet calls for a food or similar food not to be eaten again within at least four to seven days. If it is eaten sooner, it could promote sensitivity, according to the theory.

If eaten any further out, however, it could also cause sensitivity due to the body no longer recognizing it. This later point has been confirmed in peanut allergy SOTI research, as discussed earlier. Foods must be eaten somewhat regularly to remain recognizable, in other words.

Dr. Rinkel's rotary diet also included slowly introducing foods that the body was previously sensitive to. He proposed these sensitive foods are gradually introduced into the cycle in small increments: like SOTI.

The rotary diet proposed by Dr. Rinkel and modified by others is quite difficult for most people to maintain because of the discipline required. Quite simply, most people have certain foods that are more available seasonally, and there are foods we simply like to eat more frequently than others.

Also we should add that the author is aware of no hard evidence that consistently eating a certain food – or within four or seven days – will result in a sensitivity to that food. On the contrary, we can look to the Asian continent and other regions where people eat the same foods multiple times a day without becoming sensitive to those foods.

Among billions of Chinese and Indian nationals, for example – who have had one of the lowest disease rates worldwide – every meal through the day is often similar. Every meal will often contain a rice and a bread.

These indigenous populations typically do not have enough wealth to rotate their diet daily, let alone by the meal. Seasonal rotation due to the availability of certain crops – yes. But even a seasonal food might still be eaten at every meal during and shortly after harvest.

Furthermore, among these traditional populations, food allergy rates have been some of the lowest in the world.

The research provided in this text reveals the benfits of such a strategy: Embracing those foods that are seasonal and local when available.

Eating primarily seasonal and mostly locally grown foods renders a natural dietary rotation. Staple foods can still be shipped in, but locally grown seasonal foods provide phytonutrients that fit our environment and ecosystem.

It is no coincidence that the body works better on slower-digesting foods such as grains and oils during the winter, and faster-digesting foods such as fruits and vegetables during the summer months.

This doesn't mean that we avoid fruits and vegetables during the winter, or avoid eating grains in the summer however. But it may mean that we are eating more grains and oils during the winter than we do during the summer.

And it is no coincidence there are more fruits and vegetables available locally during the summer. This indicates our biological history. Often it is too hot in the summer to eat a heavy meal, while lighter foods such as fruits, grains and vegetables digest more easily.

In the fall and cooler months, meals with more nuts, grains, squash, potatoes and legumes provide increased protein and healthy fats. This natural rotation with the seasons has been a part of the human diet for millions of years.

Genetically, our bodies and our digestive tracts have been tuned to seasonal eating. When we embrace those foods that grow around us seasonally we accommodate our metabolic rhythms, which also rotate with the seasons.

Inside of this seasonal rotation, we can also eat a varied diet that is naturally rotated. This will often suit our tastes and our body's nutritional needs as well. One dinner can feature root-oriented foods such as yams, sweet potatoes or potatoes, while the next dinner can feature grains. The next dinner can feature a nut-based, or a bean-based dish.

Other meals can be rotated in the same way. Breakfasts can rotate between a variety of combinations of grains, dairy, fruits and nuts. Beans, vegetables, nuts, dairy and fruits can be rotated at lunch: according to our dietary liking, the foods' local availability and seasonal availability.

The rotary diet concept is still useful for working in foods we have been sensitive to. We can slowly and gradually work in small amounts of a particular food as documented in the SOTI section. The first rotation might include an amount as small as a tiny speck of the food. Assuming little or no reaction, the amount would be gradually increased as documented in the research, depending upon our level of sensitivity and the supervision of our health professional.

After a period of consistent gradual increase, the food can be added to a weekly rotation of the food, and the quantity of the food could be increased weekly or monthly until achieving the desired (moderate) dose.

The exact protocol needs to be highly unique, depending upon the food, the level of sensitivity, and the goal. If the goal is to be able to eat the food regularly, then this process must continue with increasing doses. If the goal is to be able to tolerate a small amount of the food in the case of accidental ingestion, the same small amount can be consumed periodically to continue the tolerance.

Again, for anyone with a severe allergy response, this process should be supervised by a trained health professional.

Keeping Track: The Food Diary

The biggest pitfall in any food sensitivity is ignorance. Many studies on food sensitivities have illustrated a common issue: Many assume they are allergic or intolerant to a food without adequate confirmation.

Even with professional diagnosis a food diary is the key to confirmation.

It is one thing to have a negative reaction after eating. But pinpointing that food that produced the reaction can be extremely difficult.

The key is the food diary. A food diary simply allows for jotting down what foods are eaten at each meal and what (if any) responses followed. If there is any negative response later, that is also written into the food diary, along with the time and the severity. A sample diary format is given on the following page:

Food Diary

Meal Date/ Time	Foods Eaten	Reaction Time	Reaction Description	Reaction Severity (1-10)

Over some time, this diary should pinpoint those foods we might be sensitive to. The diary will also be an invaluable tool for any diagnostician to use as they investigate our sensitivity. The food diary will also help give us historical context, as we begin to adjust our diet, strengthen our immune system and explore oral tolerance strategies.

The Gluten Cure

The primary conventional treatment completely left out of this discussion is the *avoidance diet* – the complete and *permanent* removal of the particular food from the diet – in this case, avoiding every food containing gluten.

Admittedly, the permanent gluten-free diet is actually probably the most clinically applied treatment for gluten sensitivities around the world by conventional medicine. And it has provided great success among those who have embraced it.

And not unexpectedly, many people report great success and many benefits from eliminating gluten from their diet permanently.

For these folks, the author supports you. Eliminating a food that once bothered you is a logical course of action. And power to you for sticking to such a difficult diet.

But for those of us who would like to continue partaking of gluten-containing foods, and/or those of us who see the health advantages of eating whole grains – including preventing colon cancer, maintaining artery health and achieving healthy cholesterol levels – this book offers significant and proven strategies to reverse gluten sensitivities.

And these strategies are not simply for those with a non-celiac, non-wheat allergy gluten sensitivity. These strategies such as SOTI, are in fact more geared to those with wheat allergies and celiac disease.

This doesn't mean a gluten elimination diet doesn't have an important role to play – it certainly does. In fact, gluten elimination is being suggested in this text throughout the strategies explained above related to:

- ✓ *cleaning* up the diet and converting to organic foods
- ✓ *strengthening* the immune system with herbs and foods
- ✓ *revitalizing* intestinal health and the mucosal membranes
- ✓ *colonizing* probiotic species in the gut

During an elimination phase, these strategies will prepare our physiology to not only digest and break down gluten proteins as we eat them, but will protect our intestinal cells from being exposed to undigested gluten proteins.

And this, in turn, will dramatically decrease the chances of undigested gluten macromolecules penetrating our intestinal cell matrix or entering our blood system.

Following this period one can continue the *Adams Gluten Protocol* with the gradual and careful addition of healthy gluten foods back into the diet. Utilizing the oral immunotherapy tools provided here, we can add healthy gluten foods back starting with extremely small portions, gradually increasing from there.

This therapeutic process as illustrated by the research in this text, can work for both intolerant and allergic individuals – noting the more severe the allergic symptoms, the greater the need for supervision will be.

We have in fact proven that contrary to popular theory, celiac disease sufferers can indeed eat bread and many other gluten-containing foods as long as these protocols are followed.

And we can say with confidence that those with a non-celiac, non-wheat allergy gluten sensitivity who would like to be able to eat healthy gluten-containing grains can also likely benefit greatly from employing some of these strategies.

We can also state with confidence that by following the protocol here, we will also be able to tolerate – and vitalize from – those healthy FODMAPs that may also (or instead) be resulting in unwanted symptoms.

Furthermore, a gluten intolerant person will benefit greatly from those strategies that employ probiotics and dietary strategies that rebuild intestinal mucosal membranes and probiotic colonies through the consumption of prebiotic foods.

These are critical because probiotics and the enzymes they produce will neutralize gliadin and glutenin proteins by breaking them down into their amino components before those macromolecules can produce sensitivity within the digestive tract. They will break down proteins and lectins into amino acids or absorbable small peptides. And they will neutralize any lectin activity that can produce reactivity in some.

We cannot ignore the health of the intestinal tract in this equation. In fact, the health of the intestines is interwoven into the ability of the intestinal probiotics to be colonized enough to supply the enzymes to break down gluten proteins.

But getting there is the trick. For a typical Western foodie who has been given periodic doses of antibiotics, some other changes may be necessary to rebuild the health of the intestinal tract. Yes, there are some supplement strategies that can accelerate the process. This has been discussed thoroughly in this chapter.

These strategies, when employed with sensible gluten-food consumption – replacing junk foods with whole grain gluten foods that are organic whenever possible – have a good chance of bringing our intestinal tracts back to a healthy state.

Those junk foods that threaten probiotic populations with refined sugars – feeding their enemies and decimating the liver's health – must be cut back to achieve digestive health.

This doesn't mean that we can't eat cake or a donut or some other junk food now and again. It simply means they should no longer remain a central part of our grain diet.

And certainly, there are strategies to mitigate the effects of junk food. Say we're at a party and junk food is being provided as *h'orderves.* Do we have to make a scene? Not necessarily. Assuming we follow the junk food with a real food containing fiber – say a salad, some nuts or some whole grains shortly thereafter – we can mitigate most negative effects of the junk food.

In other words, we must be sensible. Going radical with our diet just doesn't make sense. Even going from five grams of fiber a day to the recommended 40 grams would be a mistake that can result in bloating and even cramping.

Better to begin now and build to that level gradually. Incorporate healthy foods into each meal, and then gradually increase their portion of the meal as we go. This will provide a sensible approach.

And the fiber doesn't have to all be gluten-grain based. There are many other choices of fiber to mix in, including oats, psyllium, apples, leafy greens and others. But remember that including some whole wheat fiber will help feed those probiotics that will colonize and produce the enzymes that will in turn break down the gluten.

Speaking of probiotics, we have laid out some good strategies for increasing colonies and species. These should dramatically help us break down gliadins and glutenins. But the process is not necessarily immediate. Pathogenic bacteria can still dominate our intestines and damper the activities of healthier bacteria. In such a state exists, we must make dramatic changes in our diet, incorporating a much larger proportion of plant-based foods which will feed and strengthen the healthier probiotic populations.

And if we augment that by supplementing probiotics and consuming probiotic foods as discussed in the research, over time they will help turn around our gut environment.

In other words, a celiac patient shouldn't expect to be able to eat gluten by popping a few probiotic supplements.

But should a celiac or wheat allergy sufferer undergo – under close supervision – a thorough supplementation plan with considerable prebiotics and probiotic foods – while rebuilding the immune system to allow for better tolerance response – while rebuilding the health of the intestinal wall and its mucosal membranes – and then using SOTI to become immunologically more tolerant – the research indicates there is a significant chance of being able to resume eating whole gluten-containing foods.

The non-allergic gluten intolerant person can also employ these very same strategies, though the immunotherapy phase may not require the same drawn out process. In fact, the employment of many of the elements discussed in this chapter may be speeded up because the sensitivity is not as great.

Just employing most of the nutritional, probiotic and mucosal membrane strategies may in themselves resolve the issues that lie at the root of a gluten intolerant person's sensitivity.

Yet it can also be said with accuracy that the majority of food sensitivity sufferers in Western countries have been told by their health professionals that there is no other option: *'You have a food sensitivity and that's that. You're stuck with it. So live with it.'*

Yet simply the scientific fact that many children eventually outgrow their food sensitivity says something extremely important: *We can outgrow food sensitivities.* Our sensitivity is not a foregone conclusion.

And not only is it possible, but the research shows that a very large segment of the population that contracts a food sensitivity at some point in their life *will* outgrow it.

The point that Western physicians seem to be missing is that since the body *can* outgrow it, there must be a *mechanism* for outgrowing an allergy. After all, the body is not a lottery system, where some people just so happen to get lucky while others are not so lucky. This sort of mind-set would also lead us to the conclusion that it wouldn't matter if we dropped an atomic bomb on a city, because everything is simply luck anyway.

The fact is, those who have outgrown their sensitivities experienced a modulation of their immune system. Their immune system began tolerating something they were previously sensitive to. How does this occur?

We have discussed the mechanics of this at length in this book. By strengthening the immune system, *we increase the ability of the immune system to adapt to and tolerate what is not inherently dangerous.*

By strengthening our immune system, we give our bodies the *ability* to recognize that a particular food protein is not really life-threatening. We give the immune system the *ability* to re-adjust its priorities: to determine what is life-threatening and what is not.

Furthermore, we have shown how a burdened, weakened immune system can become hypersensitive to those foods a healthier person will easily break down and become nourished by. This of course explains why billions of extremely healthy people have continued to eat wheat products – some living beyond the age of 100.

All of the nutritional, herbal, probiotic and lifestyle information in this text illustrates *scientifically proven* methods to unburden and strengthen the immune system. These methods are not simply the opinions of the author. These methods are not simply a particular fad diet or innovative therapy. They are *peer-reviewed, tried-and-true* methods that have been proven to strengthen the immune system and/or specifically help the immune system adapt to those foods that our immune systems might have mistakenly become sensitive to.

Rather, what the author has done is put together this information – collate it and transform it into a cohesive protocol.

This doesn't mean, however, that we will not have to partake in an elimination diet while we work on strengthening our immune system. No part of this text has suggested that a person simply ignore the body's responses and arbitrarily begin to gorge on gluten or any other food they are sensitive to. While eating the offending food might be a reasonable goal, there is a safe approach, as we've discussed.

Remember also that this discussion is intended for investigative purposes, and the gluten-sensitive person should consult with their health professional before making radical changes to their diet, supplementation and/or lifestyle. Especially if they have a diagnosed allergy or celiac condition.

We've discussed a number of herbs, formulas, foods and lifestyle strategies that can be implemented to help the body learn to tolerate gluten. Some may apply to a particular situation while others won't apply or could even worsen the condition. This depends largely upon the type of gluten sensitivity, ones particular constitution, and the manner of application of the strategy. This is one reason to be in consultation with a health professional who has expertise in these areas, especially for a person with severe reactions.

For example, choosing the right herbal formulation of herbs can be downright complex. The reader may have noticed that there were several Chinese and Ayurvedic formulations discussed in this chapter. In other words, not even a Traditional Chinese Medicine doctor or Ayurvedic doctor will necessarily recommend the same thing to different people. Doctors of Chinese medicine and Ayurvedic medicine will carefully review the constitution of the patient and specify those herbs that apply to the particular constitution of the patient.

One way to utilize this text might be to present the book to ones health professional. Perhaps they already know how to apply many of these strategies. Or perhaps they are unaware of some of them. Or they are unaware of the research showing how efficacious some of these methods are. At the very least, they may be open enough to look through the research and suggest a program that integrates some of these with their current treatment strategy.

This does not mean that a person cannot, assuming they are not anaphylactic or celiac, commence to employ some of these strategies. Perhaps they have some education on employing alternative health strategies – one that permits them to select those herbs and foods that most apply to their constitution. But the reader must understand this text is not a prescription. It is an educational reference.

We each have different constitutions and different histories, families, habits and metabolisms. And there are multiple food sensitivities and single gluten sensitivities. And there are a host of different scenarios that can create a food sensitivity.

We can almost say that practically every food sensitivity case is as unique as each person. Therefore, to offer the same precise prescriptive scenario for dealing with this expanse of uniqueness would be seriously short-sighted, and misleading to the reader.

What we have done is offered well-founded and tested techniques that have been peer-reviewed by modern scientists and/or traditional healers over the centuries. We have provided the background and research on techniques that have been effective for more than a few people, and have been clinically applied repeatedly.

This provides the foundation for part of our solution to gluten sensitivities both personally and globally: Converting our diets and food production to organic and eliminating the use of toxins within our foods and lifestyles.

The bottom line of this text is that we should not give up on our body's ability to heal itself. We must not assume that our body is a static machine programmed forever to have certain food sensitivities. We should not assume that a food sensitivity is a life sentence.

But we also cannot ignore the inclination our body has to nature: The fact that our gut bacteria and our bodies thrive from the foods and the environment that nature provides. And nature has rejuvenation responses.

Yes, we can see from the research provided here that the human body is a highly adaptive machine. The immune system and its relative tolerances can quite often change. The immune system might be able to easily fight off a rhinovirus exposure immediately with no cold symptoms one day, and yet succumb to a 3-5 day hold-down of fever, sneezing and coughing to the same type of exposure another day. What was the difference? Was the rhinovirus stronger in the latter case?

Possibly, but not likely. What is more likely is that the immune system was weaker in the latter case. The immune system had to resort to a more urgent inflammatory process to remove the virus infection, due to its weakened state or the level of exposure. The immune system was weaker than the exposure, in other words.

The body is also a fluid mechanism. We know that every cell in the body will die and be replaced by a new cell within about every seven years. Intestinal cells will be replaced within just a few days. Some nerve and stem cells may live a bit longer. But every other cell – within every organ and tissue system in the body – will be replaced within weeks or months. Furthermore, the cells are constantly recycling molecules and nutrients over their life spans. In fact, researchers have determined that the body will have an entirely new molecular constitution at least every five years.

This also means the molecules within our body are constantly being replaced by new molecules. The old molecules are purged and sent into the environment, and new ones are coming in from our foods, water and environment. This means, from a molecular basis, even if we don't have a complete turnover of cells during that period, within five years we will have a different body: A body replaced by new molecules.

This might be compared to looking at a waterfall: The waterfall might look the same, but the water that makes up the waterfall is constantly changing.

Therefore, there is no reason why our bodies cannot undergo change. There is no reason why the body's immune cells cannot become tolerant to something they were previously sensitive to. The research supports this. And epigenetic research has illustrated that our DNA can change as we adapt to our environment and foods.

The message here is quite simple: Consider the body a changing, fluid molecular machine. Is it well-oiled? Are we putting the best molecular fuel into it? Just as in any machine, the better the fuel, the better it runs. The body is no different. The body's appropriate fuel is provided by nature.

Let's encourage our body to change for the better by feeding it better molecular fuel. The reward will be more than just becoming tolerant to a few foods. The bigger reward will be more resistance to disease, clearer thinking, a stronger heart, more stamina, and a more-productive life.

References and Bibliography

Abbott M, Hayward S, Ross W, Godefroy SB, Ulberth F, Van Hengel AJ, Roberts J, Akiyama H, Popping B, Yeung JM, Wehling P, Taylor SL, Poms RE, Delahaut P. Validation procedures for quantitative food allergen ELISA methods: community guidance and best practices. *J AOAC Int.* 2010 Mar-Apr;93(2):442-50.

Adel-Patient K, Ah-Leung S, Creminon C, Nouaille S, Chatel JM, Langella P, Wal JM. Oral administration of recombinant Lactococcus lactis expressing bovine beta-lactoglobulin partially prevents mice from sensitization. *Clin Exp Allergy.* 2005 Apr;35(4):539-46.

Adlercreutz H. Can rye intake decrease risk of human breast cancer? Food Nutr Res. 2010 Nov 10;54.

Aggarwal BB, Harikumar KB. Potential therapeutic effects of curcumin, the anti-inflammatory agent, against neurodegenerative, cardiovascular, pulmonary, metabolic, autoimmune and neoplastic diseases. *Int J Biochem Cell Biol.* 2009 Jan;41(1):40-59.

Aggarwal BB, Sung B. Pharmacological basis for the role of curcumin in chronic diseases: an age-old spice with modern targets. *Trends Pharmacol Sci.* 2009 Feb;30(2):85-94.

Agne PS, Bidat E, Agne PS, Rance F, Paty E. Sesame seed allergy in children. *Eur Ann Allergy Clin Immunol.* 2004 Oct;36(8):300-5.

Agostoni C, Fiocchi A, Riva E, Terracciano L, Sarratud T, Martelli A, Lodi F, D'Auria E, Zuccotti G, Giovannini M. Growth of infants with IgE-mediated cow's milk allergy fed different formulas in the complementary feeding period. *Pediatr Allergy Immunol.* 2007 Nov;18(7):599-606.

Ahmed T, Fuchs GJ. Gastrointestinal allergy to food: a review. *J Diarrhoeal Dis Res.* 1997 Dec;15(4):211-23.

Aho K, Koskenvuo M, Tuominen J, Kaprio J. Occurrence of rheumatoid arthritis in a nationwide series of twins. *J Rheumatol.* 1986 Oct;13(5):899-902.

Airola P. *How to Get Well.* Phoenix, AZ: Health Plus, 1974.

Akkol EK, Güvenç A, Yesilada E. A comparative study on the antinociceptive and anti-inflammatory activities of five Juniperus taxa. *J Ethnopharmacol.* 2009 Jun 6.

Alemán A, Sastre J, Quirce S, de las Heras M, Carnés J, Fernández-Caldas E, Pastor C, Blázquez AB, Vivanco F, Cuesta-Herranz J. Allergy to kiwi: a double-blind, placebo-controlled food challenge study in patients from a birch-free area. *J Allergy Clin Immunol.* 2004 Mar;113(3):543-50.

Alexander DD, Cabana MD. Partially hydrolyzed 100% whey protein infant formula and reduced risk of atopic dermatitis: a meta-analysis. *J Pediatr Gastroenterol Nutr.* 2010 Apr;50(4):422-30.

Alexandrakis M, Letourneau R, Kempuraj D, Kandere-Grzybowska K, Huang M, Christodoulou S, Boucher W, Seretakis D, Theoharides TC. Flavones inhibit Proliferation and increase mediator content in human leukemic mast cells (HMC-1). *Eur J Haematol.* 2003 Dec;71(6):448-54.

Al-Harrasi A, Al-Saidi S. Phytochemical analysis of the essential oil from botanically certified oleogum resin of Boswellia sacra (Omani Luban). *Molecules.* 2008 Sep 16;13(9):2181-9.

Almqvist C, Garden F, Xuan W, Mihrshahi S, Leeder SR, Oddy W, Webb K, Marks GB; CAPS team. Omega-3 and omega-6 fatty acid exposure from early life does not affect atopy and asthma at age 5 years. *J Allergy Clin Immunol.* 2007 Jun;119(6):1438-44.

Al-Mustafa AH, Al-Thunibat OY. Antioxidant activity of some Jordanian medicinal plants used traditionally for treatment of diabetes. *Pak J Biol Sci.* 2008 Feb 1;11(3):351-8.

Altman RD, Marcussen KC. Effects of a ginger extract on knee pain in patients with osteoarthritis. *Arthritis Rheum.* 2001 Nov;44(11):2531-8.

Alvarez-Sieiro P, Martin MC, Redruello B, Del Rio B, Ladero V, Palanski BA, Khosla C, Fernandez M, Alvarez MA. Generation of food-grade recombinant Lactobacillus casei delivering Myxococcus xanthus prolyl endopeptidase. Appl Microbiol Biotechnol. 2014 Apr 22.

Aman P, Pettersson D, Zhang JX, Tidehag P, Hallmans G. Starch and dietary fiber components are excreted and degraded to variable extents in ileostomy subjects consuming mixed diets with wheat- or oat-bran bread. J Nutr. 1995 Sep;125(9):2341-7.

Amato R, Pinelli M, Monticelli A, Miele G, Cocozza S. Schizophrenia and Vitamin D Related Genes Could Have Been Subject to Latitude-driven Adaptation. *BMC Evol Biol.* 2010 Nov 11;10(1):351.

American College of Gastroenterology Task Force on Irritable Bowel Syndrome, Brandt LJ, Chey WD, Foxx-Orenstein AE, Schiller LR, Schoenfeld PS, Spiegel BM, Talley NJ, Quigley EM. An evidence-based position statement on the management of irritable bowel syndrome. Am J Gastroenterol. 2009 Jan;104 Suppl 1:S1-35.

American Conference of Governmental Industrial Hygienists. *Threshold limit values for chemical substances and physical agents in the work environment.* Cincinnati, OH: ACGIH, 1986.

American Dietetic Association; Dietitians of Canada. Position of the American Dietetic Association and Dietitians of Canada: vegetarian diets. *Can J Diet Pract Res.* 2003 Summer;64(2):62-81.

Ammon HP. Boswellic acids in chronic inflammatory diseases. *Planta Med.* 2006 Oct;72(12):1100-16.

Anand P, Thomas SG, Kunnumakkara AB, Sundaram C, Harikumar KB, Sung B, Tharakan ST, Misra K, Priyadarsini IK, Rajasekharan KN, Aggarwal BB. Biological activities of curcumin and its analogues (Congeners) made by man and Mother Nature. *Biochem Pharmacol.* 2008 Dec 1;76(11):1590-611.

Anderson JL, May HT, Horne BD, Bair TL, Hall NL, Carlquist JF, Lappé DL, Muhlestein JB; Intermountain Heart Collaborative (IHC) Study Group. Relation of vitamin D deficiency to cardiovascular risk factors, disease status, and incident events in a general healthcare population. *Am J Cardiol.* 2010 Oct 1;106(7):963-8.

Anderson JW, Baird P, Davis RH Jr, Ferreri S, Knudtson M, Koraym A, Waters V, Williams CL. Health benefits of dietary fiber. Nutr Rev. 2009 Apr;67(4):188-205.

Anderson LA, McMillan SA, Watson RG, Monaghan P, Gavin AT, Fox C, Murray LJ. Malignancy and mortality in a population-based cohort of patients with coeliac disease or "gluten sensitivity". World J Gastroenterol. 2007 Jan 7;13(1):146-51.

Anderson RC, Anderson JH. Acute toxic effects of fragrance products. *Arch Environ Health.* 1998 Mar-Apr;53(2):138-46.

Anderson RP, Degano P, Godkin AJ, Jewell DP, Hill AV. In vivo antigen challenge in celiac disease identifies a single transglutaminase-modified peptide as the dominant A-gliadin T-cell epitope. Nat Med. 2000 Mar;6(3):337-42.

Andersson AA, Kamal-Eldin A, Aman P. Effects of environment and variety on alkylresorcinols in wheat in the HEALTHGRAIN diversity screen. J Agric Food Chem. 2010 Sep 8;58(17):9299-305.

Andersson U, Dey ES, Holm C, Degerman E. Rye bran alkylresorcinols suppress adipocyte lipolysis and hormone-sensitive lipase activity. Mol Nutr Food Res. 2011 Sep;55 Suppl 2:S290-3.

Andoh T, Zhang Q, Yamamoto T, Tayama M, Hattori M, Tanaka K, Kuraishi Y. Inhibitory Effects of the Methanol Extract of Ganoderma lucidum on Mosquito Allergy-Induced Itch-Associated Responses in Mice. *J Pharmacol Sci.* 2010 Oct 8.

Andre C, Andre F, Colin L, Cavagna S. Measurement of intestinal permeability to mannitol and lactulose as a means of diagnosing food allergy and evaluating therapeutic effectiveness of disodium cromoglycate. Ann Allergy. 1987 Nov;59(5 Pt 2):127-30.

André C, André F, Colin L. Effect of allergen ingestion challenge with and without cromoglycate cover on intestinal permeability in atopic dermatitis, urticaria and other symptoms of food allergy. *Allergy.* 1989;44 Suppl 9:47-51.

André C. Food allergy. Objective diagnosis and test of therapeutic efficacy by measuring intestinal permeability. *Presse Med.* 1986 Jan 25;15(3):105-8.

Andre F, Andre C, Feknous M, Colin L, Cavagna S. Digestive permeability to different-sized molecules and to sodium cromoglycate in food allergy. *Allergy Proc.* 1991 Sep-Oct;12(5):293-8.

Angeli JP, Ribeiro LR, Bellini MF, Mantovanil. Anti-clastogenic effect of beta-glucan extracted from barley towards chemically induced DNA damage in rodent cells. Hum Exp Toxicol. 2006 Jun;25(6):319-24.

Angioni A, Barra A, Russo MT, Coroneo V, Dessi S, Cabras P. Chemical composition of the essential oils of Juniperus from ripe and unripe berries and leaves and their antimicrobial activity. *J Agric Food Chem.* 2003 May 7;51(10):3073-8.

Anim-Nyame N, Sooranna SR, Johnson MR, Gamble J, Steer PJ. Garlic supplementation increases peripheral blood flow: a role for interleukin-6? *J Nutr Biochem.* 2004 Jan;15(1):30-6.

Annweiler C, Schott AM, Berrut G, Chauviré V, Le Gall D, Inzitari M, Beauchet O. Vitamin D and ageing: neurological issues. *Neuropsychobiology.* 2010 Aug;62(3):139-50.

Anthimidou E, Mossialos D. Antibacterial activity of Greek and Cypriot honeys against Staphylococcus aureus and Pseudomonas aeruginosa in comparison to manuka honey. J Med Food. 2013 Jan;16(1):42-7.

Aoki T, Usuda Y, Miyakoshi H, Tamura K, Herberman RB. Low natural killer syndrome: clinical and immunologic features. *Nat Immun Cell Growth Regul.* 1987;6(3):116-28.

Apáti P, Houghton PJ, Kite G, Steventon GB, Kéry A. In-vitro effect of flavonoids from Solidago canadensis extract on glutathione S-transferase. *J Pharm Pharmacol.* 2006 Feb;58(2):251-6.

APHA (American Public Health Association). Opposition to the Use of Hormone Growth Promoters in Beef and Dairy Cattle Production. Policy Date: 11/10/2009. Policy Number: 20098. http://www.apha.org/advocacy/policy /id=1379. Accessed Nov. 24, 2010.

Apr;71(4):625-31.

Araki K, Shinozaki T, Irie Y, Miyazawa Y. Trial of oral administration of Bifidobacterium breve for the prevention of rotavirus infections. *Kansenshogaku Zasshi.* 1999 Apr;73(4):305-10.

Argento A, Tiraferri E, Marzaloni M. Oral anticoagulants and medicinal plants. An emerging interaction. *Ann Ital Med Int.* 2000 Apr-Jun;15(2):139-43.

Argenzio RA, Meuten DJ. Short-chain fatty acids induce reversible injury of porcine colon. Dig Dis Sci. 1991;36:1459–1468.

Arshad SH, Bateman B, Sadeghnejad A, Gant C, Matthews SM. Prevention of allergic disease during childhood by allergen avoidance: the Isle of Wight prevention study. *J Allergy Clin Immunol.* 2007 Feb;119(2):307-13.

Arslan G, Kahrs GE, Lind R, Frøyland L, Florvaag E, Berstad A. Patients with subjective food hypersensitivity: the value of analyzing intestinal permeability and inflammation markers in gut lavage fluid. *Digestion.* 2004;70(1):26-35.

Arslanoglu S, Moro GE, Schmitt J, Tandoi L, Rizzardi S, Boehm G. Early dietary intervention with a mixture of prebiotic oligosaccharides reduces the incidence of allergic manifestations and infections during the first two years of life. *J Nutr.* 2008 Jun;138(6):1091-5.

Arterburn LM, Oken HA, Bailey Hall E, Hamersley J, Kuratko CN, Hoffman JP. Algal-oil capsules and cooked salmon: nutritionally equivalent sources of docosahexaenoic acid. *J Am Diet Assoc.* 2008 Jul;108(7):1204-9.

Arterburn LM, Oken HA, Hoffman JP, Bailey-Hall E, Chung G, Rom D, Hamersley J, McCarthy D. Bioequivalence of Docosahexaenoic acid from different algal oils in capsules and in a DHA-fortified food. *Lipids.* 2007 Nov;42(11):1011-24.

Asero R, Antonicelli L, Arena A, Bommarito L, Caruso B, Colombo G, Crivellaro M, De Carli M, Della Torre E, Della Torre F, Heffler E, Lodi Rizzini F, Longo R, Manzotti G, Marcotulli M, Melchiorre A, Minale P, Morandi P, Moreni B, Moschella A, Murzilli F, Nebiolo F, Poppa M, Randazzo S, Rossi G, Senna GE. Causes of food-induced anaphylaxis in Italian adults: a multi-centre study. *Int Arch Allergy Immunol.* 2009;150(3):271-7.

Asero R, Antonicelli L, Arena A, Bommarito L, Caruso B, Crivellaro M, De Carli M, Della Torre E, Della Torre F, Heffler E, Lodi Rizzini F, Longo R, Manzotti G, Marcotulli M, Melchiorre A, Minale P, Morandi P, Moreni B, Moschella A, Murzilli F, Nebiolo F, Poppa M, Randazzo S, Rossi G, Senna GE. EpidemAAITO: features of food allergy in Italian adults attending allergy clinics: a multi-centre study. *Clin Exp Allergy.* 2009 Apr;39(4):547-55.

Asero R, Mistrello G, Roncarolo D, Amato S, Caldironi G, Barocci F, van Ree R. Immunological cross-reactivity between lipid transfer proteins from botanically unrelated plant-derived foods: a clinical study. *Allergy.* 2002 Oct;57(10):900-6.

Ashrafi K, Chang FY, Watts JL, Fraser AG, Kamath RS, Ahringer J, Ruvkun G. Genome-wide RNAi analysis of Caenorhabditis elegans fat regulatory genes. *Nature.* 2003 Jan 16;421(6920):268-72.

Atkinson W, Sheldon TA, Shaath N, Whorwell PJ. Food elimination based on IgG antibodies in irritable bowel syndrome: a randomised controlled trial. *Gut.* 2004 Oct;53(10):1459-64.

Atsumi T, Tonosaki K. Smelling lavender and rosemary increases free radical scavenging activity and decreases cortisol level in saliva. *Psychiatry Res.* 2007 Feb 28;150(1):89-96.

Aubertin-Leheudre M, Koskela A, Samaletdin A, Adlercreutz H. Plasma and urinary alkylresorcinol metabolites as potential biomarkers of breast cancer risk in Finnish women: a pilot study. Nutr Cancer. 2010;62(6):759-64.

Aune D, Norat T, Romundstad P, Vatten LJ. Whole grain and refined grain consumption and the risk of type 2 diabetes: a systematic review and dose-response meta-analysis of cohort studies. Eur J Epidemiol. 2013 Nov;28(11):845-58.

Bachas-Daunert S, Deo SK. Should genetically modified foods be abandoned on the basis of allergenicity? *Anal Bioanal Chem.* 2008 Oct;392(3):341-6.

Badar VA, Thawani VR, Wakode PT, Shrivastava MP, Gharpure KJ, Hingorani LL, Khiyani RM. Efficacy of Tinospora cordifolia in allergic rhinitis. *J Ethnopharmacol.* 2005 Jan 15;96(3):445-9.

Bai JC, Fried M, Corazza GR, Schuppan D, Farthing M, Catassi C, Greco L, Cohen H, Ciacci C, Eliakim R, Fasano A, González A, Krabshuis JH, LeMair A; World Gastroenterology Organization. World Gastroenterology Organisation global guidelines on celiac disease. J Clin Gastroenterol. 2013 Feb;47(2):121-6.

Bai YH, Pak SC, Lee SH, Bae CS, Prosser C, Stelwagen K, Lee JH, Park SD. Assessment of a bioactive compound for its potential antiinflammatory property by tight junction permeability. Phytother Res. 2005 Dec;19(12):1009-12.

Baker DH. Comparative nutrition and metabolism: explication of open questions with emphasis on protein and amino acids. *Proc Natl Acad Sci U S A.* 2005 Dec 13;102(50):17897-902.

Baker SM. *Detoxification and Healing.* Chicago: Contemporary Books, 2004.

Bakshi A, Stephen S, Borum ML, Doman DB. Emerging therapeutic options for celiac disease: potential alternatives to a gluten-free diet. Gastroenterol Hepatol (N Y). 2012 Sep;8(9):582-8.

Balch P, Balch J. *Prescription for Nutritional Healing.* New York: Avery, 2000.

Ballentine R. *Diet & Nutrition: A holistic approach.* Honesdale, PA: Himalayan Int., 1978.

Ballentine R. *Radical Healing.* New York: Harmony Books, 1999.

Ballmer-Weber BK, Hoffmann A, Wüthrich B, Lüttkopf D, Pompei C, Wangorsch A, Kästner M, Vieths S. Influence of food processing on the allergenicity of celery: DBPCFC with celery spice and cooked celery in patients with celery allergy. *Allergy.* 2002 Mar;57(3):228-35.

Ballmer-Weber BK, Holzhauser T, Scibilia J, Mittag D, Zisa G, Ortolani C, Oesterballe M, Poulsen LK, Vieths S, Bindslev-Jensen C. Clinical characteristics of soybean allergy in Europe: a double-blind, placebo-controlled food challenge study. *J Allergy Clin Immunol.* 2007 Jun;119(6):1489-96.

Ballmer-Weber BK, Vieths S, Lüttkopf D, Heuschmann P, Wüthrich B. Celery allergy confirmed by double-blind, placebo-controlled food challenge: a clinical study in 32 subjects with a history of adverse reactions to celery root. *J Allergy Clin Immunol.* 2000 Aug;106(2):373-8.

Banno N, Akihisa T, Yasukawa K, Tokuda H, Tabata K, Nakamura Y, Nishimura R, Kimura Y, Suzuki T. Anti-inflammatory activities of the triterpene acids from the resin of Boswellia carteri. *J Ethnopharmacol.* 2006 Sep 19;107(2):249-53.

Bant A, Kruszewski J. Increased sensitization prevalence to common inhalant and food allergens in young adult Polish males. *Ann Agric Environ Med.* 2008 Jun;15(1):21-7.

Barau E, Dupont C. Modifications of intestinal permeability during food provocation procedures in pediatric irritable bowel syndrome. *J Pediatr Gastroenterol Nutr.* 1990 Jul;11(1):72-7.

Barnes M, Cullinan P, Athanasaki P, MacNeill S, Hole AM, Harris J, Kalogeraki S, Chatzinikolaou M, Drakonakis N, Bibaki-Liakou V, Newman Taylor AJ, Bibakis I. Crete: does farming explain urban and rural differences in atopy? *Clin Exp Allergy.* 2001 Dec;31(12):1822-8.

Barnetson RS, Drummond H, Ferguson A. Precipitins to dietary proteins in atopic eczema. *Br J Dermatol.* 1983 Dec;109(6):653-5.

Barone MV, Gimigliano A, Castoria G, Paolella G, Maurano F, Paparo F, Maglio M, Mineo A, Miele E, Nanayakkara M, Troncone R, Auricchio S. Growth factor-like activity of gliadin, an alimentary protein: implications for coeliac disease. Gut. 2007 Apr;56(4):480-8.

Barrager E, Veltmann JR Jr, Schauss AG, Schiller RN. A multicentered, open-label trial on the safety and efficacy of methylsulfonylmethane in the treatment of seasonal allergic rhinitis. *J Altern Complement Med.* 2002 Apr;8(2):167-73.

Bartłomiej S, Justyna RK, Ewa N. Bioactive compounds in cereal grains – occurrence, structure, technological significance and nutritional benefits – a Food Sci Technol Int. 2012 Dec;18(6):559-68.

Basu A, Devaraj S, Jialal I. Dietary factors that promote or retard inflammation. *Arterioscler Thromb Vasc Biol.* 2006 May;26(5):995-1001.

Bateman B, Warner JO, Hutchinson E, Dean T, Rowlandson P, Gant C, Grundy J, Fitzgerald C, Stevenson J. The effects of a double blind, placebo controlled, artificial food colourings and benzoate preservative challenge on hyperactivity in a general population sample of preschool children. *Arch Dis Child.* 2004 Jun;89(6):506-11.

Batista R, Martins I, Jeno P, Ricardo CP, Oliveira MM. A proteomic study to identify soya allergens – the human response to transgenic versus non-transgenic soya samples. Int *Arch Allergy Immunol.* 2007;144(1):29-38.

Batmanghelidj F. Neurotransmitter histamine: an alternative view point, *Science in Medicine Simplified.* Falls Church, VA: Foundation for the Simple in Medicine, 1990.

Batmanghelidj F. Pain: a need for paradigm change. *Anticancer Res.* 1987 Sep-Oct;7(5B):971-89.

Batmanghelidj F. *Your Body's Many Cries for Water.* 2nd Ed. Vienna, VA: Global Health, 1997.

Beasley R, Clayton T, Crane J, von Mutius E, Lai CK, Montefort S, Stewart A; ISAAC Phase Three Study Group. Association between paracetamol use in infancy and childhood, and risk of asthma, rhinoconjunctivitis, and eczema in children aged 6-7 years: analysis from Phase Three of the ISAAC programme. *Lancet.* 2008 Sep. 20;372(9643):1039-48.

Becker KG, Simon RM, Bailey-Wilson JE, Freidlin B, Biddison WE, McFarland HF, Trent JM. Clustering of non-major histocompatibility complex susceptibility candidate loci in human autoimmune diseases. *Proc Natl Acad Sci U S A.* 1998 Aug 18;95(17):9979-84.

Beddoe AF. *Biologic Ionization as Applied to Human Nutrition.* Warsaw: Wendell Whitman, 2002.

Beecher GR. Phytonutrients' role in metabolism: effects on resistance to degenerative processes. *Nutr Rev.* 1999 Sep;57(9 Pt 2):S3-6.

Belcaro G, Cesarone MR, Errichi S, Zulli C, Errichi BM, Vinciguerra G, Ledda A, Di Renzo A, Stuard S, Dugall M, Pellegrini L, Gizzi G, Ippolito E, Ricci A, Cacchio M, Cipollone G, Ruffini I, Fano F, Hosoi M, Rohdewald P. Variations in C-reactive protein, plasma free radicals and fibrinogen values in patients with osteoarthritis treated with Pycnogenol. *Redox Rep.* 2008;13(6):271-6.

Belderok B. Developments in bread-making processes. Plant Foods Hum Nutr. 2000;55(1):1-86.

Bell IR, Baldwin CM, Schwartz GE, Illness from low levels of environmental chemicals: relevance to chronic fatigue syndrome and fibromyalgia. *Am J Med.* 1998;105 (suppl 3A).:74-82. S.

Bell SJ, Potter PC. Milk whey-specific immune complexes in allergic and non-allergic subjects. *Allergy.* 1988 Oct;43(7):497-503.

Bellanti JA, Zeligs BJ, Malka-Rais J, Sabra A. Abnormalities of Th1 function in non-IgE food allergy, celiac disease, and ileal lymphonodular hyperplasia: a new relationship? Ann *Allergy Asthma Immunol.* 2003 Jun;90(6 Suppl 3):84-9.

Ben, X.M., Zhou, X.Y., Zhao, W.H., Yu, W.L., Pan, W., Zhang, W.L., Wu, S.M., Van Beusekom, C.M., Schaafsma, A. (2004) Supplementation of milk formula with galactooligosaccharides improves intestinal micro-flora and fermentation in term infants. *Chin Med J.* 117(6):927-931, 2004.

Benard A, Desreumeaux P, Huglo D, Hoorelbeke A, Tonnel AB, Wallaert B. Increased intestinal permeability in bronchial asthma. *J Allergy Clin Immunol.* 1996 Jun;97(6):1173-8.

Bender L. Childhood schizophrenia. Psychiatr Q. 1953 Oct;27(4):663-81.

Bengmark S. Curcumin, an atoxic antioxidant and natural NFkappaB, cyclooxygenase-2, lipooxygenase, and inducible nitric oxide synthase inhibitor: a shield against acute and chronic diseases. *JPEN J Parenter Enteral Nutr.* 2006 Jan-Feb;30(1):45-51.

Bengmark S. Immunonutrition: role of biosurfactants, fiber, and probiotic bacteria. Nutrition. 1998 Jul-Aug;14(7-8):585-94.

Benlounes N, Dupont C, Candalh C, Blaton MA, Darmon N, Desjeux JF, Heyman M. The threshold for immune cell reactivity to milk antigens decreases in cow's milk allergy with intestinal symptoms. *J Allergy Clin Immunol.* 1996 Oct;98(4):781-9.

Ben-Shoshan M, Harrington DW, Soller L, Fragapane J, Joseph L, St Pierre Y, Godefroy SB, Elliot SJ, Clarke AE. A population-based study on peanut, tree nut, fish, shellfish, and sesame allergy prevalence in Canada. *J Allergy Clin Immunol.* 2010 Jun;125(6):1327-35.

Ben-Shoshan M, Kagan R, Primeau MN, Alizadehfar R, Turnbull E, Harada L, Dufresne C, Allen M, Joseph L, St Pierre Y, Clarke A. Establishing the diagnosis of peanut allergy in children never exposed to peanut or with an uncertain history: a cross-Canada study. *Pediatr Allergy Immunol.* 2010 Sep;21(6):920-6.

Bensky D, Gable A, Kaptchuk T (transl.). *Chinese Herbal Medicine Materia Medica.* Seattle: Eastland Press, 1986.

Bentz S, Hausmann M, Piberger H, Kellermeier S, Paul S, Held L, Falk W, Obermeier F, Fried M, Schölmerich J, Rogler G. Clinical relevance of IgG antibodies against food antigens in Crohn's disease: a double-blind cross-over diet intervention study. *Digestion.* 2010;81(4):252-64.

Bergner P. *The Healing Power of Garlic.* Prima Publishing, Rocklin CA 1996.

Berin MC, Yang PC, Ciok L, Waserman S, Perdue MH. Role for IL-4 in macromolecular transport across human intestinal epithelium. Am J Physiol. 1999 May;276(5 Pt 1):C1046-52.

Berkow R., (Ed.) *The Merck Manual of Diagnosis and Therapy.* 16th Edition. Rahway, N.J.: Merck Research Labs, 1992.

Berseth CL, Mitmesser SH, Ziegler EE, Marunycz JD, Vanderhoof J. Tolerance of a standard intact protein formula versus a partially hydrolyzed formula in healthy, term infants. Nutr J. 2009 Jun 19;8:27.

Berteau O and Mulloy B. 2003. Sulfated fucans, fresh perspectives: structures, functions, and biological properties of sulfated fucans and an overview of enzymes active toward this class of polysaccharide. *Glycobiology.* Jun;13(6):29R-40R.

Beyer K, Morrow E, Li XM, Bardina L, Bannon GA, Burks AW, Sampson HA. Effects of cooking methods on peanut allergenicity. *J Allergy Clin Immunol.* 2001;107:1077-81.

Bhandari U, Sharma JN, Zafar R. The protective action of ethanolic ginger (Zingiber officinale) extract in cholesterol fed rabbits. *J Ethnopharmacol.* 1998 Jun;61(2):167-71.

Bhuja P, McLachlan K, Stephens J, Taylor G. Accumulation of 1,3-beta-D-glucans, in response to aluminum and cytosolic calcium in Triticum aestivum. Plant Cell Physiol. 2004 May;45(5):543-9.

Bielory BP, Perez VL, Bielory L. Treatment of seasonal allergic conjunctivitis with ophthalmic corticosteroids: in search of the perfect ocular corticosteroids in the treatment of allergic conjunctivitis. *Curr Opin Allergy Clin Immunol.* 2010 Oct;10(5):469-77.

Bielory L, Lupoli K. Herbal interventions in asthma and allergy. *J Asthma.* 1999;36:1–65.

Bielory L, Russin J, Zuckerman GB. Clinical efficacy, mechanisms of action, and adverse effects of complementary and alternative medicine therapies for asthma. *Allergy Asthma Proc.* 2004;25:283–91.

Biesiekierski JR, Muir JG, Gibson PR. Is gluten a cause of gastrointestinal symptoms in people without celiac disease? Curr Allergy Asthma Rep. 2013 Dec;13(6):631-8.

Biesiekierski JR, Newnham ED, Irving PM, Barrett JS, Haines M, Doecke JD, Shepherd SJ, Muir JG, Gibson PR. Gluten causes gastrointestinal symptoms in subjects without celiac disease: a double-blind randomized placebo-controlled trial. Am J Gastroenterol. 2011 Mar;106(3):508-14; quiz 515.

Biesiekierski JR, Newnham ED, Shepherd SJ, Muir JG, Gibson PR. Characterization of Adults With a Self-Diagnosis of Nonceliac Gluten Sensitivity. Nutr Clin Pract. 2014 Apr 16.

Biesiekierski JR, Peters SL, Newnham ED, Rosella O, Muir JG, Gibson PR. No effects of gluten in patients with self-reported non-celiac gluten sensitivity after dietary reduction of fermentable, poorly absorbed, short-chain carbohydrates. Gastroenterology. 2013;145(2):320–328.

Biesiekierski JR, Rosella O, Rose R, Liels K, Barrett JS, Shepherd SJ, Gibson PR, Muir JG. Quantification of fructans, galacto-oligosacharides and other short-chain carbohydrates in processed grains and cereals. J Hum Nutr Diet. 2011 Apr;24(2):154-76.

Bindslev-Jensen C, Skov PS, Roggen EL, Hvass P, Brinch DS. Investigation on possible allergenicity of 19 different commercial enzymes used in the food industry. *Food Chem Toxicol.* 2006 Nov;44(11):1909-15.

Binita R, Khetarpaul N. Probiotic fermentation: effect on antinutrients and digestibility of starch and protein of indigenously developed food mixture. Nutr Health. 1997;11(3):139-47.

Biro FM, Galvez MP, Greenspan LC, Succop PA, Vangeepuram N, Pinney SM, Teitelbaum S, Windham GC, Kushi LH, Wolff MS. Pubertal assessment method and baseline characteristics in a mixed longitudinal study of girls. *Pediatrics.* 2010 Sep;126(3):e583-90.

Bischoff SC. Food allergy and eosinophilic gastroenteritis and colitis. *Curr Opin Allergy Clin Immunol.* 2010 Jun;10(3):238-45.

Bjarnason I, MacPherson A, Hollander D. Intestinal permeability: an overview. *Gastroenterology.* 1995 May;108(5):1566-81.

Bjornsson E, Janson C, Plaschke P, Norrman E, Sjoberg O (1996) Prevalence of sensitization to food allergies in adult Swedes. *Ann Allergy Asthma Immunol.* 77: 327–332.

Blázquez AB, Mayer L, Berin MC. Thymic Stromal Lymphopoietin Is Required for Gastrointestinal Allergy but Not Oral Tolerance. *Gastroenterology.* 2010 Jun 23.

Boccafogli A, Vicentini L, Camerani A, Cogliati P, D'Ambrosi A, Scolozzi R. Adverse food reactions in patients with grass pollen allergic respiratory disease. *Ann Allergy.* 1994 Oct;73(4):301-8.

Bode C, Bode JC. Effect of alcohol consumption on the gut. *Best Pract Res Clin Gastroenterol.* 2003 Aug;17(4):575-92.

Bodinier M, Legoux MA, Pineau F, Triballeau S, Segain JP, Brossard C, Denery-Papini S. Intestinal translocation capabilities of wheat allergens using the Caco-2 cell line. *J Agric Food Chem.* 2007 May 30;55(11):4576-83.

Boehm, G., Lidestri, M., Casetta, P., Jelinek, J., Negretti, F., Stahl, B., Martini, A. (2002) Supplementation of a bovine milk formula with an oligosaccharide mixture increases counts of faecal bifidobacteria in preterm infants. *Arch Dis Child Fetal Neonatal Ed.* 86: F178-F181

Bolhaar ST, Tiemessen MM, Zuidmeer L, van Leeuwen A, Hoffmann-Sommergruber K, Bruijnzeel-Koomen CA, Taams LS, Knol EF, van Hoffen E, van Ree R, Knulst AC. Efficacy of birch-pollen immunotherapy on cross-reactive food allergy confirmed by skin tests and double-blind food challenges. *Clin Exp Allergy.* 2004 May;34(5):761-9.

Bolleddula J, Goldfarb J, Wang R, Sampson H, Li XM. Synergistic Modulation Of Eotaxin And Il-4 Secretion By Constituents Of An Anti-asthma Herbal Formula (ASHMI) In Vitro. *J Allergy Clin Immunol.* 2007;119:S172.

Bongaerts GP, Severijnen RS. Preventive and curative effects of probiotics in atopic patients. *Med Hypotheses.* 2005;64(6):1089-92.

Bongartz D, Hesse A. Selective extraction of quercetrin in vegetable drugs and urine by off-line coupling of boronic acid affinity chromatography and high-performance liquid chromatography. *J Chromatogr B Biomed Appl.* 1995 Nov 17;673(2):223-30.

Bonomi F, D'Egidio MG, Iametti S, Marengo M, Marti A, Pagani MA, Ragg EM. Structure-quality relationship in commercial pasta: a molecular glimpse. Food Chem. 2012 Nov 15;135(2):348-55.

Borchers AT, Hackman RM, Keen CL, Stern JS, Gershwin ME. Complementary medicine: a review of immunomodulatory effects of Chinese herbal medicines. *Am J Clin Nutr.* 1997 Dec;66(6):1303-12.

Borchert VE, Czyborra P, Fetscher C, Goepel M, Michel MC. Extracts from Rhois aromatica and Solidaginis virgaurea inhibit rat and human bladder contraction. *Naunyn Schmiedebergs Arch Pharmacol.* 2004 Mar;369(3):281-6.

Böttcher MF, Jenmalm MC, Voor T, Julge K, Holt PG, Björkstén B. Cytokine responses to allergens during the first 2 years of life in Estonian and Swedish children. *Clin Exp Allergy.* 2006 May;36(5):619-28.

Bouchez-Mahiout I, Pecquet C, Kerre S, Snégaroff J, Raison-Peyron N, Laurière M. High molecular weight entities in industrial wheat protein hydrolysates are immunoreactive with IgE from allergic patients. *J Agric Food Chem.* 2010 Apr 14;58(7):4207-15.

Bouchier PJ, FitzGerald RJ, O'Cuinn G. Hydrolysis of alphas1- and beta-casein-derived peptides with a broad specificity aminopeptidase and proline specific aminopeptidases from Lactococcus lactis subsp. cremoris AM2. FEBS Lett. 1999 Feb 26;445(2-3):321-4.

Boverhof DR, Gollapudi BB, Hotchkiss JA, Osterloh-Quiroz M, Woolhiser MR. A draining lymph node assay (DLNA) for assessing the sensitizing potential of proteins. *Toxicol Lett.* 2010 Mar 15;193(2):144-51.

Boyce JA, Assa'ad A, Burks AW, Jones SM, Sampson HA, Wood RA, Plaut M, Cooper SF, Fenton MJ. Guidelines for the Diagnosis and Management of Food Allergy in the United State. *Natl Instit of Health.* 2010 Dec. NIH Publ No. 11-7700.

Bradette-Hébert ME, Legault J, Lavoie S, Pichette A. A new labdane diterpene from the flowers of Solidago canadensis. *Chem Pharm Bull.* 2008 Jan;56(1):82-4.

Brandtzaeg P. Food allergy: separating the science from the mythology. Nat Rev Gastroenterol Hepatol. 2010;7(7):380–400.

Brandtzaeg P. Food allergy: separating the science from the mythology. *Nat Rev Gastroenterol Hepatol.* 2010 Jul;7(7):380-400.

Bratt K, Sunnerheim K, Bryngelsson S, Fagerlund A, Engman L, Andersson RE, Dimberg LH. Avenanthramides in oats (Avena sativa L.) and structure-antioxidant activity relationships. J Agric Food Chem. 2003 Jan 29;51(3):594-600.

Breuer K, Heratizadeh A, Wulf A, Baumann U, Constien A, Tetau D, Kapp A, Werfel T. Late eczematous reactions to food in children with atopic dermatitis. *Clin Exp Allergy.* 2004 May;34(5):817-24.

Brewster DR, Manary MJ, Menzies IS, Henry RL, O'Loughlin EV. Comparison of milk and maize based diets in kwashiorkor. *Arch Dis Child.* 1997 Mar;76(3):242-8.

Brighenti F, Valtueña S, Pellegrini N, Ardigò D, Del Rio D, Salvatore S, Piatti P, Serafini M, Zavaroni I. Total antioxidant capacity of the diet is inversely and independently related to plasma concentration of high-sensitivity C-reactive protein in adult Italian subjects. *Br J Nutr.* 2005 May;93(5):619-25.

Brody J. *Jane Brody's Nutrition Book.* New York: WW Norton, 1981.

Brostoff J, Gamlin L, Brostoff J. *Food Allergies and Food Intolerance: The Complete Guide to Their Identification and Treatment.* Rochester, VT: Healing Arts, 2000.

Brownstein D. *Salt: Your Way to Health.* West Bloomfield, MI: Medical Alternatives, 2006.

Brown-Whitehorn TF, Spergel JM. The link between allergies and eosinophilic esophagitis: implications for management strategies. *Expert Rev Clin Immunol.* 2010 Jan;6(1):101-9.

Bublin M, Pfister M, Radauer C, Oberhuber C, Bulley S, Dewitt AM, Lidholm J, Reese G, Vieths S, Breiteneder H, Hoffmann-Sommergruber K, Ballmer-Weber BK. Component-resolved diagnosis of kiwifruit allergy with purified natural and recombinant kiwifruit allergens. *J Allergy Clin Immunol.* 2010 Mar;125(3):687-94, 694.e1.

Bucci C, Zingone F, Russo I, Morra I, Tortora R, Pogna N, Scalia G, Iovino P, Ciacci C. Gliadin does not induce mucosal inflammation or basophil activation in patients with nonceliac gluten sensitivity. Clin Gastroenterol Hepatol. 2013 Oct;11(10):1294-1299.e1.

Buchanan AD, Green TD, Jones SM, Scurlock AM, Christie L, Althage KA, Steele PH, Pons L, Helm RM, Lee LA, Burks AW. Egg oral immunotherapy in nonanaphylactic children with egg allergy. *J Allergy Clin Immunol.* 2007 Jan;119(1):199-205.

Bucher X, Pichler WJ, Dahinden CA, Helbling A. Effect of tree pollen specific, subcutaneous immunotherapy on the oral allergy syndrome to apple and hazelnut. *Allergy.* 2004 Dec;59(12):1272-6.

Budzianowski J. Coumarins, caffeoyltartaric acids and their artifactual methyl esters from Taraxacum officinale leaves. *Planta Med.* 1997 Jun;63(3):288.

Bueno L. Protease activated receptor 2: a new target for IBS treatment. *Eur Rev Med Pharmacol Sci.* 2008 Aug;12 Suppl 1:95-102.

Bundy R, Walker AF, Middleton RW, Booth J. Turmeric extract may improve irritable bowel syndrome symptomology in otherwise healthy adults: a pilot study. *J Altern Complement Med.* 2004 Dec;10(6):1015-8.

Burdge GC, Jones AE, Wootton SA. Eicosapentaenoic and docosapentaenoic acids are the principal products of alpha-linolenic acid metabolism in young men. *B J Nutr.* 2002 Oct;88(4):355-63.

Buret AG. How stress induces intestinal hypersensitivity. *Am J Pathol.* 2006 Jan;168(1):3-5.

Burits M, Asres K, Bucar F. The antioxidant activity of the essential oils of Artemisia afra, Artemisia abyssinica and Juniperus procera. *Phytother Res.* 2001 Mar;15(2):103-8.

Burks AW, James JM, Hiegel A, Wilson G, Wheeler JG, Jones SM, Zuerlein N. Atopic dermatitis and food hypersensitivity reactions. *J Pediatr.* 1998;132(1):132-6.

Burks W, Jones SM, Berseth CL, Harris C, Sampson HA, Scalabrin DM. Hypoallergenicity and effects on growth and tolerance of a new amino acid-based formula with docosahexaenoic acid and arachidonic acid. *J Pediatr.* 2008 Aug;153(2):266-71.

Burney PG, Luczynska C, Chinn S, Jarvis D (1994) The European Community Respiratory Health Survey. *Eur Respir J.* 7: 954–960.

Busse PJ, Wen MC, Huang CK, Srivastava K, Zhang TF, Schofield B, Sampson HA, Li XM. Therapeutic effects of the Chinese herbal formula, MSSM-03d, on persistent airway hyperreactivity and airway remodeling. *J Allergy Clin Immunol.* 2004;113:S220.

Bustos MC, Pérez GT, León AE. Effect of four types of dietary fiber on the technological quality of pasta. Food Sci Technol Int. 2011 Jun;17(3):213-21.

Butani L, Afshinnik A, Johnson J, Javaheri D, Peck S, German JB, Perez RV. Amelioration of tacrolimus-induced nephrotoxicity in rats using juniper oil. *Transplantation.* 2003 Jul 27;76(2):306-11.

Butkus SN, Mahan LK. Food allergies: immunological reactions to food. *J Am Diet Assoc.* 1986 May;86(5):601-8.

Byrne AM, Malka-Rais J, Burks AW, Fleischer DM. How do we know when peanut and tree nut allergy have resolved, and how do we keep it resolved? *Clin Exp Allergy.* 2010 Sep;40(9):1303-11.

Cabanillas B, Pedrosa MM, Rodríguez J, González A, Muzquiz M, Cuadrado C, Crespo JF, Burbano C. Effects of enzymatic hydrolysis on lentil allergenicity. *Mol Nutr Food Res.* 2010 Mar 19.

Caffarelli C, Coscia A, Baldi F, Borghi A, Capra L, Cazzato S, Migliozzi L, Pecorari L, Valenti A, Cavagni G. Characterization of irritable bowel syndrome and constipation in children with allergic diseases. *Eur J Pediatr.* 2007 Dec;166(12):1245-52.

Caffarelli C, Petroccione T. False-negative food challenges in children with suspected food allergy. *Lancet.* 2001 Dec 1;358(9296):1871-2.

Cahn J, Borzeix MG. Administration of procyanidolic oligomers in rats. Observed effects on changes in the permeability of the blood-brain barrier. *Sem Hop.* 1983 Jul 7;59(27-28):2031-4.

Caio G, Volta U. Coeliac disease: changing diagnostic criteria. Gastroenterol Hepatol Bed Bench. 2011;5:119–22.

Calder PC. Dietary modification of inflammation with lipids. *Proc Nutr Soc.* 2002 Aug;61(3):345-58.

Calvani M, Giorgio V, Miceli Sopo S. Specific oral tolerance induction for food. A systematic review. *Eur Ann Allergy Clin Immunol.* 2010 Feb;42(1):11-9.

Caminiti L, Passalacqua G, Barberi S, Vita D, Barberio G, De Luca R, Pajno GB. A new protocol for specific oral tolerance induction in children with IgE-mediated cow's milk allergy. *Allergy Asthma Proc.* 2009 Jul-Aug;30(4):443-8.

Campbell TC, Campbell TM. *The China Study.* Dallas, TX: Benbella Books, 2006.

Canani RB, Ruotolo S, Auricchio L, Caldore M, Porcaro F, Manguso F, Terrin G, Troncone R. Diagnostic accuracy of the atopy patch test in children with food allergy-related gastrointestinal symptoms. *Allergy*. 2007 Jul;62(7):738-43.

Canonica GW, Passalacqua G. Noninjection routes for immunotherapy. *J Allergy Clin Immunol.* 2003 Mar;111(3):437-48; quiz 449.

Cantani A, Micera M. Natural history of cow's milk allergy. An eight-year follow-up study in 115 atopic children. *Eur Rev Med Pharmacol Sci.* 2004 Jul-Aug;8(4):153-64.

Cantani A, Micera M. The prick by prick test is safe and reliable in 58 children with atopic dermatitis and food allergy. *Eur Rev Med Pharmacol Sci.* 2006 May-Jun;10(3):115-20.

Cao G, Alessio HM, Cutler RG. Oxygen-radical absorbance capacity assay for antioxidants. *Free Radic Biol Med.* 1993 Mar;14(3):303-11.

Cao G, Shukitt-Hale B, Bickford PC, Joseph JA, McEwen J, Prior RL. Hyperoxia-induced changes in antioxidant capacity and the effect of dietary antioxidants. *J Appl Physiol.* 1999 Jun;86(6):1817-22.

Cara L, Dubois C, Borel P, Armand M, Senft M, Portugal H, Pauli AM, Bernard PM, Lairon D. Effects of oat bran, rice bran, wheat fiber, and wheat germ on postprandial lipemia in healthy adults. Am J Clin Nutr. 1992 Jan;55(1):81-8.

Caramia G. The essential fatty acids omega-6 and omega-3: from their discovery to their use in therapy. *Minerva Pediatr.* 2008 Apr;60(2):219-33.

Carroccio A, Brusca I, Mansueto P, D'alcamo A, Barrale M, Soresi M, *et al.* A comparison between two different in vitro basophil activation tests for gluten- and cow's milk protein sensitivity in irritable bowel syndrome (IBS)-like patients. Clin Chem Lab Med. 2013;51(6):1257–63.

Carroccio A, Brusca I, Mansueto P, D'alcamo A, Barrale M, Soresi M, Seidita A, La Chiusa SM, Iacono G, Sprini D. A comparison between two different in vitro basophil activation tests for gluten- and cow's milk protein sensitivity in irritable bowel syndrome (IBS)-like patients. Clin Chem Lab Med. 2013 Jun;51(6):1257-63.

Carroccio A, Brusca I, Mansueto P, Pirrone G, Barrale M, Di Prima L, Ambrosiano G, Iacono G, Lospalluti ML, La Chiusa SM, Di Fede G. A cytologic assay for diagnosis of food hypersensitivity in patients with irritable bowel syndrome. Clin Gastroenterol Hepatol. 2010 Mar;8(3):254-60.

Carroccio A, Cavataio F, Montalto G, D'Amico D, Alabrese L, Iacono G. Intolerance to hydrolysed cow's milk proteins in infants: clinical characteristics and dietary treatment. *Clin Exp Allergy.* 2000 Nov;30(11):1597-603.

Carroccio A, Iacono G, Di Prima L, Pirrone G, Cavataio F, Ambrosiano G, Sciumè C, Geraci G, Florena A, Teresi S, Barbaria F, Pepe I, Campisi G, Mansueto P, Soresi M, Di Fede G. Antiendomysium antibodies assay in the culture medium of intestinal mucosa: an accurate method for celiac disease diagnosis. Eur J Gastroenterol Hepatol. 2011 Nov;23(11):1018-23.

Carroccio A, Mansueto P, Iacono G, Soresi M, D'Alcamo A, Cavataio F, Brusca I, Florena AM, Ambrosiano G, Seidita A, Pirrone G, Rini GB. Non-celiac wheat sensitivity diagnosed by double-blind placebo-controlled challenge: exploring a new clinical entity. Am J Gastroenterol. 2012 Dec;107(12):1898-906; quiz 1907.

Carroll D. *The Complete Book of Natural Medicines.* New York: Summit, 1980.

Caruso M, Frasca G, Di Giuseppe PL, Pennisi A, Tringali G, Bonina FP. Effects of a new nutraceutical ingredient on allergen-induced sulphidoleukotrienes production and CD63 expression in allergic subjects. *Int Immunopharmacol.* 2008 Dec 20;8(13-14):1781-6.

Cascella NG, Kryszak D, Bhatti B, Gregory P, Kelly DL, Mc Evoy JP, Fasano A, Eaton WW. Prevalence of celiac disease and gluten sensitivity in the United States clinical antipsychotic trials of intervention effectiveness study population. Schizophr Bull. 2011 Jan;37(1):94-100.

Cash BD, Rubenstein JH, Young PE, Gentry A, Nojkov B, Lee D, Andrews AH, Dobhan R, Chey WD. The prevalence of celiac disease among patients with nonconstipated irritable bowel syndrome is similar to controls. Gastroenterology. 2011 Oct;141(4):1187-93.

Cash BD, Schoenfeld P, Chey WD. The utility of diagnostic tests in irritable bowel syndrome patients: a systematic Am J Gastroenterol. 2002;97:2812–2819.

Cataldo F, Accomando S, Fragapane ML, Montaperto D; SIGENP and GLNBI Working Groups on Food Intolerances. Are food intolerances and allergies increasing in immigrant children coming from developing countries? *Pediatr Allergy Immunol.* 2006 Aug;17(5):364-9.

Catassi C, Anderson RP, Hill ID, Koletzko S, Lionetti E, Mouane N, Schumann M, Yachha SK. World perspective on celiac disease. J Pediatr Gastroenterol Nutr 2012;55(5):494–9.

Catassi C, Bai JC, Bonaz B, Bouma G, Calabrò A, Carroccio A, Castillejo G, Ciacci C, Cristofori F, Dolinsek J, Francavilla R, Elli L, Green P, Holtmeier W, Koehler P, Koletzko S, Meinhold C, Sanders D, Schumann M, Schuppan D, Ullrich R, Vécsei A, Volta U, Zevallos V, Sapone A, Fasano A. Non-Celiac Gluten sensitivity: the new frontier of gluten related disorders. Nutrients. 2013 Sep 26;5(10):3839-53.

Catassi C, Fabiani E, Iacono G, D'Agate C, Francavilla R, Biagi F, Volta U, Accomando S, Picarelli A, De Vitis I, Pianelli G, Gesuita R, Carle F, Mandolesi A, Bearzi I, Fasano A. A prospective, double-blind, placebo-controlled trial to establish a safe gluten threshold for patients with celiac disease. Am J Clin Nutr. 2007 Jan;85(1):160-6.

Catassi C, Kryszak D, Bhatti B, Sturgeon C, Helzlsouer K, Clipp SL, Gelfond D, Puppa E, Sferruzza A, Fasano A. Natural history of celiac disease autoimmunity in a USA cohort followed since 1974. Ann Med. 2010 Oct;42(7):530-8.

Cats A, Kuipers EJ, Bosschaert MA, Pot RG, Vandenbroucke-Grauls CM, Kusters JG. Effect of frequent consumption of a Lactobacillus casei-containing milk drink in Helicobacter pylori-colonized subjects. *Aliment Pharmacol Ther.* 2003 Feb;17(3):429-35.

Cavaleiro C, Pinto E, Gonçalves MJ, Salgueiro L. Antifungal activity of Juniperus essential oils against dermatophyte, Aspergillus and Candida strains. *J Appl Microbiol.* 2006 Jun;100(6):1333-8.

Celakovská J, Van□cková J, Ettlerová K, Ettler K, Bukac J. The role of atopy patch test in diagnosis of food allergy in atopic eczema/dermatitis syndrom in patients over 14 years of age. *Acta Medica (Hradec Kralove).* 2010;53(2):101-8.

Celikel S, Karakaya G, Yurtsever N, Sorkun K, Kalyoncu AF. Bee and bee products allergy in Turkish beekeepers: determination of risk factors for systemic reactions. *Allergol Immunopathol (Madr).* 2006 Sep-Oct;34(5):180-4.

Cereijido M, Contreras RG, Flores-Benítez D, Flores-Maldonado C, Larre I, Ruiz A, Shoshani L. New diseases derived or associated with the tight junction. *Arch Med Res.* 2007 Jul;38(5):465-78.

Céspedes CL, Sampietro DA, Seigler DS, Rai MK. Natural Antioxidants and Biocides from Wild Medicinal Plants. CABI, 2013.

Chafen JJ, Newberry SJ, Riedl MA, Bravata DM, Maglione M, Suttorp MJ, Sundaram V, Paige NM, Towfigh A, Hulley BJ, Shekelle PG. Diagnosing and managing common food allergies: a systematic review. *JAMA.* 2010 May 12;303(18):1848-56.

Chahine BG, Bahna SL. The role of the gut mucosal immunity in the development of tolerance versus development of allergy to food. *Curr Opin Allergy Clin Immunol.* 2010 Aug;10(4):394-9.

Chaitow L, Trenev N. *ProBiotics.* New York: Thorsons, 1990.

Chaitow L. *Conquer Pain the Natural Way.* San Francisco: Chronicle Books, 2002.

Chakurski I, Matev M, Kouchev A, Angelova I, Stefanov G. Treatment of chronic colitis with an herbal combination of Taraxacum officinale, Hipericum perforatum, Melissa officinaliss, Calendula officinalis and Foeniculum vulgare. *Vutr Boles.* 1981;20(6):51-4.

Chan CK, Kuo ML, Shen JJ, See LC, Chang HH, Huang JL. Ding Chuan Tang, a Chinese herb decoction, could improve airway hyper-responsiveness in stabilized asthmatic children: a randomized, double-blind clinical trial. *Pediatr Allergy Immunol.* 2006;17:316–22.

Chandra RK. Prospective studies of the effect of breast feeding on incidence of infection and allergy. *Acta Paediatr Scand.* 1979 Sep;68(5):691-4.

Chaney M, Ross M. *Nutrition.* New York: Houghton Mifflin, 1971.

Chang CI, Chen WC, Shao YY, Yeh GR, Yang NS, Chiang W, Kuo YH. A new labdane-type diterpene from the bark of Juniperus chinensis Linn. *Nat Prod Res.* 2008;22(13):1158-62.

Chang TT, Huang CC, Hsu CH. Clinical evaluation of the Chinese herbal medicine formula STA-1 in the treatment of allergic asthma. *Phytother Res.* 2006;20:342–7.

Chang TT, Huang CC, Hsu CH. Inhibition of mite-induced immunoglobulin E synthesis, airway inflammation, and hyperreactivity by herbal medicine STA-1. *Immunopharmacol Immunotoxicol.* 2006;28:683–95.

Chao A, Thun MJ, Connell CJ, McCullough ML, Jacobs EJ, Flanders WD, Rodriguez C, Sinha R, Calle EE. Meat consumption and risk of colorectal cancer. *JAMA.* 2005 Jan 12;293(2):172-82.

Chapat L, Chemin K, Dubois B, Bourdet-Sicard R, Kaiserlian D. Lactobacillus casei reduces CD8+ T cell-mediated skin inflammation. *Eur J Immunol.* 2004 Sep;34(9):2520-8.

Characterization and quantitation of Antioxidant Constituents of Sweet Pepper (Capsicum annuum - Cayenne). *J Agric Food Chem.* 2004 Jun 16;52(12):3861-9.

Charles K. Food allergies are becoming more common. *N.Y. Daily News.* 2008. May 20.

Chatzi L, Apostolaki G, Bibakis I, Skypala I, Bibaki-Liakou V, Tzanakis N, Kogevinas M, Cullinan P. Protective effect of fruits, vegetables and the Mediterranean diet on asthma and allergies among children in Crete. *Thorax.* 2007 Aug;62(8):677-83.

Chatzi L, Torrent M, Romieu I, Garcia-Esteban R, Ferrer C, Vioque J, Kogevinas M, Sunyer J. Mediterranean diet in pregnancy is protective for wheeze and atopy in childhood. *Thorax.* 2008 Jun;63(6):507-13.

Chavali SR, Weeks CE, Zhong WW, Forse RA. Increased production of TNF-alpha and decreased levels of dienoic eicosanoids, IL-6 and IL-10 in mice fed menhaden oil and juniper oil diets in response to an intraperitoneal lethal dose of LPS. *Prostaglandins Leukot Essent Fatty Acids.* 1998 Aug;59(2):89-93.

Chehade M, Aceves SS. Food allergy and eosinophilic esophagitis. *Curr Opin Allergy Clin Immunol.* 2010 Jun;10(3):231-7.

Chen CY, Milbury PE, Collins FW, Blumberg JB. Avenanthramides are bioavailable and have antioxidant activity in humans after acute consumption of an enriched mixture from oats. J Nutr. 2007 Jun;137(6):1375-82.

Chen G, Jia JF, Hao JG. [In vitro selection and characterization of methionine-resistant variant in Astragalus melilotoides Pall]. Shi Yan Sheng Wu Xue Bao. 2003 Apr;36(2):118-22.

Chen HJ, Shih CK, Hsu HY, Chiang W. Mast cell-dependent allergic responses are inhibited by ethanolic extract of adlay (Coix lachryma-jobi L. var. ma-yuen Stapf) testa. *J Agric Food Chem.* 2010 Feb 24;58(4):2596-601.
Chen SJ, Chao YL, Chen CY, Chang CM, Wu EC, Wu CS, Yeh HH, Chen CH, Tsai HJ. Prevalence of autoimmune diseases in in-patients with schizophrenia: nationwide population-based study. Br J Psychiatry. 2012 May;200(5):374-80.
Cheney G, Waxler SH, Miller IJ. Vitamin U therapy of peptic ulcer; experience at San Quentin Prison. *Calif Med.* 1956 Jan;84(1):39-42.
Chevrier MR, Ryan AE, Lee DY, Zhongze M, Wu-Yan Z, Via CS. Boswellia carterii extract inhibits TH1 cytokines and promotes TH2 cytokines in vitro. *Clin Diagn Lab Immunol.* 2005 May;12(5):575-80.
Chey WD, Olden K, Carter E, Boyle J, Drossman D, Chang L. Utility of the Rome I and Rome II criteria for irritable bowel syndrome in U.S. women. Am J Gastroenterol. 2002;97:2803–2811.
Chihara G. Recent progress in immunopharmacology and therapeutic effects of polysaccharides. Dev Biol Stand. 1992;77:191-7.
Chilton FH, Rudel LL, Parks JS, Arm JP, Seeds MC. Mechanisms by which botanical lipids affect inflammatory disorders. *Am J Clin Nutr.* 2008 Feb;87(2):498S-503S.
Chilton FH, Tucker L. *Win the War Within.* New York: Rodale, 2006.
Chin A Paw MJ, de Jong N, Pallast EG, Kloek GC, Schouten EG, Kok FJ. Immunity in frail elderly: a randomized controlled trial of exercise and enriched foods. *Med Sci Sports Exerc.* 2000 Dec;32(12):2005-11.
Choi SY, Sohn JH, Lee YW, Lee EK, Hong CS, Park JW. Characterization of buckwheat 19-kD allergen and its application for diagnosing clinical reactivity. *Int Arch Allergy Immunol.* 2007;144(4):267-74.
Choi SZ, Choi SU, Lee KR. Phytochemical constituents of the aerial parts from Solidago virga-aurea var. gigantea. *Arch Pharm Res.* 2004 Feb;27(2):164-8.
Chopra RN, Nayar SL, Chopra IC, eds. *Glossary of Indian Medicinal plants.* New Delhi: CSIR, 1956.
Christensen U, Alonso-Simon A, Scheller HV, Willats WG, Harholt J. Characterization of the primary cell walls of seedlings of Brachypodium distachyon – a potential model plant for temperate grasses. Phytochemistry. 2010 Jan;71(1):62-9.
Christopher J. *School of Natural Healing.* Springville UT: Christopher Publ, 1976.
Chrubasik S, Pollak S. Pain management with herbal antirheumatic drugs. *Wien Med Wochenschr.* 2002;152(7-8):198-203.
Chu YF, Liu RH. Cranberries inhibit LDL oxidation and induce LDL receptor expression in hepatocytes. *Life Sci.* 2005;77(15):1892-1901. 27.
Chung SY, Butts CL, Maleki SJ, Champagne ET (2003) Linking peanut allergenicity to the processes of maturation, curing, and roasting. *J Agric Food Chem.* 51: 4273–4277.
Cianferoni A, Khullar K, Saltzman R, Fiedler J, Garrett JP, Naimi DR, Spergel JM. Oral food challenge to wheat: a near-fatal anaphylaxis and review of 93 food challenges in children. World Allergy Organ J. 2013 Aug 21;6(1):14.
Ciccocioppo R, Camarca A, Cangemi GC, Radano G, Vitale S, Betti E, Ferrari D, Visai L, Strada E, Badulli C, Locatelli F, Klersy C, Gianfrani C, Corazza GR. Tolerogenic effect of mesenchymal stromal cells on gliadin-specific T lymphocytes in celiac disease. Cytotherapy. 2014 May 13.
Cingi C, Demirbas D, Songu M. Allergic rhinitis caused by food allergies. *Eur Arch Otorhinolaryngol.* 2010 Sep;267(9):1327-35.
Clark AT, Islam S, King Y, Deighton J, Anagnostou K, Ewan PW. Successful oral tolerance induction in severe peanut allergy. *Allergy.* 2009 Aug;64(8):1218-20.
Clark AT, Mangat JS, Tay SS, King Y, Monk CJ, White PA, Ewan PW. Facial thermography is a sensitive and specific method for assessing food challenge outcome. *Allergy.* 2007 Jul;62(7):744-9.
Cloetens L, Broekaert WF, Delaedt Y, Ollevier F, Courtin CM, Delcour JA, Rutgeerts P, Verbeke K. Tolerance of arabinoxylan-oligosaccharides and their prebiotic activity in healthy subjects: a randomised, placebo-controlled cross-over study. Br J Nutr. 2010 Mar;103(5):703-13.
Cobo Sanz JM, Mateos JA, Muñoz Conejo A. Effect of Lactobacillus casei on the incidence of infectious conditions in children. *Nutr Hosp.* 2006 Jul-Aug;21(4):547-51.
Codispoti CD, Levin L, LeMasters GK, Ryan P, Reponen T, Villareal M, Burkle J, Stanforth S, Lockey JE, Khurana Hershey GK, Bernstein DI. Breast-feeding, aeroallergen sensitization, and environmental exposures during infancy are determinants of childhood allergic rhinitis. *J Allergy Clin Immunol.* 2010 May;125(5):1054-1060.e1.
Cohen A, Goldberg M, Levy B, Leshno M, Katz Y. Sesame food allergy and sensitization in children: the natural history and long-term follow-up. *Pediatr Allergy Immunol.* 2007 May;18(3):217-23.
Comin-Anduix B, Boros LG, Marin S, Boren J, Callol-Massot C, Centelles JJ, Torres JL, Agell N, Bassilian S, Cascante M. Fermented wheat germ extract inhibits glycolysis/pentose cycle enzymes and induces apoptosis through poly(ADP-ribose) polymerase activation in Jurkat T-cell leukemia tumor cells. *J Biol Chem.* 2002 Nov 29;277(48):46408-14.
Conquer JA, Holub BJ. Dietary docosahexaenoic acid as a source of eicosapentaenoic acid in vegetarians and omnivores. *Lipids.* 1997 Mar;32(3):341-5.

Coombs RR, McLaughlan P. Allergenicity of food proteins and its possible modification. Ann Allergy. 1984 Dec;53(6 Pt 2):592-6.

Cooper BT, Holmes GK, Ferguson R, Thompson RA, Allan RN, Cooke WT. Gluten-sensitive diarrhea without evidence of celiac disease. Gastroenterology. 1980;79:801–6.

Cooper GS, Miller FW, Germolec DR: Occupational exposures and autoimmune diseases. *Int Immunopharm* 2002, 2:303-313.

Cooper K. *The Aerobics Program for Total Well-Being.* New York: Evans, 1980.

Corbe C, Boissin JP, Siou A. Light vision and chorioretinal circulation. Study of the effect of procyanidolic oligomers (Endotelon). *J Fr Ophtalmol.* 1988;11(5):453-60.

Courtois P, Nsimba G, Jijakli H, Sener A, Scott FW, Malaisse WJ. Gut permeability and intestinal mucins, invertase, and peroxidase in control and diabetes-prone BB rats fed either a protective or a diabetogenic diet. Dig Dis Sci. 2005 Feb;50(2):266-75.

Couzy F, Kastenmayer P, Vigo M, Clough J, Munoz-Box R, Barclay DV. Calcium bioavailability from a calcium- and sulfate-rich mineral water, compared with milk, in young adult women. *Am J Clin Nutr.* 1995 Dec;62(6):1239-44.

Crescente M, Jessen G, Momi S, Höltje HD, Gresele P, Cerletti C, de Gaetano G. Interactions of gallic acid, resveratrol, quercetin and aspirin at the platelet cyclooxygenase-1 level. Functional and modelling studies. *Thromb Haemost.* 2009 Aug;102(2):336-46.

Cuesta-Herranz J, Barber D, Blanco C, Cistero-Bahíma A, Crespo JF, Fernández-Rivas M, Fernández-Sánchez J, Florido JF, Ibáñez MD, Rodríguez R, Salcedo G, Garcia BE, Lombardero M, Quiralte J, Rodriguez J, Sánchez-Monge R, Vereda A, Villalba M, Alonso Díaz de Durana MD, Basagaña M, Carrillo T, Fernández-Nieto M, Tabar AI. Differences among Pollen-Allergic Patients with and without Plant Food Allergy. *Int Arch Allergy Immunol.* 2010 Apr 23;153(2):182-192.

Cummings M. *Human Heredity: Principles and Issues.* St. Paul, MN: West, 1988.

Dahl R. Wheat sensitive - but not coeliac. Lancet. 1979;1:43–44.

Dalla Pellegrina C, Perbellini O, Scupoli MT, Tomelleri C, Zanetti C, Zoccatelli G, Fusi M, Peruffo A, Rizzi C, Chignola R. Effects of wheat germ agglutinin on human gastrointestinal epithelium: insights from an experimental model of immune/epithelial cell interaction. Toxicol Appl Pharmacol. 2009 Jun 1;237(2):146-53.

Damen B, Cloetens L, Broekaert WF, François I, Lescroart O, Trogh I, Arnaut F, Welling GW, Wijffels J, Delcour JA, Verbeke K, Courtin CM. Consumption of breads containing in situ-produced arabinoxylan oligosaccharides alters gastrointestinal effects in healthy volunteers. J Nutr. 2012 Mar;142(3):470-7.

D'Auria E, Sala M, Lodi F, Radaelli G, Riva E, Giovannini M. Nutritional value of a rice-hydrolysate formula in infants with cows' milk protein allergy: a randomized pilot study. *J Int Med Res.* 2003 May-Jun;31(3):215-22.

Davies G. *Timetables of Medicine.* New York: Black Dog & Leventhal, 2000.

Davin JC, Forget P, Mahieu PR. Increased intestinal permeability to (51 Cr) EDTA is correlated with IgA immune complex-plasma levels in children with IgA-associated nephropathies. *Acta Paediatr Scand.* 1988 Jan;77(1):118-24.

Davis JM, Murphy EA, Brown AS, Carmichael MD, Ghaffar A, Mayer EP. Effects of oat beta-glucan on innate immunity and infection after exercise stress. Med Sci Sports Exerc. 2004 Aug;36(8):1321-7.

De Angelis M, Rizzello CG, Fasano A, Clemente MG, De Simone C, Silano M, De Vincenzi M, Losito I, Gobbetti M. VSL#3 probiotic preparation has the capacity to hydrolyze gliadin polypeptides responsible for Celiac Sprue. Biochim Biophys Acta. 2006 Jan;1762(1):80-93.

de Boissieu D, Dupont C, Badoual J. Allergy to nondairy proteins in mother's milk as assessed by intestinal permeability tests. *Allergy.* 1994 Dec;49(10):882-4.

de Boissieu D, Matarazzo P, Rocchiccioli F, Dupont C. Multiple food allergy: a possible diagnosis in breastfed infants. *Acta Paediatr.* 1997 Oct;86(10):1042-6.

De Knop KJ, Hagendorens MM, Bridts CH, Stevens WJ, Ebo DG. Macadamia nut allergy: 2 case reports and a review of the literature. *Acta Clin Belg.* 2010 Mar-Apr;65(2):129-32.

De Lucca AJ, Bland JM, Vigo CB, Cushion M, Selitrennikoff CP, Peter J, Walsh TJ. CAY-I, a fungicidal saponin from Capsicum sp. fruit. *Med Mycol.* 2002 Apr;40(2):131-7.

de Magistris L, Picardi A, Siniscalco D, Riccio MP, Sapone A, Cariello R, Abbadessa S, Medici N, Lammers KM, Schiraldi C, Iardino P, Marotta R, Tolone C, Fasano A, Pascotto A, Bravaccio C. Antibodies against food antigens in patients with autistic spectrum disorders. Biomed Res Int. 2013;2013:729349.

de Martino M, Novembre E, Galli L, de Marco A, Botarelli P, Marano E, Vierucci A. Allergy to different fish species in cod-allergic children: in vivo and in vitro studies. *J Allergy Clin Immunol.* 1990;86:909-914.

De Mejia EG, Del Carmen Valadez-Vega M, Reynoso-Camacho R, Loarca-Pina G. Tannins, trypsin inhibitors and lectin cytotoxicity in tepary (Phaseolus acutifolius) and common (Phaseolus vulgaris) beans. Plant Foods Hum Nutr. 2005 Sep;60(3):137-45.

de Noni I, Pagani MA. Cooking properties and heat damage of dried pasta as influenced by raw material characteristics and processing conditions. Crit Rev Food Sci Nutr. 2010 May;50(5):465-72.

de Punder K, Pruimboom L. The dietary intake of wheat and other cereal grains and their role in inflammation. Nutrients. 2013 Mar 12;5(3):771-87.

De Santis A, Addolorato G, Romito A, Caputo S, Giordano A, Gambassi G, Taranto C, Manna R, Gasbarrini G. Schizophrenic symptoms and SPECT abnormalities in a coeliac patient: regression after a gluten-free diet. J Intern Med. 1997 Nov;242(5):421-3.

De Smet PA. Herbal remedies. *N Engl J Med.* 2002;347:2046–2056.

Dean C. *Death by Modern Medicine.* Belleville, ON: Matrix Verite-Media, 2005.

del Giudice MM, Leonardi S, Maiello N, Brunese FP. Food allergy and probiotics in childhood. *J Clin Gastroenterol.* 2010 Sep;44 Suppl 1:S22-5.

Delcour JA, Vansteelandt J, Hythier M, Abécassis J, Sindic M, Deroanne C. Fractionation and reconstitution experiments provide insight into the role of gluten and starch interactions in pasta quality. J Agric Food Chem. 2000 Sep;48(9):3767-73.

Delcour JA, Vansteelandt J, Hythier M, Abécassis J. Fractionation and reconstitution experiments provide insight into the role of starch gelatinization and pasting properties in pasta quality. J Agric Food Chem. 2000 Sep;48(9):3774-8.

D'Elia L, Iannotta C, Sabino P, Ippolito R. Potassium-rich diet and risk of stroke: updated meta-analysis. Nutr Metab Cardiovasc Dis. 2014 Mar 18. pii: S0939-4753(14)00106-9.

DeMeo MT, Mutlu EA, Keshavarzian A, Tobin MC. Intestinal permeation and gastrointestinal disease. *J Clin Gastroenterol.* 2002 Apr;34(4):385-96.

Demidov LV, Manziuk LV, Kharkevitch GY, Pirogova NA, Artamonova EV. Adjuvant fermented wheat germ extract (Avemar) nutraceutical improves survival of high-risk skin melanoma patients: a randomized, pilot, phase II clinical study with a 7-year follow-up. Cancer Biother Radiopharm. 2008 Aug;23(4):477-82.

Dengate S, Ruben A. Controlled trial of cumulative behavioural effects of a common bread preservative. *J Paediatr Child Health.* 2002 Aug;38(4):373-6.

Derebery MJ, Berliner KI. Allergy and its relation to Meniere's disease. *Otolaryngol Clin North Am.* 2010 Oct;43(5):1047-58.

Desjeux JF, Heyman M. Milk proteins, cytokines and intestinal epithelial functions in children. *Acta Paediatr Jpn.* 1994 Oct;36(5):592-6.

DesRoches A, Infante-Rivard C, Paradis L, Paradis J, Haddad E. Peanut allergy: is maternal transmission of antigens during pregnancy and breastfeeding a risk factor? *J Investig Allergol Clin Immunol.* 2010;20(4):289-94.

Deutsche Gesellschaft für Ernährung. Drink distilled water? *Med. Mo. Pharm.* 1993;16:146.

Devaraj TL. *Speaking of Ayurvedic Remedies for Common Diseases.* New Delhi: Sterling, 1985.

Dewar DH, Amato M, Ellis HJ, Pollock EL, Gonzalez-Cinca N, Wieser H, Ciclitira PJ. The toxicity of high molecular weight glutenin subunits of wheat to patients with coeliac disease. Eur J Gastroenterol Hepatol. 2006 May;18(5):483-91.

Di Cagno R, De Angelis M, Auricchio S, Greco L, Clarke C, De Vincenzi M, Giovannini C, D'Archivio M, Landolfo F, Parrilli G, Minervini F, Arendt E, Gobbetti M. Sourdough bread made from wheat and nontoxic flours and started with selected lactobacilli is tolerated in celiac sprue patients. Appl Environ Microbiol. 2004 Feb;70(2):1088-96.

Di Cagno R, De Angelis M, Lavermicocca P, De Vincenzi M, Giovannini C, Faccia M, Gobbetti M. Proteolysis by sourdough lactic acid bacteria: effects on wheat flour protein fractions and gliadin peptides involved in human cereal intolerance. Appl Environ Microbiol. 2002 Feb;68(2):623-33.

Dickerson F, Stallings C, Origoni A, Vaughan C, Khushalani S, Alaedini A, Yolken R. Markers of gluten sensitivity and celiac disease in bipolar disorder. Bipolar Disord. 2011 Feb;13(1):52-8.

Dickerson F, Stallings C, Origoni A, Vaughan C, Khushalani S, Leister F, Yang S, Krivogorsky B, Alaedini A, Yolken R. Markers of gluten sensitivity and celiac disease in recent-onset psychosis and multi-episode schizophrenia. Biol Psychiatry. 2010 Jul 1;68(1):100-4.

Dickerson F, Stallings C, Origoni A, Vaughan C, Khushalani S, Yolken R. Markers of gluten sensitivity in acute mania: a longitudinal study. Psychiatry Res. 2012 Mar 30;196(1):68-71.

Dickerson JWT, Ballantine L, Hastrop K. Food allergy. Lancet. 1978;1:773.

Dickey W, Hughes DF, McMillan SA. Patients with serum IgA endomysial antibodies and intact duodenal villi: clinical characteristics and management options. Scand J Gastroenterol. 2005;40:1240–43.

Dickey W, Kearney N. Overweight in celiac disease: prevalence, clinical characteristics, and effect of a gluten-free diet. Am J Gastoenterol. 2006;101(10):2356–9.

Diesner SC, Untersmayr E, Pietschmann P, Jensen-Jarolim E. Food Allergy: Only a Pediatric Disease? *Gerontology.* 2010 Jan 29.

Dieterich W, Ehnis T, Bauer M, Donner P, Volta U, Riecken EO, Schuppan D. Identification of tissue transglutaminase as the autoantigen of celiac disease. Nat Med. 1997 Jul;3(7):797-801.

DiGiacomo DV, Tennyson CA, Green PH, Demmer RT. Prevalence of gluten-free diet adherence among individuals without celiac disease in the USA: results from the Continuous National Health and Nutrition Examination Survey 2009-2010. Scand J Gastroenterol. 2013 Aug;48(8):921-5.

Diğrak M, Ilçim A, Hakki Alma M. Antimicrobial activities of several parts of Pinus brutia, Juniperus oxycedrus, Abies cilicia, Cedrus libani and Pinus nigra. *Phytother Res.* 1999 Nov;13(7):584-7.

Din FV, Theodoratou E, Farrington SM, Tenesa A, Barnetson RA, Cetnarskyj R, Stark L, Porteous ME, Campbell H, Dunlop MG. Effect of aspirin and NSAIDs on risk and survival from colorectal cancer. *Gut.* 2010 Dec;59(12):1670-9.

Diop L, Guillou S, Durand H. Probiotic food supplement reduces stress-induced gastrointestinal symptoms in volunteers: a double-blind, placebo-controlled, randomized trial. *Nutr Res.* 2008 Jan;28(1):1-5.

Do Nascimento AB, Fiates GM, Dos Anjos A, Teixeira E. Gluten-free is not enough - perception and suggestions of celiac consumers. Int J Food Sci Nutr. 2014 Jun;65(4):394-8.

Dobrotvorskaia TV, Martynov SP. Analysis of diversity of Russian and Ukrainian bread wheat (Triticum aestivum L.) cultivars for high-molecular-weight glutenin subunits. Genetika. 2011 Jul;47(7):905-19.

Dona A, Arvanitoyannis IS. Health risks of genetically modified foods. *Crit Rev Food Sci Nutr.* 2009 Feb;49(2):164-75.

Donato F, Monarca S, Premi S., and Gelatti, U. Drinking water hardness and chronic degenerative diseases. Part III. Tumors, urolithiasis, fetal malformations, deterioration of the cognitive function in the aged and atopic eczema. *Ann. Ig.* 2003;15:57-70.

Dooley, M.A. and Hogan S.L. Environmental epidemiology and risk factors for autoimmune disease. *Curr Opin Rheum.* 2003;15(2):99-103.

D'Orazio N, Ficoneri C, Riccioni G, Conti P, Theoharides TC, Bollea MR. Conjugated linoleic acid: a functional food? *Int J Immunopathol Pharmacol.* 2003 Sep-Dec;16(3):215-20.

Dotolo Institute. *The Study of Colon Hydrotherapy.* Pinellas Park, FL: Dotolo, 2003.

Drago S, El Asmar R, Di Pierro M, Grazia Clemente M, Tripathi A, Sapone A, Thakar M, Iacono G, Carroccio A, D'Agate C, Not T, Zampini L, Catassi C, Fasano A. Gliadin, zonulin and gut permeability: Effects on celiac and non-celiac intestinal mucosa and intestinal cell lines. Scand J Gastroenterol. 2006 Apr;41(4):408-19.

Drouault-Holowacz S, Bieuvelet S, Burckel A, Cazaubiel M, Dray X, Marteau P. A double blind randomized controlled trial of a probiotic combination in 100 patients with irritable bowel syndrome. *Gastroenterol Clin Biol.* 2008 Feb;32(2):147-52.

Ducrotté P. Irritable bowel syndrome: from the gut to the brain-gut. *Gastroenterol Clin Biol.* 2009 Aug-Sep;33(8-9):703-12.

Duke J. *The Green Pharmacy.* New York: St. Martins, 1997.

Dunlop SP, Hebden J, Campbell E, Naesdal J, Olbe L, Perkins AC, Spiller RC. Abnormal intestinal permeability in subgroups of diarrhea-predominant irritable bowel syndromes. Am J Gastroenterol. 2006 Jun;101(6):1288-94.

Dunstan JA, Hale J, Breckler L, Lehmann H, Weston S, Richmond P, Prescott SL. Atopic dermatitis in young children is associated with impaired interleukin-10 and interferon-gamma responses to allergens, vaccines and colonizing skin and gut bacteria. *Clin Exp Allergy.* 2005 Oct;35(10):1309-17.

Dunstan JA, Roper J, Mitoulas L, Hartmann PE, Simmer K, Prescott SL. The effect of supplementation with fish oil during pregnancy on breast milk immunoglobulin A, soluble CD14, cytokine levels and fatty acid composition. *Clin Exp Allergy.* 2004 Aug;34(8):1237-42.

Dupont C, Barau E, Molkhou P, Raynaud F, Barbet JP, Dehennin L. Food-induced alterations of intestinal permeability in children with cow's milk-sensitive enteropathy and atopic dermatitis. *J Pediatr Gastroenterol Nutr.* 1989 May;8(4):459-65.

Dupont C, Barau E, Molkhou P. Intestinal permeability disorders in children. *Allerg Immunol (Paris).* 1991 Mar;23(3):95-103.

Dupont C, Barau E. Diagnosis of food allergy in children. *Ann Pediatr (Paris).* 1992 Jan;39(1):5-12.

Dupont C, Soulaines P, Lapillonne A, Donne N, Kalach N, Benhamou P. Atopy patch test for early diagnosis of cow's milk allergy in preterm infants. *J Pediatr Gastroenterol Nutr.* 2010 Apr;50(4):463-4.

Dupuy P, Cassé M, André F, Dhivert-Donnadieu H, Pinton J, Hernandez-Pion C. Low-salt water reduces intestinal permeability in atopic patients. *Dermatology.* 1999;198(2):153-5.

Duran-Tauleria E, Vignati G, Guedan MJ, Petersson CJ. The utility of specific immunoglobulin E measurements in primary care. *Allergy.* 2004 Aug;59 Suppl 78:35-41.

D'Urbano LE, Pellegrino K, Artesani MC, Donnanno S, Luciano R, Riccardi C, Tozzi AE, Ravà L, De Benedetti F, Cavagni G. Performance of a component-based allergen-microarray in the diagnosis of cow's milk and hen's egg allergy. *Clin Exp Allergy.* 2010 Jul 13.

Duwiejua M, Zeitlin IJ, Waterman PG, Chapman J, Mhango GJ, Provan GJ. Anti-inflammatory activity of resins from some species of the plant family Burseraceae. *Planta Med.* 1993 Feb;59(1):12-6.

Dykewicz MS, Lemmon JK, Keaney DL. Comparison of the Multi-Test II and Skintestor Omni allergy skin test devices. *Ann Allergy Asthma Immunol.* 2007 Jun;98(6):559-62.

Eastham EJ, Walker WA. Effect of cow's milk on the gastrointestinal tract: a persistent dilemma for the pediatrician. *Pediatrics*. 1977 Oct;60(4):477-81.

Eaton KK, Howard M, Howard JM. Gut permeability measured by polyethylene glycol absorption in abnormal gut fermentation as compared with food intolerance. *J R Soc Med.* 1995 Feb;88(2):63-6.

Eaton W, Mortensen PB, Agerbo E, Byrne M, Mors O, Ewald H. Coeliac disease and schizophrenia: population based case control study with linkage of Danish national registers. BMJ. 2004 Feb 21;328(7437):438-9.

Ebers GC, Kukay K, Bulman DE, Sadovnick AD, Rice G, Anderson C, Armstrong H, Cousin K, Bell RB, Hader W, Paty DW, Hashimoto S, Oger J, Duquette P, Warren S, Gray T, O'Connor P, Nath A, Auty A, Metz L, Francis G, Paulseth JE, Murray TJ, Pryse-Phillips W, Nelson R, Freedman M, Brunet D, Bouchard JP, Hinds D, Risch N. A full genome search in multiple sclerosis. *Nat Genet.* 1996 Aug;13(4):472-6.

ECRHS (2002) The European Community Respiratory Health Survey II. *Eur Respir J.* 20: 1071–1079.

Ege MJ, Herzum I, Büchele G, Krauss-Etschmann S, Lauener RP, Roponen M, Hyvärinen A, Vuitton DA, Riedler J, Brunekreef B, Dalphin JC, Braun-Fahrländer C, Pekkanen J, Renz H, von Mutius E; Protection Against Allergy Study in Rural Environments (PASTURE) Study group. Prenatal exposure to a farm environment modifies atopic sensitization at birth. *J Allergy Clin Immunol.* 2008 Aug;122(2):407-12, 412.e1-4.

Egeberg R, Olsen A, Loft S, Christensen J, Johnsen NF, Overvad K, Tjønneland A. Intake of wholegrain products and risk of colorectal cancers in the Diet, Cancer and Health cohort study. Br J Cancer. 2010 Aug 24;103(5):730-4.

Eggermont E. Cow's milk protein allergy. *Tijdschr Kindergeneeskd.* 1981 Feb;49(1):16-20.

Ehling S, Hengel M, and Shibamoto T. Formation of acrylamide from lipids. *Adv Exp Med Biol* 2005, 561:223-233.

Ehren J, Morón B, Martin E, Bethune MT, Gray GM, Khosla C. A food-grade enzyme preparation with modest gluten detoxification properties. PLoS One. 2009 Jul 21;4(7):e6313.

Ehren J, Morón B, Martin E, Bethune MT, Gray GM, Khosla C. A food-grade enzyme preparation with modest gluten detoxification properties. *PLoS One.* 2009 Jul 21;4(7):e6313.

el-Ghazaly M, Khayyal MT, Okpanyi SN, Arens-Corell M. Study of the anti-inflammatory activity of Populus tremula, Solidago virgaurea and Fraxinus excelsior. *Arzneimittelforschung.* 1992 Mar;42(3):333-6.

El-Ghorab A, Shaaban HA, El-Massry KF, Shibamoto T. Chemical composition of volatile extract and biological activities of volatile and less-volatile extracts of juniper berry (Juniperus drupacea L.) fruit. *J Agric Food Chem.* 2008 Jul 9;56(13):5021-5.

El-Khouly F, Lewis SA, Pons L, Burks AW, Hourihane JO. IgG and IgE avidity characteristics of peanut allergic individuals. *Pediatr Allergy Immunol.* 2007 Nov;18(7):607-13.

Ellingwood F. *American Materia Medica, Therapeutics and Pharmacognosy.* Portland: Eclectic Medical Publ., 1983.

Elliott RB, Harris DP, Hill JP, Bibby NJ, Wasmuth HE. Type I (insulin-dependent) diabetes mellitus and cow milk: casein variant consumption. *Diabetologia.* 1999 Mar;42(3):292-6. Erratum in: Diabetologia 1999 Aug;42(8):1032.

Ellis A, Linaker BD. Non-coeliac gluten sensitivity? Lancet. 1978;1(8061):1358.

Elwood PC. Epidemiology and trace elements. *Clin Endocrinol Metab.* 1985 Aug;14(3):617-28.

Engel, M.F., Dimethyl sulfoxide in the treatment of scleroderma. *South Med J.* 1972;65:71.

Engler RJ. Alternative and complementary medicine: a source of improved therapies for asthma? A challenge for redefining the specialty? J Allergy Clin Immunol. 2000;106:627–9.

Environmental Working Group. *Human Toxome Project.* 2007. http://www.ewg.org/sites/ humantoxome/. Accessed: 2007 Sep.

EPA. *A Brief Guide to Mold, Moisture and Your Home.* Environmental Protection Agency, Office of Air and Radiation/Indoor Environments Division. EPA 2002;402-K-02-003.

Ernst E. Frankincense: systematic review. *BMJ.* 2008 Dec 17;337:a2813.

Erwin EA, James HR, Gutekunst HM, Russo JM, Kelleher KJ, Platts-Mills TA. Serum IgE measurement and detection of food allergy in pediatric patients with eosinophilic esophagitis. *Ann Allergy Asthma Immunol.* 2010 Jun;104(6):496-502.

Estévez AM, Castillo E, Figuerola F, Yáñez E. Effect of processing on some chemical and nutritional characteristics of pre-cooked and dehydrated legumes. Plant Foods Hum Nutr. 1991 Jul;41(3):193-201.

Eswaran S, Goel A, Chey WD. What role does wheat play in the symptoms of irritable bowel syndrome? Gastroenterol Hepatol (N Y). 2013 Feb;9(2):85-91.

Eswaran S, Muir J, Chey WD. Fiber and functional gastrointestinal disorders. Am J Gastroenterol. 2013;108:718–27. Up-to-date review of fibre and its potential in symptom induction and therapy in functionial gastrointestinsl disorders.

Eswaran S, Tack J, Chey WD. Food: the forgotten factor in the irritable bowel syndrome. Gastroenterol Clin North Am. 2011;40:141–162.

European Society for Pediatric Gastroenterology, Hepatology, and Nutrition guidelines for the diagnosis of coeliac disease. J Pediatr Gastroenterol Nutr. 2012;54(1):136–60.

EuroPrevall. *WP 1.1 Birth Cohort Update.* 1st Quarter 2006. Berlin, Germany: Charité University Medical Centre.

Eutamene H, Lamine F, Chabo C, Theodorou V, Rochat F, Bergonzelli GE, Corthésy-Theulaz I, Fioramonti J, Bueno L. Synergy between Lactobacillus paracasei and its bacterial products to counteract stress-induced gut permeability and sensitivity increase in rats. *J Nutr.* 2007 Aug;137(8):1901-7.

Evans P, Forte D, Jacobs C, Fredhoi C, Aitchison E, Hucklebridge F, Clow A. Cortisol secretory activity in older people in relation to positive and negative well-being. *Psychoneuroendocrinology.* 2007 Aug 7

Everhart JE. *Digestive Diseases in the United States.* Darby, PA: Diane Pub, 1994.

Exl BM, Deland U, Secretin MC, Preysch U, Wall M, Shmerling DH. Improved general health status in an unselected infant population following an allergen reduced dietary intervention programme. The ZUFF-study-programme. Part I: Study design and 6-month nutritional behaviour. *Eur J Nutr.* 2000 Jun;39(3):89-102.

FAAN. *Public Comment on 2005 Food Safety Survey: Docket No. 2004N-0516 (2005 FSS).* Fairfax, VA: Food Allergy & Anaphylaxis Network.

Faeste CK, Christians U, Egaas E, Jonscher KR. Characterization of potential allergens in fenugreek (Trigonella foenum-graecum) using patient sera and MS-based proteomic analysis. *J Proteomics.* 2010 May 7;73(7):1321-33.

Faeste CK, Jonscher KR, Sit L, Klawitter J, Løvberg KE, Moen LH. Differentiating cross-reacting allergens in the immunological analysis of celery (Apium graveolens) by mass spectrometry. *J AOAC Int.* 2010 Mar-Apr;93(2):451-61.

Fajac I, Frossard N. Neuropeptides of the nasal innervation and allergic rhinitis. *Rev Mal Respir.* 1994;11(4):357-67.

Falchuk ZM. Gluten-sensitive diarrhea without enteropathy: fact of fancy? Gastroenterology. 1980;79:953–55.

Fälth-Magnusson K, Kjellman NI, Magnusson KE, Sundqvist T. Intestinal permeability in healthy and allergic children before and after sodium-cromoglycate treatment assessed with different-sized polyethyleneglycols (PEG 400 and PEG 1000). *Clin Allergy.* 1984 May;14(3):277-86.

Fälth-Magnusson K, Kjellman NI, Odelram H, Sundqvist T, Magnusson KE. Gastrointestinal permeability in children with cow's milk allergy: effect of milk challenge and sodium cromoglycate as assessed with polyethyleneglycols (PEG 400 and PEG 1000). *Clin Allergy.* 1986 Nov;16(6):543-51.

Famularo G, De Simone C, Pandey V, Sahu AR, Minisola G . Probiotic lactobacilli: an innovative tool to correct the malabsorption syndrome of vegetarians? Med. Hypotheses. 2005:65(6):1132–5.

Fan AY, Lao L, Zhang RX, Zhou AN, Wang LB, Moudgil KD, Lee DY, Ma ZZ, Zhang WY, Berman BM. Effects of an acetone extract of Boswellia carterii Birdw. (Burseraceae) gum resin on adjuvant-induced arthritis in lewis rats. *J Ethnopharmacol.* 2005 Oct 3;101(1-3):104-9.

Fanaro S, Marten B, Bagna R, Vigi V, Fabris C, Peña-Quintana, Argüelles F, Scholz-Ahrens KE, Sawatzki G, Zelenka R, Schrezenmeir J, de Vrese M and Bertino E. Galacto-oligosaccharides are bifidogenic and safe at weaning: A double-blind Randomized Multicenter study. *J Pediatr Gastroent Nutr.* 2009 48; 82-88

Fang SP, Tanaka T, Tago F, Okamoto T, Kojima S. Immunomodulatory effects of gyokuheifusan on INF-gamma/IL-4 (Th1/Th2) balance in ovalbumin (OVA)-induced asthma model mice. *Biol Pharm Bull.* 2005;28:829–33.

Faniglíulo L, Comparato G, Aragona G, Cavallaro L, Iori V, Maino M, Cavestro GM, Soliani P, Sianesi M, Franzè A, Di Mario F. Role of gut microflora and probiotic effects in the irritable bowel syndrome. *Acta Biomed.* 2006 Aug;77(2):85-9.

FAO/WHO Expert Committee. *Fats and Oils in Human Nutrition.* Food and Nutrition Paper. 1994;(57).

Fardet A. New hypotheses for the health-protective mechanisms of whole-grain cereals: what is beyond fibre? Nutr Res Rev. 2010 Jun;23(1):65-134.

Fasano A, Berti I, Gerarduzzi T, Not T, Colletti RB, Drago S, Elitsur Y, Green PH, Guandalini S, Hill ID, Pietzak M, Ventura A, Thorpe M, Kryszak D, Fornaroli F, Wasserman SS, Murray JA, Horvath K. Prevalence of celiac disease in at-risk and not-at-risk groups in the United States: a large multicenter study. *Arch Intern Med.* 2003 Feb 10;163(3):286-92.

Fasano A, Not T, Wang W, Uzzau S, Berti I, Tommasini A, Goldblum SE. Zonulin, a newly discovered modulator of intestinal permeability, and its expression in coeliac disease. Lancet. 2000 Apr 29;355(9214):1518-9.

Fasano A. Zonulin and its regulation of intestinal barrier function: the biological door to inflammation, autoimmunity, and cancer. Physiol Rev. 2011 Jan;91(1):151-75.

Fasano A. Zonulin, regulation of tight junctions, and autoimmune diseases. Ann N Y Acad Sci. 2012 Jul;1258:25-33.

Fawell J, Nieuwenhuijsen MJ. Contaminants in drinking water. *Br Med Bull.* 2003;68:199-208.

Felley CP, Corthésy-Theulaz I, Rivero JL, Sipponen P, Kaufmann M, Bauerfeind P, Wiesel PH, Brassart D, Pfeifer A, Blum AL, Michetti P. Favourable effect of an acidified milk (LC-1) on Helicobacter pylori gastritis in man. *Eur J Gastroenterol Hepatol.* 2001 Jan;13(1):25-9.

Fernandez-Feo M, Wei G, Blumenkranz G, Dewhirst FE, Schuppan D, Oppenheim FG, Helmerhorst EJ. The cultivable human oral gluten-degrading microbiome and its potential implications in coeliac disease and gluten sensitivity. Clin Microbiol Infect. 2013 Sep;19(9):E386-94.

Fernández-Moya V, Martínez-Force E, Garcés R. Temperature effect on a high stearic acid sunflower mutant. Phytochemistry. 2002 Jan;59(1):33-7.1.

Fernández-Rivas M, Garrido Fernández S, Nadal JA, Díaz de Durana MD, García BE, González-Mancebo E, Martín S, Barber D, Rico P, Tabar AI. Randomized double-blind, placebo-controlled trial of sublingual immunotherapy with a Pru p 3 quantified peach extract. *Allergy.* 2009 Jun;64(6):876-83.

Fernández-Rivas M, González-Mancebo E, Rodríguez-Pérez R, Benito C, Sánchez-Monge R, Salcedo G, Alonso MD, Rosado A, Tejedor MA, Vila C, Casas ML. Clinically relevant peach allergy is related to peach lipid transfer protein, Pru p 3, in the Spanish population. *J Allergy Clin Immunol.* 2003 Oct;112(4):789-95.
Ferreira M, Davies SL, Butler M, Scott D, Clark M, Kumar P. Endomysial antibody: is it the best screening test for coeliac disease? Gut. 1992 Dec;33(12):1633-7.
Ferrier L, Berard F, Debrauwer L, Chabo C, Langella P, Bueno L, Fioramonti J. Impairment of the intestinal barrier by ethanol involves enteric microflora and mast cell activation in rodents. *Am J Pathol.* 2006 Apr;168(4):1148-54.
Filipowicz N, Kamiński M, Kurlenda J, Asztemborska M, Ochocka JR. Antibacterial and antifungal activity of juniper berry oil and its selected components. *Phytother Res.* 2003 Mar;17(3):227-31.
Finkelman FD, Boyce JA, Vercelli D, Rothenberg ME. Key advances in mechanisms of asthma, allergy, and immunology in 2009. *J Allergy Clin Immunol.* 2010 Feb;125(2):312-8.
Fiocchi A, Restani P, Bernardo L, Martelli A, Ballabio C, D'Auria E, Riva E. Tolerance of heat-treated kiwi by children with kiwifruit allergy. *Pediatr Allergy Immunol.* 2004 Oct;15(5):454-8.
Fiocchi A, Travaini M, D'Auria E, Banderali G, Bernardo L, Riva E. Tolerance to a rice hydrolysate formula in children allergic to cow's milk and soy. *Clin Exp Allergy.* 2003 Nov;33(11):1576-80.
Fiocchi, A; Restani, P; Riva, E; Qualizza, R; Bruni, P; Restelli, AR; Galli, CL. Meat allergy: I. Specific IgE to BSA and OSA in atopic, beef sensitive children. *J Am Coll Nutr.* 1995 14: 239-244.
Flammarion S, Santos C, Guimber D, Jouannic L, Thumerelle C, Gottrand F, Deschildre A. Diet and nutritional status of children with food allergies. *Pediatr Allergy Immunol.* 2010 Jun 14.
Flandrin, J, Montanari M. (eds.). *Food: A Culinary History from Antiquity to the Present.* New York: Penguin Books, 1999.
Fleischer DM, Conover-Walker MK, Christie L, Burks AW, Wood RA. Peanut allergy: recurrence and its management. *J Allergy Clin Immunol.* 2004 Nov;114(5):1195-201.
Flinterman AE, Pasmans SG, den Hartog Jager CF, Hoekstra MO, Bruijnzeel-Koomen CA, Knol EF, van Hoffen E. T cell responses to major peanut allergens in children with and without peanut allergy. *Clin Exp Allergy.* 2010 Apr;40(4):590-7.
Flinterman AE, van Hoffen E, den Hartog Jager CF, Koppelman S, Pasmans SG, Hoekstra MO, Bruijnzeel-Koomen CA, Knulst AC, Knol EF. Children with peanut allergy recognize predominantly Ara h2 and Ara h6, which remains stable over time. *Clin Exp Allergy.* 2007 Aug;37(8):1221-8.
Folkes BF, Yemm EW. The amino acid content of the proteins of barley grains. Biochem J. 1956 Jan;62(1):4-11.
Food allergy continues to increase. *Child Health Alert.* 2010 Jan;28:2.
Food and Drug Administration, HHS. Food labeling: health claims; soluble dietary fiber from certain foods and coronary heart disease. Interim final rule. Fed Regist. 2002 Oct 2;67(191):61773-83.
Forbes EE, Groschwitz K, Abonia JP, Brandt EB, Cohen E, Blanchard C, Ahrens R, Seidu L, McKenzie A, Strait R, Finkelman FD, Foster PS, Matthaei KI, Rothenberg ME, Hogan SP. IL-9- and mast cell-mediated intestinal permeability predisposes to oral antigen hypersensitivity. *J Exp Med.* 2008 Apr 14;205(4):897-913.
Ford AC, Chey WD, Talley NJ, Malhotra A, Spiegel BM. Moayyedi P Yield of diagnostic tests for celiac disease in individuals with symptoms suggestive of irritable bowel syndrome: systematic review and meta-analysis. Arch Intern Med. 2009;169:651–658.
Forestier C, Guelon D, Cluytens V, Gillart T, Sirot J, De Champs C. Oral probiotic and prevention of Pseudomonas aeruginosa infections: a randomized, double-blind, placebo-controlled pilot study in intensive care unit patients. *Crit Care.* 2008;12(3):R69.
Forget P, Sodoyez-Goffaux F, Zappitelli A. Permeability of the small intestine to 51Cr EDTA in children with acute gastroenteritis or eczema. *J Pediatr Gastroenterol Nutr.* 1985 Jun;4(3):393-6.
Forget-Dubois N, Boivin M, Dionne G, Pierce T, Tremblay RE, Pérusse D. A longitudinal twin study of the genetic and environmental etiology of maternal hostile-reactive behavior during infancy and toddlerhood. *Infant Behav Dev.* 2007
Forsberg G, Fahlgren A, Hörstedt P, Hammarström S, Hernell O, Hammarström ML. Presence of bacteria and innate immunity of intestinal epithelium in childhood celiac disease. Am J Gastroenterol. 2004 May;99(5):894-904.
Foster S, Hobbs C. *Medicinal Plants and Herbs.* Boston: Houghton Mifflin, 2002.
Fox RD, *Algoculture.* Doctorate Disseration, 1983 Jul.
Francavilla R, Lionetti E, Castellaneta SP, Magistà AM, Maurogiovanni G, Bucci N, De Canio A, Indrio F, Cavallo L, Ierardi E, Miniello VL. Inhibition of Helicobacter pylori infection in humans by Lactobacillus reuteri ATCC 55730 and effect on eradication therapy: a pilot study. *Helicobacter.* 2008 Apr;13(2):127-34.
François IE, Lescroart O, Veraverbeke WS, Marzorati M, Possemiers S, Hamer H, Windey K, Welling GW, Delcour JA, Courtin CM, Verbeke K, Broekaert WF. Effects of a Wheat Bran Extract Containing Arabinoxylan Oligosaccharides on Gastrointestinal Parameters in Healthy Preadolescent Children: A Double-Blind, Randomized, Placebo-Controlled, Crossover Trial. J Pediatr Gastroenterol Nutr. 2013 Dec 22.
François IE, Lescroart O, Veraverbeke WS, Marzorati M, Possemiers S, Evenepoel P, Hamer H, Houben E, Windey K, Welling GW, Delcour JA, Courtin CM, Verbeke K, Broekaert WF. Effects of a wheat bran extract containing ara-

binoxylan oligosaccharides on gastrointestinal health parameters in healthy adult human volunteers: a double-blind, randomised, placebo-controlled, cross-over trial. Br J Nutr. 2012 Dec 28;108(12):2229-42.

Frank J. Beyond vitamin E supplementation: an alternative strategy to improve vitamin E status. J Plant Physiol. 2005 Jul;162(7):834-43.

Frawley D, Lad V. *The Yoga of Herbs.* Sante Fe: Lotus Press, 1986.

Fremont S, Moneret-Vautrin DA, Franck P, Morisset M, Croizier A, Codreanu F, Kanny G. Prospective study of sensitization and food allergy to flaxseed in 1317 subjects. *Eur Ann Allergy Clin Immunol.* 2010 Jun;42(3):103-11.

Frias J, Song YS, Martínez-Villaluenga C, González de Mejia E, Vidal-Valverde C. Immunoreactivity and amino acid content of fermented soybean products. *J Agric Food Chem.* 2008 Jan 9;56(1):99-105.

Frič P, Zavoral M, Dvořáková T. Gluten induced diseases. Vnitr Lek. 2013 May;59(5):376-82.

Friedman M, Brandon DL. Nutritional and health benefits of soy proteins. J Agric Food Chem. 2001 Mar;49(3):1069-86.

Fry L. Dermatitis herpetiformis. In: Marsh M, editor. Coeliac disease. Oxford: Blackwell Scientific Publications; 1992.

Fu G, Zhong Y, Li C, Li Y, Lin X, Liao B, Tsang EW, Wu K, Huang S. Epigenetic regulation of peanut allergen gene Ara h 3 in developing embryos. *Planta.* 2010 Apr;231(5):1049-60.

Fujimori S, Gudis K, Mitsui K, Seo T, Yonezawa M, Tanaka S, Tatsuguchi A, Sakamoto C. A randomized controlled trial on the efficacy of synbiotic versus probiotic or prebiotic treatment to improve the quality of life in patients with ulcerative colitis. *Nutrition.* 2009 May;25(5):520-5.

Furrie E, Macfarlane S, Kennedy A, Cummings JH, Walsh SV, O'neil DA, Macfarlane GT. Synbiotic therapy (Bifidobacterium longum/Synergy 1) initiates resolution of inflammation in patients with active ulcerative colitis: a randomised controlled pilot trial. *Gut.* 2005 Feb;54(2):242-9.

Furuhjelm C, Warstedt K, Larsson J, Fredriksson M, Böttcher MF, Fälth-Magnusson K, Duchén K. Fish oil supplementation in pregnancy and lactation may decrease the risk of infant allergy. *Acta Paediatr.* 2009 Sep;98(9):1461-7.

Gagnier JJ, DeMelo J, Boon H, Rochon P, Bombardier C. Quality of reporting of randomized controlled trials of herbal medicine interventions. *Am J Med.* 2006;119:1–11.

Galli E, Ciucci A, Cersosimo S, Pagnini C, Avitabile S, Mancino G, Delle Fave G, Corleto VD. Eczema and food allergy in an Italian pediatric cohort: no association with TLR-2 and TLR-4 polymorphisms. *Int J Immunopathol Pharmacol.* 2010 Apr-Jun;23(2):671-5.

Gamboa PM, Cáceres O, Antepara I, Sánchez-Monge R, Ahrazem O, Salcedo G, Barber D, Lombardero M, Sanz ML. Two different profiles of peach allergy in the north of Spain. *Allergy.* 2007 Apr;62(4):408-14.

Gan Z, Ellis PR, Vaughan JG, Galliard T. Some effects of non-endosperm components of wheat and of added gluten on wholemeal bread microstructure. J Cer Sci. 1989; Sept: 81-91.

Gao X, Wang W, Wei S, Li W. Review of pharmacological effects of Glycyrrhiza radix and its bioactive compounds. *Zhongguo Zhong Yao Za Zhi.* 2009 Nov;34(21):2695-700.

Garakani A, Win T, Virk S, Gupta S, Kaplan D, Masand PS. Comorbidity of irritable bowel syndrome in psychiatric patients: a review. Am J Ther. 2003 Jan-Feb;10(1):61-7.

Garcia Gomez LJ, Sanchez-Muniz FJ. Review: cardiovascular effect of garlic (Allium sativum). *Arch Latinoam Nutr.* 2000 Sep;50(3):219-29.

Gardner ML. Gastrointestinal absorption of intact proteins. Annu Rev Nutr. 1988;8:329-50.

Gareau MG, Jury J, Yang PC, MacQueen G, Perdue MH. Neonatal maternal separation causes colonic dysfunction in rat pups including impaired host resistance. *Pediatr Res.* 2006 Jan;59(1):83-8.

Garzi A, Messina M, Frati F, Carfagna L, Zagordo L, Belcastro M, Parmiani S, Sensi L, Marcucci F. An extensively hydrolysed cow's milk formula improves clinical symptoms of gastroesophageal reflux and reduces the gastric emptying time in infants. *Allergol Immunopathol (Madr).* 2002 Jan-Feb;30(1):36-41.

Gass J, Bethune MT, Siegel M, Spencer A, Khosla C. Combination enzyme therapy for gastric digestion of dietary gluten in patients with celiac sprue. Gastroenterology. 2007;133:472–80.

Gastrointestinal permeability in food-allergic children. *Nutr Rev.* 1985 Aug;43(8):233-5.

Gawrońska A, Dziechciarz P, Horvath A, Szajewska H. A randomized double-blind placebo-controlled trial of Lactobacillus GG for abdominal pain disorders in children. *Aliment Pharmacol Ther.* 2007 Jan 15;25(2):177-84.

Geha RS, Beiser A, Ren C, Patterson R, Greenberger PA, Grammer LC, Ditto AM, Harris KE, Shaughnessy MA, Yarnold PR, Corren J, Saxon A. Multicenter, double-blind, placebo-controlled, multiple-challenge evaluation of reported reactions to monosodium glutamate. *J Allergy Clin Immunol.* 2000 Nov;106(5):973-80.

Genuis SJ, Lobo RA. Gluten Sensitivity Presenting as a Neuropsychiatric Disorder. Gastroenterol Res Pract. 2014;2014:293206.

Georget DM, Underwood-Toscano C, Powers SJ, Shewry PR, Belton PS. Effect of variety and environmental factors on gluten proteins: an analytical, spectroscopic, and rheological study. J Agric Food Chem. 2008 Feb 27;56(4):1172-9.

Gerez CL, Rollan GC, de Valdez GF. Gluten breakdown by lactobacilli and pediococci strains isolated from sourdough. Lett Appl Microbiol. 2006;42:459–64.

Gerez IF, Shek LP, Chng HH, Lee BW. Diagnostic tests for food allergy. Singapore Med J. 2010 Jan;51(1):4-9.

Ghadioungui P. (transl.) *The Ebers Papyrus*. Academy of Scientific Research. Cairo, 1987.
Ghayur MN, Gilani AH. Ginger lowers blood pressure through blockade of voltage-dependent calcium Channels acting as a cardiotonic pump activator in mice, rabbit and dogs. *J Cardiovasc Pharmacol.* 2005 Jan;45(1):74-80.
Giampietro PG, Kjellman NI, Oldaeus G, Wouters-Wesseling W, Businco L. Hypoallergenicity of an extensively hydrolyzed whey formula. *Pediatr Allergy Immunol.* 2001 Apr;12(2):83-6.
Gibbons E. *Stalking the Healthful Herbs.* New York: David McKay, 1966.
Gibson PR, Shepherd SJ. Evidence-based dietary management of functional gastrointestinal symptoms: the FODMAP approach. J Gastroenterol Hepatol. 2010;25:252–258.
Gibson RA. Docosa-hexaenoic acid (DHA) accumulation is regulated by the polyunsaturated fat content of the diet: Is it synthesis or is it incorporation? *Asia Pac J Clin Nutr.* 2004;13(Suppl):S78.
Gibson, G.R., McCartney, A.L., Rastall, R.A. (2005) Prebiotics and resistance to gastrointestinal infections. *Br J of Nutr.* 93, Suppl. 1, pp31-34.
Gill HS, Rutherfurd KJ, Cross ML, Gopal PK. Enhancement of immunity in the elderly by dietary supplementation with the probiotic Bifidobacterium lactis HN019. *Am J Clin Nutr.* 2001 Dec;74(6):833-9.
Gillman A, Douglass JA. What do asthmatics have to fear from food and additive allergy? *Clin Exp Allergy.* 2010 Sep;40(9):1295-302.
Gionchetti P, Rizzello F, Venturi A, Brigidi P, Matteuzzi D, Bazzocchi G, Poggioli G, Miglioli M, Campieri M. Oral bacteriotherapy as maintenance treatment in patients with chronic pouchitis: a double-blind, placebo-controlled trial. *Gastroenterology.* 2000 Aug;119(2):305-9.
Giovannini C, Sanchez M, Straface E, Scazzocchio B, Silano M, De Vincenzi M. Induction of apoptosis in Caco-2 cells by wheat gliadin peptides. Toxicology. 2000;145(1):63–71.
Glavas-Dodov M, Steffansen B, Crcarevska MS, Geskovski N, Dimchevska S, Kuzmanovska S, Goracinova K. Wheat germ agglutinin-functionalised crosslinked polyelectrolyte microparticles for local colon delivery of 5-FU: in vitro efficacy and in vivo gastrointestinal distribution. J Microencapsul. 2013;30(7):643-56.
Gliwa J, Gunenc A, Ames N, Willmore WG, Hosseinian FS. Antioxidant activity of alkylresorcinols from rye bran and their protective effects on cell viability of PC-12 AC cells. J Agric Food Chem. 2011 Nov 9;59(21):11473-82.
Glück U, Gebbers J. Ingested probiotics reduce nasal colonization with pathogenic bacteria (Staphylococcus aureus, Streptococcus pneumoniae, and b-hemolytic streptococci. *Am J. Clin. Nutr.* 2003;77:517-520.
Gobbetti M, Smacchi E, Corsetti A. The proteolytic system of Lactobacillus sanfrancisco CB1: purification and characterization of a proteinase, a dipeptidase, and an aminopeptidase. Appl Environ Microbiol. 1996 Sep;62(9):3220-6.
Gohil K, Packer L. Bioflavonoid-Rich Botanical Extracts Show Antioxidant and Gene Regulatory Activity. *Ann N Y Acad Sci.* 2002:957:70-7.
Goldin BR, Adlercreutz H, Dwyer JT, Swenson L, Warram JH, Gorbach SL. Effect of diet on excretion of estrogens in pre- and postmenopausal women. *Cancer Res.* 1981 Sep;41(9 Pt 2):3771-3.
Goldin BR, Adlercreutz H, Gorbach SL, Warram JH, Dwyer JT, Swenson L, Woods MN. Estrogen excretion patterns and plasma levels in vegetarian and omnivorous women. *N Engl J Med.* 1982 Dec 16;307(25):1542-7.
Goldin BR, Swenson L, Dwyer J, Sexton M, Gorbach SL. Effect of diet and Lactobacillus acidophilus supplements on human fecal bacterial enzymes. *J Natl Cancer Inst.* 1980 Feb;64(2):255-61.
Goldstein JL, Aisenberg J, Zakko SF, Berger MF, Dodge WE. Endoscopic ulcer rates in healthy subjects associated with use of aspirin (81 mg q.d.) alone or coadministered with celecoxib or naproxen: a randomized, 1-week trial. *Dig Dis Sci.* 2008 Mar;53(3):647-56.
Golub E. *The Limits of Medicine.* New York: Times Books, 1994.
Gonipeta B, Parvataneni S, Paruchuri P, Gangur V. Long-term characteristics of hazelnut allergy in an adjuvant-free mouse model. *Int Arch Allergy Immunol.* 2010;152(3):219-25.
Gonlachanvit S. Are rice and spicy diet good for functional gastrointestinal disorders? *J Neurogastroenterol Motil.* 2010 Apr;16(2):131-8.
González Alvarez R, Arruzazabala ML. Current views of the mechanism of action of prophylactic antiallergic drugs. *Allergol Immunopathol (Madr).* 1981 Nov-Dec;9(6):501-8.
González-Pérez A, Aponte Z, Vidaurre CF, Rodríguez LA. Anaphylaxis epidemiology in patients with and patients without asthma: a United Kingdom database review. *J Allergy Clin Immunol.* 2010 May;125(5):1098-1104.e1.
Goossens DA, Jonkers DM, Russel MG, Stobberingh EE, Stockbrügger RW. The effect of a probiotic drink with Lactobacillus plantarum 299v on the bacterial composition in faeces and mucosal biopsies of rectum and ascending colon. *Aliment Pharmacol Ther.* 2006 Jan 15;23(2):255-63.
Gordan DT, Lucia S. Chao. Relationship of components in wheat bran and spinach to iron bioavailability in the anemic rat. Journal of Nutrition. 1984; Mar: 114.
Gordon BR. Patch testing for allergies. *Curr Opin Otolaryngol Head Neck Surg.* 2010 Jun;18(3):191-4.
Gotteland M, Poliak L, Cruchet S, Brunser O. Effect of regular ingestion of Saccharomyces boulardii plus inulin or Lactobacillus acidophilus LB in children colonized by Helicobacter pylori. *Acta Paediatr.* 2005 Dec;94(12):1747-51.

Graff H, Handford A. Celiac syndrome in the case histories of five schizophrenics. Psychiatr Q. 1961 Apr;35:306-13.
Graff H, Handford A. Celiac syndrome in the case histories of five schizophrenics. Psychiatr Q. 1961 Apr;35:306-13.
Grant WB, Holick MF. Benefits and requirements of vitamin D for optimal health: a review. *Altern Med Rev.* 2005 Jun;10(2):94-111.

Grant WB. Solar ultraviolet irradiance and cancer incidence and mortality. *Adv Exp Med Biol.* 2008;624:16-30.

Graveland, A., Bosveld, P., Lichtendonk, W. J., Marseille, J. P., Moonen, J. H. E., & Scheepstra, A. (1985). A model for the molecular structure of the glutenins from wheat flour. Journal of cereal science, 3(1), 1-16.

Gray H. *Anatomy, Descriptive and Surgical.* 15th Edition. New York: Random House, 1977.

Gray-Davison F. *Ayurvedic Healing.* New York: Keats, 2002.

Greco L, D'Adamo G, Truscelli A, Parrilli G, Mayer M, Budillon G. Intestinal permeability after single dose gluten challenge in coeliac disease. Arch Dis Child. 1991 Jul;66(7):870-2.

Griffith HW. *Healing Herbs: The Essential Guide.* Tucson: Fisher Books, 2000.

Grimshaw KE, King RM, Nordlee JA, Hefle SL, Warner JO, Hourihane JO. Presentation of allergen in different food preparations affects the nature of the allergic reaction – a case series. *Clin Exp Allergy.* 2003 Nov;33(11):1581-5.

Grob M, Reindl J, Vieths S, Wüthrich B, Ballmer-Weber BK. Heterogeneity of banana allergy: characterization of allergens in banana-allergic patients. *Ann Allergy Asthma Immunol.* 2002 Nov;89(5):513-6.

Groschwitz KR, Ahrens R, Osterfeld H, Gurish MF, Han X, Abrink M, Finkelman FD, Pejler G, Hogan SP. Mast cells regulate homeostatic intestinal epithelial migration and barrier function by a chymase/Mcpt4-dependent mechanism. *Proc Natl Acad Sci U S A.* 2009 Dec 29;106(52):22381-6.

Grzanna R, Lindmark L, Frondoza CG. Ginger – an herbal medicinal product with broad anti-inflammatory actions. *J Med Food.* 2005 Summer;8(2):125-32.

Grzybowska-Chlebowczyk U, Woś H, Sieroń AL, Wiecek S, Auguściak-Duma A, Koryciak-Komarska H, Kasznia-Kocot J. Serologic investigations in children with inflammatory bowel disease and food allergy. *Mediators Inflamm.* 2009;2009:512695.

Guandalini S. The influence of gluten: weaning recommendations for healthy children and children at risk for celiac disease. *Nestle Nutr Workshop Ser Pediatr Program.* 2007;60:139-51; discussion 151-5.

Guerin M, Huntley ME, Olaizola M. Haematococcus astaxanthin: applications for human health and nutrition. *Trends Biotechnol.* 2003 May;21(5):210-6.

Gundermann KJ, Müller J. Phytodolor – effects and efficacy of a herbal medicine. *Wien Med Wochenschr.* 2007;157(13-14):343-7.

Güngör S, Celiloğlu OS, Ozcan OO, Raif SG, Selimoğlu MA. Frequency of celiac disease in attention-deficit/hyperactivity disorder. J Pediatr Gastroenterol Nutr. 2013 Feb;56(2):211-4.

Gupta R, Sheikh A, Strachan DP, Anderson HR (2006) Time trends in allergic disorders in the UK. *Thorax,* published online. doi: 10.1136/thx.2004.038844.

Guslandi M, Giollo P, Testoni PA. A pilot trial of Saccharomyces boulardii in ulcerative colitis. *Eur J Gastroenterol Hepatol.* 2003 Jun;15(6):697-8.

Gutmanis J. *Hawaiian Herbal Medicine.* Waipahu, HI: Island Heritage, 2001.

Guyonnet D, Woodcock A, Stefani B, Trevisan C, Hall C. Fermented milk containing Bifidobacterium lactis DN-173 010 improved self-reported digestive comfort amongst a general population of adults. A ran-domized, open-label, controlled, pilot study. *J Dig Dis.* 2009 Feb;10(1):61-70.

H Molina-Infante J, Santolaria S, Montoro M, Esteve M, Fernández-Bañares F. [Non-celiac gluten sensitivity: A critical review of current evidence.]. Gastroenterol Hepatol. 2014 Mar 22. pii: S0210-5705(14)00051-X.

Hadjivassiliou M, Davies-Jones GA, Sanders DS, Grünewald RA. Dietary treatment of gluten ataxia. *J Neurol Neurosurg Psychiatry.* 2003 Sep;74(9):1221-4.

Hadjivassiliou M, Grunewald RA, Davies-Jones GAB. Gluten sensitivity as a neurological illness. J Neurol Neurosurg Psychiatry. 2002;72(5):560–3.

Hadjivassiliou M, Williamson CA, Woodroofe N. The immunology of gluten sensitivity: Beyond the gut. Trends Immunol. 2004;25(11):578–82.

Hadley SK, Gaarder SM. Treatment of irritable bowel syndrome. Am Fam Physician. 2005;72(12):2501–6

Hafström I, Ringertz B, Spångberg A, von Zweigbergk L, Brannemark S, Nylander I, Rönnelid J, Laasonen L, Klareskog L. A vegan diet free of gluten improves the signs and symptoms of rheumatoid arthritis: the effects on arthritis correlate with a reduction in antibodies to food antigens. *Rheumatology (Oxford).* 2001 Oct;40(10):1175-9.

Haines JL, Ter-Minassian M, Bazyk A, Gusella JF, Kim DJ, Terwedow H, Pericak-Vance MA, Rimmler JB, Haynes CS, Roses AD, Lee A, Shaner B, Menold M, Seboun E, Fitoussi RP, Gartioux C, Reyes C, Ribierre F, Gyapay G, Weissenbach J, Hauser SL, Goodkin DE, Lincoln R, Usuku K, Oksenberg JR, *et al.* A complete genomic screen for multiple sclerosis underscores a role for the major histocompatability complex. The Multiple Sclerosis Genetics Group. *Nat Genet.* 1996 Aug;13(4):469-71..

Haines ML, Anderson RP, Gibson PR. Systematic review: the evidence base for long-term management of coeliac disease. Aliment Pharmacol Ther. 2008;28(9):1042–66.

Halken S, Hansen KS, Jacobsen HP, Estmann A, Faelling AE, Hansen LG, Kier SR, Lassen K, Lintrup M, Mortensen S, Ibsen KK, Osterballe O, Høst A. Comparison of a partially hydrolyzed infant formula with two extensively hydrolyzed formulas for allergy prevention: a prospective, randomized study. *Pediatr Allergy Immunol.* 2000 Aug;11(3):149-61.

Halmos EP, Power VA, Shepherd SJ, Gibson PR, Muir JG. A diet low in FODMAPs reduces symptoms of irritable bowel syndrome. Gastroenterology. 2014 Jan;146(1):67-75.e5.

Halpern GM, Miller AH. *Medicinal Mushrooms: Ancient Remedies for Modern Ailments.* New York: M. Evans, 2002.

Hamelmann E, Beyer K, Gruber C, Lau S, Matricardi PM, Nickel R, Niggemann B, Wahn U. Primary prevention of allergy: avoiding risk or providing protection? *Clin Exp Allergy.* 2008 Feb;38(2):233-45.

Hamilton RG. Clinical laboratory assessment of immediate-type hypersensitivity. *J Allergy Clin Immunol.* 2010 Feb;125(2 Suppl 2):S284-96.

Hammond BG, Mayhew DA, Kier LD, Mast RW, Sander WJ. Safety assessment of DHA-rich microalgae from Schizochytrium sp. *Regul Toxicol Pharmacol.* 2002 Apr;35(2 Pt 1):255-65.

Han SN, Leka LS, Lichtenstein AH, Ausman LM, Meydani SN. Effect of a therapeutic lifestyle change diet on immune functions of moderately hypercholesterolemic humans. *J Lipid Res.* 2003 Dec;44(12):2304-10.

Hansen KS, Ballmer-Weber BK, Lüttkopf D, Skov PS, Wüthrich B, Bindslev-Jensen C, Vieths S, Poulsen LK. Roasted hazelnuts – allergenic activity evaluated by double-blind, placebo-controlled food challenge. *Allergy.* 2003 Feb;58(2):132-8.

Hansen KS, Ballmer-Weber BK, Sastre J, Lidholm J, Andersson K, Oberhofer H, Lluch-Bernal M, Ostling J, Mattsson L, Schocker F, Vieths S, Poulsen LK. Component-resolved in vitro diagnosis of hazelnut allergy in Europe. *J Allergy Clin Immunol.* 2009 May;123(5):1134-41, 1141.e1-3.

Hansen KS, Khinchi MS, Skov PS, Bindslev-Jensen C, Poulsen LK, Malling HJ. Food allergy to apple and specific immunotherapy with birch pollen. *Mol Nutr Food Res.* 2004 Nov;48(6):441-8.

Harris KA, Kris-Etherton PM. Effects of whole grains on coronary heart disease risk. Curr Atheroscler Rep. 2010 Nov;12(6):368-76.

Hartz C, Lauer I, Del Mar San Miguel Moncin M, Cistero-Bahima A, Foetisch K, Lidholm J, Vieths S, Scheurer S. Comparison of IgE-Binding Capacity, Cross-Reactivity and Biological Potency of Allergenic Non-Specific Lipid Transfer Proteins from Peach, Cherry and Hazelnut. *Int Arch Allergy Immunol.* 2010 Jun 17;153(4):335-346.

Harvald B, Hauge M: Hereditary factors elucidated by twin studies. *In Genetics and the Epidemiology of Chronic Disease.* Edited by Neel JV, Shaw MV, Schull WJ. Washington, DC: Department of Health, Education and Welfare, 1965:64-76.

Hashem MM, Atta AH, Arbid MS, Nada SA, Asaad GF. Immunological studies on Amaranth, Sunset Yellow and Curcumin as food colouring agents in albino rats. *Food Chem Toxicol.* 2010 Jun;48(6):1581-6.

Hata K, Ishikawa K, Hori K, Konishi T. Differentiation-inducing activity of lupeol, a lupane-type triterpene from Chinese dandelion root (Hokouei-kon), on a mouse melanoma cell line. *Biol Pharm Bull.* 2000 Aug;23(8):962-7.

Hatakka K, Holma R, El-Nezami H, Suomalainen T, Kuisma M, Saxelin M, Poussa T, Mykkänen H, Korpela R. The influence of Lactobacillus rhamnosus LC705 together with Propionibacterium freudenreichii ssp. shermanii JS on potentially carcinogenic bacterial activity in human colon. Int J Food Microbiol. 2008 Dec 10;128(2):406-10.

Hattori K, Sasai M, Yamamoto A, Taniuchi S, Kojima T, Kobayashi Y, Iwamoto H, Yaeshima T, Hayasawa H. Intestinal flora of infants with cow milk hypersensitivity fed on casein-hydrolyzed formula supplemented raffinose. *Arerugi.* 2000 Dec;49(12):1146-55.

Hausch F, Shan L, Santiago NA, Gray GM, Khosla C. Intestinal digestive resistance of immunodominant gliadin peptides. Am J Physiol Gastrointest Liver Physiol. 2002;283:G996–1003.

Hawkes CP, Mulcair S, Hourihane JO. Is hospital based MMR vaccination for children with egg allergy here to stay? *Ir Med J.* 2010 Jan;103(1):17-9.

He J, Penson S, Powers SJ, Hawes C, Shewry PR, Tosi P. Spatial patterns of gluten protein and polymer distribution in wheat grain. J Agric Food Chem. 2013 Jul 3;61(26):6207-15.

Heaney RP, Dowell MS. Absorbability of the calcium in a high-calcium mineral water. *Osteoporos Int.* 1994 Nov;4(6):323-4.

Heap GA, van Heel DA. Genetics and pathogenesis of coeliac disease. *Semin Immunol.* May 13 2009.

Helin T, Haahtela S, Haahtela T. No effect of oral treatment with an intestinal bacterial strain, Lactobacillus rhamnosus (ATCC 53103), on birch-pollen allergy: a placebo-controlled double-blind study. *Allergy.* 2002 Mar;57(3):243-6.

Helmerhorst EJ, Zamakhchari M, Schuppan D, Oppenheim FG. Discovery of a novel and rich source of gluten-degrading microbial enzymes in the oral cavity. PLoS One. 2010 Oct 11;5(10):e13264.

Hemmer W, Focke M, Marzban G, Swoboda I, Jarisch R, Laimer M. Identification of Bet v 1-related allergens in fig and other Moraceae fruits. *Clin Exp Allergy.* 2010 Apr;40(4):679-87.

Hendel B, Ferreira P. *Water & Salt: The Essence of Life.* Gaithersburg: Natural Resources, 2003.

Herbert V. Vitamin B12: Plant sources, requirements, and assay. *Am J Clin Nutr.* 1988;48:852-858.

Herfarth HH, Martin CF, Sandler RS, Kappelman MD, Long MD. Prevalence of a Gluten-free Diet and Improvement of Clinical Symptoms in Patients with Inflammatory Bowel Diseases. Inflamm Bowel Dis. 2014 May 23.

Herman PM, Drost LM. Evaluating the clinical relevance of food sensitivity tests: a single subject experiment. *Altern Med Rev.* 2004 Jun;9(2):198-207.

Heyman M, Grasset E, Ducroc R, Desjeux JF. Antigen absorption by the jejunal epithelium of children with cow's milk allergy. *Pediatr Res.* 1988 Aug;24(2):197-202.

Hidalgo A, Brandolini A. Nutritional properties of einkorn wheat (Triticum monococcum L.). J Sci Food Agric. 2014 Mar 15;94(4):601-12.

Hiemori M, Eguchi Y, Kimoto M, Yamasita H, Takahashi K, Takahashi K, Tsuji H. Characterization of new 18-kDa IgE-binding proteins in beer. *Biosci Biotechnol Biochem.* 2008 Apr;72(4):1095-8.

Hieta N, Hasan T, Mäkinen-Kiljunen S, Lammintausta K. Sweet lupin – a new food allergen. *Duodecim.* 2010;126(12):1393-9.

Hinton JJ. The chemistry of wheat germ with particular reference to the scutellum. Biochem J. 1944;38(3):214-7.

Hirose Y, Murosaki S, Yamamoto Y, Yoshikai Y, Tsuru T. Daily intake of heat-killed Lactobacillus plantarum L-137 augments acquired immunity in healthy adults. *J Nutr.* 2006 Dec;136(12):3069-73.

Hobbs C. *Medicinal Mushrooms.* Summertown, TN: Botanica Press, 2003.

Hobbs C. *Stress & Natural Healing.* Loveland, CO: Interweave Press, 1997.

Hoffmann D. *Holistic Herbal.* London: Thorsons, 1983-2002.

Hofmann AM, Scurlock AM, Jones SM, Palmer KP, Lokhnygina Y, Steele PH, Kamilaris J, Burks AW. Safety of a peanut oral immunotherapy protocol in children with peanut allergy. *J Allergy Clin Immunol.* 2009 Aug;124(2):286-91, 291.e1-6.

Holick MF. Sunlight and vitamin D for bone health and prevention of autoimmune diseases, cancers, and cardiovascular disease. *Am J Clin Nutr.* 2004 Dec;80(6 Suppl):1678S-88S.

Holick MF. The vitamin D deficiency pandemic and consequences for nonskeletal health: mechanisms of action. *Mol Aspects Med.* 2008 Dec;29(6):361-8

Holick MF. Vitamin D status: measurement, interpretation, and clinical application. *Ann Epidemiol.* 2009 Feb;19(2):73-8.

Holick MF. Vitamin D: importance in the prevention of cancers, type 1 diabetes, heart disease, and osteoporosis. *Am J Clin Nutr.* 2004 Mar;79(3):362-71.

Holladay, S.D. Prenatal Immunotoxicant Exposure and Postnatal Autoimmune Disease. *Environ Health Perspect.* 1999; 107(suppl 5):687-691.

Holmes G. Non coeliac gluten sensitivity. Gastroenterol Hepatol Bed Bench. 2013 Summer;6(3):115-9.

Holmes GK, Asquith P, Stokes PL, Cooke WT. Cellular infiltrate of jejunal biopsies in adult coeliac disease in relation to gluten withdrawal. Gut. 1974;15:278–83.

Holtmeier W, Caspary WF. Celiac disease. Orphanet J Rare Dis. 2006;1:3.

Hönscheid A, Rink L, Haase H. T-lymphocytes: a target for stimulatory and inhibitory effects of zinc ions. *Endocr Metab Immune Disord Drug Targets.* 2009 Jun;9(2):132-44.

Hooper R, Calvert J, Thompson RL, Deetlefs ME, Burney P. Urban/rural differences in diet and atopy in South Africa. *Allergy.* 2008 Apr;63(4):425-31.

Horrobin DF. Effects of evening primrose oil in rheumatoid arthritis. *Ann Rheum Dis.* 1989 Nov;48(11):965-6.

Hospers IC, de Vries-Vrolijk K, Brand PL. Double-blind, placebo-controlled cow's milk challenge in children with alleged cow's milk allergies, performed in a general hospital: diagnosis rejected in two-thirds of the children. *Ned Tijdschr Geneeskd.* 2006 Jun 10;150(23):1292-7.

Houle CR, Leo HL, Clark NM. A developmental, community, and psychosocial approach to food allergies in children. *Curr Allergy Asthma Rep.* 2010 Sep;10(5):381-6.

Hourihane JO, Grimshaw KE, Lewis SA, Briggs RA, Trewin JB, King RM, Kilburn SA, Warner JO. Does severity of low-dose, double-blind, placebo-controlled food challenges reflect severity of allergic reactions to peanut in the community? *Clin Exp Allergy.* 2005 Sep;35(9):1227-33.

Howdle PR. Gliadin, glutenin or both? The search for the Holy grail in celiac disease. Eur J Gastroenterol Hepatol. 2006;18:703–6.

Hsu CH, Lu CM, Chang TT. Efficacy and safety of modified Mai-Men-Dong-Tang for treatment of allergic asthma. *Pediatr Allergy Immunol.* 2005;16:76–81.

Hu C, Kitts DD. Antioxidant, prooxidant, and cytotoxic activities of solvent-fractionated dandelion (Taraxacum officinale) flower extracts in vitro. *J Agric Food Chem.* 2003 Jan 1;51(1):301-10.

Hu C, Kitts DD. Dandelion (Taraxacum officinale) flower extract suppresses both reactive oxygen species and nitric oxide and prevents lipid oxidation in vitro. *Phytomedicine.* 2005 Aug;12(8):588-97.

Hu C, Kitts DD. Luteolin and luteolin-7-O-glucoside from dandelion flower suppress iNOS and COX-2 in RAW264.7 cells. *Mol Cell Biochem.* 2004 Oct;265(1-2):107-13.

Hu FB, Malik VS. Sugar-sweetened beverages and risk of obesity and type 2 diabetes: epidemiologic evidence. Physiol Behav. 2010 Apr 26;100(1):47-54.

Huang D, Ou B, Prior RL. The chemistry behind antioxidant capacity assays. *J Agric Food Chem.* 2005 Mar 23;53(6):1841-56.

Huang M, Wang W, Wei S. Investigation on medicinal plant resources of Glycyrrhiza uralensis in China and chemical assessment of its underground part. *Zhongguo Zhong Yao Za Zhi.* 2010 Apr;35(8):947-52.

Hüe S, Mention JJ, Monteiro RC, Zhang S, Cellier C, Schmitz J, Verkarre V, Fodil N, Bahram S, Cerf-Bensussan N, Caillat-Zucman S. A direct role for NKG2D/MICA interaction in villous atrophy during celiac disease. Immunity. 2004 Sep;21(3):367-77.

Huebner FR, Lieberman KW, Rubino RP, Wall JS. Demonstration of high opioid-like activity in isolated peptides from wheat gluten hydrolysates. Peptides. 1984 Nov-Dec;5(6):1139-47.

Hun L. Bacillus coagulans significantly improved abdominal pain and bloating in patients with IBS. *Postgrad Med.* 2009 Mar;121(2):119-24.

Hunter JO. Do horses suffer from irritable bowel syndrome? *Equine Vet J.* 2009 Dec;41(9):836-40.

Hur YM, Rushton JP. Genetic and environmental contributions to prosocial behaviour in 2- to 9-year-old South Korean twins. *Biol Lett.* 2007 Dec 22;3(6):664-6.

Husby S, Koletzko S, Korponay-Szabó IR, Mearin ML, Phillips A, Shamir R, Troncone R, Giersiepen K, Branski D, Catassi C, Lelgeman M, Mäki M, Ribes-Koninckx C, Ventura A, Zimmer KP; ESPGHAN Working Group on Coeliac Disease Diagnosis; ESPGHAN Gastroenterology Committee; European Society for Pediatric Gastroenterology, Hepatology, and Nutrition. European Society for Pediatric Gastroenterology, Hepatology, and Nutrition guidelines for the diagnosis of coeliac disease. J Pediatr Gastroenterol Nutr. 2012 Jan;54(1):136-60.

Husby S. Dietary antigens: uptake and humoral immunity in man. *APMIS Suppl.* 1988;1:1-40.

Ibero M, Boné J, Martín B, Martínez J. Evaluation of an extensively hydrolysed casein formula (Damira 2000) in children with allergy to cow's milk proteins. *Allergol Immunopathol (Madr).* 2010 Mar-Apr;38(2):60-8.

Iida N, Inatomi Y, Murata H, Inada A, Murata J, Lang FA, Matsuura N, Nakanishi T. A new flavone xyloside and two new flavan-3-ol glucosides from Juniperus communis var. depressa. *Chem Biodivers.* 2007 Jan;4(1):32-42.

Indrio F, Ladisa G, Mautone A, Montagna O. Effect of a fermented formula on thymus size and stool pH in healthy term infants. *Pediatr Res.* 2007 Jul;62(1):98-100.

Innis SM, Hansen JW. Plasma fatty acid responses, metabolic effects, and safety of microalgal and fungal oils rich in arachidonic and docosahexaenoic acids in adults. *Am J Clin Nutr.* 1996 Aug;64(2):159-67.

Innocenti M, Michelozzi M, Giaccherini C, Ieri F, Vincieri FF, Mulinacci N. Flavonoids and biflavonoids in Tuscan berries of Juniperus communis L.: detection and quantitation by HPLC/DAD/ESI/MS. *J Agric Food Chem.* 2007 Aug 8;55(16):6596-602.

Int J Toxicol. Final report on the safety assessment of Juniperus communis Extract, Juniperus oxycedrus Extract, Juniperus oxycedrus Tar, Juniperus phoenicea extract, and Juniperus virginiana Extract. *Int J Toxicol.* 2001;20 Suppl 2:41-56.

Ionescu JG. New insights in the pathogenesis of atopic disease. *J Med Life.* 2009 Apr-Jun;2(2):146-54.

Iribarren C, Tolstykh IV, Miller MK, Eisner MD. Asthma and the prospective risk of anaphylactic shock and other allergy diagnoses in a large integrated health care delivery system. *Ann Allergy Asthma Immunol.* 2010 May;104(5):371-7.

Ishida Y, Nakamura F, Kanzato H, Sawada D, Hirata H, Nishimura A, Kajimoto O, Fujiwara S. Clinical effects of Lactobacillus acidophilus strain L-92 on perennial allergic rhinitis: a double-blind, placebo-controlled study. *J Dairy Sci.* 2005 Feb;88(2):527-33.

Ishida Y, Nakamura F, Kanzato H, Sawada D, Yamamoto N, Kagata H, Oh-Ida M, Takeuchi H, Fujiwara S. Effect of milk fermented with Lactobacillus acidophilus strain L-92 on symptoms of Japanese cedar pollen allergy: a randomized placebo-controlled trial. *Biosci Biotechnol Biochem.* 2005 Sep;69(9):1652-60.

Ivory K, Chambers SJ, Pin C, Prieto E, Arqués JL, Nicoletti C. Oral delivery of Lactobacillus casei Shirota modifies allergen-induced immune responses in allergic rhinitis. *Clin Exp Allergy.* 2008 Aug;38(8):1282-9.

Iwańczak B, Mowszet K, Iwańczak F. Feeding disorders, ALTE syndrome, Sandifer syndrome and gastroesophageal reflux disease in the course of food hypersensitivity in 8-month old infant. *Pol Merkur Lekarski.* 2010 Jul;29(169):44-6.

Izumi K, Aihara M, Ikezawa Z. Effects of non steroidal antiinflammatory drugs (NSAIDs) on immediate-type food allergy analysis of Japanese cases from 1998 to 2009. *Arerugi.* 2009 Dec;58(12):1629-39.

Jackson LS, Al-Taher F. Effects of consumer food preparation on acrylamide formation. Adv Exp Med Biol. 2005;561:447-65.

Jackson PG, Lessof MH, Baker RW, Ferrett J, MacDonald DM. Intestinal permeability in patients with eczema and food allergy. *Lancet.* 1981 Jun 13;1(8233):1285-6.

Jagetia GC, Aggarwal BB. "Spicing up" of the immune system by curcumin. *J Clin Immunol.* 2007 Jan;27(1):19-35.

Jagetia GC, Nayak V, Vidyasagar MS. Evaluation of the antineoplastic activity of guduchi (Tinospora cordifolia) in cultured HeLa cells. *Cancer Lett.* 1998 May 15;127(1-2):71-82.

Jagetia GC, Rao SK. Evaluation of Cytotoxic Effects of Dichloromethane Extract of Guduchi (Tinospora cordifolia Miers ex Hook F & THOMS) on Cultured HeLa Cells. *Evid Based Complement Alternat Med.* 2006 Jun;3(2):267-72.

Janson C, Anto J, Burney P, Chinn S, de Marco R, Heinrich J, Jarvis D, Kuenzli N, Leynaert B, Luczynska C, Neukirch F, Svanes C, Sunyer J, Wjst M; European Community Respiratory Health Survey II. The European Community Respiratory Health Survey: what are the main results so far? European Community Respiratory Health Survey II. *Eur Respir J.* 2001 Sep;18(3):598-611.

Jappe U, Vieths S. Lupine, a source of new as well as hidden food allergens. *Mol Nutr Food Res.* 2010 Jan;54(1):113-26.

Jarocka-Cyrta E, Baniukiewicz A, Wasilewska J, Pawlak J, Kaczmarski M. Focal villous atrophy of the duodenum in children who have outgrown cow's milk allergy. Chromoendoscopy and magnification endoscopy evaluation. *Med Wieku Rozwoj.* 2007 Apr-Jun;11(2 Pt 1):123-7.

Järvinen KM, Amalanayagam S, Shreffler WG, Noone S, Sicherer SH, Sampson HA, Nowak-Wegrzyn A. Epinephrine treatment is infrequent and biphasic reactions are rare in food-induced reactions during oral food challenges in children. *J Allergy Clin Immunol.* 2009 Dec;124(6):1267-72.

Jauregi-Miguel A, Fernandez-Jimenez N, Irastorza I, Plaza-Izurieta L, Vitoria JC, Bilbao JR. Alteration of Tight Junction Gene Expression in Celiac Disease. J Pediatr Gastroenterol Nutr. 2014 Feb 14.

Jazani NH, Karimzad M, Mazloomi E, Sohrabpour M, Hassan ZM, Ghasemnejad H, Roshan-Milani S, Shahabi S. Evaluation of the adjuvant activity of naloxone, an opioid receptor antagonist, in combination with heat-killed Listeria monocytogenes vaccine. *Microbes Infect.* 2010 May;12(5):382-8.

Jenkins M, Vickers A. Unreliability of IgE/IgG4 antibody testing as a diagnostic tool in food intolerance. Clin Exp Allergy. 1998 Dec;28(12):1526-9.

Jennings S, Prescott SL. Early dietary exposures and feeding practices: role in pathogenesis and prevention of allergic disease? *Postgrad Med J.* 2010 Feb;86(1012):94-9.

Jensen B. *Foods that Heal.* Garden City Park, NY: Avery Publ, 1988, 1993.

Jensen B. *Nature Has a Remedy.* Los Angeles: Keats, 2001.

Jeon HJ, Kang HJ, Jung HJ, Kang YS, Lim CJ, Kim YM, Park EH. Anti-inflammatory activity of Taraxacum officinale. J *Ethnopharmacol.* 2008 Jan 4;115(1):82-8.

Johansson G, Holmén A, Persson L, Högstedt B, Wassén C, Ottova L, Gustafsson JA. Long-term effects of a change from a mixed diet to a lacto-vegetarian diet on human urinary and faecal mutagenic activity. *Mutagenesis.* 1998 Mar;13(2):167-71.

Johansson G, Holmén A, Persson L, Högstedt B, Wassén C, Ottova L, Gustafsson JA. Dietary influence on some proposed risk factors for colon cancer: fecal and urinary mutagenic activity and the activity of some intestinal bacterial enzymes. *Cancer Detect Prev.* 1997;21(3):258-66.

Johansson G, Holmén A, Persson L, Högstedt R, Wassén C, Ottova L, Gustafsson JA. The effect of a shift from a mixed diet to a lacto-vegetarian diet on human urinary and fecal mutagenic activity. *Carcinogenesis.* 1992 Feb;13(2):153-7.

Johansson G, Ravald N. Comparison of some salivary variables between vegetarians and omnivores. *Eur J Oral Sci.* 1995 Apr;103(2 (Pt 1)):95-8.

Johari H. *Ayurvedic Massage: Traditional Indian Techniques for Balancing Body and Mind.* Rochester, VT: Healing Arts, 1996.

Johnson LM. Gitksan medicinal plants – cultural choice and efficacy. *J Ethnobiol Ethnomed.* 2006 Jun 21;2:29.

Jonas A. Wheat sensitive - but not coeliac. Lancet. 1978;1:1047.

Jones MA, Silman AJ, Whiting S, *et al.* Occurrence of rheumatoid arthritis is not increased in the first degree relatives of a population based inception cohort of inflammatory polyarthritis. *Ann Rheum Dis.* 1996;55(2): 89-93.

Jones SM, Zhong Z, Enomoto N, Schemmer P, Thurman RG. Dietary juniper berry oil minimizes hepatic reperfusion injury in the rat. *Hepatology.* 1998 Oct;28(4):1042-50.

Jones VA. Food intolerance: A major factor in the pathogenesis of irritable bowel syndrome. Lancet. 1982;2(8308):1115–7.

Judson PL, Al Sawah E, Marchion DC, Xiong Y, Bicaku E, Bou Zgheib N, Chon HS, Stickles XB, Hakam A, Wenham RM, Apte SM, Gonzalez-Bosquet J, Chen DT, Lancaster JM. Characterizing the efficacy of fermented wheat germ extract against ovarian cancer and defining the genomic basis of its activity. Int J Gynecol Cancer. 2012 Jul;22(6):960-7.

Juillerat-Jeanneret L, Robert MC, Juillerat MA. Peptides from Lactobacillus hydrolysates of bovine milk caseins inhibit prolyl-peptidases of human colon cells. J Agric Food Chem. 2011 Jan 12;59(1):370-7.

Julkunen-Tiitto R. A chemotaxonomic survey of phenolics in leaves of northern Salicaceae species. Phytochemistry. 1986;25(3):663-667.

Jung HA, Yokozawa T, Kim BW, Jung JH, Choi JS. Selective inhibition of prenylated flavonoids from Sophora flavescens against BACE1 and cholinesterases. *Am J Chin Med.* 2010;38(2):415-29.

Junker Y, Zeissig S, Kim SJ, Barisani D, Wieser H, Leffler DA, Zevallos V, Libermann TA, Dillon S, Freitag TL, Kelly CP, Schuppan D. Wheat amylase trypsin inhibitors drive intestinal inflammation via activation of toll-like receptor 4. J Exp Med. 2012 Dec 17;209(13):2395-408.

Jurakić Toncić R, Lipozencić J. Role and significance of atopy patch test. *Acta Dermatovenerol Croat.* 2010;18(1):38-55.

Jurenka JS. Anti-inflammatory properties of curcumin, a major constituent of Curcuma longa: a review of preclinical and clinical research. *Altern Med Rev.* 2009 Feb;14(2):141-153.

Kagnoff MF. Two genetic loci control the murine immune response to A-gliadin, a wheat protein that activates coeliac sprue. Nature. 1982;296(5853):158–60.

Kähkönen MP, Hopia AI, Vuorela HJ, Rauha JP, Pihlaja K, Kujala TS, Heinonen M. Antioxidant activity of plant extracts containing phenolic compounds. *J Agric Food Chem.* 1999 Oct;47(10):3954-62.

Kaila M, Vanto T, Valovirta E, Koivikko A, Juntunen-Backman K. Diagnosis of food allergy in Finland: survey of pediatric practices. *Pediatr Allergy Immunol.* 2000 Nov;11(4):246-9.

Kajander K, Hatakka K, Poussa T, Färkkilä M, Korpela R. A probiotic mixture alleviates symptoms in irritable bowel syndrome patients: a controlled 6-month intervention. *Aliment Pharmacol Ther.* 2005 Sep 1;22(5):387-94.

Kajander K, Krogius-Kurikka L, Rinttilä T, Karjalainen H, Palva A, Korpela R. Effects of multispecies probiotic supplementation on intestinal microbiota in irritable bowel syndrome. *Aliment Pharmacol Ther.* 2007 Aug 1;26(3):463-73.

Kajander K, Myllyluoma E, Rajilić-Stojanović M, Kyrönpalo S, Rasmussen M, Järvenpää S, Zoetendal EG, de Vos WM, Vapaatalo H, Korpela R. Clinical trial: multispecies probiotic supplementation alleviates the symptoms of irritable bowel syndrome and stabilizes intestinal microbiota. *Aliment Pharmacol Ther.* 2008 Jan 1;27(1):48-57.

Kalach N, Benhamou PH, Campeotto F, Dupont Ch. Anemia impairs small intestinal absorption measured by intestinal permeability in children. *Eur Ann Allergy Clin Immunol.* 2007 Jan;39(1):20-2.

Kalach N, Rocchiccioli F, de Boissieu D, Benhamou PH, Dupont C. Intestinal permeability in children: variation with age and reliability in the diagnosis of cow's milk allergy. *Acta Paediatr.* 2001 May;90(5):499-504.

Kalaydjian AE, Eaton W, Cascella N, Fasano A. The gluten connection: the association between schizophrenia and celiac disease. Acta Psychiatr Scand. 2006 Feb;113(2):82-90.

Kalaydjian AE, Eaton W, Cascella N, Fasano A. The gluten connection: the association between schizophrenia and celiac disease. Acta Psychiatr Scand. 2006 Feb;113(2):82-90.

Kalliomäki M, Salminen S, Arvilommi H, Kero P, Koskinen P, Isolauri E. Probiotics in primary prevention of atopic disease: a randomised placebo-controlled trial. *Lancet.* 2001 Apr 7;357(9262):1076-9.

Kamdar T, Bryce PJ. Immunotherapy in food allergy. Immunotherapy. 2010 May;2(3):329-38.

Kang SK, Kim JK, Ahn SH, Oh JE, Kim JH, Lim DH, Son BK. Relationship between silent gastroesophageal reflux and food sensitization in infants and young children with recurrent wheezing. *J Korean Med Sci.* 2010 Mar;25(3):425-8.

Kanny G, Grignon G, Dauca M, Guedenet JC, Moneret-Vautrin DA. Ultrastructural changes in the duodenal mucosa induced by ingested histamine in patients with chronic urticaria. *Allergy.* 1996 Dec;51(12):935-9.

Kapil A, Sharma S. Immunopotentiating compounds from Tinospora cordifolia. *J Ethnopharmacol.* 1997 Oct;58(2):89-95.

Kaptan K, Beyan C, Ural AU, Cetin T, Avcu F, Gülşen M, Finci R, Yalçín A. Helicobacter pylori – is it a novel causative agent in Vitamin B12 deficiency? *Arch Intern Med.* 2000 May 8;160(9):1349-53.

Karaman I, Sahin F, Güllüce M, Ogütçü H, Sengül M, Adigüzel A. Antimicrobial activity of aqueous and methanol extracts of Juniperus oxycedrus L. *J Ethnopharmacol.* 2003 Apr;85(2-3):231-5.

Karkoulias K, Patouchas D, Alahiotis S, Tsiamita M, Vrodakis K, Spiropoulos K. Specific sensitization in wheat flour and contributing factors in traditional bakers. *Eur Rev Med Pharmacol Sci.* 2007 May-Jun;11(3):141-8.

Karpińska J, Mikołuć B, Motkowski R, Piotrowska-Jastrzebska J. HPLC method for simultaneous determination of retinol, alpha-tocopherol and coenzyme Q10 in human plasma. *J Pharm Biomed Anal.* 2006 Sep 18;42(2):232-6.

Kashiwada Y, Takanaka K, Tsukada H, Miwa Y, Taga T, Tanaka S, Ikeshiro Y. Sesquiterpene glucosides from anti-leukotriene B4 release fraction of Taraxacum officinale. *J Asian Nat Prod Res.* 2001;3(3):191-7.

Kattan JD, Srivastava KD, Sampson HA, Li XM. Pharmacologic and Immunologic Effects of Individual Herbs of Food Allergy Herbal Formula 2 in a Murine Model of Peanut Allergy. *J Allergy Clin Immunol.* 2006;117(2):S34.

Kattan JD, Srivastava KD, Zou ZM, Goldfarb J, Sampson HA, Li XM. Pharmacological and immunological effects of individual herbs in the Food Allergy Herbal Formula-2 (FAHF-2) on peanut allergy. *Phytother Res.* 2008 May;22(5):651-9.

Katz Y, Rajuan N, Goldberg MR, Eisenberg E, Heyman E, Cohen A, Leshno M. Early exposure to cow's milk protein is protective against IgE-mediated cow's milk protein allergy. *J Allergy Clin Immunol.* 2010 Jul;126(1):77-82.e1.

Kaukinen K, Maki M, Partanen J, Sievanen H, Collin P. Celiac disease without villous atrophy: revision of criteria called for. Dig Dis Sci. 2001;46:879–887.

Kazansky DB. MHC restriction and allogeneic immune responses. *J Immunotoxicol.* 2008 Oct;5(4):369-84.

Kazłowska K, Hsu T, Hou CC, Yang WC, Tsai GJ. Anti-inflammatory properties of phenolic compounds and crude extract from Porphyra dentata. *J Ethnopharmacol.* 2010 Mar 2;128(1):123-30.

Keenan JM, Goulson M, Shamliyan T, Knutson N, Kolberg L, Curry L. The effects of concentrated barley beta-glucan on blood lipids in a population of hypercholesterolaemic men and women. Br J Nutr. 2007 Jun;97(6):1162-8.

Keita AV, Söderholm JD. The intestinal barrier and its regulation by neuroimmune factors. *Neurogastroenterol Motil.* 2010 Jul;22(7):718-33.

Kekkonen RA, Sysi-Aho M, Seppanen-Laakso T, Julkunen I, Vapaatalo H, Oresic M, Korpela R. Effect of probiotic Lactobacillus rhamnosus GG intervention on global serum lipidomic profiles in healthy adults. *World J Gastroenterol.* 2008 May 28;14(20):3188-94.

Kelder P. *Ancient Secret of the Fountain of Youth.* New York: Doubleday, 1998.

Kelly G. Inulin-type prebiotics: a (Part 2). Altern Med Rev. 2009;14:36–55. Gibson PR, Newnham E, Barrett JS, Shepherd SJ, Muir JG. Review article: fructose malabsorption and the bigger picture. Aliment Pharmacol Ther. 2007;25(4):349–63.

Kelly SA, Summerbell CD, Brynes A, Whittaker V, Frost G. Wholegrain cereals for coronary heart disease. Cochrane Database Syst Rev. 2007 Apr 18;(2):CD005051.

Keogh JB, Grieger JA, Noakes M, Clifton PM. Flow-Mediated Dilatation Is Impaired by a High-Saturated Fat Diet but Not by a High-Carbohydrate Diet. *Arterioscler Thromb Vasc Biol.* 2005 Mar 17

Kerckhoffs DA, Brouns F, Hornstra G, Mensink RP. Effects on the human serum lipoprotein profile of beta-glucan, soy protein and isoflavones, plant sterols and stanols, garlic and tocotrienols. *J Nutr.* 2002 Sep;132(9):2494-505.

Key T, Appleby P, Davey G, Allen N, Spencer E, Travis R. Mortality in British vegetarians: review and preliminary results from EPIC-Oxford. *Amer. Jour. Clin. Nutr. Suppl.* 2003;78(3): 533S-538S.

Kiefte-de Jong JC, Escher JC, Arends LR, Jaddoe VW, Hofman A, Raat H, Moll HA. Infant nutritional factors and functional constipation in childhood: the Generation R study. *Am J Gastroenterol.* 2010 Apr;105(4):940-5.

Kim DC, Choi SY, Kim SH, Yun BS, Yoo ID, Reddy NR, Yoon HS, Kim KT. Isoliquiritigenin selectively inhibits H(2) histamine receptor signaling. *Mol Pharmacol.* 2006 Aug;70(2):493-500.

Kim HM, Shin HY, Lim KH, Ryu ST, Shin TY, Chae HJ, Kim HR, Lyu YS, An NH, Lim KS. Taraxacum officinale inhibits tumor necrosis factor-alpha production from rat astrocytes. *Immunopharmacol Immunotoxicol.* 2000 Aug;22(3):519-30.

Kim JH, An S, Kim JE, Choi GS, Ye YM, Park HS. Beef-induced anaphylaxis confirmed by the basophil activation test. *Allergy Asthma Immunol Res.* 2010 Jul;2(3):206-8.

Kim JY, Kim DY, Lee YS, Lee BK, Lee KH, Ro JY. DA-9601, Artemisia asiatica herbal extract, ameliorates airway inflammation of allergic asthma in mice. *Mol Cells.* 2006;22:104–12.

Kim MN, Kim N, Lee SH, Park YS, Hwang JH, Kim JW, Jeong SH, Lee DH, Kim JS, Jung HC, Song IS. The effects of probiotics on PPI-triple therapy for Helicobacter pylori eradication. Helicobacter. 2008 Aug;13(4):261-8.

Kim NI, Jo Y, Ahn SB, Son BK, Kim SH, Park YS, Kim SH, Ju JE. A case of eosinophilic esophagitis with food hypersensitivity. *J Neurogastroenterol Motil.* 2010 Jul;16(3):315-8.

Kim SJ, Jung JY, Kim HW, Park T. Anti-obesity effects of Juniperus chinensis extract are associated with increased AMP-activated protein kinase expression and phosphorylation in the visceral adipose tissue of rats. *Biol Pharm Bull.* 2008 Jul;31(7):1415-21.

Kim TE, Park SW, Noh G, Lee S. Comparison of skin prick test results between crude allergen extracts from foods and commercial allergen extracts in atopic dermatitis by double-blind placebo-controlled food challenge for milk, egg, and soybean. *Yonsei Med J.* 2002 Oct;43(5):613-20.

Kim YG, Moon JT, Lee KM, Chon NR, Park H. The effects of probiotics on symptoms of irritable bowel syndrome. *Korean J Gastroenterol.* 2006 Jun;47(6):413-9.

Kim YH, Kim KS, Han CS, Yang HC, Park SH, Ko KI, Lee SH, Kim KH, Lee NH, Kim JM, Son K. Inhibitory effects of natural plants of Jeju Island on elastase and MMP-1 expression. *Int J Cosmet Sci.* 2007 Dec;29(6):487-8.

Kimata M, Inagaki N, Nagai H. Effects of luteolin and other flavonoids on IgE-mediated allergic reactions. *Planta Med.* 2000 Feb;66(1):25-9.

Kimata M, Shichijo M, Miura T, Serizawa I, Inagaki N, Nagai H. Effects of luteolin, quercetin and baicalein on immunoglobulin E-mediated mediator release from human cultured mast cells. *Clin Exp Allergy.* 2000 Apr;30(4):501-8.

Kimber I, Dearman RJ. Factors affecting the development of food allergy. *Proc Nutr Soc.* 2002 Nov;61(4):435-9.

Kimmatkar N, Thawani V, Hingorani L, Khiyani R. Efficacy and tolerability of Boswellia serrata extract in treatment of osteoarthritis of knee – a randomized double blind placebo controlled trial. *Phytomedicine.* 2003 Jan;10(1):3-7.

Kinaciyan T, Jahn-Schmid B, Radakovics A, Zwölfer B, Schreiber C, Francis JN, Ebner C, Bohle B. Successful sublingual immunotherapy with birch pollen has limited effects on concomitant food allergy to apple and the immune response to the Bet v 1 homolog Mal d 1. *J Allergy Clin Immunol.* 2007 Apr;119(4):937 43.

Kiran KS, Padmaja G. Inactivation of trypsin inhibitors in sweet potato and taro tubers during processing. Plant Foods Hum Nutr. 2003 Spring;58(2):153-63.

Kirjavainen PV, Salminen SJ, Isolauri E. Probiotic bacteria in the management of atopic disease: underscoring the importance of viability. *J Pediatr Gastroenterol Nutr.* 2003 Feb;36(2):223-7.

Kisiel W, Barszcz B. Further sesquiterpenoids and phenolics from Taraxacum officinale. *Fitoterapia.* 2000 Jun;71(3):269-73.

Kisiel W, Michalska K. Sesquiterpenoids and phenolics from Taraxacum hondoense. *Fitoterapia*. 2005 Sep;76(6):520-4.

Kjellman NI, Björkstén B, Hattevig G, Fälth-Magnusson K. Natural history of food allergy. *Ann Allergy*. 1988 Dec;61(6 Pt 2):83-7.

Klein R, Landau MG. *Healing: The Body Betrayed*. Minneapolis: DCI:Chronimed, 1992.

Klein-Galczinsky C. Pharmacological and clinical effectiveness of a fixed phytogenic combination trembling poplar (Populus tremula), true goldenrod (Solidago virgaurea) and ash (Fraxinus excelsior) in mild to moderate rheumatic complaints. *Wien Med Wochenschr*. 1999;149(8-10):248-53.

Klemola T, Vanto T, Juntunen-Backman K, Kalimo K, Korpela R, Varjonen E. Allergy to soy formula and to extensively hydrolyzed whey formula in infants with cow's milk allergy: a prospective, randomized study with a follow-up to the age of 2 years. *J Pediatr*. 2002 Feb;140(2):219-24.

Klepacka J, Fornal Ł. Ferulic acid and its position among the phenolic compounds of wheat. Crit Rev Food Sci Nutr. 2006;46(8):639-47.

Klingberg TD, Pedersen MH, Cencic A, Budde BB. Application of measurement of transepithelial electrical resistance of intestinal epithelial cell monolayers to evaluate probiotic activity. Appl Environ Microbiol. 2005;71:7528–30.

Kloss J. *Back to Eden*. Twin Oaks, WI: Lotus Press, 1939-1999.

Knutson TW, Bengtsson U, Dannaeus A, Ahlstedt S, Knutson L. Effects of luminal antigen on intestinal albumin and hyaluronan permeability and ion transport in atopic patients. *J Allergy Clin Immunol*. 1996 Jun;97(6):1225-32.

Ko J, Busse PJ, Shek L, Noone SA, Sampson HA, Li XM. Effect of Chinese Herbal Formulas on T Cell Responses in Patients with Peanut Allergy or Asthma. *J Allergy Clin Immunol* .2005;115:S34.

Ko J, Lee JI, Munoz-Furlong A, Li XM, Sicherer SH. Use of complementary and alternative medicine by food-allergic patients. *Ann Allergy Asthma Immunol*. 2006;97:365–9.

Koo HN, Hong SH, Song BK, Kim CH, Yoo YH, Kim HM. Taraxacum officinale induces cytotoxicity through TNF-alpha and IL-1alpha secretion in Hep G2 cells. *Life Sci*. 2004 Jan 16;74(9):1149-57.

Kootstra HS, Vlieg-Boerstra BJ, Dubois AE. Assessment of the reduced allergenic properties of the Santana apple. *Ann Allergy Asthma Immunol*. 2007 Dec;99(6):522-5.

Korkina LG. Phenylpropanoids as naturally occurring antioxidants: from plant defense to human health. Cell Mol Biol (Noisy-le-grand). 2007 Apr 15;53(1):15-25.

Kotzampassi K, Giamarellos-Bourboulis EJ, Voudouris A, Kazamias P, Eleftheriadis E. Benefits of a synbiotic formula (Synbiotic 2000Forte) in critically Ill trauma patients: early results of a randomized controlled trial. *World J Surg*. 2006 Oct;30(10):1848-55.

Kovács T, Mette H, Per B, Kun L, Schmelczer M, Barta J, Jean-Claude D, Nagy J. Relationship between intestinal permeability and antibodies against food antigens in IgA nephropathy. *Orv Hetil*. 1996 Jan 14;137(2):65-9.

Kowalchik C, Hylton W (eds). *Rodale's Illustrated Encyclopedia of Herbs*. Emmaus, PA: 1987.

Kowalczyk E, Krzesiński P, Kura M, Niedworok J, Kowalski J, Błaszczyk J. Pharmacological effects of flavonoids from Scutellaria baicalensis. *Przegl Lek*. 2006;63(2):95-6.

Kozlowski LT, Mehta NY, Sweeney CT, Schwartz SS, Vogler GP, Jarvis MJ, West RJ. Filter ventilation and nicotine content of tobacco in cigarettes from Canada, the United Kingdom, and the United States. *Tob Control*. 1998 Winter;7(4):369-75.

Kreig M. *Black Market Medicine*. New York: Bantam, 1968.

Kristjansson I, Ardal B, Jonsson JS, Sigurdsson JA, Foldevi M, Bjorksten B (1999) Adverse reactions to food and food allergy in young children in Iceland and Sweden. *Scand J Prim Health Care*. 17: 30–34.

Krogulska A, Wasowska-Królikowska K, Dynowski J. Evaluation of bronchial hyperreactivity in children with asthma undergoing food challenges. *Pol Merkur Lekarski*. 2007 Jul;23(133):30-5.

Krogulska A, Wasowska-Królikowska K, Trzeźwińska B. Food challenges in children with asthma. *Pol Merkur Lekarski*. 2007 Jul;23(133):22-9.

Krüger P, Kanzer J, Hummel J, Fricker G, Schubert-Zsilavecz M, Abdel-Tawab M. Permeation of Boswellia extract in the Caco-2 model and possible interactions of its constituents KBA and AKBA with OATP1B3 and MRP2. *Eur J Pharm Sci*. 2009 Feb 15;36(2-3):275-84.

Krull LF, Wall JS. Relationship of Amino Acid Composition and Wheat Protein Properties. USDA ARS/Bakers Dig. 1969; 43(4):38-39.

Kueh JS, Bright SW. Proline accumulation in a barley mutant resistant to trans-4-hydroxy-L-proline. Planta. 1981 Oct;153(2):166-71.

Kuitunen M, Kukkonen K, Juntunen-Backman K, Korpela R, Poussa T, Tuure T, Haahtela T, Savilahti E. Probiotics prevent IgE-associated allergy until age 5 years in cesarean-delivered children but not in the total cohort. *J Allergy Clin Immunol*. 2009 Feb;123(2):335-41.

Kuitunen M, Savilahti E, Sarnesto A. Human alpha-lactalbumin and bovine beta-lactoglobulin absorption in infants. *Allergy*. 1994 May;49(5):354-60.

Kuitunen M, Savilahti E. Mucosal IgA, mucosal cow's milk antibodies, serum cow's milk antibodies and gastrointestinal permeability in infants. *Pediatr Allergy Immunol.* 1995 Feb;6(1):30-5.

Kukkonen K, Kuitunen M, Haahtela T, Korpela R, Poussa T, Savilahti E. High intestinal IgA associates with reduced risk of IgE-associated allergic diseases. *Pediatr Allergy Immunol.* 2010 Feb;21(1 Pt 1):67-73.

Kukkonen K, Savilahti E, Haahtela T, Juntunen-Backman K, Korpela R, Poussa T, Tuure T, Kuitunen M. Probiotics and prebiotic galacto-oligosaccharides in the prevention of allergic diseases: a randomized, double-blind, placebo-controlled trial. *J Allergy Clin Immunol.* 2007 Jan;119(1):192-8.

Kulka M. The potential of natural products as effective treatments for allergic inflammation: implications for allergic rhinitis. *Curr Top Med Chem.* 2009;9(17):1611-24.

Kull I, Bergström A, Lilja G, Pershagen G, Wickman M. Fish consumption during the first year of life and development of allergic diseases during childhood. *Allergy.* 2006 Aug;61(8):1009-15.

Kull I, Melen E, Alm J, Hallberg J, Svartengren M, van Hage M, Pershagen G, Wickman M, Bergström A. Breast-feeding in relation to asthma, lung function, and sensitization in young schoolchildren. *J Allergy Clin Immunol.* 2010 May;125(5):1013-9.

Kumar R, Singh BP, Srivastava P, Sridhara S, Arora N, Gaur SN. Relevance of serum IgE estimation in allergic bronchial asthma with special reference to food allergy. *Asian Pac J Allergy Immunol.* 2006 Dec;24(4):191-9.

Kummeling I, Mills EN, Clausen M, Dubakiene R, Pérez CF, Fernández-Rivas M, Knulst AC, Kowalski ML, Lidholm J, Le TM, Metzler C, Mustakov T, Popov T, Potts J, van Ree R, Sakellariou A, Töndury B, Tzannis K, Burney P. The EuroPrevall surveys on the prevalence of food allergies in children and adults: background and study methodology. *Allergy.* 2009 Oct;64(10):1493-7.

Kung HC, Hoyert DL, Xu J, Murphy SL. Deaths: Final Data for 2005. *National Vital Statistics Reports.* 2008;56(10). http://www.cdc.gov/nchs/data/ nvsr/nvsr56/nvsr56_10.pdf. Accessed: 2008 Jun.

Kunisawa J, Kiyono H. Aberrant interaction of the gut immune system with environmental factors in the development of food allergies. *Curr Allergy Asthma Rep.* 2010 May;10(3):215-21.

Kupfer SS, Jabri B. Pathophysiology of celiac disease. Gastrointest Endosc Clin N Am. 2012;22:639–60.

Kurppa K, Collin P, Viljamaa M, Haimila K, Saavalainen P, Partanen J, Laurila K, Huhtala H, Paasikivi K, Mäki M, Kaukinen K. Diagnosing mild enteropathy celiac disease: a randomized, controlled clinical study. Gastroenterology. 2009 Mar;136(3):816-23.

Kusano M, Zai H, Hosaka H, Shimoyama Y, Nagoshi A, Maeda M, Kawamura O, Mori M. New frontiers in gut nutrient sensor research: monosodium L-glutamate added to a high-energy, high-protein liquid diet promotes gastric emptying: a possible therapy for patients with functional dyspepsia. *J Pharmacol Sci.* 2010 Jan;112(1):33-6.

Kusunoki T, Miyanomae T, Inoue Y, Itoh M, Yoshioka T, Okafuji I, Nishikomori R, Heike T, Nakahata T. Changes in food allergen sensitization rates of Japanese allergic children during the last 15 years. *Arerugi.* 2004 Jul;53(7):683-8.

Kusunoki T, Morimoto T, Nishikomori R, Yasumi T, Heike T, Mukaida K, Fujii T, Nakahata T. Breastfeeding and the prevalence of allergic diseases in schoolchildren: Does reverse causation matter? *Pediatr Allergy Immunol.* 2010 Feb;21(1 Pt 1):60-6.

Kuvaeva IB. Permeability of the gastronintestinal tract for macromolecules in health and disease. *Hum Physiol.* 1979 Mar-Apr;4(2):272-83.

Kuznetsova TA, Shevchenko NM, Zviagintseva TN, Besednova NN. Biological activity of fucoidans from brown algae and the prospects of their use in medicine]. *Antibiot Khimioter.* 2004;49(5):24-30..

Kyrø C, Olsen A, Bueno-de-Mesquita HB, *et al.* Plasma alkylresorcinol concentrations, biomarkers of whole-grain wheat and rye intake, in the European Prospective Investigation into Cancer and Nutrition (EPIC) cohort. Br J Nutr. 2014 May;111(10):1881-90.

Kyrø C, Olsen A, Landberg R, *et al.* Plasma alkylresorcinols, biomarkers of whole-grain wheat and rye intake, and incidence of colorectal cancer. J Natl Cancer Inst. 2014 Jan;106(1):djt352.

Kyrø C, Skeie G, Loft S, Landberg R, Christensen J, Lund E, Nilsson LM, Palmqvist R, Tjønneland A, Olsen A. Intake of whole grains from different cereal and food sources and incidence of colorectal cancer in the Scandinavian HELGA cohort. Cancer Causes Control. 2013 Jul;24(7):1363-74.

Lachance LR, McKenzie K. Biomarkers of gluten sensitivity in patients with non-affective psychosis: a meta-analysis. Schizophr Res. 2014 Feb;152(2-3):521-7.

Lad V. *Ayurveda: The Science of Self-Healing.* Twin Lakes, WI: Lotus Press.

Ladd SL, Sommer, SA, LaBerge S, Toscano W. Brief Report: Effect of Phosphatidylcholine on Explicit Memory. Clin Neuroph. 1993 Dec. 16(6).

Lamaison JL, Carnat A, Petitjean-Freytet C. Tannin content and inhibiting activity of elastase in Rosaceae. *Ann Pharm Fr.* 1990;48(6):335-40.

Lambert MT, Bjarnason I, Connelly J, Crow TJ, Johnstone EC, Peters TJ, Smethurst P. Small intestine permeability in schizophrenia. Br J Psychiatry. 1989 Nov;155:619-22.

Lammers KM, Lu R, Brownley J, Lu B, Gerard C, Thomas K, Rallabhandi P, Shea-Donohue T, Tamiz A, Alkan S, Netzel-Arnett S, Antalis T, Vogel SN, Fasano A. Gliadin induces an increase in intestinal permeability and zonulin release by binding to the chemokine receptor CXCR3. Gastroenterology. 2008 Jul;135(1):194-204.e3.

Landberg R, Kamal-Eldin A, Andersson R, Aman P. Alkylresorcinol content and homologue composition in durum wheat (Triticum durum) kernels and pasta products. J Agric Food Chem. 2006 Apr 19;54(8):3012-4.

Lappe FM. *Diet for a Small Planet.* New York: Ballantine, 1971.

Lau BH, Riesen SK, Truong KP, Lau EW, Rohdewald P, Barreta RA. Pycnogenol as an adjunct in the management of childhood asthma. *J Asthma.* 2004;41(8):825-32.

Lau NM, Green PH, Taylor AK, Hellberg D, Ajamian M, Tan CZ, Kosofsky BE, Higgins JJ, Rajadhyaksha AM, Alaedini A. Markers of Celiac Disease and Gluten Sensitivity in Children with Autism. PLoS One. 2013 Jun 18;8(6):e66155. Print 2013.

Laubereau B, Filipiak-Pittroff B, von Berg A, Grübl A, Reinhardt D, Wichmann HE, Koletzko S; GINI Study Group. Caesarean section and gastrointestinal symptoms, atopic dermatitis, and sensitisation during the first year of life. *Arch Dis Child.* 2004 Nov;89(11):993-7.

Laudat A, Arnaud P, Napoly A, Brion F. The intestinal permeability test applied to the diagnosis of food allergy in paediatrics. West Indian Med J. 1994 Sep;43(3):87-8.

Laugesen M, Elliott R. Ischaemic heart disease, Type 1 diabetes, and cow milk A1 beta-casein. *N Z Med J.* 2003 Jan 24;116(1168):U295.

Laurière M, Pecquet C, Bouchez-Mahiout I, Snégaroff J, Bayrou O, Raison-Peyron N, Vigan M. Hydrolysed wheat proteins present in cosmetics can induce immediate hypersensitivities. *Contact Dermatitis.* 2006 May;54(5):283-9.

LaValle JB. *The Cox-2 Connection.* Rochester, VT: Healing Arts, 2001.

Law MH, Bradford M, McNamara N, Gajda A, Wei J. No association observed between schizophrenia and non-HLA coeliac disease genes: integration with the initial MYO9B association with coeliac disease. Am J Med Genet B Neuropsychiatr Genet. 2011 Sep;156B(6):709-19.

Lean G. US study links more than 200 diseases to pollution. *London Independent.* 2004 Nov 14.

Lee AA, McKibbin CL, Bourassa KA, Wykes TL, Kitchen Andren KA. Depression, Diabetic Complications and Disability Among Persons With Comorbid Schizophrenia and Type 2 Diabetes. Psychosomatics. 2013 Dec 31. pii: S0033-3182(13)00247-8.

Lee BJ, Park HS. Common whelk (Buccinum undatum) allergy: identification of IgE-binding components and effects of heating and digestive enzymes. *J Korean Med Sci.* 2004 Dec;19(6):793-9.

Lee CK, Cheng YS. Diterpenoids from the leaves of Juniperus chinensis var. kaizuka. *J Nat Prod.* 2001 Apr;64(4):511-4.

Lee JH, Noh J, Noh G, Kim HS, Mun SH, Choi WS, Cho S, Lee S. Allergen-specific B cell subset responses in cow's milk allergy of late eczematous reactions in atopic dermatitis. *Cell Immunol.* 2010;262(1):44-51.

Lee JY, Kim CJ. Determination of allergenic egg proteins in food by protein-, mass spectrometry-, and DNA-based methods. *J AOAC Int.* 2010 Mar-Apr;93(2):462-77.

Lee YS, Kim SH, Jung SH, Kim JK, Pan CH, Lim SS. Aldose reductase inhibitory compounds from Glycyrrhiza uralensis. *Biol Pharm Bull.* 2010;33(5):917-21.

Leenhardt F, Levrat-Verny MA, Chanliaud E, Rémésy C. Moderate decrease of pH by sourdough fermentation is sufficient to reduce phytate content of whole wheat flour through endogenous phytase activity. J Agric Food Chem. 2005 Jan 12;53(1):98-102.

Leffler DA, Schuppan D. Update on serologic testing in celiac disease. *Am J Gastroenterol.* 2010 Dec;105(12):2520-4.

Lehmann B. The vitamin D3 pathway in human skin and its role for regulation of biological processes. *Photochem Photobiol.* 2005 Nov-Dec;81(6):1246-51.

Lehto M, Airaksinen L, Puustinen A, Tillander S, Hannula S, Nyman T, Toskala E, Alenius H, Lauerma A. Thaumatin-like protein and baker's respiratory allergy. *Ann Allergy Asthma Immunol.* 2010 Feb;104(2):139-46.

Lehto M, Airaksinen L, Puustinen A, Tillander S, Hannula S, Nyman T, Toskala E, Alenius H, Lauerma A. Thaumatin-like protein and baker's respiratory allergy. *Ann Allergy Asthma Immunol.* 2010 Feb;104(2):139-46.

Leitzmann C. Vegetarian diets: what are the advantages? *Forum Nutr.* 2005;(57):147-56.

Leu YL, Shi LS, Damu AG. Chemical constituents of Taraxacum formosanum. Chem *Pharm Bull.* 2003 May;51(5):599-601.

Leu YL, Wang YL, Huang SC, Shi LS. Chemical constituents from roots of Taraxacum formosanum. *Chem Pharm Bull.* 2005 Jul;53(7):853-5.

Leucci MR, Lenucci MS, Piro G, Dalessandro G. Water stress and cell wall polysaccharides in the apical root zone of wheat cultivars varying in drought tolerance. J Plant Physiol. 2008 Jul 31;165(11):1168-80.

Leung DY, Sampson HA, Yunginger JW, Burks AW Jr, Schneider LC, Wortel CH, Davis FM, Hyun JD, Shanahan WR Jr; Avon Longitudinal Study of Parents and Children Study Team. Effect of anti-IgE therapy in patients with peanut allergy. *N Engl J Med.* 2003 Mar 13;348(11):986-93.

Leung DY, Shanahan WR Jr, Li XM, Sampson HA. New approaches for the treatment of anaphylaxis. *Novartis Found Symp.* 2004;257:248-60; discussion 260-4, 276-85.

Lewerin C, Jacobsson S, Lindstedt G, Nilsson-Ehle H. Serum biomarkers for atrophic gastritis and antibodies against Helicobacter pylori in the elderly: Implications for vitamin B12, folic acid and iron status and response to oral vitamin therapy. *Scand J Gastroenterol.* 2008;43(9):1050-6.

Lewis SA, Grimshaw KE, Warner JO, Hourihane JO. The promiscuity of immunoglobulin E binding to peanut allergens, as determined by Western blotting, correlates with the severity of clinical symptoms. *Clin Exp Allergy.* 2005 Jun;35(6):767-73.

Lewis WH, Elvin-Lewis MPF. *Medical Botany: Plants Affecting Man's Health.* New York: Wiley, 1977.

Lewontin R. *The Genetic Basis of Evolutionary Change.* New York: Columbia Univ Press, 1974.

Leyel CF. *Culpeper's English Physician & Complete Herbal.* Hollywood, CA: Wilshire, 1971.

Leynadier F. Mast cells and basophils in asthma. Ann Biol Clin (Paris). 1989;47(6):351-6.

Li H, Tan G, Jiang X, Qiao H, Pan S, Jiang H, Kanwar JR, Sun X. Therapeutic effects of matrine on primary and metastatic breast cancer. *Am J Chin Med.* 2010;38(6):1115-30.

Li N, DeMarco VG, West CM, Neu J. Glutamine supports recovery from loss of transepithelial resistance and increase of permeability induced by media change in Caco-2 cells. J Nutr Biochem. 2003;14:947–9.

Li S, Li W, Wang Y, Asada Y, Koike K. Prenylflavonoids from Glycyrrhiza uralensis and their protein tyrosine phosphatase-1B inhibitory activities. *Bioorg Med Chem Lett.* 2010 Sep 15;20(18):5398-401.

Li W, Cui SW, Wang Q. Solution and conformational properties of wheat beta-D-glucans studied by light scattering and viscometry. Biomacromolecules. 2006 Feb;7(2):446-52.

Li XM, Huang CK, Zhang TF, Teper AA, Srivastava K, Schofield BH, Sampson HA. The chinese herbal medicine formula MSSM-002 suppresses allergic airway hyperreactivity and modulates TH1/TH2 responses in a murine model of allergic asthma. *J Allergy Clin Immunol.* 2000;106:660–8.

Li XM, Schofield BH, Huang CK, Kleiner GA, Sampson HA. A Murine Model of IgE Mediated Cow Milk Hypersensitivity. *J Allergy Clin Immunol.* 1999;103:206–14.

Li XM, Serebrisky D, Lee SY, Huang CK, Bardina L, Schofield BH, Stanley JS, Burks AW, Bannon GA, Sampson HA. A murine model of peanut anaphylaxis: T- and B-cell responses to a major peanut allergen mimic human responses. *J Allergy Clin Immunol.* 2000;106:150–8.

Li XM, Zhang TF, Huang CK, Srivastava K, Teper AA, Zhang L, Schofield BH, Sampson HA. Food Allergy Herbal Formula-1 (FAHF-1) blocks peanut-induced anaphylaxis in a murine model. *J Allergy Clin Immunol.* 2001;108:639–46.

Li XM, Zhang TF, Sampson H, Zou ZM, Beyer K, Wen MC, Schofield B. The potential use of Chinese herbal medicines in treating allergic asthma. *Ann Allergy Asthma Immunol.* 2004;93:S35–S44.

Li XM. Beyond allergen avoidance: update on developing therapies for peanut allergy. *Curr Opin Allergy Clin Immunol.* 2005;5:287–92.

Lidén M, Kristjánsson G, Valtysdottir S, Venge P, Hällgren R. Cow's milk protein sensitivity assessed by the mucosal patch technique is related to irritable bowel syndrome in patients with primary Sjögren's syndrome. *Clin Exp Allergy.* 2008 Jun;38(6):929-35.

Lidén M, Kristjánsson G, Valtysdottir S, Venge P, Hällgren R. Self-reported food intolerance and mucosal reactivity after rectal food protein challenge in patients with rheumatoid arthritis. *Scand J Rheumatol.* 2010 Aug;39(4):292-8.

Lied GA, Lillestøl K, Valeur J, Berstad A. Intestinal B cell-activating factor: an indicator of non-IgE-mediated hypersensitivity reactions to food? *Aliment Pharmacol Ther.* 2010 Jul;32(1):66-73.

Liggins J, Mulligan A, Runswick S, Bingham SA. Daidzein and genistein content of cereals. Eur J Clin Nutr. 2002 Oct;56(10):961-6.

Lillestøl K, Berstad A, Lind R, Florvaag E, Arslan Lied G, Tangen T. Anxiety and depression in patients with self-reported food hypersensitivity. *Gen Hosp Psychiatry.* 2010 Jan-Feb;32(1):42-8.

Lillestøl K, Helgeland L, Arslan Lied G, Florvaag E, Valeur J, Lind R, Berstad A. Indications of 'atopic bowel' in patients with self-reported food hypersensitivity. *Aliment Pharmacol Ther.* 2010 May;31(10):1112-22.

Lillioja S, Neal AL, Tapsell L, Jacobs DR Jr. Whole grains, type 2 diabetes, coronary heart disease, and hypertension: links to the aleurone preferred over indigestible fiber. Biofactors. 2013 May-Jun;39(3):242-58.

Lim JP, Song YC, Kim JW, Ku CH, Eun JS, Leem KH, Kim DK. Free radical scavengers from the heartwood of Juniperus chinensis. *Arch Pharm Res.* 2002 Aug;25(4):449-52.

Lindfors K, Blomqvist T, Juuti-Uusitalo K, Stenman S, Venäläinen J, Mäki M, Kaukinen K. Live probiotic Bifidobacterium lactis bacteria inhibit the toxic effects induced by wheat gliadin in epithelial cell culture. Clin Exp Immunol. 2008 Jun;152(3):552-8.

Ling WH, Hänninen O. Shifting from a conventional diet to an uncooked vegan diet reversibly alters fecal hydrolytic activities in humans. *J Nutr.* 1992 Apr;122(4):924-30.

Lininger S, Gaby A, Austin S, Brown D, Wright J, Duncan A. *The Natural Pharmacy.* New York: Three Rivers, 1999.

Linko-Parvinen AM, Landberg R, Tikkanen MJ, Adlercreutz H, Peñalvo JL. Alkylresorcinols from whole-grain wheat and rye are transported in human plasma lipoproteins. J Nutr. 2007 May;137(5):1137-42.

Linsalata M, Russo F, Berloco P, Caruso ML, Matteo GD, Cifone MG, Simone CD, Ierardi E, Di Leo A. The influence of Lactobacillus brevis on ornithine decarboxylase activity and polyamine profiles in Helicobacter pylori-infected gastric mucosa. Helicobacter. 2004 Apr;9(2):165-72. Madden JA, Plummer SF, Tang J, Garaiova I, Plummer NT, Herbison M, Hunter JO, Shimada T, Cheng L, Shirakawa T. Effect of probiotics on preventing disruption of the intestinal microflora following antibiotic therapy: a double-blind, placebo-controlled pilot study. *Int Immunopharmacol.* 2005 Jun;5(6):1091-7.

Lipozencić J, Wolf R. The diagnostic value of atopy patch testing and prick testing in atopic dermatitis: facts and controversies. *Clin Dermatol.* 2010 Jan-Feb;28(1):38-44.

Lipski E. *Digestive Wellness.* Los Angeles, CA: Keats, 2000.

Liu GM, Cao MJ, Huang YY, Cai QF, Weng WY, Su WJ. Comparative study of in vitro digestibility of major allergen tropomyosin and other food proteins of Chinese mitten crab (Eriocheir sinensis). *J Sci Food Agric.* 2010 Aug 15;90(10):1614-20.

Liu HY, Giday Z, Moore BF. Possible pathogenetic mechanisms producing bovine milk protein inducible malabsorption: a hypothesis. *Ann Allergy.* 1977 Jul;39(1):1-7.

Liu JY, Hu JH, Zhu QG, Li FQ, Wang J, Sun HJ. Effect of matrine on the expression of substance P receptor and inflammatory cytokines production in human skin keratinocytes and fibroblasts. *Int Immunopharmacol.* 2007 Jun;7(6):816-23.

Liu L, Zubik L, Collins FW, Marko M, Meydani M. The antiatherogenic potential of oat phenolic compounds. Atherosclerosis. 2004 Jul;175(1):39-49.

Liu X, Beaty TH, Deindl P, Huang SK, Lau S, Sommerfeld C, Fallin MD, Kao WH, Wahn U, Nickel R. Associations between specific serum IgE response and 6 variants within the genes IL4, IL13, and IL4RA in German children: the German Multicenter Atopy Study. *J Allergy Clin Immunol.* 2004 Mar;113(3):489-95.

Liu XJ, Cao MA, Li WH, Shen CS, Yan SQ, Yuan CS. Alkaloids from Sophora flavescens Aition. *Fitoterapia.* 2010 Sep;81(6):524-7.

Lloyd JU. *American Materia Medica, Therapeutics and Pharmacognosy.* Portland, OR: Eclectic Medical Publications, 1989-1983.

Lloyd-Still JD, Powers CA, Hoffman DR, Boyd-Trull K, Lester LA, Benisek DC, Arterburn LM. Bioavailability and safety of a high dose of docosahexaenoic acid triacylglycerol of algal origin in cystic fibrosis patients: a randomized, controlled study. *Nutrition.* 2006 Jan;22(1):36-46.

Loft DE, Nwokolo CU, Ciclitira PJ. The diagnosis of gluten sensitivity and coeliac disease – the two are not mutually inclusive. Eur J Gastroenterol Hepatol. 1998;10:911–913.

Loizzo MR, Saab AM, Tundis R, Statti GA, Menichini F, Lampronti I, Gambari R, Cinatl J, Doerr HW. Phytochemical analysis and in vitro antiviral activities of the essential oils of seven Lebanon species. *Chem Biodivers.* 2008 Mar;5(3):461-70.

Lomax AR, Calder PC. Probiotics, immune function, infection and inflammation: a review of the evidence from studies conducted in humans. *Curr Pharm Des.* 2009;15(13):1428-518.

Longo G, Barbi E, Berti I, Meneghetti R, Pittalis A, Ronfani L, Ventura A. Specific oral tolerance induction in children with very severe cow's milk-induced reactions. *J Allergy Clin Immunol.* 2008 Feb;121(2):343-7.

Longstreth GF, Thompson WG, Chey WD, Houghton LA, Mearin F, Spiller RC. Functional bowel disorders. Gastroenterology. 2006;130:1480–1491.

López N, de Barros-Mazón S, Vilela MM, Silva CM, Ribeiro JD. Genetic and environmental influences on atopic immune response in early life. *J Investig Allergol Clin Immunol.* 1999 Nov-Dec;9(6):392-8.

Lopez-Garcia E, Schulze MB, Meigs JB, Manson JE, Rifai N, Stampfer MJ, Willett WC, Hu FB. Consumption of trans fatty acids is related to plasma biomarkers of inflammation and endothelial dysfunction. *J Nutr.* 2005 Mar;135(3):562-6.

Lorea Baroja M, Kirjavainen PV, Hekmat S, Reid G. Anti-inflammatory effects of probiotic yogurt in inflammatory bowel disease patients. *Clin Exp Immunol.* 2007 Sep;149(3):470-9.

Lorenz W, Buhrmann C, Mobasheri A, Lueders C, Shakibaei M. Bacterial lipopolysaccharides form procollagen-endotoxin complexes that trigger cartilage inflammation and degeneration: implications for the development of rheumatoid arthritis. Arthritis Res Ther. 2013;15(5):R111.

Lovchik MA, Fráter G, Goeke A, Hug W. Total synthesis of junionone, a natural monoterpenoid from Juniperus communis L., and determination of the absolute configuration of the naturally occurring enantiomer by ROA spectroscopy. *Chem Biodivers.* 2008 Jan;5(1):126-39.

Lu MK, Shih YW, Chang Chien TT, Fang LH, Huang HC, Chen PS. □-Solanine inhibits human melanoma cell migration and invasion by reducing matrix metalloproteinase-2/9 activities. Biol Pharm Bull. 2010;33(10):1685-91.

Lu W, Gwee KA, Siah KT, Kang JY, Lee R, Ngan CC. Prevalence of Anti-deamidated Gliadin Peptide Antibodies in Asian Patients With Irritable Bowel Syndrome. J Neurogastroenterol Motil. 2014 Apr 30;20(2):236-41.

Lucarelli S, Frediani T, Zingoni AM, Ferruzzi F, Giardini O, Quintieri F, Barbato M, D'Eufemia P, Cardi E. Food allergy and infantile autism. Panminerva Med. 1995 Sep;37(3):137-41.

Ludvigsson JF, Leffler DA, Bai JC, Biagi F, Fasano A, Green PH, Hadjivassiliou M, Kaukinen K, Kelly CP, Leonard JN, Lundin KE, Murray JA, Sanders DS, Walker MM, Zingone F, Ciacci C. The Oslo definitions for coeliac disease and related terms. Gut. 2013 Jan;62(1):43-52.

Lundin KE, Alaedini A. Non-celiac gluten sensitivity. Gastrointest Endosc Clin N Am. 2012 Oct;22(4):723-34.

Lundin KE, Gjertsen HA, Scott H, Sollid LM, Thorsby E. T cells from the small intestinal mucosa of a DR4, DQ7/DR4, DQ8 celiac disease patient preferentially recognize gliadin when presented by DQ8. Hum Immunol. 1994;41(4):285–91.

Lundin KE, Scott H, Hansen T, Paulsen G, Halstensen TS, Fausa O, Thorsby E, Sollid LM. Gliadin-specific, HLA-DQ(alpha 1*0501,beta 1*0201) restricted T cells isolated from the small intestinal mucosa of celiac disease patients. J Exp Med. 1993 Jul 1;178(1):187-96.

Lustig RH, Schmidt LA, Brindis CD. Public health: The toxic truth about sugar. Nature. 2012 Feb 1;482(7383):27-9.

Lykken DT, Tellegen A, DeRubeis R: Volunteer bias in twin research: the rule of two-thirds. *Soc Biol* 1978, 25(1): 1-9. Phillips DI: Twin studies in medical research: can they tell us whether diseases are genetically determined? *Lancet* 1993;341(8851): 1008-1009.

Ma J, Ross AB, Shea MK, Bruce SJ, Jacques PF, Saltzman E, Lichtenstein AH, Booth SL, McKeown NM. Plasma alkylresorcinols, biomarkers of whole-grain intake, are related to lower BMI in older adults. J Nutr. 2012 Oct;142(10):1859-64.

Mabey R, ed. *The New Age Herbalist.* New York: Simon & Schuster, 1941.

Macdonald TT, Monteleone G. Immunity, inflammation, and allergy in the gut. *Science.* 2005 Mar 25;307(5717):1920-5. Review. PubMed PMID: 15790845.

Macfarlane BJ, Bezwoda WR, Bothwell TH, Baynes, RD, Bothwell JE, MacPhail AP, Lamparelli RD, Mayet F. Inhibitory effect of nuts on iron absorption. The American Journal of Clinical Nutrition. 1988: Feb; 47 (2): 270–274.

Maciorkowska E, Kaczmarski M, Andrzej K. Endoscopic evaluation of upper gastrointestinal tract mucosa in children with food hypersensitivity. *Med Wieku Rozwoj.* 2000 Jan-Mar;4(1):37-48.

Maeda N, Inomata N, Morita A, Kirino M, Ikezawa Z. Correlation of oral allergy syndrome due to plant-derived foods with pollen sensitization in Japan. *Ann Allergy Asthma Immunol.* 2010 Mar;104(3):205-10.

Maes HH, Silberg JL, Neale MC, Eaves LJ. Genetic and cultural transmission of antisocial behavior: an extended twin parent model. *Twin Res Hum Genet.* 2007 Feb;10(1):136-50.

Magnusdottir OK, Landberg R, Gunnarsdottir I, Cloetens L, Akesson B, Landin-Olsson M, Rosqvist F, Iggman D, Schwab U, Herzig KH, Savolainen MJ, Brader L, Hermansen K, Kolehmainen M, Poutanen K, Uusitupa M, Thorsdottir I, Risérus U. Plasma alkylresorcinols C17:0/C21:0 ratio, a biomarker of relative whole-grain rye intake, is associated to insulin sensitivity: a randomized study. Eur J Clin Nutr. 2014 Apr;68(4):453-8.

Mahady GB, Pendland SL, Stoia A, Hamill FA, Fabricant D, Dietz BM, Chadwick LR. In vitro susceptibility of Helicobacter pylori to botanical extracts used traditionally for the treatment of gastrointestinal disorders. *Phytother Res.* 2005 Nov;19(11):988-91.

Mai XM, Kull I, Wickman M, Bergström A. Antibiotic use in early life and development of allergic diseases: respiratory infection as the explanation. *Clin Exp Allergy.* 2010 Aug;40(8):1230-7.

Maiuri L, Ciacci C, Ricciardelli I, Vacca L, Raia V, Auricchio S, Picard J, Osman M, Quaratino S, Londei M. Association between innate response to gliadin and activation of pathogenic T cells in coeliac disease. Lancet. 2003 Jul 5;362(9377):30-7.

Maiuri L, Ciacci C, Ricciardelli I, Vacca L, Raia V, Rispo A, Griffin M, Issekutz T, Quaratino S, Londei M. Unexpected role of surface transglutaminase type II in celiac disease. Gastroenterology. 2005 Nov;129(5):1400-13.

Majamaa H, Isolauri E. Probiotics: a novel approach in the management of food allergy. *J Allergy Clin Immunol.* 1997 Feb;99(2):179-85.

Maki KC, Gibson GR, Dickmann RS, Kendall CW, Chen CY, Costabile A, Comelli EM, McKay DL, Almeida NG, Jenkins D, Zello GA, Blumberg JB. Digestive and physiologic effects of a wheat bran extract, arabino-xylan-oligosaccharide, in breakfast cereal. Nutrition. 2012 Nov-Dec;28(11-12):1115-21.

Makrides M, Neumann M, Gibson R. Effect of maternal docosahexaenoic acid (DHA) supplementation on breast milk composition. *Europ Jrnl of Clin Nutr.* 1996;50:352-357.

Maliakal PP, Wanwimolruk S. Effect of herbal teas on hepatic drug metabolizing enzymes in rats. *J Pharm Pharmacol.* 2001 Oct;53(10):1323-9.

Mälkönen T, Alanko K, Jolanki R, Luukkonen R, Aalto-Korte K, Lauerma A, Susitaival P. Long-term follow-up study of occupational hand eczema. Br J Dermatol. 2010 Aug 13.

Månsson HL. Fatty acids in bovine milk fat. *Food Nutr Res.* 2008;52. doi: 10.3402/fnr.v52i0.1821.

Mansueto P, Seidita A, D'Alcamo A, Carroccio A. Non-celiac gluten sensitivity: literature review. J Am Coll Nutr. 2014;33(1):39-54.

Manz F. Hydration and disease. *J Am Coll Nutr.* 2007 Oct;26(5 Suppl):535S-541S.

Marcucci F, Duse M, Frati F, Incorvaia C, Marseglia GL, La Rosa M. The future of sublingual immunotherapy. *Int J Immunopathol Pharmacol.* 2009 Oct-Dec;22(4 Suppl):31-3.

Margioris AN. Fatty acids and postprandial inflammation. *Curr Opin Clin Nutr Metab Care.* 2009 Mar;12(2):129-37.

Martinez M. Docosahexaenoic acid therapy in docosahexaenoic acid-deficient patients with disorders of peroxisomal biogenesis. *Versicherungsmedizin.* 1996;31 Suppl:145-152

Martínez-Augustin O, Boza JJ, Del Pino JI, Lucena J, Martínez-Valverde A, Gil A. Dietary nucleotides might influence the humoral immune response against cow's milk proteins in preterm neonates. *Biol Neonate.* 1997;71(4):215-23.

Martin-Venegas R, Roig-Perez S, Ferrer R, Moreno JJ. Arachidonic acid cascade and epithelial barrier function during Caco-2 cell differentiation. J Lipid Res. 2006 Apr;3.

Massey DG, Chien YK, Fournier-Massey G. Mamane: scientific therapy for asthma? *Hawaii Med J.* 1994;53:350–1. 363.

Massicot JG, Cohen SG. Epidemiologic and socioeconomic aspects of allergic diseases. *J Allergy Clin Immunol.* 1986 Nov;78(5 Pt 2):954-8.

Matheson MC, Haydn Walters E, Burgess JA, Jenkins MA, Giles GG, Hopper JL, Abramson MJ, Dharmage SC. Childhood immunization and atopic disease into middle-age – a prospective cohort study. *Pediatr Allergy Immunol.* 2010 Mar;21(2 Pt 1):301-6.

Matricardi PM, Bockelbrink A, Beyer K, Keil T, Niggemann B, Grüber C, Wahn U, Lau S. Primary versus secondary immunoglobulin E sensitization to soy and wheat in the Multi-Centre Allergy Study cohort. *Clin Exp Allergy.* 2008 Mar;38(3):493-500.

Matsuda T, Maruyama T, Iizuka H, Kondo A, Tamai T, Kurohane K, Imai Y. Phthalate esters reveal skin-sensitizing activity of phenethyl isothiocyanate in mice. *Food Chem Toxicol.* 2010 Jun;48(6):1704-8.

Mattila P, Pihlava JM, Hellström J. Contents of phenolic acids, alkyl- and alkenylresorcinols, and avenanthramides in commercial grain products. J Agric Food Chem. 2005 Oct 19;53(21):8290-5.

Matuccia A, Gianluca Venerib, Chiara Dalla Pellegrinab, Gianni Zoccatellib, Simone Vincenzib, Roberto Chignolab, Angelo D.B. Peruffob, Corrado Rizzib. Temperature-dependent decay of wheat germ agglutinin activity and its implications for food processing and analysis. Food Control. Volume 15, Issue 5, July 2004, Pages 391–395.

Mayes MD. Epidemiologic studies of environmental agents and systemic autoimmune diseases. *Environ Health Perspect.* 1999 Oct;107 Suppl 5:743-8.

McAlindon TE. Nutraceuticals: do they work and when should we use them? *Best Pract Res Clin Rheumatol.* 2006 Feb;20(1):99-115.

McBride C, McBride-Henry K, Wissen K. Parenting a child with medically diagnosed severe food allergies in New Zealand: The experience of being unsupported in keeping their children healthy and safe. *Contemp Nurse.* 2010 Apr;35(1):77-87.

McConnaughey E. *Sea Vegetables.* Happy Camp, CA: Naturegraph, 1985.

McCune LM, Johns T. Antioxidant activity in medicinal plants associated with the symptoms of diabetes mellitus used by the indigenous peoples of the North American boreal forest. *J Ethnopharmacol.* 2002 Oct;82(2-3):197-205.

McDougall J, McDougall M. *The McDougal Plan.* Clinton, NJ: New Win, 1983.

McKenzie H, Main J, Pennington CR, Parratt D. Antibody to selected strains of Saccharomyces cerevisiae (baker's and brewer's yeast) and Candida albicans in Crohn's disease. *Gut.* 1990 May;31(5):536-8.

McKeown NM, Meigs JB, Liu S, Wilson PW, Jacques PF. Whole-grain intake is favorably associated with metabolic risk factors for type 2 diabetes and cardiovascular disease in the Framingham Offspring Study. Am J Clin Nutr. 2002 Aug;76(2):390-8.

McLachlan CN. beta-casein A1, ischaemic heart disease mortality, and other illnesses. *Med Hypotheses.* 2001 Feb;56(2):262-72.

McLean S, Sheikh A. Does avoidance of peanuts in early life reduce the risk of peanut allergy? *BMJ.* 2010 Mar 11;340:c424. doi: 10.1136/bmj.c424.

McNally ME, Atkinson SA, Cole DE. Contribution of sulfate and sulfoesters to total sulfur intake in infants fed human milk. *J Nutr.* 1991 Aug;121(8):1250-4.

Meglio P, Bartone E, Plantamura M, Arabito E, Giampietro PG. A protocol for oral desensitization in children with IgE-mediated cow's milk allergy. Allergy. 2004 Sep;59(9):980-7.

Mehra PN, Puri HS. Studies on Gaduchi satwa. *Indian J Pharm.* 1969;31:180-2.

Meier B, Shao Y, Julkunen-Tiitto R, Bettschart A, Sticher O. A chemotaxonomic survey of phenolic compounds in Swiss willow species. Planta Med. 1992;58:A698.

Meier B, Sticher O, Julkunen-Tiitto R. Pharmaceutical aspects of the use of willows in herbal remedies. Planta Med. 1988;54(6):559-560.

Melcion C, Verroust P, Baud L, Ardaillou N, Morel-Maroger L, Ardaillou R. Protective effect of procyanidolic oligomers on the heterologous phase of glomerulonephritis induced by anti-glomerular basement membrane antibodies. *C R Seances Acad Sci III.* 1982 Dec 6;295(12):721-6.

Melzig MF. Goldenrod – a classical exponent in the urological phytotherapy. *Wien Med Wochenschr.* 2004 Nov;154(21-22):523-7.

Merchant RE and Andre CA. 2001. A review of recent clinical trials of the nutritional supplement Chlorella pyrenoidosa in the treatment of fibromyalgia, hypertension, and ulcerative colitis. *Altern Ther Health Med.* May-Jun;7(3):79-91.

Metsälä J, Lundqvist A, Kaila M, Gissler M, Klaukka T, Virtanen SM. Maternal and perinatal characteristics and the risk of cow's milk allergy in infants up to 2 years of age: a case-control study nested in the Finnish population. *Am J Epidemiol.* 2010 Jun 15;171(12):1310-6.

Meyer A, Kirsch H, Domergue F, Abbadi A, Sperling P, Bauer J, Cirpus P, Zank TK, Moreau H, Roscoe TJ, Zahringer U, Heinz E. Novel fatty acid elongases and their use for the reconstitution of docosahexaenoic acid biosynthesis. *J Lipid Res.* 2004 Oct;45(10):1899-909.

Miceli N, Trovato A, Dugo P, Cacciola F, Donato P, Marino A, Bellinghieri V, La Barbera TM, Güvenç A, Taviano MF. Comparative Analysis of Flavonoid Profile, Antioxidant and Antimicrobial Activity of the Berries of Juniperus communis L. var. communis and Juniperus communis L. var. saxatilis Pall. *J Agric Food Chem.* 2009 Jul 6.

Michaelsen KF. Probiotics, breastfeeding and atopic eczema. *Acta Derm Venereol Suppl (Stockh).* 2005 Nov;(215):21-4.

Michalska K, Kisiel W. Sesquiterpene lactones from Taraxacum obovatum. *Planta Med.* 2003 Feb;69(2):181-3.

Michetti P, Dorta G, Wiesel PH, Brassart D, Verdu E, Herranz M, Felley C, Porta N, Rouvet M, Blum AL, Corthésy-Theulaz I. Effect of whey-based culture supernatant of Lactobacillus acidophilus (johnsonii) La1 on Helicobacter pylori infection in humans. *Digestion.* 1999;60(3):203-9.

Mikoluc B, Motkowski R, Karpinska J, Piotrowska-Jastrzebska J. Plasma levels of vitamins A and E, coenzyme Q10, and anti-ox-LDL antibody titer in children treated with an elimination diet due to food hypersensitivity. *Int J Vitam Nutr Res.* 2009 Sep;79(5-6):328-36.

Miller GT. *Living in the Environment.* Belmont, CA: Wadsworth, 1996.

Miller K. Cholesterol and In-Hospital Mortality in Elderly Patients. *Am Family Phys.* 2004 May.

Miller MJ, Zhang XJ, Gu X, Tenore E, Clark DA. Exaggerated intestinal histamine release by casein and casein hydrolysate but not whey hydrolysate. Scand J Gastroenterol. 1991 Apr;26(4):379-84.

Mindell E, Hopkins V. *Prescription Alternatives.* New Canaan, CT: Keats, 1998.

Miranda H, Outeiro TF. The sour side of neurodegenerative disorders: the effects of protein glycation. J Pathol. 2010 May;221(1):13-25.

Mitchell AE, Hong YJ, Koh E, Barrett DM, Bryant DE, Denison RF, Kaffka S. Ten-year comparison of the influence of organic and conventional crop management practices on the content of flavonoids in tomatoes. *J Agric Food Chem.* 2007 Jul 25;55(15):6154-9.

Mitea C, Havenaar R, Drijfhout JW, Edens L, Dekking L, Koning F. Efficient degradation of gluten by a prolyl endopeptidase in a gastrointestinal model: implications for celiac disease. Gut. 2008;57:25–32.

Mittag D, Akkerdaas J, Ballmer-Weber BK, Vogel L, Wensing M, Becker WM, Koppelman SJ, Knulst AC, Helbling A, Hefle SL, Van Ree R, Vieths S. Ara h 8, a Bet v 1-homologous allergen from peanut, is a major allergen in patients with combined birch pollen and peanut allergy. *J Allergy Clin Immunol.* 2004 Dec;114(6):1410-7.

Mittag D, Vieths S, Vogel L, Becker WM, Rihs HP, Helbling A, Wüthrich B, Ballmer-Weber BK. Soybean allergy in patients allergic to birch pollen: clinical investigation and molecular characterization of allergens. *J Allergy Clin Immunol.* 2004 Jan;113(1):148-54.

Miyazaki T, Kohno S, Mitsutake K, Maesaki S, Tanaka K, Ishikawa N, Hara K. Plasma (1 – >3)-beta-D-glucan and fungal antigenemia in patients with candidemia, aspergillosis, and cryptococcosis. J Clin Microbiol. 1995 Dec;33(12):3115-8.

Miyazawa T, Itahashi K, Imai T. Management of neonatal cow's milk allergy in high-risk neonates. *Pediatr Int.* 2009 Aug;51(4):544-7.

Mofidi A, Ferraro ZM, Stewart KA, Tulk HM, Robinson LE, Duncan AM, Graham TE. The acute impact of ingestion of sourdough and whole-grain breads on blood glucose, insulin, and incretins in overweight and obese men. J Nutr Metab. 2012;2012:184710.

Molkhou P, Dupont C. Ketotifen in prevention and therapy of food allergy. *Ann Allergy.* 1987 Nov;59(5 Pt 2):187-93.

Monarca S. Zerbini I, Simonati C, Gelatti U. Drinking water hardness and chronic degenerative diseases. Part II. Cardiovascular diseases. *Ann. Ig.* 2003;15:41-56.

Moneret-Vautrin DA, Kanny G, Thévenin F. Asthma caused by food allergy. *Rev Med Interne.* 1996;17(7):551-7.

Moneret-Vautrin DA, Morisset M. Adult food allergy. *Curr Allergy Asthma Rep.* 2005 Jan;5(1):80-5.

Monks H, Gowland MH, Mackenzie H, Erlewyn-Lajeunesse M, King R, Lucas JS, Roberts G. How do teenagers manage their food allergies? *Clin Exp Allergy.* 2010 Aug 2.

Monsbakken KW, Vandvik PO, Farup PG. Perceived food intolerance in subjects with irritable bowel syndrome – etiology, prevalence, and consequences. Eur J Clin Nutr. 2006;60:667–672.

Montalto M, Maggiano N, Ricci R, Curigliano V, Santoro L, Di Nicuolo F, Vecchio FM, Gasbarrini A, Gasbarrini G. Lactobacillus acidophilus protects tight junctions from aspirin damage in HT-29 cells. Digestion. 2004;69(4):225-8.

Moorhead KJ, Morgan HC. *Spirulina: Nature's Superfood.* Kailua-Kona, HI: Nutrex, 1995.

Morales de León JC, Bourges Rodríguez H, Zardain MI. Cooking procedures for direct consumption of whole soybeans. Arch Latinoam Nutr. 1985 Jun;35(2):326-36.

Morel AF, Dias GO, Porto C, Simionatto E, Stuker CZ, Dalcol II. Antimicrobial activity of extractives of Solidago microglossa. *Fitoterapia.* 2006 Sep;77(6):453-5.

Moreno-Franco B, García-González Á, Montero-Bravo AM, Iglesias-Gutiérrez E, Úbeda N, Maroto-Núñez L, Adlercreutz H, Peñalvo JL. Dietary alkylresorcinols and lignans in the Spanish diet: development of the alignia database. J Agric Food Chem. 2011 Sep 28;59(18):9827-34.

Morgan JE, Daul CB, Hughes J, McCants M, Lehrer SB. Food specific skin-test reactivity in atopic subjects. *Clin Exp Allergy.* 1989 Jul;19(4):431-5.

Mori F, Bianchi L, Pucci N, Azzari C, De Martino M, Novembre E. CD4+CD25+Foxp3+ T regulatory cells are not involved in oral desensitization. *Int J Immunopathol Pharmacol.* 2010 Jan-Mar;23(1):359-61.

Morisset M, Moneret-Vautrin DA, Guenard L, Cuny JM, Frentz P, Hatahet R, Hanss Ch, Beaudouin E, Petit N, Kanny G. Oral desensitization in children with milk and egg allergies obtains recovery in a significant proportion of cases. A randomized study in 60 children with cow's milk allergy and 90 children with egg allergy. *Eur Ann Allergy Clin Immunol.* 2007 Jan;39(1):12-9.

Morisset M, Moneret-Vautrin DA, Kanny G, Guénard L, Beaudouin E, Flabbée J, Hatahet R. Thresholds of clinical reactivity to milk, egg, peanut and sesame in immunoglobulin E-dependent allergies: evaluation by double-blind or single-blind placebo-controlled oral challenges. *Clin Exp Allergy.* 2003 Aug;33(8):1046-51.

Morisset M, Moneret-Vautrin DA, Kanny G; Allergo-Vigilance Network. Prevalence of peanut sensitization in a population of 4,737 subjects – an Allergo-Vigilance Network enquiry carried out in 2002. *Eur Ann Allergy Clin Immunol.* 2005 Feb;37(2):54-7.

Morisset M, Moneret-Vautrin DA, Maadi F, Frémont S, Guénard L, Croizier A, Kanny G. Prospective study of mustard allergy: first study with double-blind placebo-controlled food challenge trials (24 cases). *Allergy.* 2003 Apr;58(4):295-9.

Morley JE, Levine AS, Yamada T, Gebhard RL, Prigge WF, Shafer RB, Goetz FC, Silvis SE. Effect of exorphins on gastrointestinal function, hormonal release, and appetite. Gastroenterology. 1983 Jun;84(6):1517-23.

Mortensen PB, Pedersen CB, Westergaard T, Wohlfahrt J, Ewald H, Mors O, Andersen PK, Melbye M. Effects of family history and place and season of birth on the risk of schizophrenia. N Engl J Med. 1999 Feb 25;340(8):603-8.

Moujir L, Seca AM, Silva AM, Barreto MC. Cytotoxic activity of diterpenes and extracts of Juniperus brevifolia. *Planta Med.* 2008 Jun;74(7):751-3.

Moussaieff A, Shein NA, Tsenter J, Grigoriadis S, Simeonidou C, Alexandrovich AG, Trembovler V, Ben-Neriah Y, Schmitz ML, Fiebich BL, Munoz E, Mechoulam R, Shohami E. Incensole acetate: a novel neuroprotective agent isolated from Boswellia carterii. *J Cereb Blood Flow Metab.* 2008 Jul;28(7):1341-52.

Mozaffarian D, Aro A, Willett WC. Health effects of trans-fatty acids: experimental and observational evidence. *Eur J Clin Nutr.* 2009 May;63 Suppl 2:S5-21.

Mrowietz-Ruckstuhl B. Bacteriological stool examinations. *Dtsch Arztebl Int.* 2010 Jan;107(3):40; author reply 40-1.

Mullin GE, Swift KM, Lipski L, Turnbull LK, Rampertab SD. Testing for food reactions: the good, the bad, and the ugly. Nutr Clin Pract. 2010 Apr;25(2):192-8.

Mullin GE, Swift KM, Lipski L, Turnbull LK, Rampertab SD. Testing for food reactions: the good, the bad, and the ugly. *Nutr Clin Pract.* 2010 Apr;25(2):192-8.

Muralikrishna G, Rao MV. Cereal non-cellulosic polysaccharides: structure and function relationship - an overview. Crit Rev Food Sci Nutr. 2007;47(6):599-610.

Murphy EA, Davis JM, Brown AS, Carmichael MD, Ghaffar A, Mayer EP. Oat beta-glucan effects on neutrophil respiratory burst activity following exercise. Med Sci Sports Exerc. 2007 Apr;39(4):639-44.

Murray JA, Watson T, Clearman B, Mitros F. Effect of a gluten-free diet on gastrointestinal symptoms in celiac disease. Am J Clin Nutr. 2004 Apr;79(4):669-73.

Murray M, Pizzorno J. *Encyclopedia of Natural Medicine.* 2nd Edition. Roseville, CA: Prima Publishing, 1998.

Murtaugh MA, Jacobs DR Jr, Jacob B, Steffen LM, Marquart L. Epidemiological support for the protection of whole grains against diabetes. Proc Nutr Soc. 2003 Feb;62(1):143-9.

Muthusamy A, Jayabalan N. Variations in seed protein content of cotton (Gossypium hirsutum L.) mutant lines by in vivo and in vitro mutagenesis. J Environ Biol. 2013 Jan;34(1):11-6.

Mykletun A, Jacka F, Williams L, Pasco J, Henry M, Nicholson GC, Kotowicz MA, Berk M. Prevalence of mood and anxiety disorder in self reported irritable bowel syndrome (IBS). An epidemiological population based study of women. BMC Gastroenterol. 2010 Aug 5;10:88.

Myléus A, Hernell O, Gothefors L, Hammarström ML, Persson LÅ, Stenlund H, Ivarsson A. Early infections are associated with increased risk for celiac disease: an incident case-referent study. BMC Pediatr. 2012 Dec 19;12:194.

Na HJ, Koo HN, Lee GG, Yoo SJ, Park JH, Lyu YS, Kim HM. Juniper oil inhibits the heat shock-induced apoptosis via preventing the caspase-3 activation in human astrocytes CCF-STTG1 cells. *Clin Chim Acta.* 2001 Dec;314(1-2):215-20.

Nadkarni AK, Nadkarni KM. *Indian Materia Medica.* (Vols 1 and 2). Bombay, India: Popular Pradashan, 1908, 1976.

Nagel G, Weinmayr G, Kleiner A, Garcia-Marcos L, Strachan DP; ISAAC Phase Two Study Group. Effect of diet on asthma and allergic sensitisation in the International Study on Allergies and Asthma in Childhood (ISAAC) Phase Two. *Thorax.* 2010 Jun;65(6):516-22.

Naghii MR, Samman S. The role of boron in nutrition and metabolism. *Prog Food Nutr Sci.* 1993 Oct-Dec;17(4):331-49.

Nair PK, Rodriguez S, Ramachandran R, Alamo A, Melnick SJ, Escalon E, Garcia PI Jr, Wnuk SF, Ramachandran C. Immune stimulating properties of a novel polysaccharide from the medicinal plant Tinospora cordifolia. *Int Immunopharmacol.* 2004 Dec 15;4(13):1645-59.

Najjar AM, Parsons PM, Duncan AM, Robinson LE, Yada RY, Graham TE. The acute impact of ingestion of breads of varying composition on blood glucose, insulin and incretins following first and second meals. Br J Nutr. 2009 Feb;101(3):391-8.

Nakamura M, Yagami A, Hara K, Sano A, Kobayashi T, Aihara M, Hide M, Chinuki Y, Morita E, Teshima R, Matsunaga K. A New Reliable Method for Detecting Specific IgE Antibodies in the Patients with Immediate Type Wheat Allergy due to Hydrolyzed Wheat Protein: Correlation of Its Titer and Clinical Severity. Allergol Int. 2014 Apr 25.

Nakano T, Shimojo N, Morita Y, Arima T, Tomiita M, Kohno Y. Sensitization to casein and beta-lactoglobulin (BLG) in children with cow's milk allergy (CMA). *Arerugi.* 2010 Feb;59(2):117-22.

Napoli, J.E., Brand-Miller, J.C., Conway, P. (2003) Bifidogenic effects of feeding infant formula containing galactooligosaccharides in healthy formula-fed infants. *Asia Pac J Clin Nutr.* 12(Suppl): S60

Nariya M, Shukla V, Jain S, Ravishankar B. Comparison of enteroprotective efficacy of triphala formulations (Indian Herbal Drug) on methotrexate-induced small intestinal damage in rats. *Phytother Res.* 2009 Aug;23(8):1092-8.

Naruszewicz M, Johansson ML, Zapolska-Downar D, Bukowska H. Effect of Lactobacillus plantarum 299v on cardiovascular disease risk factors in smokers. *Am J Clin Nutr.* 2002 Dec;76(6):1249-55.

Natural Foods Merchandiser. 10 Lessons to better serve customers who follow gluten-free and other special diets. 2014 April;21-22.

NDL, BHNRC, ARS, USDA. *Oxygen Radical Absorbance Capacity (ORAC) of Selected Foods - 2007.* Beltsville, MD: USDA-ARS. 2007.

Nehra V. New clinical issues in celiac disease. *Gastroenterol Clin North Am.* 1998 Jun;27(2):453-65.

Neilan NA, Dowling PJ, Taylor DL, Ryan P, Schurman JV, Friesen CA. Useful biomarkers in pediatric eosinophilic duodenitis and their existence: a case-control, single-blind, observational pilot study. *J Pediatr Gastroenterol Nutr.* 2010 Apr;50(4):377-84.

Nentwich I, Michková E, Nevoral J, Urbanek R, Szépfalusi Z. Cow's milk-specific cellular and humoral immune responses and atopy skin symptoms in infants from atopic families fed a partially (pHF) or extensively (eHF) hydrolyzed infant formula. *Allergy.* 2001 Dec;56(12):1144-56.

Nermes M, Karvonen H, Sarkkinen E, Isolauri E. Safety of barley starch syrup in patients with allergy to cereals. *Br J Nutr.* 2009 Jan;101(2):165-8.

Newall CA, Anderson LA, Philpson JD. *Herbal Medicine: A Guide for Healthcare Professionals.* London: Pharmaceutical Press, 1996.

Newby PK, Maras J, Bakun P, Muller D, Ferrucci L, Tucker KL. Intake of whole grains, refined grains, and cereal fiber measured with 7-d diet records and associations with risk factors for chronic disease. Am J Clin Nutr. 2007 Dec;86(6):1745-53.

Newhouse KE, Smith WA, Starrett MA, Schaefer TJ, Singh BK. Tolerance to imidazolinone herbicides in wheat. Plant Physiol. 1992 Oct;100(2):882-6.

Newmark T, Schulick P. *Beyond Aspirin.* Prescott, AZ: Holm, 2000.

Neyestani TR, Shariatzadeh N, Gharavi A, Kalayi A, Khalaji N. Physiological dose of lycopene suppressed oxidative stress and enhanced serum levels of immunoglobulin M in patients with Type 2 diabetes mellitus: a possible role in the prevention of long-term complications. *J Endocrinol Invest.* 2007 Nov;30(10):833-8.

Ngemakwe PN, Le Roes-Hill M, Jideani V. Advances in gluten-free bread technology. Food Sci Technol Int. 2014 May 16. pii: 1082013214531425.

Nicholls SJ, Lundman P, Harmer JA, Cutri B, Griffiths KA, Rye KA, Barter PJ, Celermajer DS. Consumption of saturated fat impairs the anti-inflammatory properties of high-density lipoproteins and endothelial function. *J Am Coll Cardiol.* 2006 Aug 15;48(4):715-20.

Nicolaou N, Poorafshar M, Murray C, Simpson A, Winell H, Kerry G, Härlin A, Woodcock A, Ahlstedt S, Custovic A. Allergy or tolerance in children sensitized to peanut: prevalence and differentiation using component-resolved diagnostics. *J Allergy Clin Immunol.* 2010 Jan;125(1):191-7.e1-13.

Nie L, Wise M, Peterson D, Meydani M. Mechanism by which avenanthramide-c, a polyphenol of oats, blocks cell cycle progression in vascular smooth muscle cells. Free Radic Biol Med. 2006 Sep 1;41(5):702-8.

Nie L, Wise ML, Peterson DM, Meydani M. Avenanthramide, a polyphenol from oats, inhibits vascular smooth muscle cell proliferation and enhances nitric oxide production. Atherosclerosis. 2006 Jun;186(2):260-6. 25. Sur R, Nigam A, Grote D, Liebel F, Southall MD. Avenanthramides, polyphenols from oats, exhibit anti-inflammatory and anti-itch activity. Arch Dermatol Res. 2008 May 7.

Niederau C, Göpfert E. The effect of chelidonium- and turmeric root extract on upper abdominal pain due to functional disorders of the biliary system. Results from a placebo-controlled double-blind study. *Med Klin.* 1999 Aug 15;94(8):425-30.

Niederberger V, Horak F, Vrtala S, Spitzauer S, Krauth MT, Valent P, Reisinger J, Pelzmann M, Hayek B, Kronqvist M, Gafvelin G, Grönlund H, Purohit A, Suck R, Fiebig H, Cromwell O, Pauli G, van Hage-Hamsten M, Valenta R.

Vaccination with genetically engineered allergens prevents progression of allergic disease. *Proc Natl Acad Sci U S A.* 2004 Oct 5;101 Suppl 2:14677-82.

Niederhofer H. Association of attention-deficit/hyperactivity disorder and celiac disease: a brief report. Prim Care Companion CNS Disord. 2011;13(3). pii: PCC.10br01104.

Niedzielin K, Kordecki H, Birkenfeld B. A controlled, double-blind, randomized study on the efficacy of Lactobacillus plantarum 299V in patients with irritable bowel syndrome. *Eur J Gastroenterol Hepatol.* 2001 Oct;13(10):1143-7.

Nielsen RG, Bindslev-Jensen C, Kruse-Andersen S, Husby S. Severe gastroesophageal reflux disease and cow milk hypersensitivity in infants and children: disease association and evaluation of a new challenge procedure. *J Pediatr Gastroenterol Nutr.* 2004 Oct;39(4):383-91.

Nielsen WW, Lindsey K. When there is no school nurse – are teachers prepared for students with peanut allergies? *School Nurse News.* 2010 Jan;27(1):12-5.

Niggemann B, Binder C, Dupont C, Hadji S, Arvola T, Isolauri E. Prospective, controlled, multi-center study on the effect of an amino-acid-based formula in infants with cow's milk allergy/intolerance and atopic dermatitis. *Pediatr Allergy Immunol.* 2001 Apr;12(2):78-82.

Niggemann B, Celik-Bilgili S, Ziegert M, Reibel S, Sommerfeld C, Wahn U. Specific IgE levels do not indicate persistence or transience of food allergy in children with atopic dermatitis. *J Investig Allergol Clin Immunol.* 2004;14(2):98-103.

Niggemann B, von Berg A, Bollrath C, Berdel D, Schauer U, Rieger C, Haschke-Becher E, Wahn U. Safety and efficacy of a new extensively hydrolyzed formula for infants with cow's milk protein allergy. *Pediatr Allergy Immunol.* 2008 Jun;19(4):348-54.

Nikulina M, Habich C, Flohe SB, Scott FW, Kolb H. Wheat gluten causes dendritic cell maturation and chemokine secretion. J Immunol. 2004;173:1925–31.

Nilsson AC, Ostman EM, Holst JJ, Björck IM. Including indigestible carbohydrates in the evening meal of healthy subjects improves glucose tolerance, lowers inflammatory markers, and increases satiety after a subsequent standardized breakfast. J Nutr. 2008 Apr;138(4):732-9.

Nobaek S, Johansson ML, Molin G, Ahrné S, Jeppsson B. Alteration of intestinal microflora is associated with reduction in abdominal bloating and pain in patients with irritable bowel syndrome. *Am J Gastroenterol.* 2000 May;95(5):1231-8.

Nodake Y, Fukumoto S, Fukasawa M, Sakakibara R, Yamasaki N. Reduction of the immunogenicity of beta-lactoglobulin from cow's milk by conjugation with a dextran derivative. *Biosci Biotechnol Biochem.* 2010;74(4):721-6.

Noh J, Lee JH, Noh G, Bang SY, Kim HS, Choi WS, Cho S, Lee SS. Characterisation of allergen-specific responses of IL-10-producing regulatory B cells (Br1) in Cow Milk Allergy. *Cell Immunol.* 2010;264(2):143-9.

Noorbakhsh R, Mortazavi SA, Sankian M, Shahidi F, Assarehzadegan MA, Varasteh A. Cloning, expression, characterization, and computational approach for cross-reactivity prediction of manganese superoxide dismutase allergen from pistachio nut. *Allergol Int.* 2010 Sep;59(3):295-304.

Nowak-Wegrzyn A, Fiocchi A. Is oral immunotherapy the cure for food allergies? *Curr Opin Allergy Clin Immunol.* 2010 Jun;10(3):214-9.

Nowak-Wegrzyn A, Muraro A. Food protein-induced enterocolitis syndrome. *Curr Opin Allergy Clin Immunol.* 2009 Aug;9(4):371-7.

Nowak-Wegrzyn A, Sampson HA, Wood RA, Sicherer SH. Food protein-induced enterocolitis syndrome caused by solid food proteins. *Pediatrics.* 2003 Apr;111(4 Pt 1):829-35.

Nuñez YO, Salabarria IS, Collado IG, Hernández-Galán R. Sesquiterpenes from the wood of Juniperus lucayana. *Phytochemistry.* 2007 Oct;68(19):2409-14.

Nurmi T, Lampia AM, Nyströma L, Hemery Y, Rouaub X, Piironena V. Distribution and composition of phytosterols and steryl ferulates in wheat grain and bran fractions. Journal of Cereal Sci. 2012:56(2); Sept, 379–388.

Nyström L, Lampi AM, Rita H, Aura AM, Oksman-Caldentey KM, Piironen V. Effects of processing on availability of total plant sterols, steryl ferulates and steryl glycosides from wheat and rye bran. J Agric Food Chem. 2007 Oct 31;55(22):9059-65.

O'Connor J., Bensky D. (ed). *Shanghai College of Traditional Chinese Medicine: Acupuncture: A Comprehensive Text.* Seattle: Eastland Press, 1981.

O'Connor MI. Warming strengthens an herbivore-plant interaction. *Ecology.* 2009 Feb;90(2):388-98.

Odamaki T, Xiao JZ, Iwabuchi N, Sakamoto M, Takahashi N, Kondo S, Miyaji K, Iwatsuki K, Togashi H, Enomoto T, Benno Y. Influence of Bifidobacterium longum BB536 intake on faecal microbiota in individuals with Japanese cedar pollinosis during the pollen season. *J Med Microbiol.* 2007 Oct;56(Pt 10):1301-8.

Oehme FW (ed.). *Toxicity of heavy metals in the environment. Part 1.* New York: M.Dekker, 1979.

Oh CK, Lücker PW, Wetzelsberger N, Kuhlmann F. The determination of magnesium, calcium, sodium and potassium in assorted foods with special attention to the loss of electrolytes after various forms of food preparations. *Mag.-Bull.* 1986;8:297-302.

Oh JW, Pyun BY, Choung JT, Ahn KM, Kim CH, Song SW, Son JA, Lee SY, Lee SI. Epidemiological change of atopic dermatitis and food allergy in school-aged children in Korea between 1995 and 2000. *J Korean Med Sci.* 2004 Oct;19(5):716-23.

Oh SY, Chung J, Kim MK, Kwon SO, Cho BH. Antioxidant nutrient intakes and corresponding biomarkers associated with the risk of atopic dermatitis in young children. Eur J Clin Nutr. 2010 Mar;64(3):245-52.

Ohman L, Simren M. Pathogenesis of IBS: role of inflammation, immunity and neuroimmune interactions. Nat Rev Gastroenterol Hepatol. 2010;7:163–173.

Okasaka M, Takaishi Y, Kashiwada Y, Kodzhimatov OK, Ashurmetov O, Lin AJ, Consentino LM, Lee KH.Terpenoids from Juniperus polycarpus var. seravschanica. *Phytochemistry.* 2006 Dec;67(24):2635-40.

Okazaki Y, Isobe T, Iwata Y, Matsukawa T, Matsuda F, Miyagawa H, Ishihara A, Nishioka T, Iwamura H. Metabolism of avenanthramide phytoalexins in oats. Plant J. 2004 Aug;39(4):560-72.

Ołdak E, Kurzatkowska B, Stasiak-Barmuta A. Natural course of sensitization in children: follow-up study from birth to 6 years of age, I. Evaluation of total serum IgE and specific IgE antibodies with regard to atopic family history. *Rocz Akad Med Bialymst.* 2000;45:87-95.

Olivieri M, Biscardo CA, Palazzo P, Pahr S, Malerba G, Ferrara R, Zennaro D, Zanoni G, Xumerle L, Valenta R, Mari A. Wheat IgE profiling and wheat IgE levels in bakers with allergic occupational phenotypes. Occup Environ Med. 2013 Sep;70(9):617-22.

O'Mahony L, McCarthy J, Kelly P, Hurley G, Luo F, Chen K, O'Sullivan GC, Kiely B, Collins JK, Shanahan F, Quigley EM. Lactobacillus and bifidobacterium in irritable bowel syndrome: symptom responses and relationship to cytokine profiles. *Gastroenterology.* 2005 Mar;128(3):541-51.

O'Neil C, Helbling AA, Lehrer SB. Allergic reactions to fish. *Clin Rev Allergy.* 1993 Summer;11(2):183-200.

O'Neil C, Helbling AA, Lehrer SB. Allergic reactions to fish. *Clin Rev Allergy.* 1993;11(2):183-200.

Ong DK, Mitchell SB, Barrett JS, Shepherd SJ, Irving PM, Biesiekierski JR, Smith S, Gibson PR, Muir JG. Manipulation of dietary short chain carbohydrates alters the pattern of gas production and genesis of symptoms in irritable bowel syndrome. J Gastroenterol Hepatol. 2010 Aug;25(8):1366-73.

Orhan F, Karakas T, Cakir M, Aksoy A, Baki A, Gedik Y. Prevalence of immunoglobulin E-mediated food allergy in 6-9-year-old urban schoolchildren in the eastern Black Sea region of Turkey. *Clin Exp Allergy.* 2009 Jul;39(7):1027-35.

Ortiz-Andrellucchi A, Sánchez-Villegas A, Rodríguez-Gallego C, Lemes A, Molero T, Soria A, Peña-Quintana L, Santana M, Ramírez O, García J, Cabrera F, Cobo J, Serra-Majem L. Immunomodulatory effects of the intake of fermented milk with Lactobacillus casei DN114001 in lactating mothers and their children. Br J Nutr. 2008 Oct;100(4):834-45.

Osborne TB. The Proteins of the Wheat Kernel. Carnegie Instit. 1907

Osguthorpe JD. Immunotherapy. *Curr Opin Otolaryngol Head Neck Surg.* 2010 Jun;18(3):206-12.

Otte JM, Podolsky DK. Functional modulation of enterocytes by Gram-positive and Gram-negative microorganisms. Am J Physiol Gastrointest Liver Physiol. 2004;286:G613–26.

Otto SJ, van Houwelingen AC, Hornstra G. The effect of supplementation with docosahexaenoic and arachidonic acid derived from single cell oils on plasma and erythrocyte fatty acids of pregnant women in the second trimester. *Prostaglandins Leukot Essent Fatty Acids.* 2000 Nov;63(5):323-8.

Ou CC, Tsao SM, Lin MC, Yin MC. Protective action on human LDL against oxidation and glycation by four organosulfur compounds derived from garlic. *Lipids.* 2003 Mar;38(3):219-24.

Ou G, Hedberg M, Hörstedt P, Baranov V, Forsberg G, Drobni M, Sandström O, Wai SN, Johansson I, Hammarström ML, Hernell O, Hammarström S. Proximal small intestinal microbiota and identification of rod-shaped bacteria associated with childhood celiac disease. Am J Gastroenterol. 2009 Dec;104(12):3058-67.

Ouwehand AC, Nermes M, Collado MC, Rautonen N, Salminen S, Isolauri E. Specific probiotics alleviate allergic rhinitis during the birch pollen season. *World J Gastroenterol.* 2009 Jul 14;15(26):3261-8.

Ouwehand AC, Tiihonen K, Saarinen M, Putaala H, Rautonen N. Influence of a combination of Lactobacillus acidophilus NCFM and lactitol on healthy elderly: intestinal and immune parameters. *Br J Nutr.* 2009 Feb;101(3):367-75.

Ozdemir O. Any benefits of probiotics in allergic disorders? *Allergy Asthma Proc.* 2010 Mar;31(2):103-11.

Paajanen L, Tuure T, Poussa T, Korpela R. No difference in symptoms during challenges with homogenized and unhomogenized cow's milk in subjects with subjective hypersensitivity to homogenized milk. *J Dairy Res.* 2003 May;70(2):175-9.

Paganelli R, Pallone F, Montano S, Le Moli S, Matricardi PM, Fais S, Paoluzi P, D'Amelio R, Aiuti F. Isotypic analysis of antibody response to a food antigen in inflammatory bowel disease. *Int Arch Allergy Appl Immunol.* 1985;78(1):81-5.

Pahud JJ, Schwarz K. Research and development of infant formulae with reduced allergenic properties. *Ann Allergy.* 1984 Dec;53(6 Pt 2):609-14.

Pak CH, Oleneva VA, Agadzhanov SA. Dietetic aspects of preventing urolithiasis in patients with gout and uric acid diathesis. *Vopr Pitan.* 1985 Jan-Feb;(1):21-4.

Palacin A, Bartra J, Muñoz R, Diaz-Perales A, Valero A, Salcedo G. Anaphylaxis to wheat flour-derived foodstuffs and the lipid transfer protein syndrome: a potential role of wheat lipid transfer protein Tri a 14. *Int Arch Allergy Immunol.* 2010;152(2):178-83.

Paller AS, Nimmagadda S, Schachner L, Mallory SB, Kahn T, Willis I, Eichenfield LF. Fluocinolone acetonide 0.01% in peanut oil: therapy for childhood atopic dermatitis, even in patients who are peanut sensitive. *J Am Acad Dermatol.* 2003 Apr;48(4):569-77.

Palmer DJ, Gold MS, Makrides M. Effect of cooked and raw egg consumption on ovalbumin content of human milk: a randomized, double-blind, cross-over trial. *Clin Exp Allergy.* 2005 Feb;35(2):173-8.

Panzani R, Ariano R, Mistrello G. Cypress pollen does not cross-react to plant-derived foods. *Eur Ann Allergy Clin Immunol.* 2010 Jun;42(3):125-6.

Parcell S. Sulfur in human nutrition and applications in medicine. *Altern Med Rev.* 2002 Feb;7(1):22-44.

Parekh PI, Petro AE, Tiller JM, Feinglos MN, Surwit RS. Reversal of diet-induced obesity and diabetes in C57BL/6J mice. Metabolism. 1998 Sep;47(9):1089-96.

Parikka K, Rowland IR, Welch RW, Wähälä K. In vitro antioxidant activity and antigenotoxicity of 5-n-alkylresorcinols. J Agric Food Chem. 2006 Mar 8;54(5):1646-50.

Pastorello EA, Farioli L, Conti A, Pravettoni V, Bonomi S, Iametti S, Fortunato D, Scibilia J, Bindslev-Jensen C, Ballmer-Weber B, Robino AM, Ortolani C. Wheat IgE-mediated food allergy in European patients: alpha-amylase inhibitors, lipid transfer proteins and low-molecular-weight glutenins. Allergenic molecules recognized by double-blind, placebo-controlled food challenge. Int Arch Allergy Immunol. 2007;144(1):10-22.

Pastorello EA, Farioli L, Pravettoni V, Robino AM, Scibilia J, Fortunato D, Conti A, Borgonovo L, Bengtsson A, Ortolani C. Lipid transfer protein and vicilin are important walnut allergens in patients not allergic to pollen. *J Allergy Clin Immunol.* 2004 Oct;114(4):908-14.

Pastorello EA, Farioli L, Pravettoni V, Scibilia J, Conti A, Fortunato D, Borgonovo L, Bonomi S, Primavesi L, Ballmer-Weber B. Maize food allergy: lipid-transfer proteins, endochitinases, and alpha-zein precursor are relevant maize allergens in double-blind placebo-controlled maize-challenge-positive patients. *Anal Bioanal Chem.* 2009 Sep;395(1):93-102.

Pastorello EA, Pompei C, Pravettoni V, Farioli L, Calamari AM, Scibilia J, Robino AM, Conti A, Iametti S, Fortunato D, Bonomi S, Ortolani C. Lipid-transfer protein is the major maize allergen maintaining IgE-binding activity after cooking at 100 degrees C, as demonstrated in anaphylactic patients and patients with positive double-blind, placebo-controlled food challenge results. *J Allergy Clin Immunol.* 2003 Oct;112(4):775-83.

Pastorello EA, Vieths S, Pravettoni V, Farioli L, Trambaioli C, Fortunato D, Lüttkopf D, Calamari M, Ansaloni R, Scibilia J, Ballmer-Weber BK, Poulsen LK, Wütrich B, Hansen KS, Robino AM, Ortolani C, Conti A. Identification of hazelnut major allergens in sensitive patients with positive double-blind, placebo-controlled food challenge results. *J Allergy Clin Immunol.* 2002 Mar;109(3):563-70.

Pastuszewska B, Vitjazkova M, Swiech E, Taciak M. Composition and in vitro digestibility of raw versus cooked white- and colour-flowered peas. Nahrung. 2004 Jun;48(3):221-5.

Patriarca G, Nucera E, Pollastrini E, Roncallo C, De Pasquale T, Lombardo C, Pedone C, Gasbarrini G, Buonomo A, Schiavino D. Oral specific desensitization in food-allergic children. *Dig Dis Sci.* 2007 Jul;52(7):1662-72.

Patriarca G, Nucera E, Roncallo C, Pollastrini E, Bartolozzi F, De Pasquale T, Buonomo A, Gasbarrini G, Di Campli C, Schiavino D. Oral desensitizing treatment in food allergy: clinical and immunological results. *Aliment Pharmacol Ther.* 2003 Feb;17(3):459-65.

Patwardhan B, Gautam M. Botanical immunodrugs: scope and opportunities. *Drug Discov Today.* 2005 Apr 1;10(7):495-502.

Payment P, Franco E, Richardson L, Siemiatyck, J. Gastrointestinal health effects associated with the consumption of drinking water produced by point-of-use domestic reverse-osmosis filtration units. *Appl. Environ. Microbiol.* 1991;57:945-948.

Peeters KA, Koppelman SJ, van Hoffen E, van der Tas CW, den Hartog Jager CF, Penninks AH, Hefle SL, Bruijnzeel-Koomen CA, Knol EF, Knulst AC. Does skin prick test reactivity to purified allergens correlate with clinical severity of peanut allergy? *Clin Exp Allergy.* 2007 Jan;37(1):108-15.

Pehowich DJ, Gomes AV, Barnes JA. Fatty acid composition and possible health effects of coconut constituents. *West Indian Med J.* 2000 Jun;49(2):128-33.

Peña AS, Crusius JB. Food allergy, coeliac disease and chronic inflammatory bowel disease in man. *Vet Q.* 1998;20 Suppl 3:S49-52.

Pepeljnjak S, Kosalec I, Kalodera Z, Blazević N. Antimicrobial activity of juniper berry essential oil (Juniperus communis L., Cupressaceae). *Acta Pharm.* 2005 Dec;55(4):417-22.

Pereira B, Venter C, Grundy J, Clayton CB, Arshad SH, Dean T (2005) Prevalence of sensitization to food allergens, reported adverse reaction to foods, food avoidance, and food hypersensitivity among teenagers. *J Allergy Clin Immunol.* 116: 884–892.

Pereira MA, Jacobs DR Jr, Pins JJ, Raatz SK, Gross MD, Slavin JL, Seaquist ER. Effect of whole grains on insulin sensitivity in overweight hyperinsulinemic adults. Am J Clin Nutr. 2002 May;75(5):848-55.

Perez-Galvez A, Martin HD, Sies H, Stahl W. Incorporation of carotenoids from paprika oleoresin into human chylomicrons. *Br J Nutr.* 2003 Jun;89(6):787-93.

Perez-Pena R. Secrets of the Mummy's Medicine Chest. *NY Times.* 2005 Sept 10.

Perisic VN, Lopicic Z, Kokai G. Celiac disease and schizophrenia: family occurrence. J Pediatr Gastroenterol Nutr. 1990 Aug;11(2):279.

Permaul P, Stutius LM, Sheehan WJ, Rangsithienchai P, Walter JE, Twarog FJ, Young MC, Scott JE, Schneider LC, Phipatanakul W. Sesame allergy: role of specific IgE and skin-prick testing in predicting food challenge results. *Allergy Asthma Proc.* 2009 Nov-Dec;30(6):643-8.

Perrier C, Thierry AC, Mercenier A, Corthésy B. Allergen-specific antibody and cytokine responses, mast cell reactivity and intestinal permeability upon oral challenge of sensitized and tolerized mice. *Clin Exp Allergy.* 2010 Jan;40(1):153-62.

Pessi T, Sütas Y, Hurme M, Isolauri E. Interleukin-10 generation in atopic children following oral Lactobacillus rhamnosus GG. *Clin Exp Allergy.* 2000 Dec;30(12):1804-8.

Peterson CG, Hansson T, Skott A, Bengtsson U, Ahlstedt S, Magnussons J. Detection of local mast-cell activity in patients with food hypersensitivity. *J Investig Allergol Clin Immunol.* 2007;17(5):314-20.

Petitot M, Brossard C, Barrona C, Larréb C, Morela MH, Micard V. Modification of pasta structure induced by high drying temperatures. Effects on the in vitro digestibility of protein and starch fractions and the potential allergenicity of protein hydrolysates. Food Chem. 2009 Sept; 116 (2): 401–412.

Petlevski R, Hadzija M, Slijepcević M, Juretić D, Petrik J. Glutathione S-transferases and malondialdehyde in the liver of NOD mice on short-term treatment with plant mixture extract P-9801091. *Phytother Res.* 2003 Apr;17(4):311-4.

Petlevski R, Hadzija M, Slijepcević M, Juretić D. Toxicological assessment of P-9801091 plant mixture extract after chronic administration in CBA/HZg mice – a biochemical and histological study. *Coll Antropol.* 2008 Jun;32(2):577-81.

Pfefferle PI, Sel S, Ege MJ, Büchele G, Blümer N, Krauss-Etschmann S, Herzum I, Albers CE, Lauener RP, Roponen M, Hirvonen MR, Vuitton DA, Riedler J, Brunekreef B, Dalphin JC, Braun-Fahrländer C, Pekkanen J, von Mutius E, Renz H; PASTURE Study Group. Cord blood allergen-specific IgE is associated with reduced IFN-gamma production by cord blood cells: the Protection against Allergy-Study in Rural Environments (PASTURE) Study. *J Allergy Clin Immunol.* 2008 Oct;122(4):711-6.

Pfundstein B, El Desouky SK, Hull WE, Haubner R, Erben G, Owen RW. Polyphenolic compounds in the fruits of Egyptian medicinal plants (Terminalia bellerica, Terminalia chebula and Terminalia horrida): characterization, quantitation and determination of antioxidant capacities. *Phytochemistry.* 2010 Jul;71(10):1132-48.

Pharmacopoeia of the People's Republic of China. English. Beijing: Chemical Industry Press; 2005. The State Pharmacopoeia Commission of The People's Republic of China.Nusem D, Panasoff J. Beer anaphylaxis. *Isr Med Assoc J.* 2009 Jun;11(6):380-1.

Phillippy BQ, Bland BM, Evens TJ, Ion Chromatography of Phytate in Roots and Tubers. Journal of Agricultural and Food Chemistry. 2002; Dec:51(2): 350–3.

Physicians' Desk Reference. Montvale, NJ: Thomson, 2003-2008

Phytochemical investigation of juniper rufescens Juniperus oxycedrus L. leaves and fruits. *Georgian Med News.* 2009 Mar;(168):107-11.

Piboonpocanun S, Boonchoo S, Pariyaprasert W, Visitsunthorn N, Jirapongsananuruk O. Determination of storage conditions for shrimp extracts: analysis of specific IgE-allergen profiles. *Asian Pac J Allergy Immunol.* 2010 Mar;28(1):47-52.

Picarelli A, Maiuri L, Mazzilli MC, Coletta S, Ferrante P, Di Giovambattista F, Greco M, Torsoli A, Auricchio S. Gluten-sensitive disease with mild enteropathy. Gastroenterology. 1996 Sep;111(3):608-16.

Pierce SK, Klinman NR. Antibody-specific immunoregulation. *J Exp Med.* 1977 Aug 1;146(2):509-19.

Pierucci VR, Tilley M, Graybosch RA, Blechl AE, Bean SR, Tilley KA. Effects of overexpression of high molecular weight glutenin subunit 1Dy10 on wheat tortilla properties. J Agric Food Chem. 2009 Jul 22;57(14):6318-26.

Piirainen L, Haahtela S, Helin T, Korpela R, Haahtela T, Vaarala O. Effect of Lactobacillus rhamnosus GG on rBet v1 and rMal d1 specific IgA in the saliva of patients with birch pollen allergy. *Ann Allergy Asthma Immunol.* 2008 Apr;100(4):338-42.

Pike MG, Heddle RJ, Boulton P, Turner MW, Atherton DJ. Increased intestinal permeability in atopic eczema. *J Invest Dermatol.* 1986 Feb;86(2):101-4.

Piperno DR Host I. The Humid Neotropics: Indications of Early Tuber Use and Agriculture in Panama. Journal of Archaeological Science. 1998; 25(8) Aug. 765–776.

Pisani A, Ierardi E, Comelli MC, Barone M. Phytoestrogens/insoluble fibers and colonic estrogen receptor β: randomized, double-blind, placebo-controlled study. World J Gastroenterol. 2013 Jul 21;19(27):4325-33.

Pitt-Rivers R, Trotter WR. *The Thyroid Gland.* London: Butterworth Publ, 1954.

Plein K, Hotz J. Therapeutic effects of Saccharomyces boulardii on mild residual symptoms in a stable phase of Crohn's disease with special respect to chronic diarrhea – a pilot study. *Z Gastroenterol.* 1993 Feb;31(2):129-34.

Plohmann B, Bader G, Hiller K, Franz G. Immunomodulatory and antitumoral effects of triterpenoid saponins. *Pharmazie.* 1997 Dec;52(12):953-7.

Pobłocka-Olech L, Krauze-Baranowska M. SPE-HPTLC of procyanidins from the barks of different species and clones of Salix. *J Pharm Biomed Anal.* 2008 Nov 4;48(3):965-8.

Pochard P, Vickery B, Berin MC, Grishin A, Sampson HA, Caplan M, Bottomly K. Targeting Toll-like receptors on dendritic cells modifies the T(H)2 response to peanut allergens in vitro. *J Allergy Clin Immunol.* 2010 Jul;126(1):92-7.e5.

Pohjavuori E, Viljanen M, Korpela R, Kuitunen M, Tiittanen M, Vaarala O, Savilahti E. Lactobacillus GG effect in increasing IFN-gamma production in infants with cow's milk allergy. *J Allergy Clin Immunol.* 2004 Jul;114(1):131-6.

Pollini F, Capristo C, Boner AL. Upper respiratory tract infections and atopy. *Int J Immunopathol Pharmacol.* 2010 Jan-Mar;23(1 Suppl):32-7.

Ponsonby AL, McMichael A, van der Mei I. Ultraviolet radiation and autoimmune disease: insights from epidemiological research. *Toxicology.* 2002 Dec 27;181-182:71-8.

Poppitt SD, van Drunen JD, McGill AT, Mulvey TB, Leahy FE. Supplementation of a high-carbohydrate breakfast with barley beta-glucan improves postprandial glycaemic response for meals but not beverages. Asia Pac J Clin Nutr. 2007;16(1):16-24.

Potocki P, Hozyasz K. [Psychiatric symptoms and coeliac disease]. Psychiatr Pol. 2002 Jul-Aug;36(4):567-78. Polish.

Potocki P, Hozyasz K. Psychiatric symptoms and coeliac disease. Psychiatr Pol. 2002 Jul-Aug;36(4):567-78.

Potterton D. (Ed.) *Culpeper's Color Herbal.* New York: Sterling, 1983.

Poulos LM, Waters AM, Correll PK, Loblay RH, Marks GB. Trends in hospitalizations for anaphylaxis, angioedema, and urticaria in Australia, 1993-1994 to 2004-2005. *J Allergy Clin Immunol.* 2007 Oct;120(4):878-84.

Prescott SL, Wickens K, Westcott L, Jung W, Currie H, Black PN, Stanley TV, Mitchell EA, Fitzharris P, Siebers R, Wu L, Crane J; Probiotic Study Group. Supplementation with Lactobacillus rhamnosus or Bifidobacterium lactis probiotics in pregnancy increases cord blood interferon-gamma and breast milk transforming growth factor-beta and immunoglobin A detection. *Clin Exp Allergy.* 2008 Oct;38(10):1606-14.

Price RK, Keaveney EM, Hamill LL, Wallace JM, Ward M, Ueland PM, McNulty H, Strain JJ, Parker MJ, Welch RW. Consumption of wheat aleurone-rich foods increases fasting plasma betaine and modestly decreases fasting homocysteine and LDL-cholesterol in adults. J Nutr. 2010 Dec;140(12):2153-7.

Price RK, Wallace JM, Hamill LL, Keaveney EM, Strain JJ, Parker MJ, Welch RW. Evaluation of the effect of wheat aleurone-rich foods on markers of antioxidant status, inflammation and endothelial function in apparently healthy men and women. Br J Nutr. 2012 Nov 14;108(9):1644-51.

Prieto A, Razzak E, Lindo DP, Alvarez-Perea A, Rueda M, Baeza ML. Recurrent anaphylaxis due to lupin flour: primary sensitization through inhalation. *J Investig Allergol Clin Immunol.* 2010;20(1):76-9.

Principi M, Di Leo A, Pricci M, Scavo MP, Guido R, Tanzi S, Piscitelli D,

Prioult G, Fliss I, Pecquet S. Effect of probiotic bacteria on induction and maintenance of oral tolerance to beta-lactoglobulin in gnotobiotic mice. *Clin Diagn Lab Immunol.* 2003 Sep;10(5):787-92.

Proujansky R, Winter HS, Walker WA. Gastrointestinal syndromes associated with food sensitivity. *Adv Pediatr.* 1988;35:219-37.

Prucksunand C, Indrasukhsri B, Leethochawalit M, Hungspreugs K. Phase II clinical trial on effect of the long turmeric (Curcuma longa Linn) on healing of peptic ulcer. *Southeast Asian J Trop Med Public Health.* 2001 Mar;32(1):208-15.

Prussin C, Lee J, Foster B. Eosinophilic gastrointestinal disease and peanut allergy are alternatively associated with IL-5+ and IL-5(-) T(H)2 responses. *J Allergy Clin Immunol.* 2009 Dec;124(6):1326-32.e6.

Pruthi S, Thapa MM. Infectious and inflammatory disorders. *Magn Reson Imaging Clin N Am.* 2009 Aug;17(3):423-38, v.

Pulcini JM, Sease KK, Marshall GD. Disparity between the presence and absence of food allergy action plans in one school district. *Allergy Asthma Proc.* 2010 Mar;31(2):141-6.

Pustisek N, Jaklin-Kekez A, Frkanec R, Sikanić-Dugić N, Misak Z, Jadresin O, Kolacek S. Our experiences with the use of atopy patch test in the diagnosis of cow's milk hypersensitivity. Acta Dermatovenerol Croat. 2010;18(1):14-20. Kim JH, Kim JE, Choi GS, Hwang EK, An S, Ye YM, Park HS. A case of occupational rhinitis caused by rice powder in the grain industry. *Allergy Asthma Immunol Res.* 2010 Apr;2(2):141-3.

Pusztai A, Ewen SW, Grant G, Brown DS, Stewart JC, Peumans WJ, Van Damme EJ, Bardocz S. Antinutritive effects of wheat-germ agglutinin and other N-acetylglucosamine-specific lectins. Br J Nutr. 1993 Jul;70(1):313-21.

Pyle GG, Paaso B, Anderson BE, Allen DD, Marti T, Li Q, Siegel M, Khosla C, Gray GM. Effect of pretreatment of food gluten with prolyl endopeptidase on gluten-induced malabsorption in celiac sprue. Clin Gastroenterol Hepatol. 2005 Jul;3(7):687-94.

Pysz M, Polaszczyk S, Leszczyńska T, Piątkowska E. Effect of microwave field on trypsin inhibitors activity and protein quality of broad bean seeds (Vicia faba var. major). Acta Sci Pol Technol Aliment. 2012 Apr 2;11(2):193-8.

Qin HL, Zheng JJ, Tong DN, Chen WX, Fan XB, Hang XM, Jiang YQ. Effect of Lactobacillus plantarum enteral feeding on the gut permeability and septic complications in the patients with acute pancreatitis. *Eur J Clin Nutr.* 2008 Jul;62(7):923-30.

Qu C, Srivastava K, Ko J, Zhang TF, Sampson HA, Li XM. Induction of tolerance after establishment of peanut allergy by the food allergy herbal formula-2 is associated with up-regulation of interferon-gamma. *Clin Exp Allergy.* 2007 Jun;37(6):846-55.

Quigley EM, Abdel-Hamid H, Barbara G, Bhatia SJ, Boeckxstaens G, De Giorgio R, *et al.* A global perspective on irritable bowel syndrome: a consensus statement of the World Gastroenterology Organisation Summit Task Force on irritable bowel syndrome. J Clin Gastroenterol. 2012;46:356–66.

Rafter J, Bennett M, Caderni G, Clune Y, Hughes R, Karlsson PC, Klinder A, O'Riordan M, O'Sullivan GC, Pool-Zobel B, Rechkemmer G, Roller M, Rowland I, Salvadori M, Thijs H, Van Loo J, Watzl B, Collins JK. Dietary synbiotics reduce cancer risk factors in polypectomized and colon cancer patients. *Am J Clin Nutr.* 2007 Feb;85(2):488-96.

Raherison C, Pénard-Morand C, Moreau D, Caillaud D, Charpin D, Kopferschmitt C, Lavaud F, Taytard A, Maesano IA. Smoking exposure and allergic sensitization in children according to maternal allergies. *Ann Allergy Asthma Immunol.* 2008 Apr;100(4):351-7.

Rahman MM, Bhattacharya A, Fernandes G. Docosahexaenoic acid is more potent inhibitor of osteoclast differentiation in RAW 264.7 cells than eicosapentaenoic acid. *J Cell Physiol.* 2008 Jan;214(1):201-9.

Railey MD, Burks AW. Therapeutic approaches for the treatment of food allergy. *Expert Opin Pharmacother.* 2010 May;11(7):1045-8.

Raimondi F, Indrio F, Crivaro V, Araimo G, Capasso L, Paludetto R. Neonatal hyperbilirubinemia increases intestinal protein permeability and the prevalence of cow's milk protein intolerance. *Acta Paediatr.* 2008 Jun;97(6):751-3.

Raithel M, Weidenhiller M, Abel R, Baenkler HW, Hahn EG. Colorectal mucosal histamine release by mucosa oxygenation in comparison with other established clinical tests in patients with gastrointestinally mediated allergy. *World J Gastroenterol.* 2006 Aug 7;12(29):4699-705.

Ramagopalan SV, Dyment DA, Guimond C, Orton SM, Yee IM, Ebers GC, Sadovnick AD. Childhood cow's milk allergy and the risk of multiple sclerosis: a population based study. *J Neurol Sci.* 2010 Apr 15;291(1-2):86-8.

Rampal G, Thind TS, Vig AP, Arora S. Antimutagenic potential of glucosinolate-rich seed extracts of broccoli (Brassica oleracea L var italica Plenck). Int J Toxicol. 2010 Dec;29(6):616-24.

Rampton DS, Murdoch RD, Sladen GE. Rectal mucosal histamine release in ulcerative colitis. *Clin Sci (Lond).* 1980 Nov;59(5):389-91.

Rancé F, Abbal M, Lauwers-Cancès V. Improved screening for peanut allergy by the combined use of skin prick tests and specific IgE assays. *J Allergy Clin Immunol.* 2002 Jun;109(6):1027-33.

Rancé F, Bidat E, Bourrier T, Sabouraud D. Cashew allergy: observations of 42 children without associated peanut allergy. *Allergy.* 2003 Dec;58(12):1311-4.

Rance F, Kanny G, Dutau G, Moneret-Vautrin DA. Food allergens in children. *Arch Pediatr.* 1999;6(Suppl 1):61S-66S.

Randal Bollinger R, Barbas AS, Bush EL, Lin SS, Parker W. Biofilms in the large bowel suggest an apparent function of the human vermiform appendix. *J Theor Biol.* 2007 Dec 21;249(4):826-31.

Rao SK, Rao PS, Rao BN. Preliminary investigation of the radiosensitizing activity of guduchi (Tinospora cordifolia) in tumor-bearing mice. *Phytother Res.* 2008 Nov;22(11):1482-9.

Rapin JR, Wiernsperger N. Possible links between intestinal permeablity and food processing: A potential therapeutic niche for glutamine. *Clinics (Sao Paulo).* 2010 Jun;65(6):635-43.

Rappoport J. Both sides of the pharmaceutical death coin. *Townsend Letter for Doctors and Patients.* 2006 Oct.

Ratnayake S, Beahan CT, Callahan DL, Bacic A. The reducing end sequence of wheat endosperm cell wall arabinoxylans. Carbohydr Res. 2014 Mar 11;386:23-32.

Rauha JP, Remes S, Heinonen M, Hopia A, Kähkönen M, Kujala T, Pihlaja K, Vuorela H, Vuorela P. Antimicrobial effects of Finnish plant extracts containing flavonoids and other phenolic compounds. *Int J Food Microbiol.* 2000 May 25;56(1):3-12.

Rauma A. Antioxidant status in vegetarians versus omnivores. *Nutrition.* 2003;16(2): 111-119.

Rautava S, Isolauri E. Cow's milk allergy in infants with atopic eczema is associated with aberrant production of interleukin-4 during oral cow's milk challenge. *J Pediatr Gastroenterol Nutr.* 2004 Nov;39(5):529-35.

Rave K, Roggen K, Dellweg S, Heise I, tom Dieck H. Improvement of insulin resistance after diet with a whole-grain based dietary product: results of a randomized, controlled cross-over study in obese subjects with elevated fasting blood glucose. Br J Nutr. 2007 Nov;98(5):929-36.

Reddy, N. R.; Sathe, Shridhar K. Food Phytates. Boca Raton: CRC. ISBN 1-56676-867-5, 2001.

Reger D, Goode S, Mercer E. *Chemistry: Principles & Practice.* Fort Worth, TX: Harcourt Brace, 1993.

Reha CM, Ebru A. Specific immunotherapy is effective in the prevention of new sensitivities. *Allergol Immunopathol (Madr).* 2007 Mar-Apr;35(2):44-51.

Reichling J, Schmökel H, Fitzi J, Bucher S, Saller R. Dietary support with Boswellia resin in canine inflammatory joint and spinal disease. *Schweiz Arch Tierheilkd.* 2004 Feb;146(2):71-9.

Resta-Lenert S, Barrett KE. Live probiotics protect intestinal epithelial cells from the effects of infection with entero-invasive Escherichia coli (EIEC) Gut. 2003;52:988–97.

Reuter A, Lidholm J, Andersson K, Ostling J, Lundberg M, Scheurer S, Enrique E, Cistero-Bahima A, San Miguel-Moncin M, Ballmer-Weber BK, Vieths S. A critical assessment of allergen component-based in vitro diagnosis in cherry allergy across Europe. *Clin Exp Allergy.* 2006 Jun;36(6):815-23.

Reyna-Villasmil N, Bermúdez-Pirela V, Mengual-Moreno E, Arias N, Cano-Ponce C, Leal-Gonzalez E, Souki A, Inglett GE, Israili ZH, Hernández-Hernández R, Valasco M, Arraiz N. Oat-derived beta-glucan significantly improves HDLC and diminishes LDLC and non-HDL cholesterol in overweight individuals with mild hypercholesterolemia. Am J Ther. 2007 Mar-Apr;14(2):203-12.

Richard A, Rohrmann S, Mohler-Kuo M, Rodgers S, Moffat R, Güth U, Eichholzer M. Urinary phytoestrogens and depression in perimenopausal US women: NHANES 2005-2008. J Affect Disord. 2014 Mar;156:200-5.

Rimbaud L, Heraud F, La Vieille S, Leblanc JC, Crepet A. Quantitative risk assessment relating to adventitious presence of allergens in food: a probabilistic model applied to peanut in chocolate. *Risk Anal.* 2010 Jan;30(1):7-19.

Rinne M, Kalliomaki M, Arvilommi H, Salminen S, Isolauri E. Effect of probiotics and breastfeeding on the bifidobacterium and lactobacillus/enterococcus microbiota and humoral immune responses. *J Pediatr.* 2005 Aug;147(2):186-91.

Río ME, Zago Beatriz L, Garcia H, Winter L. The nutritional status change the effectiveness of a dietary supplement of lactic bacteria on the emerging of respiratory tract diseases in children. *Arch Latinoam Nutr.* 2002 Mar;52(1):29-34.

Rivabene R, Mancini E, DeVincenzi M. In vitro cytotoxic effect of wheat gliadin-derived peptides on the Caco-2 intestinal cell line is associated with intracellular oxidative imbalance: implications for coeliac disease. Biochim Biophys Acta. 1999;1453:152–60.

Rizzello CG, De Angelis M, Di Cagno R, Camarca A, Silano M, Losito I, De Vincenzi M, De Bari MD, Palmisano F, Maurano F, Gianfrani C, Gobbetti M. Highly efficient gluten degradation by lactobacilli and fungal proteases during food processing: new perspectives for celiac disease. Appl Environ Microbiol. 2007 Jul;73(14):4499-507.

Rizzello CG, Mueller T, Coda R, Reipsch F, Nionelli L, Curiel JA, Gobbetti M. Synthesis of 2-methoxy benzoquinone and 2,6-dimethoxybenzoquinone by selected lactic acid bacteria during sourdough fermentation of wheat germ. Microb Cell Fact. 2013 Nov 11;12(1):105.

Robert AM, Groult N, Six C, Robert L. The effect of procyanidolic oligomers on mesenchymal cells in culture II – Attachment of elastic fibers to the cells. *Pathol Biol.* 1990 Jun;38(6):601-7.

Robert AM, Groult N, Six C, Robert L. The effect of procyanidolic oligomers on mesenchymal cells in culture II – Attachment of elastic fibers to the cells. *Pathol Biol.* 1990 Jun;38(6):601-7.

Roberts G, Lack G. Diagnosing peanut allergy with skin prick and specific IgE testing. *J Allergy Clin Immunol.* 2005 Jun;115(6):1291-6.

Rodriguez J, Crespo JF, Burks W, Rivas-Plata C, Fernandez-Anaya S, Vives R, Daroca P. Randomized, double-blind, crossover challenge study in 53 subjects reporting adverse reactions to melon (Cucumis melo). *J Allergy Clin Immunol.* 2000 Nov;106(5):968-72.

Rodriguez-Fragoso L, Reyes-Esparza J, Burchiel SW, Herrera-Ruiz D, Torres E. Risks and benefits of commonly used herbal medicines in Mexico. *Toxicol Appl Pharmacol.* 2008 Feb 15;227(1):125-35.

Rodríguez-Ortiz PG, Muñoz-Mendoza D, Arias-Cruz A, González-Díaz SN, Herrera-Castro D, Vidaurri-Ojeda AC. Epidemiological characteristics of patients with food allergy assisted at Regional Center of Allergies and Clinical Immunology of Monterrey. *Rev Alerg Mex.* 2009 Nov-Dec;56(6):185-91.

Roduit C, Scholtens S, de Jongste JC, Wijga AH, Gerritsen J, Postma DS, Brunekreef B, Hoekstra MO, Aalberse R, Smit HA. Asthma at 8 years of age in children born by caesarean section. *Thorax.* 2009 Feb;64(2):107-13.

Roessler A, Friedrich U, Vogelsang H, Bauer A, Kaatz M, Hipler UC, Schmidt I, Jahreis G. The immune system in healthy adults and patients with atopic dermatitis seems to be affected differently by a probiotic intervention. *Clin Exp Allergy.* 2008 Jan;38(1):93-102.

Rollan G, De Angelis M, Gobbetti M, de Valdez GF. Proteolytic activity and reduction of gliadin-like fractions by sourdough lactobacilli. J Appl Microbiol. 2005;99:1495–502.

Rollan G, De Angelis M, Gobbetti M, de Valdez GF. Proteolytic activity and reduction of gliadin-like fractions by sourdough lactobacilli. J Appl Microbiol. 2005;99:1495–502.

Romeo J, Wärnberg J, Nova E, Díaz LE, González-Gross M, Marcos A. Changes in the immune system after moderate beer consumption. *Ann Nutr Metab.* 2007;51(4):359-66.

Rona RJ, Keil T, Summers C, Gislason D, Zuidmeer L, Sodergren E, Sigurdardottir ST, Lindner T, Goldhahn K, Dahlstrom J, McBride D, Madsen C. The prevalence of food allergy: a meta-analysis. *J Allergy Clin Immunol.* 2007 Sep;120(3):638-46.

Ronteltap A, van Schaik J, Wensing M, Rynja FJ, Knulst AC, de Vries JH. Sensory testing of recipes masking peanut or hazelnut for double-blind placebo-controlled food challenges. Allergy. 2004 Apr;59(4):457-60. Clark S, Bock

SA, Gaeta TJ, Brenner BE, Cydulka RK, Camargo CA; Multicenter Airway Research Collaboration-8 Investigators. Multicenter study of emergency department visits for food allergies. *J Allergy Clin Immunol.* 2004 Feb;113(2):347-52.

Ros E, Mataix J. Fatty acid composition of nuts – implications for cardiovascular health. *Br J Nutr.* 2006 Nov;96 Suppl 2:S29-35.

Rosa NN, Dufour C, Lullien-Pellerin V, Micard V. Exposure or release of ferulic acid from wheat aleurone: impact on its antioxidant capacity. Food Chem. 2013 Dec 1;141(3):2355-62.

Rosenfeldt V, Benfeldt E, Valerius NH, Paerregaard A, Michaelsen KF. Effect of probiotics on gastrointestinal symptoms and small intestinal permeability in children with atopic dermatitis. *J Pediatr.* 2004 Nov;145(5):612-6.

Ross AB, Becker W, Chen Y, Kamal-Eldin A, Aman P. Intake of alkylresorcinols from wheat and rye in the United Kingdom and Sweden. Br J Nutr. 2005 Oct;94(4):496-9.

Rossmeisl M, Rim JS, Koza RA, Kozak LP. Variation in type 2 diabetes – related traits in mouse strains susceptible to diet-induced obesity. Diabetes. 2003 Aug;52(8):1958-66.

Rostami K, Hogg-Kollars S. A patient's journey. Non-coeliac gluten sensitivity. BMJ. 2012;345:e7982.

Rozycki VR, Baigorria CM, Freyre MR, Bernard CM, Zannier MS, Charpentier M. Nutrient content in vegetable species from the Argentine Chaco. *Arch Latinoam Nutr.* 1997 Sep;47(3):265-70.

Rubin E., Farber JL. *Pathology.* 3rd Ed. Philadelphia: Lippincott-Raven, 1999.

Rubio-Tapia A, Hill ID, Kelly CP, Calderwood AH, Murray JA. ACG clinical guidelines: diagnosis and management of celiac disease. Am J Gastroenterol. 2013;108:656–76.

Rudders SA, Espinola JA, Camargo CA Jr. North-south differences in US emergency department visits for acute allergic reactions. *Ann Allergy Asthma Immunol.* 2010 May;104(5):413-6.

Saarinen KM, Juntunen-Backman K, Järvenpää AL, Klemetti P, Kuitunen P, Lope L, Renlund M, Siivola M, Vaarala O, Savilahti E. Breast-feeding and the development of cows' milk protein allergy. *Adv Exp Med Biol.* 2000;478:121-30.

Saggioro A. Probiotics in the treatment of irritable bowel syndrome. *J Clin Gastroenterol.* 2004 Jul;38(6 Suppl):S104-6.

Sahagún-Flores JE, López-Peña LS, de la Cruz-Ramírez Jaimes J, García-Bravo MS, Peregrina-Gómez R, de Alba-García JE. Eradication of Helicobacter pylori: triple treatment scheme plus Lactobacillus vs. triple treatment alone. *Cir Cir.* 2007 Sep-Oct;75(5):333-6.

Sahin-Yilmaz A, Nocon CC, Corey JP. Immunoglobulin E-mediated food allergies among adults with allergic rhinitis. *Otolaryngol Head Neck Surg.* 2010 Sep;143(3):379-85.

Sahyoun NR, Jacques PF, Zhang XL, Juan W, McKeown NM. Whole-grain intake is inversely associated with the metabolic syndrome and mortality in older adults. Am J Clin Nutr. 2006 Jan;83(1):124-31.

Saito-Loftus Y, Brantner T, Zimmerman J, Talley N, Murray J. The prevalence of positive serologic tests for celiac sprue does not differ between irritable bowel syndrome (IBS) patients compared with controls. Am J Gastroenterol. 2008;103:S472.

Salem N, Wegher B, Mena P, Uauy R. Arachidonic and docosahexaenoic acids are biosynthesized from their 18-carbon precursors in human infants. *Proc Natl Acad Sci.* 1996;93:49-54.

Salido S, Altarejos J, Nogueras M, Sánchez A, Pannecouque C, Witvrouw M, De Clercq E. Chemical studies of essential oils of Juniperus oxycedrus ssp. badia. *J Ethnopharmacol.* 2002 Jun;81(1):129-34.

Salim AS. Sulfhydryl-containing agents in the treatment of gastric bleeding induced by nonsteroidal anti-inflammatory drugs. *Can J Surg.* 1993 Feb;36(1):53-8.

Salim, A.S., Role of oxygen-derived free radical scavengers in the management of recurrent attacks of ulcerative colitis: A new approach. *J. Lab Clin Med.* 1992;119:740-747.

Salmi H, Kuitunen M, Viljanen M, Lapatto R. Cow's milk allergy is associated with changes in urinary organic acid concentrations. *Pediatr Allergy Immunol.* 2010 Mar;21(2 Pt 2):e401-6.

Salminen S, Isolauri E, Salminen E. Clinical uses of probiotics for stabilizing the gut mucosal barrier: successful strains and future challenges. *Antonie Van Leeuwenhoek.* 1996 Oct;70(2-4):347-58.

Salom IL, Silvis SE, Doscherholmen A. Effect of cimetidine on the absorption of vitamin B12. *Scand J Gastroenterol.* 1982;17:129-31.

Salpietro CD, Gangemi S, Briuglia S, Meo A, Merlino MV, Muscolino G, Bisignano G, Trombetta D, Saija A. The almond milk: a new approach to the management of cow-milk allergy/intolerance in infants. *Minerva Pediatr.* 2005 Aug;57(4):173-80.

Samaroo D, Dickerson F, Kasarda DD, Green PH, Briani C, Yolken RH, Alaedini A. Novel immune response to gluten in individuals with schizophrenia. Schizophr Res. 2010 May;118(1 3):248-55.

Samoylenko V, Dunbar DC, Gafur MA, Khan SI, Ross SA, Mossa JS, El-Feraly FS, Tekwani BL, Bosselaers J, Muhammad I. Antiparasitic, nematicidal and antifouling constituents from Juniperus berries. *Phytother Res.* 2008 Dec;22(12):1570-6.

Samsel A, Seneff S. Glyphosate, pathways to modern diseases II: Celiac sprue and gluten intolerance. Interdiscip Toxicol. 2013; Vol. 6(4): 159–184. doi: 10.2478/intox-2013-0026.

Sancho AI, Hoffmann-Sommergruber K, Alessandri S, Conti A, Giuffrida MG, Shewry P, Jensen BM, Skov P, Vieths S. Authentication of food allergen quality by physicochemical and immunological methods. *Clin Exp Allergy.* 2010 Jul;40(7):973-86.

Sander GR, Cummins AG, Powell BC. Rapid disruption of intestinal barrier function by gliadin involves altered expression of apical junctional proteins. FEBS Lett. 2005;579(21):4851–5.

Sandin A, Annus T, Björkstén B, Nilsson L, Riikjärv MA, van Hage-Hamsten M, Bråbäck L. Prevalence of self-reported food allergy and IgE antibodies to food allergens in Swedish and Estonian schoolchildren. *Eur J Clin Nutr.* 2005 Mar;59(3):399-403.

Santos A, Dias A, Pinheiro JA. Predictive factors for the persistence of cow's milk allergy. *Pediatr Allergy Immunol.* 2010 Apr 27.

Sanz Ortega J, Martorell Aragonés A, Michavila Gómez A, Nieto García A; Grupo de Trabajo para el Estudio de la Alergia Alimentaria. Incidence of IgE-mediated allergy to cow's milk proteins in the first year of life. *An Esp Pediatr.* 2001 Jun;54(6):536-9.

Sapone A, Bai JC, Ciacci C, Dolinsek J, Green PH, Hadjivassiliou M, Kaukinen K, Rostami K, Sanders DS, Schumann M, Ullrich R, Villalta D, Volta U, Catassi C, Fasano A. Spectrum of gluten-related disorders: consensus on new nomenclature and classification. BMC Med. 2012 Feb 7;10:13.

Sapone A, Lammers KM, Casolaro V, Cammarota M, Giuliano MT, De Rosa M, Stefanile R, Mazzarella G, Tolone C, Russo MI, Esposito P, Ferraraccio F, Cartenì M, Riegler G, de Magistris L, Fasano A. Divergence of gut permeability and mucosal immune gene expression in two gluten-associated conditions: celiac disease and gluten sensitivity. BMC Med. 2011 Mar 9;9:23.

Sapone A, Lammers KM, Mazzarella G, Mikhailenko I, Cartenì M, Casolaro V, Fasano A. Differential mucosal IL-17 expression in two gliadin-induced disorders: gluten sensitivity and the autoimmune enteropathy celiac disease. Int Arch Allergy Immunol. 2010;152(1):75-80.

Sato S, Tachimoto H, Shukuya A, Kurosaka N, Yanagida N, Utsunomiya T, Iguchi M, Komata T, Imai T, Tomikawa M, Ebisawa M. Basophil activation marker CD203c is useful in the diagnosis of hen's egg and cow's milk allergies in children. *Int Arch Allergy Immunol.* 2010;152 Suppl 1:54-61.

Sato Y, Akiyama H, Matsuoka H, Sakata K, Nakamura R, Ishikawa S, Inakuma T, Totsuka M, Sugita-Konishi Y, Ebisawa M, Teshima R. Dietary carotenoids inhibit oral sensitization and the development of food allergy. *J Agric Food Chem.* 2010 Jun 23;58(12):7180-6.

Satyanarayana S, Sushruta K, Sarma GS, Srinivas N, Subba Raju GV. Antioxidant activity of the aqueous extracts of spicy food additives – evaluation and comparison with ascorbic acid in in-vitro systems. *J Herb Pharmacother.* 2004;4(2):1-10.

Savage JH, Kaeding AJ, Matsui EC, Wood RA. The natural history of soy allergy. *J Allergy Clin Immunol.* 2010 Mar;125(3):683-6.

Savilahti EM, Karinen S, Salo HM, Klemetti P, Saarinen KM, Klemola T, Kuitunen M, Hautaniemi S, Savilahti E, Vaarala O. Combined T regulatory cell and Th2 expression profile identifies children with cow's milk allergy. *Clin Immunol.* 2010 Jul;136(1):16-20.

Savilahti EM, Rantanen V, Lin JS, Karinen S, Saarinen KM, Goldis M, Mäkelä MJ, Hautaniemi S, Savilahti E, Sampson HA. Early recovery from cow's milk allergy is associated with decreasing IgE and increasing IgG4 binding to cow's milk epitopes. *J Allergy Clin Immunol.* 2010 Jun;125(6):1315-1321.e9.

Savilahti EM, Rantanen V, Lin JS, Karinen S, Saarinen KM, Goldis M, Mäkelä MJ, Hautaniemi S, Savilahti E, Sampson HA. Early recovery from cow's milk allergy is associated with decreasing IgE and increasing IgG4 binding to cow's milk epitopes. *J Allergy Clin Immunol.* 2010 Jun;125(6):1315-1321.e9.

Sazanova NE, Varnacheva LN, Novikova AV, Pletneva NB. Immunological aspects of food intolerance in children during first years of life. *Pediatriia.* 1992;(3):14-8. Russian.

Scadding G, Bjarnason I, Brostoff J, Levi AJ, Peters TJ. Intestinal permeability to 51Cr-labelled ethylenediaminetetraacetate in food-intolerant subjects. *Digestion.* 1989;42(2):104-9.

Scalabrin DM, Johnston WH, Hoffman DR, P'Pool VL, Harris CL, Mitmesser SH. Growth and tolerance of healthy term infants receiving hydrolyzed infant formulas supplemented with Lactobacillus rhamnosus GG: randomized, double-blind, controlled trial. *Clin Pediatr (Phila).* 2009 Sep;48(7):734-44.

Schabath MB, Hernandez LM, Wu X, Pillow PC, Spitz MR. Dietary phytoestrogens and lung cancer risk. JAMA. 2005 Sep 28;294(12):1493-504.

Schabelman E, Witting M. The Relationship of Radiocontrast, Iodine, and Seafood Allergies: A Medical Myth Exposed. *J Emerg Med.* 2009 Dec 31.

Schade RP, Meijer Y, Pasmans SG, Knulst AC, Kimpen JL, Bruijnzeel-Koomen CA. Double blind placebo controlled cow's milk provocation for the diagnosis of cow's milk allergy in infants and children. *Ned Tijdschr Geneeskd.* 2002 Sep 14;146(37):1739-42.

Schauenberg P, Paris F. *Guide to Medicinal Plants.* New Canaan, CT: Keats Publ, 1977.

Schauss AG, Wu X, Prior RL, Ou B, Huang D, Owens J, Agarwal A, Jensen GS, Hart AN, Shanbrom E. Antioxidant capacity and other bioactivities of the freeze-dried Amazonian palm berry, Euterpe oleraceae mart. (acai). *J Agric Food Chem.* 2006 Nov 1;54(22):8604-10.

Schempp H, Weiser D, Elstner EF. Biochemical model reactions indicative of inflammatory processes. Activities of extracts from Fraxinus excelsior and Populus tremula. *Arzneimittelforschung.* 2000 Apr;50(4):362-72.

Schepetkin IA, Faulkner CL, Nelson-Overton LK, Wiley JA, Quinn MT. Macrophage immunomodulatory activity of polysaccharides isolated from Juniperus scopolorum. *Int Immunopharmacol.* 2005 Dec;5(13-14):1783-99.

Schilcher H, Leuschner F. The potential nephrotoxic effects of essential juniper oil. *Arzneimittelforschung.* 1997 Jul;47(7):855-8.

Schillaci D, Arizza V, Dayton T, Camarda L, Di Stefano V. In vitro anti-biofilm activity of Boswellia spp. oleogum resin essential oils. *Lett Appl Microbiol.* 2008 Nov;47(5):433-8.

Schmid B, Kötter I, Heide L. Pharmacokinetics of salicin after oral administration of a standardised willow bark extract. *Eur J Clin Pharmacol.* 2001 Aug;57(5):387-91.

Schmitt DA, Maleki SJ (2004) Comparing the effects of boiling, frying and roasting on the allergenicity of peanuts. *J Allergy Clin Immunol.* 113: S155.

Schmulson M, Chey WD. Abnormal immune regulation and low-grade inflammation in IBS: does one size fit all? Am J Gastroenterol. 2012;107:273–275.

Schnappinger M, Sausenthaler S, Linseisen J, Hauner H, Heinrich J. Fish consumption, allergic sensitisation and allergic diseases in adults. *Ann Nutr Metab.* 2009;54(1):67-74.

Schneider I, Gibbons S, Bucar F. Inhibitory activity of Juniperus communis on 12(S)-HETE production in human platelets. *Planta Med.* 2004 May;70(5):471-4.

Schönfeld P. Phytanic Acid toxicity: implications for the permeability of the inner mitochondrial membrane to ions. *Toxicol Mech Methods.* 2004;14(1-2):47-52.

Schottner M, Gansser D, Spiteller G. Lignans from the roots of Urtica dioica and their metabolites bind to human sex hormone binding globulin (SHBG). *Planta Med.* 1997;63:529–532.

Schouten B, van Esch BC, Hofman GA, Boon L, Knippels LM, Willemsen LE, Garssen J. Oligosaccharide-induced whey-specific CD25(+) regulatory T-cells are involved in the suppression of cow milk allergy in mice. *J Nutr.* 2010 Apr;140(4):835-41.

Schouten B, van Esch BC, van Thuijl AO, Blokhuis BR, Groot Kormelink T, Hofman GA, Moro GE, Boehm G, Arslanoglu S, Sprikkelman AB, Willemsen LE, Knippels LM, Redegeld FA, Garssen J. Contribution of IgE and immunoglobulin free light chain in the allergic reaction to cow's milk proteins. *J Allergy Clin Immunol.* 2010 Jun;125(6):1308-14.

Schroecksnadel S, Jenny M, Fuchs D. Sensitivity to sulphite additives. *Clin Exp Allergy.* 2010 Apr;40(4):688-9.

Schulick P. *Ginger: Common Spice & Wonder Drug.* Brattleboro, VT: Herbal Free Perss, 1996.

Schumacher P. *Biophysical Therapy Of Allergies.* Stuttgart: Thieme, 2005.

Schütz K, Carle R, Schieber A. Taraxacum – a review on its phytochemical and pharmacological profile. *J Ethnopharmacol.* 2006 Oct 11;107(3):313-23.

Schwab D, Hahn EG, Raithel M. Enhanced histamine metabolism: a comparative analysis of collagenous colitis and food allergy with respect to the role of diet and NSAID use. *Inflamm Res.* 2003 Apr;52(4):142-7.

Schwab D, Müller S, Aigner T, Neureiter D, Kirchner T, Hahn EG, Raithel M. Functional and morphologic characterization of eosinophils in the lower intestinal mucosa of patients with food allergy. *Am J Gastroenterol.* 2003 Jul;98(7):1525-34.

Schwelberger HG. Histamine intolerance: a metabolic disease? *Inflamm Res.* 2010 Mar;59 Suppl 2:S219-21.

Scibilia J, Pastorello EA, Zisa G, Ottolenghi A, Ballmer-Weber B, Pravettoni V, Scovena E, Robino A, Ortolani C. Maize food allergy: a double-blind placebo-controlled study. *Clin Exp Allergy.* 2008 Dec;38(12):1943-9.

Scott-Taylor TH, O'B Hourihane J, Strobel S. Correlation of allergen-specific IgG subclass antibodies and T lymphocyte cytokine responses in children with multiple food allergies. *Pediatr Allergy Immunol.* 2010 Sep;21(6):935-44.

Scurlock AM, Jones SM. An update on immunotherapy for food allergy. *Curr Opin Allergy Clin Immunol.* 2010 Dec;10(6):587-93.

Sealey-Voyksner JA, Khosla C, Voyksner RD, Jorgenson JW. Novel aspects of quantitation of immunogenic wheat gluten peptides by liquid chromatography-mass spectrometry/mass spectrometry. *J Chromatogr A.* 2010 Jun 18;1217(25):4167-83.

Seca AM, Silva AM, Bazzocchi IL, Jimenez IA. Diterpene constituents of leaves from Juniperus brevifolia. *Phytochemistry.* 2008 Jan;69(2):498-505.

Seca AM, Silva AM. The chemical composition of hexane extract from bark of Juniperus brevifolia. *Nat Prod Res.* 2008;22(11):975-83.

Senna G, Gani F, Leo G, Schiappoli M. Alternative tests in the diagnosis of food allergies. *Recenti Prog Med.* 2002 May;93(5):327-34.

Seo K, Jung S, Park M, Song Y, Choung S. Effects of leucocyanidines on activities of metabolizing enzymes and antioxidant enzymes. *Biol Pharm Bull.* 2001 May;24(5):592-3.

Seo SW, Koo HN, An HJ, Kwon KB, Lim BC, Seo EA, Ryu DG, Moon G, Kim HY, Kim HM, Hong SH. Taraxacum officinale protects against cholecystokinin-induced acute pancreatitis in rats. *World J Gastroenterol.* 2005 Jan 28;11(4):597-9.

Seppo L, Korpela R, Lönnerdal B, Metsäniitty L, Juntunen-Backman K, Klemola T, Paganus A, Vanto T. A follow-up study of nutrient intake, nutritional status, and growth in infants with cow milk allergy fed either a soy formula or an extensively hydrolyzed whey formula. *Am J Clin Nutr.* 2005 Jul;82(1):140-5.

Settipane RA, Siri D, Bellanti JA. Egg allergy and influenza vaccination. *Allergy Asthma Proc.* 2009 Nov-Dec;30(6):660-5.

Severance EG, Gressitt KL, Yang S, Stallings CR, Origoni AE, Vaughan C, Khushalani S, Alaedini A, Dickerson FB, Yolken RH. Seroreactive marker for inflammatory bowel disease and associations with antibodies to dietary proteins in bipolar disorder. Bipolar Disord. 2014 May;16(3):230-40.

Shahani KM, Meshbesher BF, Mangalampalli V. *Cultivate Health From Within.* Danbury, CT: Vital Health Publ, 2005.

Shakib F, Brown HM, Phelps A, Redhead R. Study of IgG sub-class antibodies in patients with milk intolerance. *Clin Allergy.* 1986 Sep;16(5):451-8.

Shan L, Molberg O, Parrot I, Hausch F, Filiz F, Gray GM. Structural basis for gluten intolerance in celiac sprue. Science. 2002;297:2275–9.

Shao J, Sheng J, Dong W, Li YZ, Yu SC. Effects of feeding intervention on development of eczema in atopy high-risk infants: an 18-month follow-up study. *Zhonghua Er Ke Za Zhi.* 2006 Sep;44(9):684-7. Chinese.

Sharma P, Sharma BC, Puri V, Sarin SK. An open-label randomized controlled trial of lactulose and probiotics in the treatment of minimal hepatic encephalopathy. *Eur J Gastroent Hepatol.* 2008 Jun;20(6):506-11.

Sharma SC, Sharma S, Gulati OP. Pycnogenol inhibits the release of histamine from mast cells. *Phytother Res.* 2003 Jan;17(1):66-9.

Sharnan J, Kumar L, Singh S. Comparison of results of skin prick tests, enzyme-linked immunosorbent assays and food challenges in children with respiratory allergy. *J Trop Pediatr.* 2001 Dec;47(6):367-8.

Shaw J, Roberts G, Grimshaw K, White S, Hourihane J. Lupin allergy in peanut-allergic children and teenagers. *Allergy.* 2008 Mar;63(3):370-3.

Shawcross DL, Wright G, Olde Damink SW, Jalan R. Role of ammonia and inflammation in minimal hepatic encephalopathy. *Metab Brain Dis.* 2007 Mar;22(1):125-38.

Shea-Donohue T, Stiltz J, Zhao A, Notari L. Mast Cells. *Curr Gastroenterol Rep.* 2010 Aug 14.

Shehata AA, Schrödl W, Aldin AA, Hafez HM, Krüger M. The effect of glyphosate on potential pathogens and beneficial members of poultry microbiota in vitro. Curr Microbiol. 2013 Apr;66(4):350-8. doi: 10.1007/s00284-012-0277-2.

Shepherd SJ, Lomer MC, Gibson PR. Short-chain carbohydrates and functional gastrointestinal disorders. Am JGastroenterol. 2013;108(5):707–17.

Shepherd SJ, Parker FC, Muir JG, Gibson PR. Dietary triggers of abdominal symptoms in patients with irritable bowel syndrome: randomized placebo-controlled evidence. Clin Gastroenterol Hepatol. 2008;6:765–71.

Sheth SS, Waserman S, Kagan R, Alizadehfar R, Primeau MN, Elliot S, St Pierre Y, Wickett R, Joseph L, Harada L, Dufresne C, Allen M, Allen M, Godefroy SB, Clarke AE. Role of food labels in accidental exposures in food-allergic individuals in Canada. *Ann Allergy Asthma Immunol.* 2010 Jan;104(1):60-5.

Shi S, Zhao Y, Zhou H, Zhang Y, Jiang X, Huang K. Identification of antioxidants from Taraxacum mongolicum by high-performance liquid chromatography-diode array detection-radical-scavenging detection-electrospray ionization mass spectrometry and nuclear magnetic resonance experiments. *J Chromatogr A.* 2008 Oct 31;1209(1-2):145-52

Shi S, Zhou H, Zhang Y, Huang K, Liu S. Chemical constituents from Neo-Taraxacum siphonathum. *Zhongguo Zhong Yao Za Zhi.* 2009 Apr;34(8):1002-4.

Shi SY, Zhou CX, Xu Y, Tao QF, Bai H, Lu FS, Lin WY, Chen HY, Zheng W, Wang LW, Wu YH, Zeng S, Huang KX, Zhao Y, Li XK, Qu J. Studies on chemical constituents from herbs of Taraxacum mongolicum. *Zhongguo Zhong Yao Za Zhi.* 2008 May;33(10):1147-57.

Shibata H, Nabe T, Yamamura H, Kohno S. l-Ephedrine is a major constituent of Mao-Bushi-Saishin-To, one of the formulas of Chinese medicine, which shows immediate inhibition after oral administration of passive cutaneous anaphylaxis in rats. *Inflamm Res.* 2000 Aug;49(8):398-403.

Shimoi T, Ushiyama H, Kan K, Saito K, Kamata K, Hirokado M. Survey of glycoalkaloids content in the various potatoes. Shokuhin Eiseigaku Zasshi. 2007 Jun;48(3):77-82.

Shishehbor F, Behroo L, Ghafouriyan Broujerdnia M, Namjoyan F, Latifi SM. Quercetin effectively quells peanut-induced anaphylactic reactions in the peanut sensitized rats. *Iran J Allergy Asthma Immunol.* 2010 Mar;9(1):27-34.

Shoaf, K., Muvey, G.L., Armstrong, G.D., Hutkins, R.W. (2006) Prebiotic galactooligosaccharides reduce adherence of enteropathogenic Escherichia coli to tissue culture cells. *Infect Immun.* Dec;74(12):6920-8.

Shwry PR, Tatham AS, Barro F, Barcelo P, Lazzeri P. Biotechnology of breadmaking: unraveling and manipulating the multi-protein gluten complex. Biotechnology (N Y). 1995 Nov;13(11):1185-90.

Sicherer SH, Muñoz-Furlong A, Godbold JH, Sampson HA. US prevalence of self-reported peanut, tree nut, and sesame allergy: 11-year follow-up. *J Allergy Clin Immunol.* 2010 Jun;125(6):1322-6.

Sicherer SH, Munoz-Furlong A, Sampson HA (2003) Prevalence of peanut and tree nut allergy in the United States determined by means of a random digit dial telephone survey: a 5-year follow-up study. *J Allergy Clin Immunol.* 112: 1203–1207.

Sicherer SH, Noone SA, Koerner CB, Christie L, Burks AW, Sampson HA. Hypoallergenicity and efficacy of an amino acid-based formula in children with cow's milk and multiple food hypersensitivities. *J Pediatr.* 2001 May;138(5):688-93.

Sicherer SH, Sampson HA. Food allergy. *J Allergy Clin Immunol.* 2010 Feb;125(2 Suppl 2):S116-25.

Sicherer SH, Wood RA, Stablein D, Burks AW, Liu AH, Jones SM, Fleischer DM, Leung DY, Grishin A, Mayer L, Shreffler W, Lindblad R, Sampson HA. Immunologic features of infants with milk or egg allergy enrolled in an observational study (Consortium of Food Allergy Research) of food allergy. *J Allergy Clin Immunol.* 2010 May;125(5):1077-1083.e8.

Sigstedt SC, Hooten CJ, Callewaert MC, Jenkins AR, Romero AE, Pullin MJ, Kornienko A, Lowrey TK, Slambrouck SV, Steelant WF. Evaluation of aqueous extracts of Taraxacum officinale on growth and invasion of breast and prostate cancer cells. *Int J Oncol.* 2008 May;32(5):1085-90.

Silman AJ, MacGregor AJ, Thomson W, Holligan S, Carthy D, Farhan A, Ollier WE. Twin concordance rates for rheumatoid arthritis: results from a nationwide study. *Br J Rheumatol.* 1993 Oct;32(10):903-7.

Silva MF, Kamphorst AO, Hayashi EA, Bellio M, Carvalho CR, Faria AM, Sabino KC, Coelho MG, Nobrega A, Tavares D, Silva AC. Innate profiles of cytokines implicated on oral tolerance correlate with low- or high-suppression of humoral response. *Immunology.* 2010 Jul;130(3):447-57.

Simeone D, Miele E, Boccia G, Marino A, Troncone R, Staiano A. Prevalence of atopy in children with chronic constipation. *Arch Dis Child.* 2008 Dec;93(12):1044-7.

Simonte SJ, Ma S, Mofidi S, Sicherer SH. Relevance of casual contact with peanut butter in children with peanut allergy. *J Allergy Clin Immunol.* 2003 Jul;112(1):180-2.

Simopoulos AP. Essential fatty acids in health and chronic disease. *Am J Clin Nutr.* 1999 Sep;70(3 Suppl):560S-569S.

Simpson AB, Yousef E, Hossain J. Association between peanut allergy and asthma morbidity. *J Pediatr.* 2010 May;156(5):777-81, 781.e1.

Sindhu SC, Khetarpaul N. Effect of probiotic fermentation on antinutrients and in vitro protein and starch digestibilities of indigenously developed RWGT food mixture. Nutr Health. 2002;16(3):173-81.

Singer P, Shapiro H, Theilla M, Anbar R, Singer J, Cohen J. Anti-inflammatory properties of omega-3 fatty acids in critical illness: novel mechanisms and an integrative perspective. *Intensive Care Med.* 2008 Sep;34(9):1580-92.

Singh S, Khajuria A, Taneja SC, Johri RK, Singh J, Qazi GN. Boswellic acids: A leukotriene inhibitor also effective through topical application in inflammatory disorders. *Phytomedicine.* 2008 Jun;15(6-7):400-7.

Sirvent S, Palomares O, Vereda A, Villalba M, Cuesta-Herranz J, Rodríguez R. nsLTP and profilin are allergens in mustard seeds: cloning, sequencing and recombinant production of Sin a 3 and Sin a 4. *Clin Exp Allergy.* 2009 Dec;39(12):1929-36.

Skamstrup Hansen K, Vieths S, Vestergaard H, Skov PS, Bindslev-Jensen C, Poulsen LK. Seasonal variation in food allergy to apple. *J Chromatogr B Biomed Sci Appl.* 2001 May 25;756(1-2):19-32.

Skripak JM, Nash SD, Rowley H, Brereton NH, Oh S, Hamilton RG, Matsui EC, Burks AW, Wood RA. A randomized, double-blind, placebo-controlled study of milk oral immunotherapy for cow's milk allergy. *J Allergy Clin Immunol.* 2008 Dec;122(6):1154-60.

Sletten GB, Halvorsen R, Egaas E, Halstensen TS. Changes in humoral responses to beta-lactoglobulin in tolerant patients suggest a particular role for IgG4 in delayed, non-IgE-mediated cow's milk allergy. *Pediatr Allergy Immunol.* 2006 Sep;17(6):435-43.

Smecuol E, Hwang HJ, Sugai E, Corso L, Cherñavsky AC, Bellavite FP, González A, Vodánovich F, Moreno ML, Vázquez H, Lozano G, Niveloni S, Mazure R, Meddings J, Mauriño E, Bai JC. Exploratory, randomized, double-blind, placebo-controlled study on the effects of Bifidobacterium infantis natren life start strain super strain in active celiac disease. J Clin Gastroenterol. 2013 Feb;47(2):139-47.

Smith J. *Genetic Roulette: The Documented Health Risks of Genetically Engineered Foods.* White River Jct, Vermont: Chelsea Green, 2007.

Smith K, Warholak T, Armstrong E, Leib M, Rehfeld R, Malone D. Evaluation of risk factors and health outcomes among persons with asthma. *J Asthma.* 2009 Apr;46(3):234-7.

Smith MM, Goodfellow L. The relationship between quality of life and coping strategies of adults with celiac disease adhering to a gluten-free diet. Gastroenterol Nurs. 2011 Nov-Dec;34(6):460-8.

Smith S, Sullivan K. Examining the influence of biological and psychological factors on cognitive performance in chronic fatigue syndrome: a randomized, double-blind, placebo-controlled, crossover study. *Int J Behav Med.* 2003;10(2):162-73.

Soares FL, de Oliveira Matoso R, Teixeira LG, Menezes Z, Pereira SS, Alves AC, Batista NV, de Faria AM, Cara DC, Ferreira AV, Alvarez-Leite JI. Gluten-free diet reduces adiposity, inflammation and insulin resistance associated with the induction of PPAR-alpha and PPAR-gamma expression. J Nutr Biochem. 2013 Jun;24(6):1105-11.

Sofic E, Denisova N, Youdim K, Vatrenjak-Velagic V, De Filippo C, Mehmedagic A, Causevic A, Cao G, Joseph JA, Prior RL. Antioxidant and pro-oxidant capacity of catecholamines and related compounds. Effects of hydrogen peroxide on glutathione and sphingomyelinase activity in pheochromocytoma PC12 cells: potential relevance to age-related diseases. *J Neural Transm.* 2001;108(5):541-57.

Soleo L, Colosio C, Alinovi R, Guarneri D, Russo A, Lovreglio P, Vimercati L, Birindelli S, Cortesi I, Flore C, Carta P, Colombi A, Parrinello G, Ambrosi L. Immunologic effects of exposure to low levels of inorganic mercury. *Med Lav.* 2002 May-Jun;93(3):225-32. Italian.

Sollid LM, Jabri B. Is celiac disease an autoimmune disorder? Curr Opin Immunol. 2005;17:1–6.

Sollid LM, Khosla C. Future therapeutic options for celiac disease. Nat Clin Pract Gastroenterol Hepatol. 2005;2:140–7.

Sollid LM, Kolberg J, Scott H, Ek J, Fausa O, Brandtzaeg P. Antibodies to wheat germ agglutinin in coeliac disease. Clin Exp Immunol. 1986 Jan;63(1):95-100.

Sollid LM. Coeliac disease: dissecting a complex inflammatory disorder. Nat Rev Immunol. 2002;2(9):647–55.

Sompamit K, Kukongviriyapan U, Nakmareong S, Pannangpetch P, Kukongviriyapan V. Curcumin improves vascular function and alleviates oxidative stress in non-lethal lipopolysaccharide-induced endotoxaemia in mice. *Eur J Pharmacol.* 2009 Aug 15;616(1-3):192-9.

Sotelo A, Argote RM, Moreno RI, Flores NI, Diaz M. Nutritive evaluation of the seed, germinated seed, and string bean of Erythrina americana and the detoxification of the material by boiling. J Agric Food Chem. 2003 Apr 23;51(9):2821-5.

Souza NC, Mendonca JN, Portari GV, Jordao Junior AA, Marchini JS, Chiarello PG. Intestinal permeability and nutritional status in developmental disorders. Altern Ther Health Med. 2012 Mar-Apr;18(2):19-24.

Søyland Wasenius AK, Halvorsen R. Oral provocation tests for adverse reactions to food. *Tidsskr Nor Laegeforen.* 2003 Jun 26;123(13-14):1829-30.

Spence A. *Basic Human Anatomy.* Menlo Park, CA: Benjamin/Commings, 1986.

Spence D. Bad medicine: food intolerance. BMJ. 2013 Jan 30;346:f529.

Spiller G. *The Super Pyramid.* New York: HRS Press, 1993.

Srivastava K, Zou ZM, Sampson HA, Dansky H, Li XM. Direct Modulation of Airway Reactivity by the Chinese Anti-Asthma Herbal Formula ASHMI. *J Allergy Clin Immunol.* 2005;115:S7.

Srivastava KD, Kattan JD, Zou ZM, Li JH, Zhang L, Wallenstein S, Goldfarb J, Sampson HA, Li XM. The Chinese herbal medicine formula FAHF-2 completely blocks anaphylactic reactions in a murine model of peanut allergy. *J Allergy Clin Immunol.* 2005;115:171–8.

Srivastava KD, Qu C, Zhang T, Goldfarb J, Sampson HA, Li XM. Food Allergy Herbal Formula-2 silences peanut-induced anaphylaxis for a prolonged posttreatment period via IFN-gamma-producing CD8+ T cells. *J Allergy Clin Immunol.* 2009 Feb;123(2):443-51.

Srivastava KD, Zhang TF, Qu C, Sampson HA, Li XM. Silencing Peanut Allergy: A Chinese Herbal Formula, FAHF-2, Completely Blocks Peanut-induced Anaphylaxis for up to 6 Months Following Therapy in a Murine Model Of Peanut Allergy. *J Allergy Clin Immunol.* 2006;117:S328.

Staden U, Rolinck-Werninghaus C, Brewe F, Wahn U, Niggemann B, Beyer K. Specific oral tolerance induction in food allergy in children: efficacy and clinical patterns of reaction. *Allergy.* 2007 Nov;62(11):1261-9.

Stahl SM. Selective histamine H1 antagonism: novel hypnotic and pharmacologic actions challenge classical notions of antihistamines. CNS Spectr. 2008 Dec;13(12):1027-38.

Stapel SO, Asero R, Ballmer-Weber BK, Knol EF, Strobel S, Vieths S, Kleine-Tebbe J; EAACI Task Force. Testing for IgG4 against foods is not recommended as a diagnostic tool: EAACI Task Force Report. Allergy. 2008 Jul;63(7):793-6.

Stapel SO, Asero R, Ballmer-Weber BK, Knol EF, Strobel S, Vieths S, Kleine-Tebbe J; EAACI Task Force. Testing for IgG4 against foods is not recommended as a diagnostic tool: EAACI Task Force Report. Allergy. 2008 Jul;63(7):793-6.

Staudacher HM, Whelan K, Irving PM, Lomer MC. Comparison of symptom response following advice for a diet low in fermentable carbohydrates (FODMAPs) versus standard dietary advice in patients with irritable bowel syndrome. J HumNutr Diet. 2011;24:487–495.

Stenberg JA, Hambäck PA, Ericson L. Herbivore-induced "rent rise" in the host plant may drive a diet breadth enlargement in the tenant. *Ecology.* 2008 Jan;89(1):126-33.

Stengler M. *The Natural Physician's Healing Therapies.* Stamford, CT: Bottom Line Books, 2008.

Stenman SM, Venäläinen JI, Lindfors K, Auriola S, Mauriala T, Kaukovirta-Norja A, Jantunen A, Laurila K, Qiao SW, Sollid LM, Männisto PT, Kaukinen K, Mäki M. Enzymatic detoxification of gluten by germinating wheat proteases: implications for new treatment of celiac disease. Ann Med. 2009;41(5):390-400.

Stevens BJ, Selvendran RR. Changes in composition and structure of wheat bran resulting from the action of human faecal bacteria in vitro. Carbohydr Res. 1988 Dec 1;183(2):311-9.

Stevens FM, Lloyd RS, Geraghty SM, Reynolds MT, Sarsfield MJ, Mcnicholl B, Fottrell PF, Wright R, Mccarthy CF. Schizophrenia and coeliac disease – the nature of the relationship. Psychol Med. 1977 May;7(2):259-63.

Stirapongsasuti P, Tanglertsampan C, Aunhachoke K, Sangasapaviliya A. Anaphylactic reaction to phuk-waan-ban in a patient with latex allergy. *J Med Assoc Thai.* 2010 May;93(5):616-9.

Stratiki Z, Costalos C, Sevastiadou S, Kastanidou O, Skouroliakou M, Giakoumatou A, Petrohilou V. The effect of a bifidobacter supplemented bovine milk on intestinal permeability of preterm infants. *Early Hum Dev.* 2007 Sep;83(9):575-9.

Strinnholm A, Brulin C, Lindh V. Experiences of double-blind, placebo-controlled food challenges (DBPCFC): a qualitative analysis of mothers' experiences. *J Child Health Care.* 2010 Jun;14(2):179-88.

Stuknytė M, Cattaneo S, Pagani MA, Marti A, Micard V, Hogenboom J, De Noni I. Spaghetti from durum wheat: effect of drying conditions on heat damage, ultrastructure and in vitro digestibility. Food Chem. 2014 Apr 15;149:40-6.

Stüsser R, Batista J, Padrón R, Sosa F, Pereztol O. Long-term therapy with policosanol improves treadmill exercise-ECG testing performance of coronary heart disease patients. Int J Clin Pharmacol Ther. 1998 Sep;36(9):469-73.

Stutius LM, Sheehan WJ, Rangsithienchai P, Bharmanee A, Scott JE, Young MC, Dioun AF, Schneider LC, Phipatanakul W. Characterizing the relationship between sesame, coconut, and nut allergy in children. *Pediatr Allergy Immunol.* 2010 Dec;21(8):1114-8.

Sugawara G, Nagino M, Nishio H, Ebata T, Takagi K, Asahara T, Nomoto K, Nimura Y. Perioperative synbiotic treatment to prevent postoperative infectious complications in biliary cancer surgery: a randomized controlled trial. *Ann Surg.* 2006 Nov;244(5):706-14.

Suh KY. Food allergy and atopic dermatitis: separating fact from fiction. *Semin Cutan Med Surg.* 2010 Jun;29(2):72-8.

Sumantran VN, Kulkarni AA, Harsulkar A, Wele A, Koppikar SJ, Chandwaskar R, Gaire V, Dalvi M, Wagh UV. Hyaluronidase and collagenase inhibitory activities of the herbal formulation Triphala guggulu. *J Biosci.* 2007 Jun;32(4):755-61.

Sumiyoshi M, Sakanaka M, Kimura Y. Effects of Red Ginseng extract on allergic reactions to food in Balb/c mice. *J Ethnopharmacol.* 2010 Aug 14.

Sung JH, Lee JO, Son JK, Park NS, Kim MR, Kim JG, Moon DC. Cytotoxic constituents from Solidago virga-aurea var. gigantea MIQ. *Arch Pharm Res.* 1999 Dec;22(6):633-7.

Suomalainen H, Isolauri E. New concepts of allergy to cow's milk. *Ann Med.* 1994 Aug;26(4):289-96.

Sütas Y, Kekki OM, Isolauri E. Late onset reactions to oral food challenge are linked to low serum interleukin-10 concentrations in patients with atopic dermatitis and food allergy. *Clin Exp Allergy.* 2000 Aug;30(8):1121-8.

Suter D, Fleming F. Cereal food allergy issues, opportunities and the way forward for industry. in 41st AIFST Convention. 2008. Sydney, Australia.

Svendsen AJ, Holm NV, Kyvik K, *et al.* Relative importance of genetic effects in rheumatoid arthritis: historical cohort study of Danish nationwide twin population. *BMJ* 2002;324(7332): 264-266.

Sweeney B, Vora M, Ulbricht C, Basch E. Evidence-based systematic review of dandelion (Taraxacum officinale) by natural standard research collaboration. *J Herb Pharmacother.* 2005;5(1):79-93.

Swiderska-Kiełbik S, Krakowiak A, Wiszniewska M, Dudek W, Walusiak-Skorupa J, Krawczyk-Szulc P, Michowicz A, Pałczyński C. Health hazards associated with occupational exposure to birds. *Med Pr.* 2010;61(2):213-22.

Szyf M, McGowan P, Meaney MJ. The social environment and the epigenome. *Environ Mol Mutagen.* 2008 Jan;49(1):46-60.

Tack GJ, van de Water JM, Bruins MJ, Kooy-Winkelaar EM, van Bergen J, Bonnet P, Vreugdenhil AC, Korponay-Szabo I, Edens L, von Blomberg BM, Schreurs MW, Mulder CJ, Koning F. Consumption of gluten with gluten-degrading enzyme by celiac patients: a pilot-study. World J Gastroenterol. 2013 Sep 21;19(35):5837-47.

Takada Y, Ichikawa H, Badmaev V, Aggarwal BB. Acetyl-11-keto-beta-boswellic acid potentiates apoptosis, inhibits invasion, and abolishes osteoclastogenesis by suppressing NF-kappa B and NF-kappa B-regulated gene expression. *J Immunol.* 2006 Mar 1;176(5):3127-40.

Takahashi N, Eisenhuth G, Lee I, Schachtele C, Laible N, Binion S. Nonspecific antibacterial factors in milk from cows immunized with human oral bacterial pathogens. *J Dairy Sci.* 1992 Jul;75(7):1810-20.

Takasaki M, Konoshima T, Tokuda H, Masuda K, Arai Y, Shiojima K, Ageta H. Anti-carcinogenic activity of Taraxacum plant. I. *Biol Pharm Bull.* 1999 Jun;22(6):602-5.

Tamura M, Shikina T, Morihana T, Hayama M, Kajimoto O, Sakamoto A, Kajimoto Y, Watanabe O, Nonaka C, Shida K, Nanno M. Effects of probiotics on allergic rhinitis induced by Japanese cedar pollen: randomized double-blind, placebo-controlled clinical trial. *Int Arch Allergy Imml.* 2007;143(1):75-82.

Tanabe S. Analysis of food allergen structures and development of foods for allergic patients. Biosci Biotechnol Biochem. 2008;72(3):649–59.

Tanpowpong P, Ingham TR, Lampshire PK, Kirchberg FF, Epton MJ, Crane J, Camargo CA Jr; New Zealand Asthma and Allergy Cohort Study Group. Coeliac disease and gluten avoidance in New Zealand children. Arch Dis Child. 2012 Jan;97(1):12-6.

Tapiero H, Ba GN, Couvreur P, Tew KD. Polyunsaturated fatty acids (PUFA) and eicosanoids in human health and pathologies. *Biomed Pharmacother.* 2002 Jul;56(5):215-22.

Tapola N, Karvonen H, Niskanen L, Mikola M, Sarkkinen E. Glycemic responses of oat bran products in type 2 diabetic patients. Nutr Metab Cardiovasc Dis. 2005 Aug;15(4):255-61.

Tapsell LC, Hemphill I, Cobiac L, Patch CS, Sullivan DR, Fenech M, Roodenrys S, Keogh JB, Clifton PM, Williams PG, Fazio VA, Inge KE. Health benefits of herbs and spices: the past, the present, the future. *Med J Aust.* 2006 Aug 21;185(4 Suppl):S4-24.

Tasli L, Mat C, De Simone C, Yazici H. Lactobacilli lozenges in the management of oral ulcers of Behçet's syndrome. *Clin Exp Rheumatol.* 2006 Sep-Oct;24(5 Suppl 42):S83-6.

Taussig SJ, Batkin S. Bromelain, the enzyme complex of pineapple (Ananas comosus) and its clinical application. An update. *J Ethnopharmacol.* 1988 Feb-Mar;22(2):191-203.

Taylor AL, Dunstan JA, Prescott SL. Probiotic supplementation for the first 6 months of life fails to reduce the risk of atopic dermatitis and increases the risk of allergen sensitization in high-risk children: a randomized controlled trial. *J Allergy Clin Immunol.* 2007 Jan;119(1):184-91.

Taylor AL, Hale J, Wiltschut J, Lehmann H, Dunstan JA, Prescott SL. Effects of probiotic supplementation for the first 6 months of life on allergen- and vaccine-specific immune responses. *Clin Exp Allergy.* 2006 Oct;36(10):1227-35.

Taylor RB, Lindquist N, Kubanek J, Hay ME. Intraspecific variation in palatability and defensive chemistry of brown seaweeds: effects on herbivore fitness. *Oecologia.* 2003 Aug;136(3):412-23.

Taylor SL, Moneret-Vautrin DA, Crevel RW, Sheffield D, Morisset M, Dumont P, Remington BC, Baumert JL. Threshold dose for peanut: Risk characterization based upon diagnostic oral challenge of a series of 286 peanut-allergic individuals. *Food Chem Toxicol.* 2010 Mar;48(3):814-9.

Teitelbaum J. *From Fatigue to Fantastic.* New York: Avery, 2001.

Terheggen-Lagro SW, Khouw IM, Schaafsma A, Wauters EA. Safety of a new extensively hydrolysed formula in children with cow's milk protein allergy: a double blind crossover study. *BMC Pediatr.* 2002 Oct 14;2:10.

Terracciano L, Bouygue GR, Sarratud T, Veglia F, Martelli A, Fiocchi A. Impact of dietary regimen on the duration of cow's milk allergy: a random allocation study. *Clin Exp Allergy.* 2010 Apr;40(4):637-42.

Tham KW, Zuraimi MS, Koh D, Chew FT, Ooi PL. Associations between home dampness and presence of molds with asthma and allergic symptoms among young children in the tropics. *Pediatr Allergy Immunol.* 2007 Aug;18(5):418-24.

Thampithak A, Jaisin Y, Meesarapee B, Chongthammakun S, Piyachaturawat P, Govitrapong P, Supavilai P, Sanvarinda Y. Transcriptional regulation of iNOS and COX-2 by a novel compound from Curcuma comosa in lipopolysaccharide-induced microglial activation. *Neurosci Lett.* 2009 Sep 22;462(2):171-5.

Theler B, Brockow K, Ballmer-Weber BK. Clinical presentation and diagnosis of meat allergy in Switzerland and Southern Germany. *Swiss Med Wkly.* 2009 May 2;139(17-18):264-70.

Theofilopoulos AN, Kono DH: The genes of systemic autoimmunity. *Proc Assoc Am Physicians.* 1999;111(3): 228-240.

Theuwissen E, Mensink RP. Water-soluble dietary fibers and cardiovascular disease. Physiol Behav. 2008 May 23;94(2):285-92.

Thomas, R.G., Gebhardt, S.E. 2008. Nutritive value of pomegranate fruit and juice. *Maryland Dietetic Association Annual Meeting, USDA-ARS.* 2008 April 11.

Thompson RL, Miles LM, Lunn J, Devereux G, Dearman RJ, Strid J, Buttriss JL. Peanut sensitisation and allergy: influence of early life exposure to peanuts. *Br J Nutr.* 2010 May;103(9):1278-86.

Thompson T, Lee AR, Grace T. Gluten contamination of grains, seeds, and flours in the United States: a pilot study. J Am Diet Assoc. 2010 Jun;110(6):937-40.

Tierra L. *The Herbs of Life.* Freedom, CA: Crossing Press, 1992.

Tierra M. *The Way of Herbs.* New York: Pocket Books, 1990.

Tisserand R. *The Art of Aromatherapy.* New York: Inner Traditions, 1979.

Tiwari M. *Ayurveda: A Life of Balance.* Rochester, VT: Healing Arts, 1995.

Tlaskalová-Hogenová H, Stepánková R, Hudcovic T, Tucková L, Cukrowska B, Lodinová-Zádníková R, Kozáková H, Rossmann P, Bártová J, Sokol D, Funda DP, Borovská D, Reháková Z, Sinkora J, Hofman J, Drastich P, Kokesová A. Commensal bacteria (normal microflora), mucosal immunity and chronic inflammatory and autoimmune diseases. *Immunol Lett.* 2004 May 15;93(2-3):97-108.

Todd GR, Acerini CL, Ross-Russell R, Zahra S, Warner JT, McCance D. Survey of adrenal crisis associated with inhaled corticosteroids in the United Kingdom. *Arch Dis Child.* 2002 Dec;87(6):457-61.

Tomičić S, Norrman G, Fälth-Magnusson K, Jenmalm MC, Devenney I, Böttcher MF. High levels of IgG4 antibodies to foods during infancy are associated with tolerance to corresponding foods later in life. *Pediatr Allergy Immunol.* 2009 Feb;20(1):35-41.

Tonkal AM, Morsy TA. An update review on Commiphora molmol and related species. *J Egypt Soc Parasitol.* 2008 Dec;38(3):763-96.

Topçu G, Erenler R, Cakmak O, Johansson CB, Celik C, Chai HB, Pezzuto JM. Diterpenes from the berries of Juniperus excelsa. *Phytochemistry.* 1999 Apr;50(7):1195-9.

Tordesillas L, Pacios LF, Palacín A, Cuesta-Herranz J, Madero M, Díaz-Perales A. Characterization of IgE epitopes of Cuc m 2, the major melon allergen, and their role in cross-reactivity with pollen profilins. *Clin Exp Allergy.* 2010 Jan;40(1):174-81.

Tosco A, Auricchio R, Aitoro R, Ponticelli D, Primario M, Miele E, Rotondi Aufiero V, Discepolo V, Greco L, Troncone R, Maglio M. In celiac disease intestinal titers of anti-tissue transglutaminase2 antibodies positively correlate with the mucosal damage degree and inversely with the gluten-free diet duration. Clin Exp Immunol. 2014 Apr 28.

Tosi P, Gritsch CS, He J, Shewry PR. Distribution of gluten proteins in bread wheat (Triticum aestivum) grain. Ann Bot. 2011 Jul;108(1):23-35.

Tovey FI, Bardhan KD, Hobsley M. Dietary phosphilipids and sterols protective against peptic ulceration. Phytother Res. 2013 Sep;27(9):1265-9.

Tovey FI. Staple diets and duodenal ulcer prevalence. Int Health. 2009 Dec;1(2):124-32.

Towers GH. FAHF-1 purporting to block peanut-induced anaphylaxis. *J Allergy Clin Immunol.* 2003 May;111(5):1140; author reply 1140-1.

Towle A. *Modern Biology.* Austin: Harcourt Brace, 1993.

Trojanová I, Rada V, Kokoska L, Vlková E. The bifidogenic effect of Taraxacum officinale root. *Fitoterapia.* 2004 Dec;75(7-8):760-3.

Troncone R, Caputo N, Florio G, Finelli E. Increased intestinal sugar permeability after challenge in children with cow's milk allergy or intolerance. *Allergy.* 1994 Mar;49(3):142-6.

Trugo LC, Donangelo CM, Trugo NM, Bach Knudsen KE. Effect of heat treatment on nutritional quality of germinated legume seeds. J Agric Food Chem. 2000 Jun;48(6):2082-6.

Truswell AS. The A2 milk case: a critical review. *Euro J Clin Nutr.* 2005:59;623–631.

Tsai JC, Tsai S, Chang WC. Comparison of two Chinese medical herbs, Huangbai and Qianniuzi, on influence of short circuit current across the rat intestinal epithelia. *J Ethnopharmacol.* 2004 Jul;93(1):21-5.

Tsong T. Deciphering the language of cells. *Trends in Biochem Sci.* 1989;14:89-92.

Tsuchiya J, Barreto R, Okura R, Kawakita S, Fesce E, Marotta F. Single-blind follow-up study on the effectiveness of a symbiotic preparation in irritable bowel syndrome. *Chin J Dig Dis.* 2004;5(4):169-74.

Tucková L, Novotná J, Novák P, Flegelová Z, Kveton T, Jelínková L, Zídek Z, Man P, Tlaskalová-Hogenová H. Activation of macrophages by gliadin fragments: isolation and characterization of active peptide. J Leukoc Biol. 2002

Tulk HM, Robinson LE. Modifying the n-6/n-3 polyunsaturated fatty acid ratio of a high-saturated fat challenge does not acutely attenuate postprandial changes in inflammatory markers in men with meta-bolic syndrome. *Metabolism.* 2009 Jul 20.

Tursi A, Brandimarte G, Giorgetti GM, Elisei W. Mesalazine and/or Lactobacillus casei in maintaining long-term remission of symptomatic uncomplicated diverticular disease of the colon. *Hepatogastroenterology.* 2008 May-Jun;55(84):916-20.

U.S. Food and Drug Administration CfDEaR. *Guidance for Industry Botanical Drug Products.* 2000

Ueno H, Yoshioka K, Matsumoto T. Usefulness of the skin index in predicting the outcome of oral challenges in children. *J Investig Allergol Clin Immunol.* 2007;17(4):207-10.

Ueno M, Adachi A, Fukumoto T, Nishitani N, Fujiwara N, Matsuo H, Kohno K, Morita E. Analysis of causative allergen of the patient with baker's asthma and wheat-dependent exercise-induced anaphylaxis (WDEIA). *Arerugi.* 2010 May;59(5):552-7.

Ukabam SO, Mann RJ, Cooper BT. Small intestinal permeability to sugars in patients with atopic eczema. *Br J Dermatol.* 1984 Jun;110(6):649-52.

Unsel M, Ardeniz O, Mete N, Ersoy R, Sin AZ, Gulbahar O, Kokuludag A. Food allergy due to olive. J Investig Allergol Clin Immunol. 2009;19(6):497-9. García BE, Gamboa PM, Asturias JA, López-Hoyos M, Sanz ML, Caballero MT, García JM, Labrador M, Lahoz C, Longo Areso N, Martínez Quesada J, Mayorga L, Monteseirín FJ; Clinical Immunology Committee; Spanish Society of Allergology and Clinical Immunology. Guidelines on the clinical usefulness of determination of specific immunoglobulin E to foods. *J Investig Allergol Clin Immunol.* 2009;19(6):423-32.

Unsel M, Sin AZ, Ardeniz O, Erdem N, Ersoy R, Gulbahar O, Mete N, Kokuludağ A. New onset egg allergy in an adult. *J Investig Allergol Clin Immunol.* 2007;17(1):55-8.

Untersmayr E, Vestergaard H, Malling HJ, Jensen LB, Platzer MH, Boltz-Nitulescu G, Scheiner O, Skov PS, Jensen-Jarolim E, Poulsen LK. Incomplete digestion of codfish represents a risk factor for anaphylaxis in patients with allergy. *J Allergy Clin Immunol.* 2007 Mar;119(3):711-7.

Upadhyay AK, Kumar K, Kumar A, Mishra HS. Tinospora cordifolia (Willd.) Hook. f. and Thoms. (Guduchi) - validation of the Ayurvedic pharmacology through experimental and clinical studies. *Int J Ayurveda Res.* 2010 Apr;1(2):112-21.

Vally H, Thompson PJ, Misso NL. Changes in bronchial hyperresponsiveness following high- and low-sulphite wine challenges in wine-sensitive asthmatic patients. *Clin Exp Allergy.* 2007 Jul;37(7):1062-6.

van Beelen VA, Roeleveld J, Mooibroek H, Sijtsma L, Bino RJ, Bosch D, Rietjens IM, Alink GM. A comparative study on the effect of algal and fish oil on viability and cell proliferation of Caco-2 cells. *Food Chem Toxicol.* 2007 May;45(5):716-24.

van Elburg RM, Uil JJ, de Monchy JG, Heymans HS. Intestinal permeability in pediatric gastroenterology. *Scand J Gastroenterol Suppl.* 1992;194:19-24.

van Kampen V, Merget R, Rabstein S, Sander I, Bruening T, Broding HC, Keller C, Muesken H, Overlack A, Schultze-Werninghaus G, Walusiak J, Raulf-Heimsoth M. Comparison of wheat and rye flour solutions for skin prick testing: a multi-centre study (Stad 1). *Clin Exp Allergy.* 2009 Dec;39(12):1896-902.

van Odijk J, Peterson CG, Ahlstedt S, Bengtsson U, Borres MP, Hulthén L, Magnusson J, Hansson T. Measurements of eosinophil activation before and after food challenges in adults with food hypersensitivity. *Int Arch Allergy Immunol.* 2006;140(4):334-41.

Vanderhoof JA. Probiotics in allergy management. *J Pediatr Gastroenterol Nutr.* 2008 Nov;47 Suppl 2:S38-40.

Vanto T, Helppilä S, Juntunen-Backman K, Kalimo K, Klemola T, Korpela R, Koskinen P. Prediction of the development of tolerance to milk in children with cow's milk hypersensitivity. *J Pediatr.* 2004 Feb;144(2):218-22.

Vassallo MF, Banerji A, Rudders SA, Clark S, Mullins RJ, Camargo CA Jr. Season of birth and food allergy in children. *Ann Allergy Asthma Immunol.* 2010 Apr;104(4):307-13.

Vazquez-Roque MI, Camilleri M, Smyrk T, Murray JA, Marietta E, O'Neill J, Carlson P, Lamsam J, Janzow D, Eckert D, Burton D, Zinsmeister AR. A controlled trial of gluten-free diet in patients with irritable bowel syndrome-diarrhea: effects on bowel frequency and intestinal function. Gastroenterology. 2013 May;144(5):903-911.e3.

Veleminský J, Silhánková L, Smiovská V, Gichner T. Mutagenesis of Saccharomyces cerevisiae by sodium azide activated in barley. Mutat Res. 1979 Jul;61(2):197-205.

Vendt N, Grünberg H, Tuure T, Malminiemi O, Wuolijoki E, Tillmann V, Sepp E, Korpela R. Growth during the first 6 months of life in infants using formula enriched with Lactobacillus rhamnosus GG: double-blind, randomized trial. *J Hum Nutr Diet.* 2006 Feb;19(1):51-8.

Venkatachalam KV. Human 3'-phosphoadenosine 5'-phosphosulfate (PAPS) synthase: biochemistry, molecular biology and genetic deficiency. *IUBMB Life.* 2003 Jan;55(1):1-11.

Venter C, Hasan Arshad S, Grundy J, Pereira B, Bernie Clayton C, Voigt K, Higgins B, Dean T. Time trends in the prevalence of peanut allergy: three cohorts of children from the same geographical location in the UK. *Allergy.* 2010 Jan;65(1):103-8.

Venter C, Meyer R. Session 1: Allergic disease: The challenges of managing food hypersensitivity. *Proc Nutr Soc.* 2010 Feb;69(1):11-24.

Venter C, Pereira B, Grundy J, Clayton CB, Arshad SH, Dean T (2006a) Prevalence of sensitization reported and objectively assessed food hypersensitivity amongst six-year-old children: A population-based study. *Pediatr Allergy Immunol.* 17: 356–363.

Venter C, Pereira B, Grundy J, Clayton CB, Roberts G, Higgins B, Dean T (2006b) Incidence of parentally reported and clinically diagnosed food hypersensitivity in the first year of life. *J Allergy Clin Immunol.* 117: 1118–1124.

Ventura MT, Polimeno L, Amoruso AC, Gatti F, Annoscia E, Marinaro M, Di Leo E, Matino MG, Buquicchio R, Bonini S, Tursi A, Francavilla A. Intestinal permeability in patients with adverse reactions to food. *Dig Liver Dis.* 2006 Oct;38(10):732-6.

Venturi A, Gionchetti P, Rizzello F, Johansson R, Zucconi E, Brigidi P, Matteuzzi D, Campieri M. Impact on the composition of the faecal flora by a new probiotic preparation: preliminary data on maintenance treatment of patients with ulcerative colitis. *Aliment Pharmacol Ther.* 1999 Aug;13(8):1103-8.

Veraverbeke WS, Delcour JA. Wheat protein composition and properties of wheat glutenin in relation to breadmaking functionality. Crit Rev Food Sci Nutr. 2002;42(3):179-208.

Verdu EF, Armstrong D, Murray JA. Between celiac disease and irritable bowel syndrome: the "no man's land" of gluten sensitivity. Am J Gastroenterol. 2009;104:1587–1594.

Verhasselt V. Oral tolerance in neonates: from basics to potential prevention of allergic disease. *Mucosal Immunol.* 2010 Jul;3(4):326-33.

Verstege A, Mehl A, Rolinck-Werninghaus C, Staden U, Nocon M, Beyer K, Niggemann B. The predictive value of the skin prick test weal size for the outcome of oral food challenges. Clin Exp Allergy. 2005 Sep;35(9):1220-6. Rolinck-Werninghaus C, Staden U, Mehl A, Hamelmann E, Beyer K, Niggemann B. Specific oral tolerance induction with food in children: transient or persistent effect on food allergy? *Allergy.* 2005 Oct;60(10):1320-2.

Vidal PJ, López-Nicolás JM, Gandía-Herrero F, García-Carmona F. Inactivation of ipoxygenase and cyclooxygenase by natural betalains and semi-synthetic analogues. Food Chem. 2014 Jul 1;154:246-54.

Vidgren HM, Agren JJ, Schwab U, Rissanen T, Hanninen O, Uusitupa MI. Incorporation of n-3 fatty acids into plasma lipid fractions, and erythrocyte membranes and platelets during dietary supplementation with fish, fish oil, and docosahexaenoic acid-rich oil among healthy young men. *Lipids.* 1997 Jul;32(7):697-705.

Vila R, Mundina M, Tomi F, Furlán R, Zacchino S, Casanova J, Cañigueral S. Composition and antifungal activity of the essential oil of Solidago chilensis. *Planta Med.* 2002 Feb;68(2):164-7.

Viljanen M, Kuitunen M, Haahtela T, Juntunen-Backman K, Korpela R, Savilahti E. Probiotic effects on faecal inflammatory markers and on faecal IgA in food allergic atopic eczema/dermatitis syndrome infants. *Pediatr Allergy Immunol.* 2005 Feb;16(1):65-71.

Viljanen M, Savilahti E, Haahtela T, Juntunen-Backman K, Korpela R, Poussa T, Tuure T, Kuitunen M. Probiotics in the treatment of atopic eczema/dermatitis syndrome in infants: a double-blind placebo-controlled trial. *Allergy.* 2005 Apr;60(4):494-500.

Vinning G,McMahon G. Gluten-free Grains. A demand-and-supply analysis of prospects for the Australian grains industry. Rural industries Research and Development Corporation: Canberra. 2006. 21(5): p. 359–65.

Vinson JA, Proch J, Bose P. MegaNatural((R)) Gold Grapeseed Extract: In Vitro Antioxidant and In Vivo Human Supplementation Studies. *J Med Food.* 2001 Spring;4(1):17-26.

Visness CM, London SJ, Daniels JL, Kaufman JS, Yeatts KB, Siega-Riz AM, Liu AH, Calatroni A, Zeldin DC. Association of obesity with IgE levels and allergy symptoms in children and adolescents: results from the National Health and Nutrition Examination Survey 2005-2006. *J Allergy Clin Immunol.* 2009 May;123(5):1163-9, 1169.e1-4.

Vivinus-Nébot M, Dainese R, Anty R, Saint-Paul MC, Nano JL, Gonthier N, Marjoux S, Frin-Mathy G, Bernard G, Hébuterne X, Tran A, Theodorou V, Piche T. Combination of allergic factors can worsen diarrheic irritable bowel syndrome: role of barrier defects and mast cells. Am J Gastroenterol. 2012 Jan;107(1):75-81.

Vlieg-Boerstra BJ, Dubois AE, van der Heide S, Bijleveld CM, Wolt-Plompen SA, Oude Elberink JN, Kukler J, Jansen DF, Venter C, Duiverman EJ. Ready-to-use introduction schedules for first exposure to allergenic foods in children at home. Allergy. 2008 Jul;63(7):903-9.

Vlieg-Boerstra BJ, van der Heide S, Bijleveld CM, Kukler J, Duiverman EJ, Dubois AE. Placebo reactions in double-blind, placebo-controlled food challenges in children. *Allergy.* 2007 Aug;62(8):905-12.

Vlieg-Boerstra BJ, van der Heide S, Bijleveld CM, Kukler J, Duiverman EJ, Wolt-Plompen SA, Dubois AE. Dietary assessment in children adhering to a food allergen avoidance diet for allergy prevention. *Eur J Clin Nutr.* 2006 Dec;60(12):1384-90.

Vojdani A. Antibodies as predictors of complex autoimmune diseases. *Int J Immunopathol Pharmacol.* 2008 Apr-Jun;21(2):267-78.

Vojdani A. The characterization of the repertoire of wheat antigens and peptides involved in the humoral immune responses in patients with gluten sensitivity and Crohn's disease. ISRN Allergy. 2011 Oct 27;2011:950104.

Volman JJ, Ramakers JD, Plat J. Dietary modulation of immune function by beta-glucans. Physiol Behav. 2008 May 23;94(2):276-84.

Volta U, Tovoli F, Cicola R, Parisi C, Fabbri A, Piscaglia M, Fiorini E, Caio G. Serological tests in gluten sensitivity (nonceliac gluten intolerance). J Clin Gastroenterol. 2012 Sep;46(8):680-5.

von Berg A, Filipiak-Pittroff B, Krämer U, Link E, Bollrath C, Brockow I, Koletzko S, Grübl A, Heinrich J, Wichmann HE, Bauer CP, Reinhardt D, Berdel D; GINIplus study group. Preventive effect of hydrolyzed infant formulas persists until age 6 years: long-term results from the German Infant Nutritional Intervention Study (GINI). *J Allergy Clin Immunol.* 2008 Jun;121(6):1442-7.

von Berg A, Koletzko S, Grübl A, Filipiak-Pittroff B, Wichmann HE, Bauer CP, Reinhardt D, Berdel D; German Infant Nutritional Intervention Study Group. The effect of hydrolyzed cow's milk formula for allergy prevention in the first year of life: the German Infant Nutritional Intervention Study, a randomized double-blind trial. J Allergy Clin Immunol. 2003 Mar;111(3):533-40.

von Kruedener S, Schneider W, Elstner EF. A combination of Populus tremula, Solidago virgaurea and Fraxinus excelsior as an anti-inflammatory and antirheumatic drug. A short review. *Arzneimittelforschung.* 1995 Feb;45(2):169-71.

Vulevic J, Drakoularakou A, Yaqoob P, Tzortzis G and Gibson GR; Modulation of the fecal microflora profile and immune function by a novel trans-galactooligosaccharide mixture (B-GOS) in healthy elderly volunteers. *Am J Clin Nutr.* 1988 88;1438-1446.

Waddell L. Food allergies in children: the difference between cow's milk protein allergy and food intolerance. *J Fam Health Care.* 2010;20(3):104.

Waglay A, Karboune S, Alli I. Potato protein isolates: recovery and characterization of their properties. Food Chem. 2014 Jan 1;142:373-82.

Wahler D, Gronover CS, Richter C, Foucu F, Twyman RM, Moerschbacher BM, Fischer R, Muth J, Prufer D. Polyphenoloxidase silencing affects latex coagulation in Taraxacum spp. *Plant Physiol.* 2009 Jul 15.

Wahn U, Warner J, Simons FE, de Benedictis FM, Diepgen TL, Naspitz CK, de Longueville M, Bauchau V; EPAAC Study Group. IgE antibody responses in young children with atopic dermatitis. *Pediatr Allergy Immunol.* 2008 Jun;19(4):332-6.

Wahnschaffe U, Schulzke JD, Zeitz M, Ullrich R. Predictors of clinical response to gluten-free diet in patients diagnosed with diarrhea-predominant irritable bowel syndrome. Clin Gastroenterol Hepatol. 2007;5:844–50.

Wahnschaffe U, Ullrich R, Riecken EO, Schulzke JD. Celiac disease-like abnormalities in a subgroup of patients with irritable bowel syndrome. Gastroen-terology. 2001;121:1329–1338.

Wainstein BK, Yee A, Jelley D, Ziegler M, Ziegler JB. Combining skin prick, immediate skin application and specific-IgE testing in the diagnosis of peanut allergy in children. Pediatr Allergy Immunol. 2007 May;18(3):231-9. Nolan RC, Richmond P, Prescott SL, Mallon DF, Gong G, Franzmann AM, Naidoo R, Loh RK. Skin prick testing predicts peanut challenge outcome in previously allergic or sensitized children with low serum peanut-specific IgE antibody concentration. *Pediatr Allergy Immunol.* 2007 May;18(3):224-30.

Wakim-Fleming J, Pagadala MR, McCullough AJ, Lopez R, Bennett AE, Barnes DS, Carey WD. Prevalence of celiac disease in cirrhosis and outcome of cirrhosis on a gluten free diet: A prospective study. J Hepatol. 2014 May 16. pii: S0168-8278(14)00361-4.

Walker JR, Ediger JP, Graff LA, Greenfeld JM, Clara I, Lix L, Rawsthorne P, Miller N, Rogala L, McPhail CM, Bernstein CN. The Manitoba IBD cohort study: a population-based study of the prevalence of lifetime and 12-month anxiety and mood disorders. Am J Gastroenterol. 2008 Aug;103(8):1989-97.

Walker S, Wing A. Allergies in children. *J Fam Health Care.* 2010;20(1):24-6.

Walker WA. Antigen absorption from the small intestine and gastrointestinal disease. *Pediatr Clin North Am.* 1975 Nov;22(4):731-46.

Walker WA. Antigen handling by the small intestine. *Clin Gastroenterol.* 1986 Jan;15(1):1-20.

Walle UK, Walle T. Transport of the cooked-food mutagen 2-amino-1-methyl-6-phenylimidazo- 4,5-b pyridine (PhIP) across the human intestinal Caco-2 cell monolayer: role of efflux pumps. *Carcinogenesis.* 1999 Nov;20(11):2153-7.

Walsh SJ, Rau LM: Autoimmune diseases: a leading cause of death among young and middle-aged women in the United States. *Am J Public Health* 2000, 90(9): 1463-1466.

Walton GE, Lu C, Trogh I, Arnaut F, Gibson GR. A randomised, double-blind, placebo controlled cross-over study to determine the gastrointestinal effects of consumption of arabinoxylanoligosaccharides enriched bread in healthy volunteers. Nutr J. 2012 Jun 1;11(1):36.

Wan KS, Yang W, Wu WF. A survey of serum specific-IgE to common allergens in primary school children of Taipei City. *Asian Pac J Allergy Immunol.* 2010 Mar;28(1):1-6.

Wang J, Lin J, Bardina L, Goldis M, Nowak-Wegrzyn A, Shreffler WG, Sampson HA. Correlation of IgE/IgG4 milk epitopes and affinity of milk-specific IgE antibodies with different phenotypes of clinical milk allergy. *J Allergy Clin Immunol.* 2010 Mar;125(3):695-702, 702.e1-702.e6.

Wang J, Patil SP, Yang N, Ko J, Lee J, Noone S, Sampson HA, Li XM. Safety, tolerability, and immunologic effects of a food allergy herbal formula in food allergic individuals: a randomized, double-blinded, placebo-controlled, dose escalation, phase 1 study. *Ann Allergy Asthma Immunol.* 2010 Jul;105(1):75-84.

Wang J. Management of the patient with multiple food allergies. *Curr Allergy Asthma Rep.* 2010 Jul;10(4):271-7.

Wang K, Hasjim J, Wu AC, Henry RJ, Gilbert RG. Variation in Amylose Fine Structure of Starches from Different Botanical Sources. J Agric Food Chem. 2014 May 1.

Wang KY, Li SN, Liu CS, Perng DS, Su YC, Wu DC, Jan CM, Lai CH, Wang TN, Wang WM. Effects of ingesting Lactobacillus- and Bifidobacterium-containing yogurt in subjects with colonized Helicobacter pylori. *Am J Clin Nutr.* 2004 Sep;80(3):737-41.

Wang Q, Ge X, Tian X, Zhang Y, Zhang J, Zhang P. Soy isoflavone: The multipurpose phytochemical (Review). Biomed Rep. 2013 Sep;1(5):697-701.

Wang WS, Li EW, Jia ZJ. Terpenes from Juniperus przewalskii and their antitumor activities. *Pharmazie.* 2002 May;57(5):343-5.

Wang YM, Huan GX. *Utilization of Classical Formulas.* Beijing, China: Chinese Medicine and Pharmacology Publishing Co, 1998.

Waring G, Levy D. Challenging adverse reactions in children with food allergies. *Paediatr Nurs.* 2010 Jul;22(6):16-22.

Waser M, Michels KB, Bieli C, Flöistrup H, Pershagen G, von Mutius E, Ege M, Riedler J, Schram-Bijkerk D, Brunekreef B, van Hage M, Lauener R, Braun-Fahrländer C; PARSIFAL Study team. Inverse association of farm milk consumption with asthma and allergy in rural and suburban populations across Europe. *Clin Exp Allergy.* 2007 May;37(5):661-70.

Watkins BA, Hannon K, Ferruzzi M, Li Y. Dietary PUFA and flavonoids as deterrents for environmental pollutants. *J Nutr Biochem.* 2007 Mar;18(3):196-205.

Watzl B, Bub A, Blockhaus M, Herbert BM, Lührmann PM, Neuhäuser-Berthold M, Rechkemmer G. Prolonged tomato juice consumption has no effect on cell-mediated immunity of well-nourished elderly men and women. *J Nutr.* 2000 Jul;130(7):1719-23.

Webber CM, England RW. Oral allergy syndrome: a clinical, diagnostic, and therapeutic challenge. *Ann Allergy Asthma Immunol.* 2010 Feb;104(2):101-8; quiz 109-10, 117.

Weber J, Cheinsong-Popov R, Callow D, Adams S, Patou G, Hodgkin K, Martin S, Gotch F, Kingsman A. Immunogenicity of the yeast recombinant p17/p24:Ty virus-like particles (p24-VLP) in healthy volunteers. Vaccine. 1995 Jun;13(9):831-4.

Webster D, Taschereau P, Belland RJ, Sand C, Rennie RP. Antifungal activity of medicinal plant extracts; preliminary screening studies. *J Ethnopharmacol.* 2008 Jan 4;115(1):140-6.

Wedge DE, Tabanca N, Sampson BJ, Werle C, Demirci B, Baser KH, Nan P, Duan J, Liu Z. Antifungal and insecticidal activity of two Juniperus essential oils. *Nat Prod Commun.* 2009 Jan;4(1):123-7.

Wei A, Shibamoto T. Antioxidant activities and volatile constituents of various essential oils. *J Agric Food Chem.* 2007 Mar 7;55(5):1737-42.

Weiner MA. *Secrets of Fijian Medicine.* Berkeley, CA: Univ. of Calif., 1969.

Weiss RF. *Herbal Medicine.* Gothenburg, Sweden: Beaconsfield, 1988.

Wen MC, Huang CK, Srivastava KD, Zhang TF, Schofield B, Sampson HA, Li XM. Ku–Shen (Sophora flavescens Ait), a single Chinese herb, abrogates airway hyperreactivity in a murine model of asthma. *J Allergy Clin Immunol.* 2004;113:218.

Wen MC, Taper A, Srivastava KD, Huang CK, Schofield B, Li XM. Immunology of T cells by the Chinese Herbal Medicine Ling Zhi (Ganoderma lucidum) *J Allergy Clin Immunol.* 2003;111:S320.

Wen MC, Wei CH, Hu ZQ, Srivastava K, Ko J, Xi ST, Mu DZ, Du JB, Li GH, Wallenstein S, Sampson H, Kattan M, Li XM. Efficacy and tolerability of anti-asthma herbal medicine intervention in adult patients with moderate-severe allergic asthma. *J Allergy Clin Immunol.* 2005;116:517–24.

Wensing M, Penninks AH, Hefle SL, Akkerdaas JH, van Ree R, Koppelman SJ, Bruijnzeel-Koomen CA, Knulst AC. The range of minimum provoking doses in hazelnut-allergic patients as determined by double-blind, placebo-controlled food challenges. *Clin Exp Allergy.* 2002 Dec;32(12):1757-62.

Werbach M. *Nutritional Influences on Illness.* Tarzana, CA: Third Line Press, 1996.

West CE, Hammarström ML, Hernell O. Probiotics during weaning reduce the incidence of eczema. *Pediatr Allergy Immunol.* 2009 Aug;20(5):430-7.

West R. Risk of death in meat and non-meat eaters. *BMJ.* 1994 Oct 8;309(6959):955.

Westerholm-Ormio M, Vaarala O, Tiittanen M, Savilahti E. Infiltration of Foxp3- and Toll-like receptor-4-positive cells in the intestines of children with food allergy. *J Pediatr Gastroenterol Nutr.* 2010 Apr;50(4):367-76.

Wheeler JG, Shema SJ, Bogle ML, Shirrell MA, Burks AW, Pittler A, Helm RM. Immune and clinical impact of Lactobacillus acidophilus on asthma. *Ann Allergy Asthma Immunol.* 1997 Sep;79(3):229-33.

Which? Food allergy tests could risk your health. 21 Aug 2008. http://www.which.co.uk/news/2008/08/food-allergy-tests-could-risk-your-health-154711. Retrieved June 20, 2014

Whitfield KE, Wiggins SA, Belue R, Brandon DT. Genetic and environmental influences on forced expiratory volume in African Americans: the Carolina African-American Twin Study of Aging. *Ethn Dis.* 2004 Spring;14(2):206-11.

WHO. *Guidelines for Drinking-water Quality.* 2nd ed, vol. 2. Geneva: World Health Organization, 1996.

WHO. Health effects of the removal of substances occurring naturally in drinking water, with special reference to demineralized and desalinated water. Report on a working group (Brussels, 20-23 March 1978). *EURO Reports and Studies.* 1979;16.

WHO. How trace elements in water contribute to health. *WHO Chronicle.* 1978;32:382-385.

WHO. *INFOSAN Food Allergies. Information Note No. 3.* Geneva, Switzerland: World Health Organization, 2006.

Whorwell PJ, Altringer L, Morel J, Bond Y, Charbonneau D, O'Mahony L, Kiely B, Shanahan F, Quigley EM. Efficacy of an encapsulated probiotic Bifidobacterium infantis 35624 in women with irritable bowel syndrome. *Am J Gastroenterol.* 2006 Jul;101(7):1581-90.

Wieser H. Chemistry of gluten proteins. Food Microbiol. 2007;24(2):115–9.

Wildt S, Munck LK, Vinter-Jensen L, Hanse BF, Nordgaard-Lassen I, Christensen S, Avnstroem S, Rasmussen SN, Rumessen JJ. Probiotic treatment of collagenous colitis: a randomized, double-blind, placebo-controlled trial with Lactobacillus acidophilus and Bifidobacterium animalis subsp. *Lactis. Inflamm Bowel Dis.* 2006 May;12(5):395-401.

Willard T, Jones K. *Reishi Mushroom: Herb of Spiritual Potency and Medical Wonder.* Issaquah, Washington: Sylvan Press, 1990.

Willard T. *Edible and Medicinal Plants of the Rocky Mountains and Neighbouring Territories.* Calgary: 1992.

Willemsen LE, Koetsier MA, Balvers M, Beermann C, Stahl B, van Tol EA. Polyunsaturated fatty acids support epithelial barrier integrity and reduce IL-4 mediated permeability in vitro. *Eur J Nutr.* 2008 Jun;47(4):183-91.

Wilson D, Evans M, Guthrie N, Sharma P, Baisley J, Schonlau F, Burki C. A randomized, double-blind, placebo-controlled exploratory study to evaluate the potential of pycnogenol for improving allergic rhinitis symptoms. *Phytother Res.* 2010 Aug;24(8):1115-9.

Wilson K, McDowall L, Hodge D, Chetcuti P, Cartledge P. Cow's milk protein allergy. *Community Pract.* 2010 May;83(5):40-1.

Wilson L. *Nutritional Balancing and Hair Mineral Analysis.* Prescott, AZ: LD Wilson, 1998.

Winchester AM. *Biology and its Relation to Mankind.* New York: Van Nostrand Reinhold, 1969.

Wise M, Doehlert D, McMullen M. Association of Avenanthramide Concentration in Oat (Avena sativa L.) Grain with Crown Rust Incidence and Genetic Resistance. Cereal Chem. 85(5):639-641.

Wittenberg JS. *The Rebellious Body*. New York: Insight, 1996.

Wöhrl S, Hemmer W, Focke M, Rappersberger K, Jarisch R. Histamine intolerance-like symptoms in healthy volunteers after oral provocation with liquid histamine. *Allergy Asthma Proc.* 2004 Sep-Oct;25(5):305-11.

Wolever TM, Jenkins DJ, Kalmusky J, Giordano C, Giudici S, Jenkins AL, Thompson LU, Wong GS, Josse RG. Glycemic response to pasta: effect of surface area, degree of cooking, and protein enrichment. Diabetes Care. 1986 Jul-Aug;9(4):401-4.

Wolf J, Hasenclever D, Petroff D, Richter T, Uhlig HH, Laa□ MW, Hauer A, Stern M, Bossuyt X, de Laffolie J, Flemming G, Villalta D, Schlumberger W, Mothes T. Antibodies in the diagnosis of coeliac disease: a biopsy-controlled, international, multicentre study of 376 children with coeliac disease and 695 controls. PLoS One. 2014 May 15;9(5):e97853.

Wolters VM, Wijmenga C. Genetic background of celiac disease and its clinical implications. J Gastroenterol. 2007;102:1–6.

Wolvers DA, van Herpen-Broekmans WM, Logman MH, van der Wielen RP, Albers R. Effect of a mixture of micronutrients, but not of bovine colostrum concentrate, on immune function parameters in healthy volunteers: a randomized placebo-controlled study. *Nutr J.* 2006 Nov 21;5:28.

Wood M. *The Book of Herbal Wisdom.* Berkeley, CA: North Atlantic, 1997.

Wood NC, Hamilton I, Axon AT, Khan SA, Quirke P, Mindham RH, McGuigan K, Prison HM. Abnormal intestinal permeability. An aetiological factor in chronic psychiatric disorders? Br J Psychiatry. 1987 Jun;150:853-6.

Wood RA, Kraynak J. *Food Allergies for Dummies.* Hoboken, NJ: Wiley Publ, 2007.

Woods RK, Abramson M, Bailey M, Walters EH (2001) International prevalences of reported food allergies and intolerances. Comparisons arising from the European Community Respiratory Health Survey (ECRHS) 1991–1994. *Eur J Clin Nutr* 55: 298–304.

Woods RK, Abramson M, Bailey M, Walters EH. International prevalences of reported food allergies and intolerances. Comparisons arising from the European Community Respiratory Health Survey (ECRHS) 1991-1994. *Eur J Clin Nutr.* 2001 Apr;55(4):298-304.

Woods RK, Abramson M, Raven JM, Bailey M, Weiner JM, Walters EH (1998) Reported food intolerance and respiratory symptoms in young adults. *Eur Respir J.* 11: 151–155.

Worm M, Hompes S, Fiedler EM, Illner AK, Zuberbier T, Vieths S. Impact of native, heat-processed and encapsulated hazelnuts on the allergic response in hazelnut-allergic patients. *Clin Exp Allergy.* 2009 Jan;39(1):159-66.

Wu BY, Wu BJ, Lee SM, Sun HJ, Chang YT, Lin MW. Prevalence and associated factors of comorbid skin diseases in patients with schizophrenia: a clinical survey and national health database study. Gen Hosp Psychiatry. 2014 Mar 5. pii: S0163-8343(14)00058-9.

Würsch P, Pi-Sunyer FX. The role of viscous soluble fiber in the metabolic control of diabetes. A review with special emphasis on cereals rich in beta-glucan. Diabetes Care. 1997 Nov;20(11):1774-80.

Xiao P, Kubo H, Ohsawa M, Higashiyama K, Nagase H, Yan YN, Li JS, Kamei J, Ohmiya S. kappa-Opioid receptor-mediated antinociceptive effects of stereoisomers and derivatives of (+)-matrine in mice. *Planta Med.* 1999 Apr;65(3):230-3.

Xu X, Zhang D, Zhang H, Wolters PJ, Killeen NP, Sullivan BM, Locksley RM, Lowell CA, Caughey GH. Neutrophil histamine contributes to inflammation in mycoplasma pneumonia. *J Exp Med.* 2006 Dec 25;203(13):2907-17.

Yadav VS, Mishra KP, Singh DP, Mehrotra S, Singh VK. Immunomodulatory effects of curcumin. *Immunopharmacol Immunotoxicol.* 2005;27(3):485-97.

Yadzir ZH, Misnan R, Abdullah N, Bakhtiar F, Arip M, Murad S. Identification of Ige-binding proteins of raw and cooked extracts of Loligo edulis (white squid). *Southeast Asian J Trop Med Public Health.* 2010 May;41(3):653-9.

Yan F, Cao H, Cover TL, Whitehead R, Washington MK, Polk DB. Soluble proteins produced by probiotic bacteria regulate intestinal epithelial cell survival and growth. Gastroenterology. 2007;132:562–75.

Yang Z. Are peanut allergies a concern for using peanut-based formulated foods in developing countries? *Food Nutr Bull.* 2010 Jun;31(2 Suppl):S147-53.

Yarnell E. Botanical medicines for the urinary tract. *World J Urol.* 2002 Nov;20(5):285-93.

Yasumatsu H, Tanabe S. The casein peptide Asn-Pro-Trp-Asp-Gln enforces the intestinal tight junction partly by increasing occludin expression in Caco-2 cells. Br J Nutr. 2010 Oct;104(7):951-6.

Yeager S. *The Doctor's Book of Food Remedies.* Emmaus, PA: Rodale Press, 1998.

Ying R, Rondeau-Mouro C, Barron C, Mabille F, Perronnet A, Saulnier L. Hydration and mechanical properties of arabinoxylans and □-D-glucans films. Carbohydr Polym. 2013 Jul 1;96(1):31-8.

Yu L. Wheat Antioxidants. Wiley, 2007.

Yu LC. The epithelial gatekeeper against food allergy. *Pediatr Neonatol.* 2009 Dec;50(6):247-54.

Yuan S, Chang SK, Liu Z, Xu B. Elimination of trypsin inhibitor activity and beany flavor in soy milk by consecutive blanching and ultrahigh-temperature (UHT) processing. J Agric Food Chem. 2008 Sep 10;56(17):7957-63.

Yuan S, Chang SK, Liu Z, Xu B. Elimination of trypsin inhibitor activity and beany flavor in soy milk by consecutive blanching and ultrahigh-temperature (UHT) processing. J Agric Food Chem. 2008 Sep 10;56(17):7957-63.

Yun CH, Estrada A, Van Kessel A, Gajadhar A, Redmond M, Laarveld B. Immunomodulatory effects of oat beta-glucan administered intragastrically or parenterally on mice infected with Eimeria vermiformis. Microbiol Immunol. 1998;42(6):457-65.

Yusoff NA, Hampton SM, Dickerson JW, Morgan JB. The effects of exclusion of dietary egg and milk in the management of asthmatic children: a pilot study. *J R Soc Promot Health.* 2004 Mar;124(2):74-80.

Zamakhchari M, Wei G, Dewhirst F, Lee J, Schuppan D, Oppenheim FG, Helmerhorst EJ. Identification of Rothia bacteria as gluten-degrading natural colonizers of the upper gastro-intestinal tract. PLoS One. 2011;6(9):e24455.

Zanjanian MH. The intestine in allergic diseases. *Ann Allergy.* 1976 Sep;37(3):208-18.

Zant-Przeworska E, Stasiuk M, Gubernator J, Kozubek A. Resorcinolic lipids improve the properties of sphingomyelin-cholesterol liposomes. Chem Phys Lipids. 2010 Sep;163(7):648-54.

Zarkadas M, Scott FW, Salminen J, Ham Pong A. Common Allergenic Foods and Their Labelling in Canada. *Can J Allerg Clin Immun.* 1999; 4:118-141.

Zarnowski R, Suzuki Y, Yamaguchi I, Pietr SJ. Alkylresorcinols in barley (Hordeum vulgare L. distichon) grains. Z Naturforsch C. 2002 Jan-Feb;57(1-2):57-62.

Zeiger RS, Heller S. The development and prediction of atopy in high-risk children: follow-up at age seven years in a prospective randomized study of combined maternal and infant food allergen avoidance. *J Allergy Clin Immunol.* 1995 Jun;95(6):1179-90.

Zeng Q, Dong SY, Wu LX, Li H, Sun ZJ, Li JB, Jiang HX, Chen ZH, Wang QB, Chen WW. Variable food-specific IgG antibody levels in healthy and symptomatic Chinese adults. PLoS One. 2013;8(1):e53612.

Zhang J, Zhang X, Lei G, Li B, Chen J, Zhou T. A new phenolic glycoside from the aerial parts of Solidago canadensis. *Fitoterapia.* 2007 Jan;78(1):69-71.

Zheng M. Experimental study of 472 herbs with antiviral action against the herpes simplex virus. *Zhong Xi Yi Jie He Za Zhi.* 1990 Jan;10(1):39-41, 6.

Zhou Q, Zhang B, Verne GN. Intestinal membrane permeability and hypersensitivity in the irritable bowel syndrome. *Pain.* 2009 Nov;146(1-2):41-6.

Zhou Y, Zhao D, Foster TJ, Liu Y, Wang Y, Nirasawa S, Tatsumi E, Cheng Y. Konjac glucomannan-induced changes in thiol/disulphide exchange and gluten conformation upon dough mixing. Food Chem. 2014 Jan 15;143:163-9.

Zhu Y, Soroka DN, Sang S. Synthesis and inhibitory activities against colon cancer cell growth and proteasome of alkylresorcinols. J Agric Food Chem. 2012 Sep 5;60(35):8624-31.

Ziemniak W. Efficacy of Helicobacter pylori eradication taking into account its resistance to antibiotics. *J Physiol Pharmacol.* 2006 Sep;57 Suppl 3:123-41.

Zizza, C. The nutrient content of the Italian food supply 1961-1992. *Euro J Clin Nutr.* 1997;51: 259-265.

Zoccatelli G, Pokoj S, Foetisch K, Bartra J, Valero A, Del Mar San Miguel-Moncin M, Vieths S, Scheurer S. Identification and characterization of the major allergen of green bean (Phaseolus vulgaris) as a non-specific lipid transfer protein (Pha v 3). *Mol Immunol.* 2010 Apr;47(7-8):1561-8.

Zotta T, Piraino P, Ricciardi A, McSweeney PL, Parente E. Proteolysis in model sourdough fermentation. J Agric Food Chem. 2006;54:2567–74.

Zuidmeer L, Goldhahn K, Rona RJ, Gislason D, Madsen C, Summers C, Sodergren E, Dahlstrom J, Lindner T, Sigurdardottir ST, McBride D, Keil T. The prevalence of plant food allergies: a systematic review. *J Allergy Clin Immunol.* 2008 May;121(5):1210-1218.e4.

Zwolińska-Wcisło M, Brzozowski T, Mach T, Budak A, Trojanowska D, Konturek PC, Pajdo R, Droz-dowicz D, Kwiecień S. Are probiotics effective in the treatment of fungal colonization of the gastroin-testinal tract? Experimental and clinical studies. *J Physiol Pharmacol.* 2006 Nov;57 Suppl 9:35-49.

Index

(foods and herbs too numerous to index)

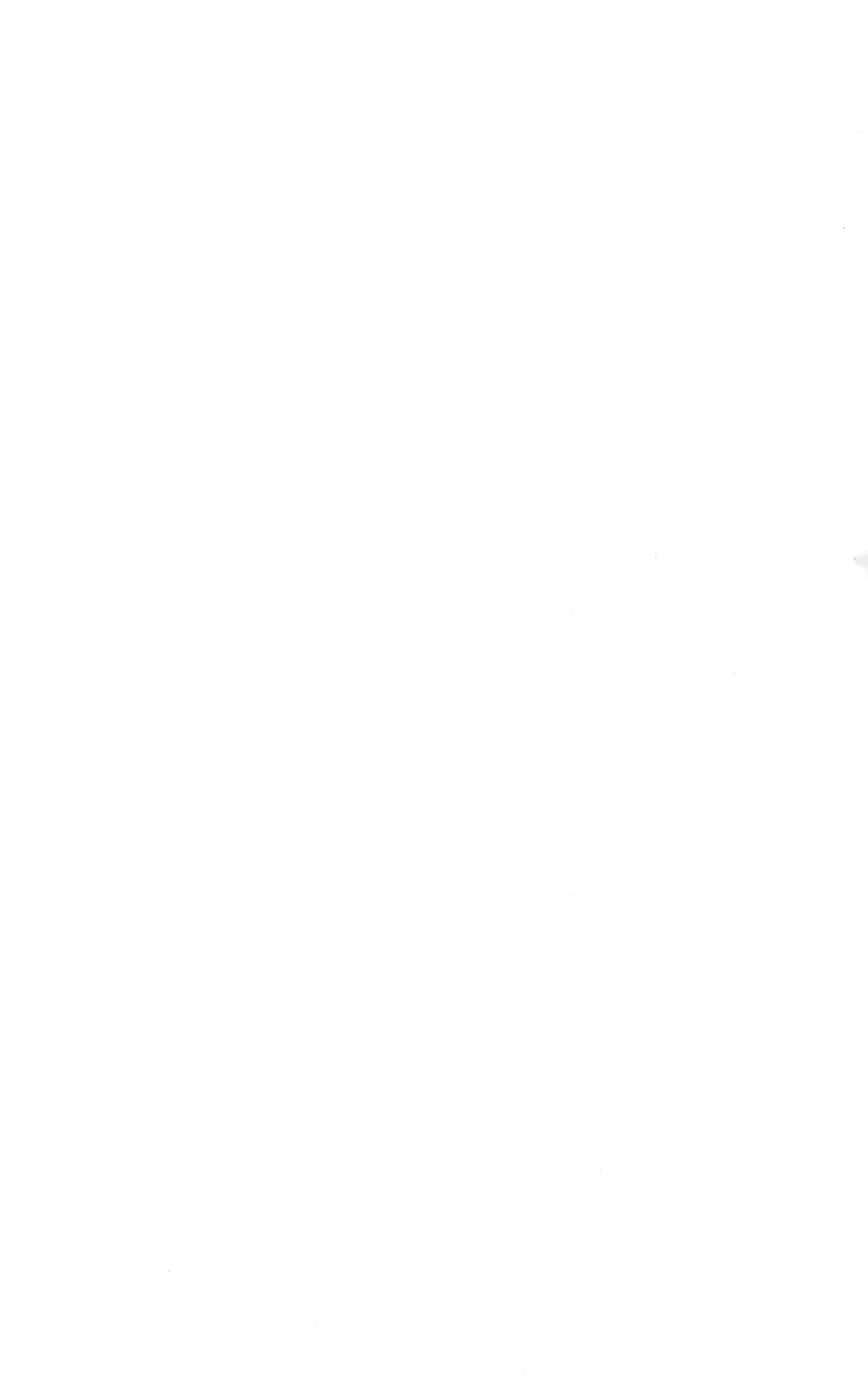